Economics of Health and Medical Care

SEVENTH EDITION

Lanis L. Hicks, PhD

Professor Emerita
Department of Health Management and Informatics
School of Medicine
University of Missouri, Columbia

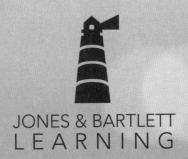

JONES & BARTLETT
L E A R N I N G

World Headquarters
Jones & Bartlett Learning
5 Wall Street
Burlington, MA 01803
978-443-5000
info@jblearning.com
www.jblearning.com

Jones & Bartlett Learning books and products are available through most bookstores and online booksellers. To contact Jones & Bartlett Learning directly, call 800-832-0034, fax 978-443-8000, or visit our website, www.jblearning.com.

21431-4

Production Credits

VP, Product Management: Amanda Martin
Director of Product Management: Laura Pagluica
Product Manager: Sophie Fleck Teague
Product Assistant: Tess Sackmann
Project Specialist: Meghan McDonagh
Digital Project Specialist: Rachel Reyes
Senior Marketing Manager: Susanne Walker
Production Services Manager: Colleen Lamy
VP, Manufacturing and Inventory Control: Therese Connell
Manufacturing and Inventory Control Supervisor: Amy Bacus

Composition: codeMantra U.S. LLC
Project Management: codeMantra U.S. LLC
Cover Design: Scott Moden
Text Design: Kristin Parker
Senior Media Development Editor: Troy Liston
Rights Specialist: Maria Leon Maimone
Cover Image (Title Page, Part Opener, Chapter Opener):
    © Gremlin/E+/Getty Images
Printing and Binding: McNaughton & Gunn
Cover Printing: McNaughton & Gunn

Library of Congress Cataloging-in-Publication Data

Names: Hicks, Lanis L., author.
Title: Economics of health and medical care / Lanis L. Hicks.
Description: Seventh edition. | Burlington, MA: Jones & Bartlett Learning, [2021] | Includes bibliographical references and index. | Summary: "Health Economics is a required course in almost every graduate program in Health Admin, though there are health econ courses (often electives) across disciplines; for example, public health, respiratory care, pharmacy, and nursing. Because of the role economics plays in finance and policy, it can also be adopted in those courses. This book is not discipline-specific, so it covers a wide breadth"—Provided by publisher.
Identifiers: LCCN 2019055950 | ISBN 9781284183535 (paperback)
Subjects: MESH: Economics, Medical | United States
Classification: LCC RA410.5 | NLM W 74 AA1 | DDC 338.4/73621—dc23
LC record available at https://lccn.loc.gov/2019055950

6048

Printed in the United States of America
24 23 22 21 20   10 9 8 7 6 5 4 3 2 1

Brief Contents

Contents

CHAPTER 17 Reform of the Healthcare Market 315

Introduction

Why Health Economics?

The healthcare sector is a major component of the economy of the United States. As expenditures on health care approach almost one-fifth of the gross domestic product (GDP) of the United States (CMS 2018), there is increasing pressure to lower costs by improving efficiency and effectiveness in the healthcare industry. As pressures mount, decision makers have to make increasingly hard decisions about how their limited resources will be used. As a result, economics, a discipline that focuses on the efficient allocation of scarce resources, has an expanded role to play at all levels of decision making in health care (Wilensky, 2010).

In this text, an examination of the factors leading to the greater involvement of economics in health care is presented, and the role, theories, models, and tools of economics as they apply to health care are discussed. As decisions are made regarding the volume and composition of healthcare goods and services produced, economics can be used to assist making these decisions more explicit and transparent. Economics can be used to facilitate a comparison among alternative uses of limited resources and make explicit the consequences associated with each of these alternatives.

The fundamental role of health economics is to provide systematic information about the costs and consequences of the available opportunities in the provision of healthcare goods and services. This role is becoming more and more crucial as focus on value-added outcomes intensifies in health care (Reinhardt, 1985). Keep in mind, value added does not always refer to its contribution to the bottom line, but may also include more intangible things, like quality and social welfare.

As health care consumes more and more resources, there is a growing recognition that there are limited resources available to society, and that as more of these resources go to the healthcare sector, there are fewer resources available for other goods and services. As a result, decision makers at all levels are seeking ways to maximize the value obtained from the use of their resources. Economics provides a mechanism to assist in making decisions regarding the use of these limited resources.

The basic objective of this text is to provide an introduction to the tools, models, and theories of economics, and to show how economics can be used to improve decision making in health care. In this world of increased pressure, all providers, support staff, suppliers, policymakers, and consumers are being asked to justify their roles in the provision of healthcare goods and services. Pressure is being placed on all participants in health care to justify why more resources should be allocated to the provision and consumption of healthcare goods and services. As participants are asked to justify their roles, economics can be used to assist in quantifying the additional value the participant brings to the healthcare system (Debrand & Dourgnon, 2010).

For example, should the local health department hire another public health worker or use its limited budget for something else, such as a mobile mammogram program? While it used to be sufficient for public health workers to simply say they do "good," this is no longer enough. Now, decision makers are asking public health workers to tell them how much "good" they do, as the decision makers try to determine whether they could get more "good" from some other use of their resources. While economics can provide important information about alternative uses of resources to decision makers, it cannot provide all the answers. It can, however, systematically contribute important information to the decision-making process.

As you read this text, the role of economics in the healthcare sector of the economy will become clearer. It will also become clearer how economics can be used by individual decision makers at all levels in healthcare organizations and the healthcare system to improve the delivery of cost-effective, high-quality health care to the population (Hicks & Boles, 1984). Hopefully, by the end of this text, you will come to appreciate the value of economics in the decision-making process in health care.

Outline of Contents

In the Introduction, why there is a need for health economics is explored. A brief explanation is provided on the increasing role of economics in decision making in the healthcare system.

In Chapter 1, this text introduces the analysis of healthcare economics in the context of three tasks: description, explanation, and evaluation. It also contains an introduction to the tools used in economics. Part I, which consists of Chapters 2 and 3, describes the output of the healthcare sector and the economic dimensions of the healthcare field. Part II, consisting of Chapters 4–11, presents explanatory analyses of a number of health-related issues. Part III, which consists of Chapters 12–17, develops evaluative analyses of several important aspects of healthcare resource use. The analyses in this text focus on three distinct markets: the medical care market, the health insurance market, and the labor market. Throughout the text, tools are developed to analyze the economic behavior of all three markets.

Chapter 2 contains a discussion of the output of the healthcare sector. Three types of output are identified: (1) health and/or medical care, which consists of activities designed to improve health; (2) health itself; and (3) health insurance coverage. Types of input, such as the hiring of healthcare personnel, are also discussed. Measurements of each type of output are presented. In Chapter 3, economic dimensions of the healthcare sector are identified and some measures of these dimensions are presented. In particular, economic flows of the various components of the healthcare system are described, and the concept of cost is analyzed.

Chapter 4, the first explanatory chapter, develops a model to explain the demand for health or medical care by consumers. A number of separate factors are identified as influences on the demand for health or medical care. These are incorporated into a single model that allows us to predict the effects of each factor when all other relevant factors are held constant. In this chapter, the demand for medical care is presented as if medical care were an ordinary good or service in the consumer's budget.

However, medical care has characteristics that combine to warrant special treatment. These include the importance of medical care in influencing health status, uncertainty when illness occurs, people's concern about others' health status and healthcare consumption, and the asymmetry in the medical knowledge possessed by providers and consumers. A number of these characteristics are introduced and analyzed in light of the standard demand model.

Chapters 5–7 focus on the behavior of healthcare providers, such as physicians, hospitals, and laboratories. Chapter 5 discusses the relationships between resource use (inputs) and output, quality of care and output, and cost of care and output. All these relationships are examined with regard to each individual provider. Chapter 6 presents an analysis of the supply behavior of individual providers and of groups of providers (i.e., market supply). The behavior of investor-owned (for-profit) providers and the behavior of tax-exempt (not-for-profit) providers are treated separately, since tax-exempt and government providers play such an important role in the healthcare field. The chapter also considers a model of the supply behavior of health insurers, as well as a model of the demand for labor (which is based on the supply model). Chapter 7 deals with one important aspect of supply analysis in health care—provider reimbursement. In health care, there are many examples of providers being paid by a third party (a health insurer or the government). The important economic concept of the principal–agent relationship is introduced and is used to analyze alternative payment schemes for physicians, hospitals, long-term care providers, and health maintenance organizations. Included here is a discussion of the additional pressures that value-based purchasing brings to health care.

Chapter 8 examines a standard textbook explanation of how the market resource allocation process works. This is the competitive market model, which has drawn a good deal of attention recently, especially in terms of fee differences among patients and quality of care. Included in this chapter is an explanation of a phenomenon that has received considerable attention in health economics: supplier-induced demand. Not all market behavior is competitive. Chapter 9 looks at the concept of market power: how it is acquired by suppliers and demanders, and how its acquisition affects market phenomena (e.g., prices, and quantity and quality of output).

Chapters 10 and 11 consider two types of markets whose functioning is closely tied to health care. Chapter 10 describes the market for health insurance and its implications for efficiency in the healthcare market. Chapter 11 presents an analysis of the labor market and of several variants of this market that are associated with health care. Budgeting and staffing decisions are also presented in this chapter.

The third part of the text focuses on economic evaluation and health policy issues. There is a great deal of controversy over whether healthcare markets can ensure that health care is delivered efficiently to consumers. One way to study this issue is to gauge whether specific interventions improve health status in an efficient way. Cost-benefit and cost-effectiveness analyses are two techniques by which we can judge the economic impact of various interventions and policies on health status. Chapter 12 offers an introduction to these tools.

Chapter 13 introduces the topic of evaluation by identifying several alternative standards that have been used in evaluating resource use in the healthcare field. These standards include efficiency and equity. Two frameworks used to evaluate efficiency are presented: the narrower efficiency framework and the broader "extra-welfarist" framework. A set of specific goals for the healthcare system is derived from these welfare analyses.

Chapter 14 discusses alternative types of healthcare finance: out-of-pocket payment, health insurance reimbursement, and taxation. Discussion also focuses on the issues of charity care and bad debt, especially in hospitals. It uses economic models to identify the burden of each type of financing. Special consideration is given to pay-for-performance initiatives and value-based purchasing.

Chapter 15 discusses two major public insurance programs, Medicare and Medicaid. It presents specific policy problems and, using the explanatory economic models developed in Chapters 3–11, evaluates the effects of policy measures in light of specific policy goals.

The role of regulation and antitrust policy in influencing the performance of the healthcare market is the topic of Chapter 16. Two views of regulation are presented there. According to the first, the public-interest approach, the government establishes regulations to ensure that providers act in the public interest. Evidence of the effectiveness of this approach has not been very convincing. The second view of regulation is based on a wider picture of the market. According to this view, the government is a participant in a marketplace that encompasses both the suppliers and demanders of the traded product as well as politicians and regulators. In this marketplace, various regulations and laws that have an impact on the supply–demand situation are "traded." The market outcome is, thus, influenced by regulation. Faced with discontent over the results of traditional market regulation, some observers have proposed that the medical market should be reshaped in the competitive mold. Also included in Chapter 16 is an analysis of antitrust regulation, a topic of considerable policy interest in recent years, and tax reform, which is always a hot political issue.

Chapter 17 focuses on methods to reform health insurance and healthcare markets. It discusses various proposals for restructuring the health insurance market so that the preferred risk selection of the health insurers might discriminate less against high-risk individuals, thereby increasing the equity of these markets. Chapter 17 also introduces the concept of "consumerism."

How to Use This Text

There is a considerable amount of material in this text, much more than would be included in a typical introductory course in healthcare economics. As a rough guide, a typical student without any prior economics background should be able to cover a chapter a week. In a 14-week course, 13 chapters could be covered comfortably. Although more advanced students could handle more, instructors will probably want to be selective in covering the subjects.

The text could be used as the main text for a basic healthcare economics course for public health students and for a similar course in which the emphasis is more on healthcare administration students or health policy and finance. The following are suggestions for coverage in each kind of course.

Orientation	Chapters
Public health	1–6, 8, 9, 11–15
Health administration/ finance and policy	1–11, 14–17

At the end of each chapter, a set of questions and problems is provided. The student is encouraged to work through these problems, as it is easier to learn and retain the material by doing actual problems and self-testing. At the end of this text, answers to the odd-numbered exercises are provided. The answers to the even-numbered exercises are contained in the instructor's manual.

Bibliography

Centers for Medicare & Medicaid. (2018). *NHE fact sheet.* Baltimore, MD: Author.Debrand, T., & Dourgnon, P. (2010). Building bridges between health economics research and public policy evaluation. *Expert Review of Pharmacoeconomics & Outcomes Research, 10*(6), 637–640.

Hicks, L. L., & Boles, K. (1984). Why health economics? *Nursing Economic$, 2*(3), 176–180.

Reinhardt, U. (1985). Future trends in the economics of medical practice and care. *American Journal of Cardiology, 56,* 50C–58C.

Wilensky, G. R. (2010). Health economics. *Studies in Health Technology & Informatics, 153,* 179–193.

CHAPTER 1

Overview of Economics

OBJECTIVES

1. Introduce the discipline of economics and its application to health care.
2. Explain the role of scarcity in health care.
3. Outline the three major tasks of economics.
4. Describe the tools used in economic analysis.

1.1 Introduction

This book is an introduction to the economic approach to understanding healthcare issues and problems. The approach is based on the identification of scarcity as a major cause of many of today's healthcare system problems. Scarcity can be defined as a deficiency in the quantity and/or quality of available goods and services compared with the amounts that people desire. Perhaps the most glaring deficiency in the United States today is the lack of affordable health insurance coverage. While the Affordable Care Act (ACA) resulted in improved access to health insurance coverage, with the number of uninsured non-elderly people decreasing from over 44 million to just below 27 million in 2016, recent changes to the ACA led to an increase in the uninsured of almost 700,000 in 2017 (Kaiser Family Foundation, 2018b). Continued changes to the ACA are likely to result in additional people becoming uninsured or underinsured. Many of the uninsured and underinsured often have difficulty obtaining adequate health care, especially primary and preventive care. Although there are other individuals as well who have inadequate access to care because of other factors, such as location, the size of the uninsured

and underinsured population in the United States has become an indicator of the access problems in the U.S. healthcare system.

Yet, the fundamental difficulty in health care is not merely that there is "not enough" to go around. Side by side with problems of scarcity are problems of "too much" (Aaron & Schwartz, 1990; Dranove, 2000). In 2017, total expenditures on health care in the United States reached over $3.5 trillion, over 17.9% of the gross domestic product (GDP), the dollar sum of all final goods and services produced in the United States. In 1965, healthcare expenditures were only 5.9% of the GDP (CMS, 2018). Included in these expenditures are high-cost services whose impact on health has been questioned, including large-volume "little ticket" items, such as radiographs and lab tests, which make up about a quarter of all hospital expenditures (Angell, 1985); high-cost procedures, such as coronary artery bypass grafting and transplants, costly intensive care services, and new drugs, whose effectiveness is often still undocumented; and some hospital services for the terminally ill, which consume a disproportionate share of the healthcare dollar (Jha, 2018; Long et al., 1984; Zook & Moore, 1980). A number of commentators have asserted that a considerable amount of "flat of the curve" medicine, that is, medical care that produces little or no improvement in health, is being practiced (Enthoven, 1980; Schoder & Zweifel, 2011). Accusations of "too much," when uttered side by side with cries of "not enough," point to the importance of studying the entire resource allocation process in health care (Arrow, 1972).

Economics is the discipline that deals with the consequences of resource scarcity, and about making choices; and, health economics deals with the consequences of resource scarcity in the healthcare industry and the necessity of making choices in health care (Hicks, 2011; Reinhardt, 1987; Wilensky, 1991). Because of its very broad scope, economics does not provide a body of rigid doctrines about scarce resources. Rather, economics offers an overall viewpoint intended to help in understanding the many problems related to various types of scarcity.

This book focuses on how to *do* economics; that is, how to think about economic problems in a systematic way. It divides the discipline into three separate areas, which can be regarded as the three main tasks of economics: description, explanation, and evaluation. The explanation of these tasks in a health context is the objective of this book; the performance of these tasks should be regarded as the objective of the reader.

Accomplishing these tasks involves asking specific questions and searching for answers to them. It should be stressed that searching for relevant questions to be asked is as critical a part of the process of analyzing economic problems as searching for answers. By formulating a problem in the context of scarcity, a deeper understanding of it can be obtained, and discovery of a solution or a means of accommodation might be the end result.

1.2 Three Major Tasks of Economics

The three major tasks of economics covered in this book—description, explanation, and evaluation—will usually not be performed in isolation from one another. Rather, descriptive economics will be used to complement explanations and evaluations of events. But even though these tasks may be intermingled in economic analysis, the specific task being performed should be kept clearly in mind.

1.2.1 Descriptive Economics

Descriptive economics involves the identification, definition, and measurement of phenomena. By performing this task, we obtain some notion of the existing facts. It should be pointed out that this task basically amounts to fact-finding. There is, at this stage, no explanation of why the facts are what they are and no evaluative pronouncement or judgment. Of course, the selection of which phenomena to describe is usually motivated by an ultimate explanatory or evaluative purpose.

The statement that, for example, in 2015, Americans 65 years and older visited physicians' offices, on the average, 6.6 times per year while those in the 18–44-year-old age group paid 2.0 visits per year (National Center for Health Statistics, 2018) falls within the realm of description. It is simply a statement of fact without any explanation or analysis.

1.2.2 Explanatory Economics

The second task of economics is explaining and predicting certain phenomena. This task involves conducting a cause-and-effect analysis. In undertaking such a task, we are moving one step beyond description; we are now identifying the causes of certain events that have occurred. This task is performed with the aid of models that classify various causal factors (assuming there is more than one) in a systematic framework. Based on this framework, hypotheses are developed about the net effect of each causal factor on the phenomena we want to explain. We do not do any further analysis at this stage. That is, we do not pass judgment on whether the phenomena we have observed are present in the desired amounts.

As an example of an explanation, suppose we want to determine why those in the 65-year-old and above age group utilized more medical care than those in the 15–44-year-old age group. First, we would develop a framework that incorporates the major causal factors relevant to this phenomenon. Let us say that our framework contains two essential causal factors: (1) the health status of each group and (2) the price paid by the members of each group for their medical care. Using these causal factors, we might then hypothesize that the quantity of medical care demanded will increase when health status is lowered and when consumers pay less for their medical care. These causal factors relate to our example because (1) the health status of the older group is lower and (2) government-sponsored health insurance for the elderly (Medicare) reduces the amount the older group pays for medical care. Assuming these facts to be true, our hypothesis would predict that the older group will demand medical care in greater quantities. Should these increased quantities also be available, then the older group will utilize more medical care.

1.2.3 Evaluative Economics

The third task of economics is evaluation. This task involves judging or ranking alternative phenomena according to some standard or relative position of alternatives. An acceptable standard is first chosen, then used to rank alternative ways of distributing scarce resources. In choosing the standard, one major criterion is acceptability. Standards are easy to come by; however, many are controversial, and the standard chosen should have some degree of acceptability.

Using the standard, alternative quantities of economic variables—that is, alternative uses of scarce resources—can be evaluated. For example, if we choose a standard that says that the more medical care one has the better off one is, then, according to this standard, the older group in our example is better off than the younger group. Furthermore, any measure that raises the utilization of the younger group (by lowering the price paid by this group and by increasing the resources available for use by this group) would, according to our standard, improve the well-being of the younger group (Hemenway, 1982; Kaiser Family Foundation, 2018a). Evaluative economics is also used to compare alternative uses of resources to achieve an identified goal or to allocate resources most efficiently in the achievement of alternative goals.

1.3 Tools Used in Economic Analysis

Several tools are used in economic analysis. One general tool is graphic analysis. The purpose of graphic analysis is to illustrate relations between economic variables. Also helpful are models that allow us to draw inferences about the relations we might expect to occur when specific underlying conditions are present. Such tools help us to be explicit about the underlying factors that are present in the workings of the resource-allocation process.

1.3.1 Economic Variables

An economic variable is an economically relevant phenomenon whose value or magnitude may vary. Examples of economic variables include prices, costs, incomes, and quantities of goods and services. An economic variable can be measured along a scale, once appropriate units of measurement have been chosen. For example, price can be measured in cents or dollars per unit, and quantities can be expressed in terms of number of visits, number of hospital days,

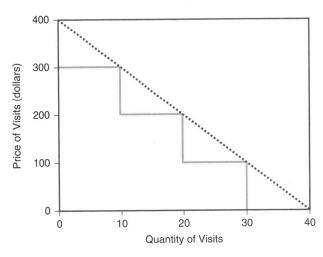

Figure 1-1 Relation between price and quantity of visits. The dashed line in the graph shows continuous values, and the solid lines show discrete values in the graph.
© Jones & Bartlett Learning.

number of hospital beds, and so on. Two examples of units of measurement are shown in **Figure 1-1**. Along the vertical axis, values of the price of medical care are shown. The price per visit to a physician, which is the economic variable being examined, is expressed in terms of dollars. Along this axis, the price can be 0, 100, 200, 300, and so on.

Along the horizontal axis are alternative values of the quantity of visits to a physician's office. These are measured in terms of the number of visits made by the population to a physician's office.

1.3.2 Relations Between Economic Variables

The next step, after the identification and measurement of economic variables, is to determine the relations between these variables. The relations show how one variable changes with respect to another variable.

These relations can be causal or noncausal. For example, we can state that one variable (total healthcare costs) has increased, while another variable (time) has also increased. This is an example of a noncausal relation, because it is not time itself that has caused the costs to increase. As time has passed, other influencing variables have changed, and these have caused the healthcare costs to increase.

In a causal relation, when the value of one economic variable changes, the value of a second economic variable also changes as a result. For example, if the price falls for a visit to the doctor, the lower price will cause more visits to be demanded or utilized. Causal relations are usually expressed in the form of hypothetical statements (e.g., "if price falls, then the quantity demanded will increase").

1.3.3 Graphic Representation of Relations

Let us start with a simple relation between price and quantity of visits: When the price is $400, the quantity of visits is 0; when the price is $300, the quantity of visits is 10; when the price is $200, the quantity of visits is 20; and when the price is $100, the quantity of visits is 30. Associated with each price is a specific quantity: 0 visits with $400, 10 visits with $300, and so on. Each of the associations can be represented by a point, as shown in Figure 1-1. All these points, together, form the relation. If we knew only these values, we could draw this relation diagrammatically as the solid line in Figure 1-1. This solid line is known as a step function and relates only to the values specified.

However, we could go further and generalize about the nature of our function by saying that the values between 0 and 100 dollars (or 100 and 200 dollars) and between 0 and 10 visits (or 10 and 20 visits) could also be specified as part of the relation. We could draw a continuous curve joining all the points specified in the relation in order to represent the values not explicitly expressed, such as 155 dollars, 5 visits, and so on (consider the dashed line in Figure 1-1). Once we have drawn a continuous curve, we have a more complete specification of the relation between price and quantity. Any value of price, within our specified ranges, has an associated quantity or number of visits.

1.3.4 The Direction of Relations

We can now be more specific about the nature of the relation between the two variables. The first characteristic to be examined is the direction of the relation. A relation can have four possible directions, as shown in **Figure 1-2**. First, the relation may be positive, as shown by curve B. Here higher values of price are associated with higher values of quantity of visits. If there was a causal relation between them, and if the direction of causation ran from price to quantity, we would hypothesize that, as price increases, so does quantity.

The opposite type of relation is shown by curve D. The relation is negative: the greater the price, the smaller the quantity. Thus, higher values of price are associated with lower values of quantity of visits. The remaining cases show where variables are unrelated.

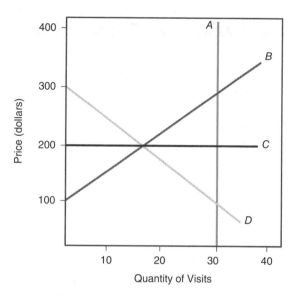

Figure 1-2 Direction of relations. Curve A, constant quantity of visits for all prices; curve B, price and quantity positively related; curve C, constant price for all quantities; and curve D, price and quantity negatively related.

© Jones & Bartlett Learning.

For curve C, whatever the quantity of visits, the price stays the same (i.e., 200 dollars). Curve A shows that, whatever the price may be, the quantity of visits will remain the same (i.e., 30 visits).

1.3.5 The Slope of Relations

The slope of a geometric relation shows how much of a change in one variable is associated with a given change in a related variable. In causal terms, slope can be expressed as the magnitude or sensitivity of response. Several examples are shown in **Figure 1-3**.

Curve F touches the price axis where the price equals $200. This price is associated with a quantity of visits of 0. If we raise the price by $50 to a level of $250, the associated new quantity of visits, as shown by F, is 10. A $50 increase in the price is associated with a 10-visit increase in quantity. The slope of F is, thus, 50/10 with regard to the quantity axis (or 10/50 with regard to the price axis). Because F is a straight line (linear), the slope remains constant at every point on the line. (Some nonlinear relations are presented later.)

The relation in curve E also has a positive slope. As can be seen in Figure 1-3, curve E shows a greater change in price associated with a given change in quantity than does curve F. From the initial price of $200 and 0 visits, a quantity change of 10 visits is associated with a price change from $200 to $300. The slope is, thus, 100/10 with regard to the quantity

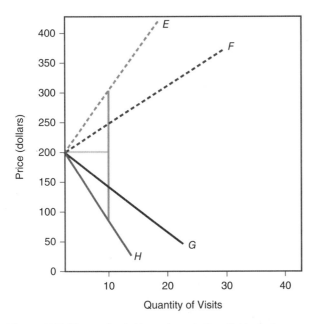

Figure 1-3 Slope of relations. In relation *E*, the price increases more than in relation *F* for a given increase in quantity. In relation *H*, the price decreases more than in relation *G* for a given increase in quantity.

© Jones & Bartlett Learning.

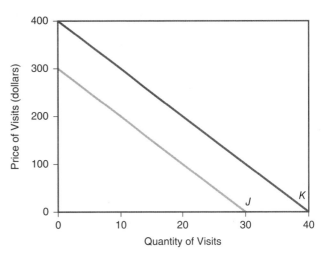

Figure 1-4 Position of relations. *K* shows a greater quantity of visits than *J* for any given price.

© Jones & Bartlett Learning.

axis (or 10/100 with regard to the price axis). Comparing curves *E* and *F*, we can say that for the same quantity change, the price change in *E* must be double that in *F*.

The relations in curves *G* and *H* can be regarded in a similar manner, but now the direction of these relations is such that a higher price is associated with a lower quantity. In relation to curve *G*, a fall in price of $50 is associated with an increase in quantity of 10 visits. The slope is, thus, the same as the slope of curve *F*, but in the opposite direction. The relation in curve *H* shows a change in price of $100 associated with a quantity change of 10—the same as the relation in curve *E*, except the slope is in the opposite direction. Where the two variables change in the same direction (as occurs in curves *E* and *F*), the slope is considered to be positive; where the change is in the opposite direction (as occurs in curves *G* and *H*), the slope is considered to be negative.

1.3.6 The Position of Relations

The next characteristic of a relation is its position. In **Figure 1-4**, two relations, *J* and *K*, are shown with similar slopes but different positions. Each relation exhibits a $100 change in price associated with a change of 10 visits. Relation *J* shows no visits at a price of $300, 10 visits at a price of $200, and so on. By comparison, *K* shows 10 visits at a price of $300, twenty visits at a price of $200, and so on. The essential point of this

figure is to show how the two relations are positioned with respect to each other. Relation *K* is higher than *J* in the sense that, at any specific price, the related quantity of visits for *K* is greater than the related quantity for *J*.

1.3.7 The Shape of Relations

The examples so far have involved only linear (straight-line) relations, in which the change in one variable with regard to a given change in another variable is fixed. This is not the only type of relation, however. Sometimes, we also encounter nonlinear relations. For this type of relation, the magnitude of the response will vary along the curve. Relations *L* and *M* in **Figure 1-5** are both nonlinear relations.

M indicates the correspondence between the total cost of production of lab tests and the number of tests produced. At a quantity of 0, the total cost is $10, reflecting the fact that the organization incurs fixed costs of $10 regardless of the production of any output; at a quantity of 1, total cost is $11; at a quantity of 2, it is $14; and at a quantity of 3, it is $19. The slope of the relation changes as more lab tests are produced. For the first test, the slope is such that a $1 change in cost is associated with a change of one lab test. The next change of one lab test is associated with a $3 change in cost, and the next with a $5 change in cost. The slope with reference to the lab test axis increases as the number of lab tests increases. *M* is a smoothed-out version of this relation.

Relation *L* shows declining slopes with increasing production. A total cost of $0 is associated with a 0 level of output. An output level of 1 is associated with a cost of $5, an output level of 2 is associated with a

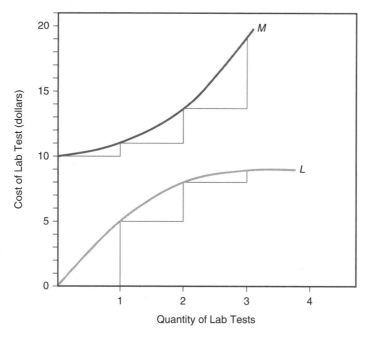

Figure 1-5 Shape of relations. *M* shows higher additional costs at successively higher levels of lab tests produced. *L* shows lower additional costs at successively higher levels of tests.

cost of $8, and an output level of 3 is associated with a cost of $9. The slope of the relation between 0 and 1 units of production, with regard to the production axis, is 5/1; for the next unit of production, it is 3/1; and for the next it is 1/1.

1.3.8 The Nature of Economic Propositions

Many statements in this book regarding the resource allocation process in the healthcare field are basically efforts to spell out the consequences of certain conditions. The propositions are hypothetical statements of the form "if . . . then . . . ."

For example, we might claim that if certain conditions x, y, and z hold, then, as a consequence, phenomenon q will occur. In making this statement, we essentially make a prediction of what will cause the phenomenon we want to explain. The "if" portions of these statements are called *conditions* or *assumptions*; the "then" portions are *conclusions*, *implications*, or *predictions*.

As an example, let us form a model to explain how much medical care an individual will demand. Our model contains several initial assumptions. The first assumption, A1, is that the price of medical care charged to an individual is $500 per visit; this $500 includes all services provided by the doctor, including transfusions, intravenous feedings (should they be needed), and so on. The second assumption,

A2, states that the individual has a monthly income of $10,000 that can be spent on any of a number of goods and services. This assumption brings the example within the realm of economics, since scarcity (limited amount of income) is now introduced. The third assumption, A3, is about the behavior of the individual; the individual has as an objective the consumption of medical care only; he does not want to consume any other good or service. We also assume, A4, that this is entirely feasible. If the individual does not consume food, for example, he would begin to starve and have to visit a physician, where, for a fee of $500, he could receive nutrition intravenously.

What are the implications of these assumptions? The main implication is that the individual will consume 20 physician office visits. Given his economic situation (income), this is all he can afford to consume, and given that he wants only medical care and can survive by consuming this service, then he will not consume less than 20 visits. This implication is a prediction of our model; the prediction is based on the initial conditions or assumptions of the model. Predictions are derivatives of the assumptions and can be regarded as the consequences that would result if the assumptions were to hold (Wilensky, 1991).

Let us now replace one of our initial assumptions, A1, with the assumption that the price of medical care is $100 per visit. Now, our model implies that the quantity of visits will be 100. With a fall in price, the quantity demanded will increase. This is a prediction of our model when we consider all the assumptions and do a comparative analysis.

We can also predict the consequences that would result if the individual's income increases. Suppose we replace assumption A2 with the assumption that the individual's monthly income is $11,000. This new assumption, coupled with the original assumptions A1, A3, and A4, yields the conclusion that the quantity of visits demanded will increase. By performing a comparative analysis of the original conditions and the new conditions, we can conclude that an increase in income will lead to an increase in the quantity of medical care demanded.

The mere predicting or deriving conclusions about the resource allocation process is not the end of our task, however. Our conclusions are implications about what would result if the assumptions we have posited in the model are adequate approximations of the conditions that exist in reality. In explanatory economics, implications are tested against actual data to see if what we predicted actually does occur. The true test of an explanatory model is how well it explains or predicts actual phenomena. In evaluative economics, our task is somewhat different: we compare actual against ideal sets of events. Nevertheless, whether we are deriving explanatory or evaluative principles, we put our propositions into a logical form that allows us to incorporate a number of variables into our analysis simultaneously.

Exercises

1. Define the discipline of economics.
2. What is scarcity?
3. What are the three major tasks of economics?
4. What are the tools of economic analysis?
5. What does the slope of a geometric relation show?

Bibliography

Aaron, H. J., & Schwartz, W. B. (1990). Rationing health care. *Science, 247*, 418–422.

Angell, M. (1985). Cost containment and the physician. *JAMA, 253*, 1203–1207.

Arrow, K. H. (1972). Problems of resource allocation in United States medical care. In R. M. Kunz & H. Fehr (Eds.), *The challenge of life* (pp. 392–410). Basel: Birkhauser-Verlag.

Centers for Medicare and Medicaid. (2018). *NHE Fact Sheet.* Baltimore, MD: Author.

Dranove, E. (2000). *The economic evolution of American health care.* Princeton, NJ: Princeton University Press.

Enthoven, A. C. (1980). *Health plan.* Reading, MA: Addison-Wesley.

Hemenway, D. (1982). The optimal location of doctors. *New England Journal of Medicine, 306*, 397–401.

Hicks, L. (2011). Making hard choices: Rationing health care services. *The Journal of Legal Medicine, 32*, 27–50.

Jha, K. J. (2018). End-of-life care, not end-of-life spending. *JAMA Forum*, July 13.

Kaiser Family Foundation. (2018a). *Employer health benefits: Summary of findings.* San Francisco, CA: Author.

Kaiser Family Foundation. (2018b). *Key facts about the uninsured population.* San Francisco, CA: Author.

Long, S. H., Gibbs, J. O., Crozier, J. P., Cooper, D. I., Jr., Newman, J. F., Jr., & Larsen, A. M. (1984). Medical expenditures of terminal cancer patients during the last year of life. *Inquiry, 21*, 315–327.

National Center for Health Statistics. (2018). *Health, United States, 2017: With special feature on mortality.* Hyattsville, MD: US Department of Health and Human Services.

Reinhardt, U. (1987). Resource allocation in health care. *Milbank Quarterly, 65*, 153–176.

Schoder, J., & Zweifel, P. (2011). The flat-of-the-curve medicine: A new perspective on the production of health. *Health Economics Review, 1*(2), 1–10.

Wilensky, G. R. (1991). The health care quadrilemma: An essay on technological change, insurance, quality of care, and cost containment. *Journal of Economic Literature, 29*, 523–552.

Zook, C., & Moore, F. D. (1980). High cost users of medical care. *New England Journal of Medicine, 302*, 996–1002.

Descriptive Economics

CHAPTER 2

Output of the Healthcare Sector

OBJECTIVES

1. Describe the product *medical care* and its components.
2. Define the concepts of *risk* and *risk shifting*, and show why they are relevant to medical care.
3. Describe the concept of *health outcome*.
4. Explain the theoretical relationship between health and medical care.
5. Demonstrate the meaning of the term *flat-of-the-curve medicine*.

2.1 Introduction

Recall that the three tasks of economics are description, explanation, and evaluation. In this chapter, the descriptive elements in the study of the healthcare system are introduced. This involves identifying the factors or phenomena of interest, defining these factors in order to know their nature precisely, and measuring the factors in order to obtain an understanding of their magnitude. At this stage of the process, the goal is to discover what factors or phenomena exist, not what causes the factors (explanation), or in what quantities the factors should exist (evaluation).

In identifying the factors of interest in the healthcare system, the processes generated within the healthcare system can be examined using two basic approaches. The first approach is to examine the factors that directly influence health. These health-influencing factors can be classified as lifestyle elements, such as diet, sleep, smoking, and other individual behaviors; social determinants, such as income, job, family, community; environmental factors, such as air and water purity; genetic factors; and medical care, such as preventive services and treatment interventions. The second approach identifies the impact that medical care has on the health status of either an individual or society.

In addressing the first approach, Section 2.2 focuses on the definition and measurement of medical care. It identifies and defines the factors or phenomena associated with medical care and discusses measures that indicate how much medical care is provided or produced. Section 2.3 describes another aspect of the healthcare system: risk shifting. Because most medical expenditures of an individual do not occur with certainty, most individuals place a value on buying insurance to cover possible financial losses from experiencing a health problem. Risk shifting provides benefits to consumers and is an important output of the healthcare sector.

The second approach stems from the assertion that the true end of the healthcare sector is not the care itself, but rather the improvements in the health status that result from the utilization (consumption) of this care. When measuring the output of health care, according to this approach, the measure should be how much health is being produced with the medical care. If it is believed that the volume of medical care provided is not necessarily a good indicator of the benefits provided by the healthcare system, a more fundamental approach would be to measure what medical care is ideally supposed to produce, that is, improvements in health.

In addressing the second approach, Section 2.4 examines issues of definition and measurement associated with health. Section 2.5 focuses on the output of the healthcare system derived from the education of healthcare personnel. The healthcare system includes the training of the professionals who work within the system, and these individuals will produce output (health care) during their training and after it is completed. In economic terms, the output of the investment in the education and training production process is called the development of "human capital."

2.2 Medical Care

Medical care is a process during which certain inputs, or factors of production (e.g., healthcare provider services, medical instruments and equipment services, physical location and structure, and pharmaceuticals), are combined in varying quantities, often under a physician's supervision, to yield an output. For example, an individual visiting a physician's office may receive an examination involving the services of the physician or a nurse practitioner, nurse, or medical technician, and the use of some equipment and supplies. The inputs in the production of medical care vary from one visit to another. One patient may receive more friendly treatment than another, and healthcare providers vary in their thoroughness, knowledge, and technique. Thus, the output of one visit may differ considerably from the output of another visit, even for patients presenting with the same medical condition. Different inputs are also used during visits by individuals with different medical conditions. For example, different inputs are used for patients with a sprained ankle than for patients with pneumonia.

Much of the difficulty in measuring the medical care process stems from the issue of defining the output of the healthcare system. If physician care is measured by the number of patient visits to a physician's office, then two cursory examinations count as two visits. However, one cursory examination followed by a more thorough examination involving a battery of tests also counts as two visits, even though more resources were used and a greater quantity of medical care was provided in the second case.

Another critical factor in medical care is the issue of quality and its measurement. It should be stressed

that *quality* is a very broad term, and its meaning is elusive (Donabedian, 1988; IOM, 2005). For example, organizations providing medical care can have substantially different characteristics. To begin with, organizations can differ in terms of structure, that is, the amount and type of training of the care providers in the organization and the type of medical equipment available and used, and in terms of ownership of the assets (public or private). Further, differences in structure are associated with the use of different techniques in the provision of care. For example, a computerized axial tomography (CT) scan machine that takes cross-sectional radiographs is generally considered to provide a higher-quality product than a standard radiology machine (Sisk, Dougherty, Ehrenhaft, Ruby, & Mitchner, 1990). In addition, a CT scan can be administered with or without contrasting materials, resulting in a different output.

A second aspect of the quality of care involves the process of providing care, in particular, the amount of personal attention providers gives to consumers, and incorporates what is actually done in the provision and receipt of care. Examples of quality-of-care measures that reflect the degree of personal attention given to consumers include the volume of services performed per individual and patients' evaluations of the performance of the physician and other providers. The Institute of Medicine identifies quality services as "the degree to which health care services for individuals and populations increase the likelihood of desired health outcomes and are consistent with current professional knowledge" (IOM, 2005).

Another set of characteristics is associated with outcomes, or the effects of care on the health status of the individual or the population. In this instance, the measure of outcomes deals with the accuracy of diagnoses and the effectiveness of treatments in producing changes in health status. Examples of measures reflecting this set of characteristics include hospital mortality rates adjusted for patient condition, the rates of other adverse events in hospitals, such as postsurgical infections, or the reduction in influenza because of immunizations.

The movement from a focus in patient care on the quantity of care provided to the quality of care provided is a major component of the transition to value-based care. This is a result of the view that outcomes for the patient are more important than the number of patients an individual provider sees in a day. The Institute of Medicine defines quality health care as "safe, effective, patient-centered, timely, efficient, and equitable" (IOM, 2005). The Agency for Healthcare Research and Quality (AHRQ) has defined quality health care as "doing the right thing for the right patient, at the right time, in the right way to achieve the best possible results" (AHRQ, 1998).

All the above characteristics, as well as others, have been identified as aspects of quality. In fact, every individual tends to have his or her own definition of what quality is in health care. The challenge of measuring quality, then, derives from the fact that there are many ways of viewing quality—many different ideas as to what constitutes quality. For this reason, the raw measure "visits" should be only guardedly used as a measure of physician care.

The measurement of hospital care requires the same caution. Hospital output has frequently been measured by bed days or by the number of cases admitted to or discharged from hospitals. Over time, however, the typical admitted patient receives a greater intensity of services as a result of advances in technology. To count an admission in 1965 as having the same output as an admission in 2018 (given the same type of case) would be to neglect the greater intensity of services likely to be provided at the later date.

Despite these objections, physician visits as a measure of the output of medical care and hospital admissions or bed days as a measure of the output of hospital care have frequently been used because of their immediate availability. Recently, efforts have been made to develop additional measures that incorporate the changing quality of inputs per admission or per bed day.

Output measurements are usually conducted to make comparisons, either against other output measures or against some standard. Basically, there are two types of output comparisons: time series and cross-sectional comparisons. A time series comparison measures the output of the same good or service at different times. A cross-sectional comparison measures the output of the good or service among different groups at the same time (e.g., the medical care provided to consumers in different age groups, ethnic groups, or geographic areas, or with different diagnoses).

Medical care output can be measured from three sources of data:

1. The providers can be surveyed to determine how much medical care they have produced.
2. The payers for medical care can be surveyed to determine for how much medical care they have paid.
3. The consumers can be surveyed to determine the quantity of consumption or utilization.

With perfect measurement, all three sources would yield the same results; however, because of measurement difficulties, considerable differences will usually arise. A continuing source of data on medical care received by consumers is the National Health Interview Survey, an annual nationwide sample survey of households on health-related matters compiled for the U.S. Public Health Service. Much of the information from this survey is summarized in the National Center for Health Statistics annual compendium of health-related data, *Health United States* (www.cdc.gov/nchs/hus.htm).

The National Health Interview Survey (www.cdc .gov/nchs/nhis.htm) is also a major source of data on medical care administered by physicians outside the hospital; this care is measured by the number of visits to physicians (the numbers of visits are often adjusted for the size of the relevant populations to yield utilization rates), with utilization defined as the amount of physician services consumed.

As an illustration of the use of time series data, comparisons can be made of physician office visits per year for individuals in the 65 and over age group. For this group, physician visits per person were 4.5 in 1975, also 4.5 in 1985, 5.3 in 1995, 7.1 in 2005, 6.7 in 2010, and 6.6 in 2015. These numbers indicate that there was no increase in the output of physician office care for this group between 1975 and 1985, but that a marked increase did occur in the following two decades, with a slight decrease in the last decade (see NCHS, *Health, United States*, 1994, 1999, 2011, 2018). Also, one visit in 1975 was counted as the equivalent of one visit in 2015, because quality difference or intensity adjustments were not made. It is very likely that quality did increase in this period because of new technology, better equipment, and better training. Unfortunately, this aspect of output is usually neglected in data collection efforts (Freiman, 1985).

An alternative way of measuring physician output is to focus on procedures or services. Procedures (e.g., an appendectomy) can be measured in a number of dimensions (e.g., average time of performance, complexity, overhead expenses), and based on these dimensions, comparable weights can be developed for each procedure (Hsiao & Stason, 1979; Hsiao et al., 1992). This approach better captures the differences among various physician tasks, but the data are much more difficult to obtain.

There are also several different measures of hospital output. One way of measuring hospital output is to examine the number of admissions to a hospital on a per population basis. In 1975, there were 153 admissions to community hospitals per 1000 population, while in 2015 there were 103 admissions.

However, the length of stay per admission in community hospitals has changed substantially in this time period, from 7.7 days per admission to 5.5 days. As a result, total days in community hospitals per 1000 population fell from 1178 to 560 between 1975 and 2015. Total days is a better measure of resources used than admissions, but even days of care does not tell the whole picture, as it leaves out the consideration of such things as quality and changes in technology, the demographics of the population, and the types of medical conditions treated (NCHS, 1994, 1999, 2011, 2018).

Because of the vast differences in types of illnesses, disease severity, and medical treatment patterns (including quality of care), hospital output is difficult to characterize from an economic viewpoint. One method of doing so that captures a mixture of illness types and severities, as well as treatment patterns, is the diagnosis-related group (DRG) patient classification system. The DRG system has many variants, but all of them are simply patient classification systems. In the 1998 version of the DRG system, which was used by the Health Care Financing Administration to reimburse hospitals for care provided to Medicare patients, hospital inpatient output was divided into 511 different groups based on the major reason for hospitalization, whether the case was medical or surgical, patient age, and the presence of significant complications and comorbidities (conditions in addition to the primary condition). In 2007, the Centers for Medicare and Medicaid introduced the Medicare Severity Diagnosis-Related Groups (MS-DRG), expanding the number of groups to 745, and in 2019 the number was 999, although not all codes are used for reimbursement. While the MS-DRGs do not measure quality, they do incorporate more data on the severity of illness of the patients within the diagnosis.

In 2016, the average annual charges for specific MS-DRGs from prospective payment hospitals were as follows: vaginal delivery without complicating diagnoses (MS-DRG 775) was $14,819.91; extracranial procedures without complications (MS-DRG 039) was $39,905.81; liver transplant without major complication or comorbidity (MS-DRG 006) was $296,743.66 (CMS, 2016). Despite the fact that the DRG system develops average costs among groups, the range of costs within, as well as between, DRGs was considerable; this variation is reduced, but not eliminated with the MS-DRG system.

DRGs do not measure "quality of care." To gather a picture of the quality of the hospital product, data reported by hospitals must be examined. Hospital output data are available from *Vital and Health Statistics* (Series 13), published by the Public Health Service; *Hospital Statistics,* the annual compendium of the American Hospital Association (AHA), and various issues of *Hospitals: Journal of the American Hospital Association.* The Hospital Compare website (http://www.hospitalcompare.hhs.gov) provides another source of measures of quality in hospitals, including patient perceptions regarding their hospital stays.

The AHA formerly published a series of indexes that extensively covered the concept of measuring quality changes in hospital care over time (Phillip, 1977). This index attempted to measure the quality change of a day of care by changes in service intensity, which was defined as the quantity of real services that go into a typical day of hospitalization. The AHA's Hospital Intensity Index (HII) incorporated 46 services, including the number of dialysis treatments, obstetric unit worker hours, and pharmacy worker hours. A weighted average of these 46 services was calculated annually on data from a sample of hospitals to derive an average number of services per patient day offered during the year. With the calculation for 1969 as a baseline (the value for that year equals 100), the annual averages formed an index that measured changes in the service intensity component of output over time. Between 1969 and 1976, this index increased from 100.0 to 168.60 (AHA, 1976). Although these data are no longer published, they did provide an excellent illustration of how important service intensity is as a component of medical care output. While the intensity of service has been associated with the quality of hospital services, there is no evidence that increased intensity always results in increased quality of care. There are a number of other factors impacting the actual quality of care delivered.

In **Table 2-1**, national data are shown for three components of hospital utilization between 1975 and 2015. The three general measures are hospital admissions per 1000 population, average length of stay (ALOS) per admission, and number of hospital patient days per 1000 population. As can be seen in Table 2-1, the utilization of hospitals has been declining since 1975. The decline was large in the 1980s and early 1990s, and has leveled off somewhat in recent years, especially in terms of the length of stay of individuals admitted to community hospitals. The number of days of care per 1000 population in 2015 was only about half of what it was in 1975 (declining from 1192 to 570 days of care during that period). The decline in days of care reflects both a decrease in the number of times individuals were admitted/discharged from hospitals and the average length of time they stayed in hospital once admitted.

Table 2-1 Hospital Utilization for Selected Years, 1975–2015

Year	Resident Population (in 000)	Hospital Admissions per 1000 Population	Average Length of Stay (ALOS)	Patient Days per 1000 Population
1975	215,973	154.8	7.7	1,192
1980	227,225	159.1	7.6	1,209
1990	249,464	125.0	7.2	900
1995	262,803	125.9	5.8	730
2000	281,422	124.9	5.4	674
2005	295,517	113.7	5.4	614
2010	308,746	107.1	5.5	589
2015	321,040	103.6	5.5	570

Data from Population: U.S. Census Bureau. Current Population Reports, Series P-25. Washington, DC: US Government Printing Office. Hospital: NCHS: Health US: 2017. Hyattsville, MD: US Department of Health and Senior Services.

The National Center for Health Statistics historically collected data with a national hospital discharge survey in which hospital utilization data were presented as both crude rates and age-adjusted rates. Crude rates are simply numbers of events that occurred. The age-adjusted rates are statistical calculations to adjust the age of the population to a "standard" distribution. Age-adjusted rates enable better comparisons among populations with different age distributions, which is particularly important in health care, since there are substantial differences in health simply because of the aging process. For example, if there is interest in comparing hospital utilization across different areas, and one area has a high rate of younger individuals (possibly because of a college town in its borders), compared to another area with an older population, the age-adjusted rate can be used to reduce the confounding impact of age differentials. These data are no longer publicly available, although crude hospital utilization data are available in the most recent issues of *Health United States*.

2.3 Risk Shifting and Health Insurance

Another type of healthcare sector output is risk shifting through the purchase of health insurance. Illnesses or injuries are often unexpected and are often accompanied by monetary losses. These losses can be in the form of medical expenses, lost earnings from work, and other expenses. Individuals can be said to face a *risk* of losing some of their wealth (or well-being) from the occurrence of an illness or injury, which means that the existence of the loss and its amount are uncertain. This risk creates concern on the part of consumers, and they are usually willing to pay something to avoid the risk.

One way of dealing with this risk is to shift it to someone else. Insurers are organizations that specialize in accepting risk. When an insurer accepts risk from a large number of enrollees, the *average* loss that will be incurred by the insurer becomes much more predictable (the law of averages of large numbers). Of course, there are costs of operating such a risk-sharing organization. These include the administrative expenses associated with determining probabilities, setting prices, selling policies, and adjudicating claims. The owners also expect a return on their investment (profits). These expenses and profits are included in the fee (called a *premium*) that each individual must pay to obtain insurance. The essential point here is that, in its own right, risk shifting is an additional output that is distinct from the output called *medical care*. Someone can obtain medical care without risk shifting (by paying for it out-of-pocket from private resources when the medical care is received). Such an individual is still faced with the risk of incurring losses, but has done nothing to shift the risk to someone else. It is the *additional* activity of shifting the risk in advance—taking action to reduce the financial loss should illness occur—that is the output of this type of transaction.

There are a variety of ways in which the risk associated with financial losses connected with medical care can be shifted. It can be done privately, by the purchase of health insurance. Insurance organizations, such as Blue Cross, Blue Shield, Prudential, Aetna, etc., sell health insurance policies, either directly to individuals (individual policies) or through groups, such as employers and professional associations (group policies). In addition, health maintenance organizations (HMOs) act as both insurers and providers of care. The revenue of the insurance organizations comes from the premiums they collect.

The government also acts as a payer of healthcare bills for large numbers of individuals, although, strictly speaking, the government is not an insurer: Most of its revenues to finance payment for health services are in the form of taxes, not premiums, and often the covered individuals are not the ones who currently pay these taxes. Thus, the government does not manage its healthcare-related expenditures on an insurance (risk assessment) basis. Government-style risk-sharing is referred to as *risk pooling*.

Health insurance can cover all medical expenses of an individual. Full insurance to cover all medical expenses has become quite costly, and so insurers have come to resort to "cost-sharing" provisions in their policies, in which insured persons pay a portion of their healthcare bills and the insurer covers the rest. These provisions allow the insurers to limit expected payouts and charge the insured persons lower premium rates. In cost-sharing arrangements, the risk shifting is not complete or total.

Cost-sharing can be done in several ways. The insurance policy can require the individual to cover the first dollars of expenses, referred to as a deductible, and the insurer then pays all, or a portion, of the balance of the bill. For example, the individual might be required to pay a deductible of $1000 before the insurer begins to pay anything towards the medical bill. The insurer can also specify a limit above which payments will cease, a maximum. For example, an insurer might cover expenses up to a lifetime limit of $5,000,000. Beyond that amount, the individual would again bear the financial risk. So-called catastrophic insurance (insurance that has a very high deductible before it begins to pay anything) can be obtained to cover very large losses.

The amount and type of insurance coverage is inextricably tied to the workings of the medical care market. Thus, although insurance and medical care should be thought of as separate products, they do affect one another. In the case of insurance coverage, distribution issues have arisen as a cause for concern. In the United States in 2017, roughly 27.4 million people under age 65, 10.2% of that population, were uninsured (KFF, 2018). Among those lacking health insurance coverage were a number of children (8.0% of those under 18), a fact that has generated a considerable amount of concern.

This number of uninsured children is much lower than it was previously, mainly because of the result of the implementations of the SCHIP (State Children's Health Insurance Program) and the expansion of Medicaid coverage in many states under the Patient Protection and Affordable Care Act (CDC, 2011).

The unemployed adult is not the major contributor to the uninsured adult population under age 65. Many employed individuals in the United States have no insurance. In 2017, of the uninsured population, 77% had at least one full-time worker in their family and another 10% had a family member who worked at least part-time (KFF, 2018). Since employment is the traditional source of health insurance in the United States, the lack of insurance among workers is viewed as a worrisome development (KFF, 2018; Monheit & Short, 1989).

The mere possession of some sort of insurance coverage does not guarantee adequate risk protection. Medicare is a government plan that covers hospital expenses and (optionally) medical and drug expenses for individuals aged 65 and older. Because of the cost-sharing arrangements incorporated into the Medicare program, many of those who are covered under Medicare still face a substantial financial risk should they become ill. While Medicare covers much of hospital, physician visits, lab tests, and prescription drug expenses, the beneficiaries can still incur major expenses. For example, basic Medicare does not cover hearing aids, opticians and eye exams, dental work, custodial stays in nursing homes, or medical costs incurred outside the United States.

While Medicare Part A (hospital coverage) does not have a premium, Part B (coverage for physician services, lab tests, etc.) had a $135.50 monthly premium in 2019 and individuals who earn more than $85,000 and couples with income over $170,000 pay a higher premium. While prescription drug coverage varies by plan, the average monthly fee for coverage in 2019 was $32.50. The deductible for Medicare Part A in 2019 was $1364 and the deductible for Part B was $185 (AARP, 2018). As these data indicate, Medicare beneficiaries face considerable risk of a financial loss. Indeed, in 2016, 95% of those aged 65 and older purchased private supplemental insurance plans, also called "Medigap" policies, to cover the risk resulting from the cost-sharing elements of Medicare (Graham, 2018).

At the same time, it should also be pointed out that a complete absence of risk on the part of insured individuals (the shifting of the entire risk onto insurers) has its problems as well. A totally riskless policy may be very expensive, since individuals are more prone to demand care when it has a zero out-of-pocket price to them (as under full insurance coverage). The costs of such care must still be covered by the insurer, and so premiums must increase to cover these costs. The difficult part is finding the appropriate balance between risk reduction through insurance and an appropriate incentive for consumers to be price sensitive in the utilization of covered healthcare services.

2.4 Health Status

2.4.1 Concepts

The concept of health seems so familiar to us that we can almost reach out and touch it. It seems easy to distinguish the 97-pound weakling from the bodybuilder who kicks sand in his face at the beach or to recognize a radiant complexion when we see one in a facial soap commercial on television. More precise measures, however, are hard to obtain. The categories "healthy" and "unhealthy" are not exact. The main reason for this is that we have not defined health precisely. Lacking such a definition, two observers can have different opinions as to whether one person is healthier than another. An essential task of the scientific method is to obtain widespread agreement about the nature of a phenomenon. If we lack an operational definition, we can hardly expect two independent observers to reach an agreement about the status of the phenomenon. A definition is useful, if it helps pinpoint the characteristics of the phenomenon we are trying to describe and eventually measure.

Health is not an easy concept to define with any degree of precision. As the English epidemiologist Sir Richard Doll remarked concerning the concept of health, "Positive health seems to be as elusive to measure as love, beauty, and happiness" (Doll, 1974). Yet, in an effort to give some hold on the concept, in the preamble to the World Health Organization's Constitution, health is defined as "a complete state of physical, mental and social well-being, and not merely the absence of illness or disease or infirmity" (WHO, 2006). This is a very broad definition, and the characteristics of health suggested by it are not easy to pinpoint and measure. The definition stresses that there are three components of health, and even if a person is physically healthy, he or she can still be lacking in the other categories. Also, in terms of health, wellness is often defined as the actions taken by individuals to obtain health.

2.4.2 Measures of Individual Health

For many years, health was identified by the presence of disease (morbidity) or by death (mortality). Individual measures, such as the diagnosis rates for certain conditions or rates of hospitalization, were used as indicators for morbidity. Mortality was usually adjusted for such population factors as age and sex. More recently, mortality has been addressed in terms of premature mortality, with the difference between expected age of death and the actual age of death being proposed as a measure of life years lost prematurely. Thus, if the expected age of death for a male aged 20 is 75, a 20-year-old man who dies in a car accident is considered to have lost 55 years of life. Healthy life expectancy is a refinement of life expectancy in that it incorporates age-specific health rates and age-specific morbidity rates to reflect the average number of healthy years a person can expect to live. Another way of viewing healthy years is to refer to them as quality of life years lived.

Researchers have been looking for other measures of health with a more positive focus. Attempts at identifying and measuring health have focused on certain characteristics expected in a healthy person. These characteristics include the physical functioning of the individual's body in relation to some norm, the physical capability of the individual to perform certain acts (e.g., getting up or dressing), the social capabilities of the individual (i.e., how well he or she interacts with others), and how the individual feels. These characteristics are, by no means, distinct from one another, a fact that has led to much disagreement among researchers who have tried to invent a unique measurement of health status. Different research efforts have focused on clinical characteristics; on individual capabilities (Boyle & Torrance, 1984; Culyer, 1976; Mitchell, Al-Janabi, Richardson, Iezzi, & Coast, 2015; Ruger, 2010); on the physical functioning of people's bodies in relation to some norm (Kass, 1975; Mitchell, Venkatapuram, Richardson, Iezzi, & Coast, 2017; Williamson, 1971;); and on a mixture of physical, mental, and social characteristics (Breslow, 1972; Streiner, Norman, & Cairney, 2015).

Despite the considerable difficulties in arriving at widely acceptable indexes of health status, the importance of the topic ensures that researchers will keep trying. One widely used measure is the 15-D (for 15 health dimensions), which categorizes health status into 15 groups, as shown in **Table 2-2**. These groups include breathing, hearing, moving, and so on. Subjects rate each dimension on a five-point scale. For

Table 2-2 Health Dimensions in the 15-D Health-Related Quality-of-Life Index

Dimension	Importance Weight
Breathing	0.075
Mental functioning	0.044
Speech	0.065
Vision	0.075
Mobility	0.046
Usual activities	0.057
Vitality	0.074
Hearing	0.104
Eating	0.040
Eliminating	0.033
Sleeping	0.090
Distress	0.079
Discomfort/symptoms	0.072
Sexual activity	0.084
Depression	0.062
Total	1.000

Data from Sintonen, H. (2001). The 15D instrument of health-related quality of life: Properties and applications. *Annals of Medicine, 33*, 328–335.

the breathing dimension, for example, a "1" would indicate normal breathing and a "5" would indicate that the individual experiences breathing difficulties almost always. Within each dimension, each point on the scale is assigned a value, which scores the functioning level. For example, normal breathing is scored as 1.000, and level 1 breathing is scored as 0.093. The 15-D investigators have assigned a second set of weights to each of the 15 dimensions. These weights were obtained from community surveys and reflect the importance of each dimension (Sintonen, 1995; Sintonen & Pekurinen, 1992). Example weights are shown in Table 2-2. For example, breathing has an importance weight of 0.075. The 15 importance weights sum to 1.0000.

Investigators can use instruments, such as the 15-D, to provide measures of an individual's quality of life. Further, a time dimension can be added to provide a measure of quality-adjusted life years (QALYs). Investigators often standardize these measures, with a score of 1.0000 being the highest level of health and 0.0000 being the lowest (or perhaps even death).

Thus, for example, a group of patients with asthma had an average overall 15-D score of 0.89 (out of a maximum possible score of 1.00) (Kauppinen, Sintonen, & Tukiainen, 1998). If the condition persisted for 1 year, then the average patient's quality-of-life index would be 0.89 QALYs for the period. The individual would have lost 0.11 QALYs due to his or her asthmatic condition. The score 0.11 represents the loss of full health over the year. If the condition persisted over 2 years, then the individual would have experienced 1.78 QALYs (0.89 × 2) during that 2-year period.

The translation of health-related quality of life (HRQOL) measures into QALYs has one very convenient benefit. By evaluating death as 0.0000, one can compare interventions, some of which result in death. For example, if one person lived for 5 years at a QALY value of 0.5 rather than being dead (QALY value is 0.0000), then the difference in QALYs would be 2.5000–0.0000, or 2.5 QALYs. Of course, there are conceptual problems with placing a 0.0000 value on death; death is beyond the conscious experience of people, and so they may have great difficulty comparing different levels of health with death.

The 15-D weights can be used both to assess the HRQOL of an individual over time and to compare different individuals or groups. For example, women with breast cancer can take different forms of chemotherapy. The 15-D can measure differences in health-related quality of life among the interventions. There are several general HRQOL measures in use (Bowling, 1997); those used mostly by economists include the Euroquol 5D (Kind, 1996) and the Health Utilities Index (Feeny et al., 1996). In addition, there are a large number of HRQOL measures for specific diseases (Bowling, 1995; McNaughton-Collins, Walker-Corkery, & Barry, 2004).

2.4.3 Population Health Measures

The most commonly used population health measures have been mortality rates and morbidity (usually hospitalization or specific types of diseases or illnesses) rates. Mortality, or death, rates are standardized by age and sometimes gender and can be expressed for the entire population or for subgroups, such as whites and blacks. In **Figure 2-1**, the trends in age-adjusted death rates for the total population are shown and for whites and blacks (or African Americans) from 1950 to 2016 in the United States (NCHS, 2018). All rates have been falling, but the death rate for blacks is still substantially above that for whites.

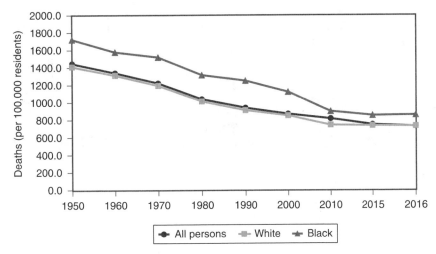

Figure 2-1 Age-adjusted death rates by group, United States 1950–2016 (deaths per 100,000 residents).
Modified from National Vital Statistics Reports 67(5). Hyattsville MD, 2018.

Table 2-3 Years of Potential Life Lost before Age 75, per 100,000 Population under 75 Years of Age, United States, Selected Years (Age Adjusted)

Year	Total	Males	Females	White	Black
1980	10,448.4	13,777.2	7350.3	9554.1	17,873.4
1990	9,085.5	11,973.5	6333.1	8159.5	16,593.0
2000	7,578.1	9,572.2	5644.6	6949.5	12,897.1
2005	7,299.8	9,206.1	5425.7	6775.6	11,890.7
2010	6,642.9	8,329.5	4994.0	6342.8	9,832.5
2015	6,757.7	8,474.7	5070.7	6514.8	9,702.3
2016	6,968.6	8,780.8	5154.1	6715.1	10,030.4

Data from National Center for Health Statistics. *Health, United States, 2010, Table 25 and Health, United States, 2017, Table 18*. Hyattsville MD, 2011 and 2018.

Death rates are also used for other subgroups; for example, the neonatal mortality rate, which expresses deaths up to the first 28 days of life as a percentage of total live births, was 3.9 in 2016, compared to 20.5 in 1950. For the white and black populations, the respective rates in 2016 were 3.3 and 7.2 (NCHS, 2018).

Increasingly, analysts have been focusing on survival time as an indicator of health status. They choose survival-time indicators because these place emphasis on the duration component of health status; a person's well-being is a function of the time spent in each health state, not merely the health state at a given moment in time. Measures that look at survival time adopt this important dimension of health. One such measure is that of potential years of life lost (PYLL) before a target age. The analyst selects a target age below which most individuals are expected to live. Deaths that occur at an age earlier than the target age are considered to be premature. The measure of premature deaths is considered to be one of the best population-level indicators of health. This indicator for males and females, whites and blacks, in the United States is shown in **Table 2-3**. The PYLL for males in 2016, expressed in terms of 100,000 persons, is 8780.8 life years, while for females it is only 5154.1 life years. The number of life years lost for blacks, on the other hand, is 10,030.4 compared to whites at 6715.1.

Of course, mortality rates do not take quality of life into account. In an effort to incorporate both mortality and quality of life into a single index, analysts at the World Health Organization have developed an index called *healthy adjusted life expectancy* (HALE) (WHO, 2018), which reflects the average number of years an individual can expect to live in "good health."

Table 2-4 Life Expectancy at Birth and Healthy Life Expectancy (HALE) at Birth, Selected Countries and World Health Organization Regions, 2016

Country	Life Expectancy at Birth, 2016			Healthy Life Expectancy (HALE) at Birth, 2016	Gap Between Life Expectancy and HALE
	Total	Males	Females	Total	Total
Argentina	76.9	73.5	77.5	68.4	8.5
Australia	82.9	81.0	84.8	73.0	9.9
Japan	84.2	81.1	87.1	74.8	9.4
New Zealand	80.2	80.5	84.0	72.8	9.4
Switzerland	83.3	81.2	85.2	73.5	9.8
United Kingdom	81.4	79.7	83.2	71.9	9.5
United States	78.5	76.0	81.0	68.5	10.0
WHO Region	**Total**	**Males**	**Females**	**Total**	**Total**
African Region	81.2	59.6	62.7	53.8	7.4
Region of the Americas	76.8	73.8	79.8	67.5	9.3
South-East Asia Region	69.5	67.9	71.3	60.4	9.1
European Region	77.5	74.2	80.8	68.4	9.1
Eastern Mediterranean Region	69.1	67.7	70.7	59.7	9.4
Western Pacific Region	76.9	75.0	78.9	68.9	8.0
Global	72.0	69.8	74.2	63.3	8.7

To estimate HALE, the investigators determine the prevalence of both fatal and nonfatal conditions in each country and adjust life years in light of disability rates due to diseases and injuries. The results for seven selected countries, the six WHO regions, and globally are displayed in **Table 2-4**. This table shows the life expectancy at birth for the population and for males and females, and the healthy life expectancy for the total population in those countries and regions. For the United States, the life expectancy at birth was 78.5 years before adjusting for disability. After making disability adjustments, this figure was reduced to 68.5 years. The difference (gap) of 10.0 disability-adjusted years is the reduction in quality of life of those who survived. The greater the gap between the two figures is a reflection of the poorer health of the surviving population. For those countries and regions shown in the table, the gap is between 7.4 and 10.0 disability years.

2.4.4 Outcome

The final output of the healthcare sector considered is health. If there is a close relationship between health and medical care, then indicators of *medical care* output can be used as indicators of the true output of the healthcare sector. It has been contended that there is not necessarily such a correspondence, and that the quantity of medical care utilized is, therefore, not a good indicator of output of the healthcare system.

Under this approach, the true output of the healthcare sector is measured by the net change in health produced by the medical care provided. That is, output is measured not by the level of the health index (e.g., by the infant mortality rate), but rather by the *change* in the index due to the medical care—in other words, the effects of the care. For example, if the infant mortality rate fell from 12.2 to 10.1 deaths per 1000 live births subsequent to a program in which a new drug was introduced, the output of the program would be that proportion of the reduction in infant mortality that was due to the new drug. It may be that other factors, such as the mothers' diets, also contributed to the change in infant mortality. The presence of such confounding factors creates difficulties in finding an accurate measure of output; medical care is seldom the only factor contributing to changes in health status. Other factors may be difficult to identify (e.g., changes in personal behaviors) and equally difficult to measure.

In addition to the identification of confounding factors, there is the problem of measuring changes in health status. The previous discussion illustrates how many difficulties are posed in trying to measure levels of health status. The measurement of changes in health status merely adds to these problems.

For example, assume that an individual with a gastrointestinal disorder will have a quality-of-life index of 0.5 for a 7-week period in the absence of any treatment. The individual, however, can be treated using one of two different drugs. The use of the less effective drug will be called Treatment A. With Treatment A, assume the individual will have a quality-of-life index of 0.7 for 2 weeks, of 0.8 for 4 additional weeks, and 1.0 for the seventh week (see **Figure 2-2**). With

Treatment B, assume the individual will have a quality of life of 0.8 for 2 weeks and will be completely cured the remaining 5 weeks (quality of life of 1.0 for weeks 3–7). Over the entire 7-week period, the individual would have a total quality-of-life measure of 3.5 quality-adjusted weeks with no treatment, 5.6 quality-adjusted weeks ([2 × 0.7] + [4 × 0.8] + 1 × 1.0) with Treatment A, and 6.6 quality-adjusted weeks with Treatment B ([2 × 0.8] + [5 × 1.0]).

The outcome measure in this example will depend on what alternative is selected. If the alternative is no care, then the outcome for Treatment A is 2.1 quality-adjusted weeks (5.6–3.5), and for Treatment B, it is 3.1 quality-adjusted weeks (6.6–3.5). That is, the outcome is the difference in the value of the index between the treatment and no treatment (Williams, 1974).

It has been contended that, in general, there is a limit to how much good medical care can do; as more medical care is provided (to the same individuals), the additional output becomes less. This is illustrated in **Figure 2-3**, where health is shown on the vertical axis and the quantity of medical care is on the horizontal axis. The medical care "outcome" curve, showing the relation between health and medical care, is drawn intersecting the health status vertical line above zero to indicate that there would be some level of health without any medical care (H_0) and that additional levels of medical care initially make contributions to health. However, the additional (marginal) contribution declines as the quantity of medical care increases.

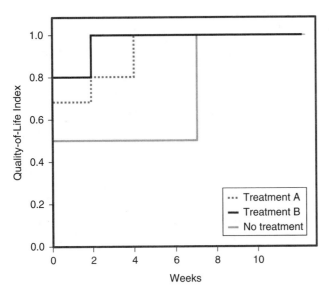

Figure 2-2 Quality-of-life indexes under three alternative treatment options. With no treatment (see thin solid line), the individual has a quality-of-life (QOL) index of 0.5 over 7 weeks and then recovers fully (QOL level 1.0). Under Treatment A (broken line), the QOL index is 0.7 for 2 weeks, 0.8 for the next 2 weeks, and 1.0 thereafter. Under Treatment B (darker solid line), the QOL index is 0.8 for 2 weeks and full recovery (1.0) thereafter.

Modified from Sintonen, H. (2001). The 15D instrument of health-related quality of life: Properties and applications. *Annals of Medicine, 33,* 328–335.

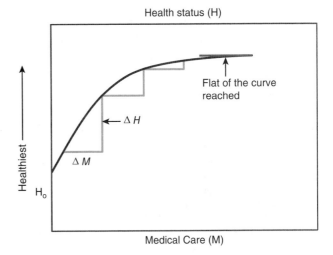

Figure 2-3 Hypothesized relationship between health and medical care. In this representation, additional doses of medical care have a diminishing impact on health status. Eventually, a situation arises of where additional medical care makes no contribution to health status, termed "the flat-of-thecurve-of-medicine".

Such an output curve assumes all other factors (environmental, genetic, social, personal) are held constant and only medical care varies. The additional output is expressed as $\Delta H/\Delta M$, where ΔM is the additional medical care and ΔH is the additional health. Note that, because of the way the curve is drawn, $\Delta H/\Delta M$ declines in value as more medical care (M) is provided, until it eventually becomes flat. This eventual flattening of the output curve has given rise to the expression "flat-of-the-curve medicine" (Culyer, 2014; Enthoven, 1980a; Fog & Mandrola, 2018; Fuchs, 2004; Schoder & Zweifel, 2011). Drawing the curve in this way illustrates, geometrically, that, as medical care provision is increased, the additional effectiveness of medical care declines until the impact reaches zero.

Researchers have attempted to establish the relation between medical care and health in different ways. Several early studies attempted to identify, statistically, a relation between mortality rates and various measures of medical input per capita using state data (Auster, Leveson, & Sarachek, 1969) and national data (Stewart, 1971). Both studies found only a small relationship or none at all. One explanation given was that we may have reached the leveling-out point on the curve. Furthermore, it was estimated that the self-care components of health care (e.g., quitting smoking, eating right, getting exercise) may, indeed, be more important than the medical care components (Newhouse & Freidlander, 1979). However, subsequent statistical research that examined specific groups, such as infants, did find significant evidence of the impact of medical care (Hadley, 1982).

Because such studies are so broadly focused, their results are often difficult to interpret, and it may be that health output is more reasonably measured only by experimental means. Setting up clinical trials, in which one group receives a certain treatment and another group with similar characteristics (a control group) does not, is an experimental method of establishing output. The difference in cure rates, if any, between the two groups could be taken as a measure of the output produced by the resources (Cochrane, 1972). Conducting experimental trials in health care often runs into ethical issues since medical treatments are withheld from the control group.

In a number of instances, less aggregated studies have sometimes failed to turn up evidence that certain medical practices impact health (e.g., no relationship was found between appendicitis death rates and appendectomies performed) (see Enthoven, 1980b, chapter 2). However, such findings should not automatically be generalized (Angell, 1985). Although it may have some analytic appeal, a broad-brush approach may pass over many situations where we are not on the "flat of the curve" of medical care.

2.5 Consumption and Investment Output

The production of any output requires the use of inputs, including human services and supplies. These inputs themselves have to be produced in order to be available for use. Many of these resources are capital inputs, which means that they are durable and last for fairly long periods of time. Capital resources are not totally consumed in the current production cycle. The totality of resources at any point in time is called a *stock* of resources. In contrast, the amount of activity that occurs during a given time period that consumes the resources is called a *flow* of resources.

An output (goods and services produced) is measured over a given period of time, such as a month or a year. Outputs fall into two classes: those that serve current wants or needs, such as the medical treatment of patients, and those that serve future wants, such as the production of capital inputs to be used in the future. The use of output for current wants is called a *consumption* activity. In health care, much of the output is used up as soon as it is produced; that is, the production of a healthcare service occurs simultaneously with its consumption by the consumer. For example, a visit to a physician for a sprained ankle is a consumption activity, because the interaction and treatment are brief, and the consumer benefits immediately from the interaction. The production of capital resources is called an *investment* activity; the effects of the activities themselves are designed to last for several years or more and are not totally consumed immediately. For example, a treatment for cancer not only has an immediate positive effect on the patient, but, if cured, the treatment has a long-term impact on the life of the consumer.

Capital inputs can be of the physical (radiological equipment) or human variety (trained radiologists and radiology technicians). Physical capital is the stock of physical means of production. Examples of physical capital include equipment and buildings. Human capital is the stock of talents, skills, and knowledge embodied in individuals. An example of investment in physical capital is the production of radiology machines. Undergraduate and postgraduate medical education, nursing education, and the education of allied health professionals, public health professionals, and administrators are examples of investment in human capital.

One feature of the healthcare sector is that much of the human capital investment activity is a byproduct of a medical care consumption activity. Much undergraduate medical education and most postgraduate medical education, for example, occur in hospitals and clinics. In many cases, education and patient care activities are inseparable, physically and financially. For many years, teaching hospitals have relied on labor from medical interns and residents to provide patient care. Because the supply of physicians, including the ratio of specialists to primary care physicians, has become such an important issue in the United States, much attention is being paid to the process by which physicians and specialists are produced.

There is a distinct relationship between capital and production activities. Imagine a given stock of capital at the beginning of 2020 (e.g., magnetic resonance imaging [MRI] machines). Net new investment is the additional stock added during the year (new machines produced minus any machines retired). The stock at the beginning of 2021 is the original capital stock plus the net new investment in MRIs. Important related concepts include the capacity of the capital equipment, actual production, and the percent utilization (or occupancy) rate. If there are 1000 MRI machines in existence, and it takes 1 hour to produce one image, then the daily capacity is 24,000 images (1000 × 24 hours) and the yearly capacity is 8.76 million images (24,000 × 365 days). If, in any year, 4.4 million images were produced, the utilization rate would be 50.2% (4.5 million/8.76 million).

Measures of capacity are particularly important in the healthcare field. Some analysts believe that the supply of resources directly influences the demand for or utilization of those resources. Commonly used terms and sayings such as "supplier-induced demand" in the physician market and "an available bed is a filled bed" in the hospital market reflect this view. One of its implications is that, in order to control consumption activity in health care, the investment in capital inputs in the healthcare system must be controlled. These issues of the relationship between supply and demand (utilization) will be discussed in greater detail in later chapters.

Exercises

1. Define medical care and discuss why it is difficult to measure it.
2. What is risk and how can people reduce it? Is there a cost to do so?
3. What is the World Health Organization's definition of health and what is a problem with using it?
4. What is a quality-adjusted life year? How can it be used to compare differences in health status between someone who is healthy and someone who is not?
5. What is the weakness of using an unadjusted mortality rate as an indicator of population health status?
6. Which issues in the measurement of population health do potential years of life lost (PYLL) and disability-adjusted life expectancy or healthy adjusted life expectancy (HALE) address?
7. Specify a hypothesized relationship between medical care and health. How does flat-of-the-curve medicine fit in with this concept?
8. Indicate at which point flat-of-the-curve medicine is experienced in the following example, assuming that influenza shots have been administered for a given population of elderly persons.

Number of Influenza Shots Administered	Number of Hospitalizations for Influenza
0	6
1	5
2	4
3	3
4	2
5	2

Bibliography

AARP. (2018). *Medicare basics*. Retrieved from www.aarp.org /health/Medicare-insurance/Medicare-basics/

Agency for Healthcare Research and Quality. (1997, September). *Statistics from the Nationwide Inpatient Sample for 1994 Hospital Inpatient Stays*. AHCPR Pub. No. 97-0056.

Agency for Healthcare Research and Quality. (1998). *Your guide to choosing quality healthcare*. Rockville, MD: Author.

American Community Survey (The American Community Survey is a nationwide survey designed to provide communities a fresh look at how they are changing). Retrieved from http:// factfinder.census.gov/servlet/DatasetMainPageServlet? _program=ACS&_submenuId=datasets_2&_lang=en

American Hospital Association. (1976). *Hospital statistics*. Chicago, IL: American Hospital Association.

Angell, M. (1985). Cost containment and the physician. *JAMA, 254*, 1203–1207.

Auster, R., Leveson, I., & Sarachek, D. (1969). The production of health, an explanatory study. *Journal of Human Resources, 4*, 412–436.

Bowling, A. (1995). Measuring disease: A review of disease specific quality measurement scales. Ann Arbor, MI: University of Michigan Press.

Bowling, A. (1997). Measuring health: A review of quality of life measurement scales. Philadelphia, PA: Open University Press.

Boyle, M. H., & Torrance, G. W. (1984). Developing multiattribute health indexes. *Medical Care, 22*, 1045–1057.

Breslow, L. (1972). A quantitative approach to the World Health Organization definition of health: Physical, mental, and social well-being. *International Journal of Epidemiology, 1*, 347–355.

Center for Disease Control. (2011). Lack of health insurance and type of coverage. *Health Insurance Coverage. Early Release of Selected Estimates*. Based on data from the January-September 2010 National Health Interview Survey. Retrieved from http://www.cdc.gov/nchs/data/nhis/earlyrelease/insur201006 .htm#footnotes8

Centers for Medicare and Medicaid Services. (2016). *DRG summary for Medicare inpatient prospective payment hospitals, CY 2016 nationally*. Baltimore, MD: Author.

Cochrane, A. (1972). *Effectiveness and efficiency*. New York, NY: Oxford University Press.

Culyer, A. J. (1976). *Need and the national health service*. London, England: Martin Robertson Co.

Culyer, A. J. (2014). *The dictionary of health economics* (3rd ed.). Cheltenham, England: Edward Elgar Publishing Limited.

Doll, R. (1974). Surveillance and monitoring. *International Journal of Epidemiology, 3*, 305–314.

Donabedian, A. (1988). The quality of care. *JAMA, 260*, 1743–1748.

Enthoven, A. C. (1980a). *Health plan*. Reading, MA: Addison-Wesley.

Enthoven, A. C. (1980b). Health planning: The only practical solution to the soaring cost of medical care. Reading, MA: Addison-Wesley.

Feeny, D. H., Torrence, G. W., & Furlong, W. J. (1996). Health utilities index. In B. Spilker (Ed.), *Quality of life and pharmacoeconomics in clinical trials*. Philadelphia, PA: Lippincott-Raven, pages, 239–252.

Fog, A. J., & Mandrola, J. M. (2018). Heavy heart: The economic burden of heart disease in the US now and in the future. *Primary Care: Clinics and Office Practice, 45*(1), 17–24.

Freiman, M. P. (1985). The rate of adoption of new procedures among physicians. *Medical Care, 23*, 939–945.

Fuchs, V. R. (2004). More variation in use of care, more flat-of-the-curve medicine. *Health Affairs, 23*(Variations Revisited Suppl2), VAR 104–VAR 107.

Graham, J. (2018, July). Here's what you need to know about medigap coverage. *Kaiser Health News*.

Hadley, J. (1982). *More medical care, better health?* Washington, DC: Urban Institute.

Hsiao, W. C., Braun, P., Dunn, D. L., Becker, E. R., Yntema, D., Verrilli, D. K., ... Chen, S. P. (1992). An overview of the development and refinement of the resource-based relative value scale. *Medical Care, 30*(suppl.), NS1.

Hsiao, W. C., & Stason, W. B. (1979). Toward developing a relative value scale for medical and surgical services. *Health Care Financing Review, 1*, 23–39.

Institute of Medicine. (2005). *Performance measurement: Accelerating improvements*. Washington, DC: National Academy Press.

Kaiser Family Foundation. (2018). Key facts about the uninsured population. *Kaiser Fact Sheet*. San Francisco, CA: Author.

Kass, L. R. (1975). The pursuit of health. *Public Interest, 40*, 11–42.

Kauppinen, R., Sintonen, H., & Tukiainen, H. (1998). One-year economic evaluation of intensive versus conventional patient education and supervision for self-management of new asthmatic patients. *Respiratory Medicine, 92*, 300–307.

Kind, P. (1996). The EUROQUOL instrument: An index of health related quality of life. In B. Spilker (ed.), *Quality of life and pharmacoeconomics in clinical trials*. Philadelphia, PA: Lippincott-Raven.

McNaughton-Collins, M., Walker-Corkery, E., & Barry, M. J. (2004). Health-related quality of life, satisfaction, and economic outcome measures in studies of prostate cancer screening and treatment, 1990–2000. *Journal of National Cancer Institute Monographs, 33*, 79–101.

Mitchell, P. M., Al-Janabi, H., Richardson, J., Iezzi, A., & Coast, J. (2015). The relative impact of disease on health status and capability well-being: A multi-country study. *PLOS ONE, 10*(12), PMCID: PNC4667875.

Mitchell, P. M., Venkatapuram, S., Richardson, J., Iezzi, A., & Coast, J. (2017). Are quality-adjusted life years a good proxy measure of individual capabilities? *Pharmacoeconomics, 35*(6), 637–646.

Monheit, A. C., & Short, P. F. (1989). Mandating health coverage for working Americans. *Health Affairs, 8*(winter), 22–38.

National Center for Health Statistics. (1994). *Health, United States, 1993*. Hyattsville, MD: Author.

National Center for Health Statistics. (1999). *Health, United States, 1998*. Hyattsville, MD: Author.

National Center for Health Statistics. (2011). *Health, United States, 2010*. Hyattsville, MD: Author.

National Center for Health Statistics. (2018). *Health, United States, 2017*. Hyattsville, MD: Author.

Newhouse, J. P., & Friedlander, L. J. (1979). The relationship between medical resources and measures of health. *Journal of Human Resources, 15*, 200–218.

Phillip, P. J. (1977, April). HCI/HII: Two new AHA indexes measure cost, intensity. *Hospital Financial Management, 31*(4), 20–22, 24, 26.

Ruger, J. P. (2010). Health capability: Conceptualization and operationalization. *American Journal of Public Health, 100*(1), 41–49.

Schoder, J., & Zweifel, P. (2011). Flat-of-curve-medicine: A new perspective on the production of health. *Health Economics Review, 2,* 1–10

Sintonen, H. (1995). The 15D-measure of health-related quality of life. II. Feasibility, reliability, and validity of its valuation system. West Heidelberg, Australia: National Centre for Health Program Evaluation.

Sintonen, H., & Pekurinen, M. (1992). A fifteen-dimensional measure of health-related quality of life and its applications. In S.R. Walker & R.M. Rosser (Eds.), *Quality of life assessment.* Dordrecht, Netherlands: Kluwer Academic.

Sisk, J. E., Dougherty, D. M., Ehrenhaft, P. M., Ruby, G., & Mitchner, B. A. (1990). Assessing information for consumers on the quality of medical care. *Inquiry, 27,* 263–272.

Stewart, C. T. (1971). Allocation of resources to health. *Journal of Human Resources, 6,* 103–122.

Streiner, D. L., Norman, G. P., & Cairney, J. (2015). *Health measurement scales: A practical guide to their development and use* (5th ed.). Oxford, NY: Oxford University Press.

Williams, A. (1974). Measuring the effectiveness of the health care system. *British Journal of the Preventive Medicine Society, 28,* 196–202.

Williamson, J. W. (1971). Evaluating quality of patient care. *JAMA, 218,* 564–569.

World Health Organization. (2006). *Constitution of the World Health Organization* (45th ed.). Geneva, Switzerland: Author.

World Health Organization. (2018). *World health statistics 2018: Monitoring health for the SDGs.* Geneva, Switzerland: Author.

CHAPTER 3

Economic Dimensions of the Healthcare System

OBJECTIVES

1. Identify the key economic units in the healthcare market.
2. Describe the flows of money and services in an uninsured and an insured healthcare market.
3. Describe the flows of money and services in a managed care environment.
4. Define the concept of cost and identify the key components in the cost of healthcare services.
5. Understand the growth of costs in the American healthcare system.
6. Understand the concepts of "cost of illness" and "economic burden of illness."

3.1 Introduction

The purpose of this chapter is twofold: to introduce readers to some basic concepts used in describing healthcare activities and to provide a description of some of the key elements of health care in the United States. To achieve its purpose, this chapter focuses on three key aspects of economic activity. First, it examines the basic economic units that participate in the healthcare economy. Second, it explains how simple flow analysis can be used to describe the economic relationships among the various units. Finally, it presents the concept of economic cost, which is used in measuring the amount of economic activity performed to produce economic output, as well as provide an overview of the potential impact of illness.

It should be pointed out that this chapter describes what happens over time as a result of activity in the healthcare economy. It identifies the economic units and their characteristics and describes the flows of money and services that occur.

Section 3.2 identifies the main "actors" in our analysis—the economic units of the healthcare

sector—and describes some of their central characteristics. It also identifies the concepts economists use to study how these units are organized. Finally, using flow diagrams, it shows how transactions among the various economic units can occur and the implications of these transactions.

Of considerable importance in understanding the implications of transactions is the measurement of the magnitude of economic activity. Section 3.3 explains the concept of "economic cost," which is a measure of economic activity in terms of money. This concept is used to measure various aspects of healthcare activity, including the total expenditures on healthcare services, the total economic costs of illness, and the burden of economic costs on various groups of the population.

3.2 Economic Units and Economic Flows

3.2.1 Economic Units

Basic units observed for economic analysis include individuals and organizations, both public and private. In examining the activity of consuming health care, the economic unit can be taken to be an individual or a household. Both of these units are commonly employed by economists, policy analysts, and others in describing and explaining economic activity. One reason the household is so frequently used in analysis is that more consistent data can usually be collected at this level. For example, if one examined housewives' consumption of healthcare services in relation to their *personal* (individual) incomes, a biased picture of the relationship might emerge, because their consumption of health care is more closely related to the income of their households than to their individual incomes. The roles that individuals take in the healthcare economy include those of demanders of healthcare goods and services and health insurance, as employees, and as taxpayers. Employers are also economic units in the healthcare system, primarily in their role as demanders of labor and of healthcare insurance for their employees.

Insurers are firms that have the function of taking on the healthcare expenditure risk of their customers. Insurance companies collect premiums from their customers and reimburse the providers for the care they provide for their enrollees. Providers of health care can include physicians, nurse practitioners, nurses, hospitals, long-term care facilities, public health agencies, mental health providers, and other providers of various forms of ambulatory care.

There has been a trend in recent years toward the integration of units. "Horizontal integration" is a term that refers to the joining together of providers (and sometimes consumers) of the same type. For example, physicians have joined group practices. Hospitals and long-term care facilities have joined chains. And there have been some instances of small businesses joining together to form group purchasing cooperatives for health insurance. There has also been a considerable movement toward "vertical integration," which is the amalgamation of providers of different types, such as hospitals purchasing physician practices and long-term care facilities. In addition, there has been an amalgamation of insurers and providers, who, for example, have joined together to create health maintenance organizations (HMOs). In addition, there has been the establishment of accountable care organizations (ACOs) and other organizational structures for managing care and healthcare costs.

3.2.2 Flows Between Units

Economic flows can involve both money and services. Generally, a flow will summarize a transaction in which

a service or good is exchanged for money. Such transactions occur in simple markets, with the degree of concentration possessed by the buyer or seller influencing the terms of the exchange. The market for lettuce is a simple market in which vendors provide lettuce to consumers in exchange for money. The exchange is at a price that is determined, in part, by how concentrated the vendor market is. In this section, the concern is with describing which flows take place, not with the terms of the transactions. Further, as shown presently, the flows in typical healthcare markets are much more complex than those in markets for lettuce, because they often contain two sets of flows—one for insurance and one for healthcare services.

3.2.2.1 Flows in a "Generic" Healthcare Market

The flows in a simple, or "generic," healthcare market are shown in **Figure 3-1**. In this market, consumers directly purchase individual health insurance policies from insurers. The cash payments to the insurance company by the consumers are called *premiums*. When a consumer uses healthcare services that are covered by the insurance policy, the insurer *reimburses* the provider the agreed-upon amount for the services provided. If the insurance does not cover the entire amount of the healthcare services used, then the individual pays the balance out of pocket.

The contract between the insurer and the consumer can have another very important dimension. The consumer can purchase varying degrees of insurance coverage. If the consumer is partially covered, and has deductibles, copayments, coinsurance, and an upper limit restriction, the insurer reimburses the provider for only a portion of the bill; the consumer must pay the remainder. The consumer's portion is

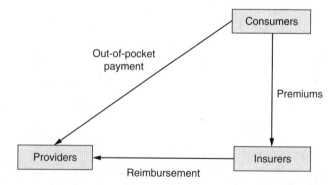

Figure 3-1 Generic healthcare market. Consumers pay premiums to insurers; insurers reimburse providers for some of the costs of the healthcare services; consumers pay the balance of the costs out of pocket to providers.

called an *out-of-pocket payment* for the services consumed. If the consumer is fully insured, there is no out-of-pocket payment by the consumer. The reimbursement provided by the insurer is payment in full for the services consumed.

The economic importance of out-of-pocket payments is that they are borne by the consumer. It is this cost that influences the consumer's decision as to how much of the healthcare service he or she demands. Among the types of direct consumer payments are deductibles, which are fixed upfront payments the consumer must pay before the insurance pays anything; copayments, which is a fixed amount paid each time a healthcare service is used, and coinsurance, which is payments related to quantity used. For example, an insurance policy might have a deductible of $500, a copayment of $50, and a coinsurance rate of 25%. This means that the consumer pays $50 each time he or she sees a healthcare provider, and, in addition, pays the first $500 charged for services received before any insurance coverage begins. After the deductible is met, the consumer pays 25% of the bill and the insurer reimburses the other 75%. The consumer still pays the $50 each time a healthcare service is used. Typically, hospital care has the highest coverage, with over 95% of expenses being covered; physician care has a lower degree of coverage (91% on average), and nursing home care has less still (71%).

With regard to insurer payments, there are numerous bases on which providers can be reimbursed. Hospitals can be reimbursed on the basis of a given budget or on a unit basis—per patient day, per case, or per service. Over the decades, there has been a movement on the part of insurers toward reimbursing hospitals on a per-case basis, recognizing differences in resource use among different case types. In this instance, hospital cases are classified into *diagnosis-related groups* (DRGs), and a separate reimbursement rate is set for each DRG. Historically, each time a patient was admitted to the hospital, the hospital was paid a rate corresponding to the patient's particular DRG. Currently, insurers are looking at readmissions within a specified period (e.g., 30 days) to determine if the admission should be considered a new admission or a continuation of the original admission before making a payment. Physicians are largely reimbursed on a fee-for-service basis, and long-term care facilities on a per diem (per day) basis.

3.2.2.2 Introducing the Employer

In 2018, only about 57% of all firms offered health benefits (health insurance) to at least some of their employees, a percent that has remained relatively stable in recent years. While only 57% of firms offer health benefits, 90% of workers are employed in firms offering health benefits because large firms usually provide health benefits (Kaiser Family Foundation, 2018). A basic set of flow relationships for employer-provided health insurance is shown in **Figure 3-2**. In these circumstances, both the employer and the employee pay a share of the premiums. In 2018, employees, on average, contributed 18% of premiums for single coverage and 29% for family coverage depending on the plan and the size of the firm.

It should be noted that the employer's share of the premiums is not a "free" benefit given to the employee;

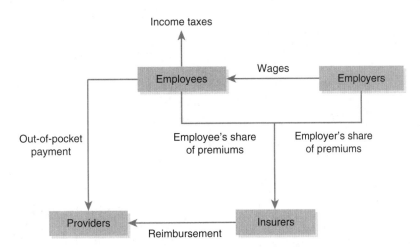

Figure 3-2 Relationships with employer-provided health insurance. Employers pay wages to employees and a share of premiums to insurers. Employees pay income taxes on wages, and pay a share of premiums to insurers and pay providers out-of-pocket for costs not covered by insurance. Insurers reimburse providers an agreed upon amount from premiums collected.

it is, rather, a form of compensation received by the employee. Total compensation to the employee takes the form of money benefits (wages or salaries) and nonmonetary benefits, such as health insurance coverage. From a financial standpoint, the employer is affected the same by either form of compensation: a dollar in wages costs the same to the employer as a dollar in noncash benefits. But the employee will have a preference because of income tax regulations. In 2018, average family premiums for health insurance were $19,616, and premiums for an individual were $6896 (Kaiser Family Foundation, 2018).

Unlike wages, many noncash benefits are not subject to income tax for the individual. Thus, noncash benefits, such as health insurance premiums, are cheaper to obtain if they are "purchased" through an employer rather than paid for out of after-tax income by the individual. As an example, assume that a family's tax rate is 20% and that the family wants to buy $1000 of health insurance. If the employee takes compensation in the form of wages, the employee must earn $1250 in order to have $1000 after paying the 20% tax (20% of $1250 is $250). The employee need earn only $1000 if compensation is taken in the form of benefits. Or put another way, $250 of compensation in the form of nontaxable benefits will buy more health insurance than the employee could with $250 in wages. The economic importance of this is that present taxation arrangements make health insurance less expensive and encourage more insurance to be bought by the individual than would be purchased with after-tax income.

When economic units are bigger or have a larger share of the market, they may be able to obtain better terms when selling or purchasing services. One type of arrangement that has been increasing in importance is the employer coalition, which is formed by businesses in local markets. Coalition members share information on provider prices, utilization trends, and so on, and they also cooperate with each other in developing benefit designs (e.g., common copayment arrangements). The original purpose of forming coalitions was to develop a sort of countervailing power in the market so that the buyers—the employers—would be able to exert some degree of market influence over price (McLauchlin, Zellers, & Brown, 1989). Another type of arrangement is the health insurance purchasing coalition (HIPC), which is a coalition of purchasers of insurance designed to garner the benefits associated with group purchasing (Reinhardt, 1993). By pooling the number of employees to be covered, the HIPC is able to negotiate a better price for premiums. HIPCs have been set up in some states to improve the access of smaller purchasers to health insurance.

The Patient Protection and Affordable Care Act, passed in 2010, provided funds to states to establish high-risk insurance pools to provide access to uninsured individuals with preexisting medical conditions who had been unable to obtain private health insurance coverage in the past because of these conditions. The intent of these temporary high-risk insurance pools (officially called the Preexisting Condition Insurance Plan) was to fill the gap until 2014, when insurance companies would no longer be able to deny coverage or charge excessive premiums to individuals because of their preexisting medical conditions. Beginning in 2014, consumers with preexisting conditions were able to access affordable care through health insurance exchanges, which were also established by the Affordable Care Act. Under the reform law, the premiums are set to not exceed 100% of the standard nongroup rate in the state and cannot vary by age by more than 4–1. While many states had offered different forms of high-risk pooled insurance plans in the past, the premiums charged by these plans (usually 125%–200% of prevailing individual market premiums) were still often prohibitive for individuals, effectively shutting them out of the insurance market. In 2019, there is a lawsuit pending that would abolish the section of the Patient Protection and Affordable Care Act that covers preexisting conditions, once more exposing these individuals to prohibitive insurance premiums.

3.2.2.3 Introducing Government Insurance

Many individuals are insured by government programs. Medicare is a program of the federal government that covers individuals 65 years old and over, certain disabled groups, individuals with certain kidney diseases, and individuals with Lou Gehrig disease. Medicare is a form of limited national health insurance. The essential flows in Medicare are shown in **Figure 3-3**.

Medicare currently has four parts. *Part A, Hospital Insurance* (HI), helps cover inpatient care in hospitals, skilled nursing facilities (for limited rehabilitative services, not long-term care or custodial care), hospice, and home health care. If an individual has paid Medicare taxes while working, there is no premium associated with enrollment in Part A (see Figure 3-3 for essential flows in Medicare). Eligible individuals are automatically enrolled in Part A upon obtaining eligible status. Part A is largely financed by a federal payroll tax paid by both employers and employees. In 2018, this tax was still 2.9% of every dollar of salary

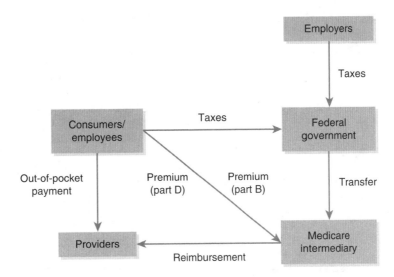

Figure 3-3 Flow of resources in Medicare market. Flow of resources: Employers and employees pay taxes to federal government. Federal government transfers resources to a Medicare intermediary who administers the Medicare program. Consumers also pay Part B and Part D premiums to Medicare and make out-of-pocket payments to providers for costs not covered by Medicare. The Medicare intermediary reimburses providers for agreed-upon costs for services provided to Medicare beneficiaries.

© Jones & Bartlett Learning.

and wages (taxable earnings); the employee's rate was 1.45%, as was the employer's rate. These taxes are placed in the Hospital Insurance Trust Fund, forming the bulk of the revenues for funding hospital and other institutional expenditures incurred by Medicare beneficiaries (Medicare Part A, 2018b).

Because of the way the Hospital Insurance Trust Fund was established, it cannot be supplemented, to any great extent, by other forms of receipt, such as general taxes, without major changes in the legislation. Because expenditures from the fund have been greater than tax revenues, there are concerns that the Trust Fund will be bankrupt soon. The projections made in the 1980s regarding potential deficits by the end of the century led to major changes in the 1990s in the method by which Medicare reimbursed hospitals, converting from a retrospective cost-based reimbursement system to the prospective payment system based on DRGs. In addition, beginning in 2013, the healthcare reform law increased the Medicare HI payroll tax for higher-income taxpayers by 0.9 percentage points, in which higher-income taxpayers are defined as earnings of more than $200,000 per individual and $250,000 per couple filing jointly or $125,000 for couples filing separately.

Although Part A Medicare has no premiums, the level of copayments is high. In 2019, there was a deductible of $1364, which covered the first 60 days of care for each spell of illness, and for anyone needing 61–90 days of hospitalization, there was a copayment of $341 for each day. If someone exceeded 90

days of care during a year, they could draw upon a lifetime reserve totaling an additional 60 days with a copayment of $682 per day. After that reserve, the beneficiary is responsible for all hospital costs. For many enrollees, the out-of-pocket payments have been considerable, and many individuals have purchased a private form of insurance called *Medigap*, which covers Medicare direct expenses not paid for by Medicare. For individuals needing long-term facility service, the first 20 days are fully covered; there was a payment required in 2018 of $170.50 per day for days 21 through 100; and for days 101 and over there is no coverage provided. Home health services that are eligible require no copayment from the beneficiary (Medicare Part A, 2018b).

Medicare Part B is the Supplementary Medical Insurance (SMI) program, which helps pay for physician, outpatient, home health, and preventive services. It also pays for ambulance services, clinical laboratory services, durable medical equipment, outpatient mental health care, kidney supplies and services, and diagnostic tests. Enrollment in Part B is voluntary and requires a monthly premium; the premium was $135.50/month in 2019 or higher depending on income. Part B has a $185 annual deductible, and typically a 20% coinsurance rate for services used. The Affordable Care Act also added a free annual comprehensive wellness visit and personalized prevention plan to the benefits. The Act also added an income-related monthly Part B premium for individuals with annual incomes greater than $85,000 and for couples with incomes of $170,000 in 2019; this premium ranged from $189.60 to $460.50 in 2019. The reform law freezes these income thresholds at 2010 levels through 2019. In addition, Part B benefits include an annual deductible ($185 in 2019), and most Part B services are subject to a coinsurance payment of 20%, although, beginning in 2011, no coinsurance and deductibles will be charged for preventive services rated as A or B by the U.S. Preventive Services Task Force (USPSTF). Revenues for Part B come from premiums, coinsurance, and general taxation (Medicare Part B, 2018c).

Part C, Medicare Advantage (MA) plans, are private health plans that pay for Medicare benefits under Parts A, B, and D. Medicare Advantage enrollees typically pay the monthly Part B premium plus an additional premium directly to their plan. While health maintenance organizations were originally an option, other private plans are now covered. These plans provide all benefits covered under traditional Medicare, plus many offer additional coverage, including prescription drugs. Plans must use any extra payment they receive (rebates) to provide additional benefits, such as lower premiums, lower cost-sharing, or vision, hearing, preventive dental care, podiatry, chiropractic, and gym memberships (Medicare Part C, 2018d).

The *Medicare Prescription Drug, Improvement, and Modernization Act* (MMA) was enacted in 2003, creating Medicare Part D, a voluntary outpatient prescription drug benefit plan that began in 2006. Enrollees in Part D generally pay a monthly premium, which is also adjusted by income, ranging from an additional $12.40 per month to $77.40 per month plus plan premiums; the plan is also funded through general revenues. Part D is very complex in terms of coverage and implementation. The law requires a standard

benefit that must be covered or an alternative equal in value (actuarially equivalent); enhanced benefits can also be offered, and most Part D plans have a coverage gap, called the "donut hole." In 2019, there could be a $415 maximum deductible and 25% coinsurance up to an initial coverage limit of $3820 in total drug costs (plan plus individual payment) under the standard benefit. Enrollees then pay 25% of their plan's drug costs and dispensing fee for brand name prescriptions and 37% of the price for generic drugs until they spend $5100 out of pocket, not including premiums. Then, the individual pays a small coinsurance for covered drugs plus dispensing fees for the rest of the year. The standard benefit amounts increase annually by the rate of per capita Part D spending growth (Medicare Part D, 2018e).

Medicaid (**Figure 3-4**) is a joint cooperative federal-state program introduced in 1966 to cover certain low-income and categorically defined individuals. Federal guidelines set basic minimum criteria for eligibility, but each state's program is unique and operates differently. Medicaid is the largest health insurance program in the country. States set their own eligibility requirements within the federal parameters; select the services that will be offered and specify the amount, duration, and scope of services; design delivery systems; determine payments for services; and administer the program.

To secure Medicaid eligibility, the person must be in one of the statutorily recognized categories or eligibility groups. There are six broad coverage categorical groups: children, pregnant women, adults in families with dependent children, adults and children with disabilities or who are blind, and older persons. In addition, Medicaid is a means-tested entitlement program, and so individuals who meet the categorical criteria must also have incomes below the income standard for

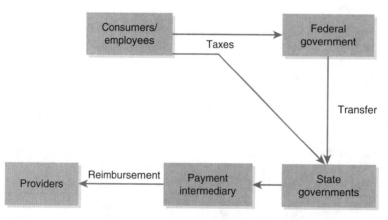

Figure 3-4 Flow of resources in Medicaid market. Consumers/employees pay taxes to the federal government and to state governments. The federal government transfers resources to states. State governments transfer resources to a payment intermediary who then transfers resources to pay providers.

the category. Because of the complicated combinations of categorical and financial factors, the mixture of mandates and options, and discretion afforded each state, eligibility varies considerably state-to-state. Federal policy, however, generally prevents Medicaid eligibility being extended to childless, nondisabled, nonelderly adults, and individuals who have primary addictive disorders, regardless of income. Currently, Medicaid covers more than two-thirds of all nursing home residents.

The Balanced Budget Act of 1997 created the State Children's Health Insurance Program (S-CHIP) to assist states in providing insurance coverage to low-income children who were not eligible for Medicaid but couldn't afford private insurance. In 2009, the Children's Health Insurance Program (CHIP) Reauthorization Act was passed and prohibits states from implementing eligibility standards, methodologies, or procedures that are more restrictive than those in place as of March 23, 2010, with the exception of waiting lists for enrolling children in CHIP. Under health reform, CHIP is maintained through 2019.

The Affordable Care Act contained provisions for dramatic expansion of the Medicaid program. Almost half of the expected gains in health insurance coverage under health reform were expected to be achieved through expansions in the Medicaid program. Historically, nonelderly adults without dependent children were not eligible for Medicaid. Under the health reform law, the categorical exclusion of these adults would end in 2014, expanding Medicaid eligibility to reach adults under 65, and provide states the option of beginning the coverage in 2010 instead of waiting until 2014. However, the mandate requiring state participation in the expansion of Medicaid was declared in violation of states' rights in the courts, and so participation by states became voluntary. Those states not participating did not receive the federal subsidies associated with the expansion, but continued to receive the subsidies for the traditional Medicaid program. Following the 2016 election, increased efforts were made to abolish the ACA.

3.2.2.4 Introducing Managed Care

Managed care refers to forms of insurance coverage in which enrollee utilization patterns and provider service patterns and costs are agreed upon and are monitored by the insurer, or an intermediary, with the aim of containing costs. There are a number of different types of managed care organization: health maintenance organizations (HMOs), preferred provider organizations (PPOs), point of service plans (POSs), and recently, accountable care organizations

(ACOs). Typically, HMOs require the most restrictive standards and cost controls on providers and enrollees.

Payment of most HMO premiums is on a "capitation" basis. That is, there is a set fee for each enrollee in the plan, and the HMO receives a single annual amount for each enrollee, regardless of the amount of care provided. This form of payment puts the HMO at risk for all expenses incurred when serving enrollees, which incidentally means that the HMO serves as an insurer as well as a provider. Enrollees in HMOs may also be expected to pay a small copayment amount (e.g., $25) each time they visit an outpatient provider.

Traditionally, an HMO had one of two forms: either it was a self-contained unit that functioned as both insurer and provider, or it was an amalgamation of private practice physicians (called an independent practice association, or IPA) who were separately reimbursed by the HMO on a discounted fee-for-service basis. Recently, several new forms of HMOs have sprung up, many owned by traditional insurance companies, such as Blue Cross or commercial companies. These new types receive the capitation fee and contract out for services with providers that the HMO enrollees use.

One of the salient features of any HMO is the restriction on access to providers. Whereas under traditional insurance coverage individuals can go to any provider they wish, enrollees in an HMO must use a group of designated providers in order for the services to be fully covered, although out-of-plan services may be covered in emergency situations. This closed-panel arrangement allows the HMO to monitor the providers and possibly have some impact on provider behavior. The providers on the panel may be employees of the HMO or contractors with the HMO; in either case, monitoring providers is more likely to be feasible than if the enrollees have an unrestricted choice of providers. Such monitoring can potentially encourage providers to practice in a more conservative, less costly manner.

Beginning in the 1980s, HMO enrollment expanded rapidly, reaching a peak in 1999. In 2017, an estimated 94.8 million individuals had HMO-type coverage (Sonofi-Aventis, 2018). HMO coverage is offered to enrollees of Medicare and Medicaid, as well as those who are traditionally covered under private insurance. Typically, HMO receipts of premiums would include employer contributions as well. It should be noted that, unlike in the case of traditional insurance coverage, there is typically no pass-through from insurer to provider; the insurer is, in essence, the provider. However, there are some types of HMOs that do contract with independent providers. Many of the characteristics of traditional HMOs have been incorporated into accountable care organizations, except for patient restriction on access to providers.

A major drawback of HMO coverage is that enrollees can only choose from a limited panel of providers to have services fully covered. In many cases, an enrollee may be attached to or prefer a specific physician before joining the HMO. If the physician is not on the HMO's provider panel, the enrollee must pay the provider's full price if he/she wishes to continue a relationship with the provider. Preferred provider organizations (PPOs) were designed to expand consumer choice while maintaining many of the monitoring benefits of HMOs.

A PPO will contract with certain providers ("preferred providers") who agree to charge lower prices and submit to utilization monitoring in exchange for being designated as a preferred provider (see **Figure 3-5**) The PPO will then contract on behalf of these providers with insurance companies to gain their business. The insurers offer their enrollees a dual pricing system— one price for those who use the preferred providers and a higher price for those who use providers outside the preferred panel. This price differential might take the form of varying copayment rates; for example, a low (or zero) copayment rate for those who use the preferred group and a higher direct payment for those who use providers outside the preferred panel. This creates an economic incentive for consumers to use the preferred group, but it allows partial coverage when a consumer chooses a provider outside the preferred panel.

Providers may join a PPO panel because of an expectation that they will likely get a greater volume of business from the enrollees of the PPO. By agreeing to submit to some form of utilization monitoring, the expectation is that, if the monitoring is successful, there will be lower utilization patterns by enrollees and lower premiums, which, in turn, translates into savings for the employer and employees.

A PPO can be a separate contractor that receives a fee from the insurer. It can be part of the insurance company itself, or it can be owned by provider groups and used as a marketing mechanism. In fact, there are many types of PPOs. What distinguishes them from HMOs is their allowance of greater choice of provider. Recently, however, HMOs have been relaxing their closed panel restrictions in favor of coverage that is more akin to PPO coverage. An HMO that allows members to seek care from non-panel providers for a differential fee is called a point-of-service (POS) plan. Under a POS plan, enrollees are required to have a primary care provider who then oversees care of the patient and provides referrals to specialty care. Out-of-network providers can be used, but at increased costs, usually in the form of higher copayments and coinsurance.

PPOs have been growing in popularity in recent years. Between 1993 and 2011, the proportion of all insured persons who were enrolled in PPOs increased from 26% to 55% (Kaiser Family Foundation, 2011). In 2017, PPOs covered 165 million people (Sonofi-Aventis, 2018). In fact, their popularity has earned them a place in a popular health insurance package now offered by many employers: the "triple option"

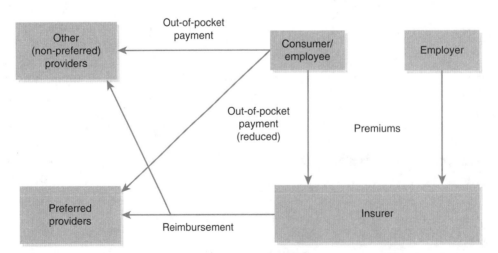

Figure 3-5 Flow of resources in a typical preferred provider organization plan. Employers, employees, and consumers pay premiums to the insurer. The insurer pays providers for services. The consumer/employee pays a reduced out-of-pocket copayment when he or she uses a preferred provider. They pay a higher copayment when they use a provider outside the preferred panel.

package. With such a package, the employer offers each employee a choice among types of coverage: traditional indemnity coverage, HMO coverage, and PPO coverage. In order to make the three types roughly comparable, the employer can alter the out-of-pocket payments and employee premiums. For example, for traditional care (the least restrictive in terms of consumer choice) the employer might set higher copayments and premiums, and enrollees who choose the more restrictive managed care options might be offered lower copayments and premiums.

Managed care is most frequently associated with HMOs and PPOs, because these types of organizations were the first to try to control the utilization of care. In a traditional HMO, providers are typically employed by the HMO or are contractually tied to it and subject to some degree of regulation. More recently, indemnity insurers have also introduced regulatory controls over providers, such as second-opinion requirements for surgery, length-of-stay reviews, and drug formularies. Providers interact with indemnity insurers at arm's length, and so indemnity insurers have had to develop such mechanisms to restrain utilization. Also, HMOs have been changing in form. In many cases, providers are more loosely tied to the HMO than has been true historically. In this type of arrangement, controlling utilization requires the establishment of contractual mechanisms. For example, providers who serve HMO members often have to obtain permission from the HMO before initiating expensive therapies.

The regulatory function of indemnity and contractual HMOs is shown in **Figure 3-6**. In this diagram, the financial flows are shown as before. The flow of services from the providers to the consumers is also shown. A dotted line from the insurer to the service flow line between providers and consumers indicates the care-management function established by the insurer. Under managed care, the service flow is regulated.

In order to set standards for providers, HMOs engage in profiling, which involves collecting comparative data on the treatment patterns of providers. Using this information, insurers can set benchmarks that can be used to regulate the utilization of care. In addition to specific controls on services, managed care organizations can also affect utilization through choosing providers to employ or with whom to contract. A cost-efficient practice style may be one characteristic such an organization is seeking when recruiting new providers.

The most recent organizational structure of managed care is the *accountable care organization* (ACO), which was created under the Affordable Care Act as a method to control rising healthcare costs. Given the rising costs of Medicare, and the number of baby boomers entering Medicare, the original focus of ACOs was Medicare, although they have expanded into the private sector. Basically, an ACO is a vertically integrated healthcare delivery system in which the network of providers (primary care physicians, specialty physicians, hospitals, and other healthcare providers, including long-term care facilities) attempt to coordinate the care provided to patients in order to provide care more efficiently (Gold, 2015).

The providers in the ACO share financial and medical responsibility for the coordinated care provided to patients. If the ACO is successful in controlling costs through cooperation and sharing of information across providers, thereby avoiding unnecessary tests, procedures, and services, then the ACO becomes eligible for bonuses and sharing the cost savings, assuming they also meet the quality standards established.

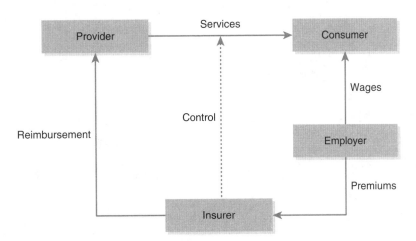

Figure 3-6 Flow of resources under regulatory function of managed care. Flow of money and resources with a control function added that enables the insurer to establish some form of control over the provider, thus regulating the flow of services from the provider to the consumer.

A major difference between an ACO and traditional managed care is that the patient does not enroll in the ACO and is not restricted in his/her choice of providers; patients can select any provider they wish without paying a higher price.

The goal of ACOs is to facilitate the delivery of more efficient and effective care through the coordination of healthcare services across providers. This coordination of care across the interdisciplinary team should increase access to appropriate care and reduce unnecessary or duplicate care. To coordinate care, the exchange of information across providers is essential. Since patients do not enroll in an ACO as they do in an HMO, attributing patients to a specific ACO can be difficult. A common way is for an insurer to examine its members' use of services and if a plurality of services of a patient is from an ACO provider, then that member is uniquely assigned to the ACO. The patient is attributed to the ACO, not to an individual provider, and the ACO is responsible for the total healthcare costs of that patient. Since the patient can elect to see any provider, the ACO can encounter difficulties in coordinating care and controlling utilization and costs (Kirschner, n.d.).

The number of ACOs is increasing and more people are covered by these organizations. As increased emphasis is placed on managing the health of the population, evolution and modifications in the structure and scope of ACOs is expected.

3.3 Cost of Activities

Having identified productive activities as efforts involving resource inputs whose aim is to create goods and services, some common measure of their creation needs to be established. The concept of *cost* is often used. In the context of a flow, cost is taken to be the magnitude of the resources devoted to an activity during a given period of time. Several different meanings can be attached to this concept.

One definition of cost is the money outlay, or expenditure, that has been paid to the providers for their services. For example, if an optometrist performs an eye pressure test, the money cost is simply what is paid for the optometrist's services. Money cost is a convenient way to measure the magnitude of an activity, but it is not always a complete measure. The same optometrist may do the same test for free for certain patients; in this case, the money cost would be zero. Yet, some activity has taken place, and this activity has used scarce resources (Monheit, 2010).

In the healthcare sector, there are many examples of free (i.e., zero money cost) services. Clinical teachers in medical schools frequently donate their efforts. Volunteer collectors for such organizations as the American Heart Association, United Way, and March of Dimes donate their time. The notion of *opportunity cost*, defined as the value of the most valuable alternative course of action given up for the chosen course of action, is used as a measure that does not depend on whether providers are paid in money for their services (Higgins & Harris, 2012).

Opportunity cost is relevant when a resource has several alternative uses. If the resource is used in activity A, the opportunity cost is what that resource would have earned if it had been used in alternative activity B, in which B is the highest valued alternative employment for that resource. The opportunity cost exists since undertaking activity A with the resources means those resources are not available to undertake activity B. For example, if an optometrist who performs a refraction for free in a clinic could have obtained a fee of $200 had he or she performed it in the office to another individual, by valuing this service at $200, we make it comparable to services performed for a fee. Whenever a service is provided at a price below its alternative value, the money cost will not take into account the portion of cost that is, in effect, subsidized; opportunity cost is a better measure of the true size of the total resources committed to an activity.

Costs can be categorized, among other ways, as direct or indirect. *Direct costs* are money expenditures, while *indirect costs* (also called *lost-productivity costs*) are unpaid resource commitments. Although these are unpaid, they may still have significant opportunity costs.

Table 3-1 shows the value of all direct national health expenditures for 1 year (2017) in the United States (Centers for Medicare and Medicaid, 2018a). These expenditures amounted to $3492.1 billion. The largest portion of funds went to hospital care (32.7%), followed by physician care (19.9%). The prescription drug portion has been growing considerably, and in 2017, it equaled 9.5% of the total. In 1980, prescription drugs had been only 4.7% of the total.

The growth in health expenditures, on a per capita (per person) basis, is shown in **Figure 3-7**. Since 1970, the growth has been steady. In 1990, health expenditures equaled $2853 per person. By 2010, they had reached $8402 per person, and by 2017, per capita expenditures were $10,739. Please note in Figure 3-7 that the first four indicators of expenditures cover 10 years and the remaining indicators of expenditures cover a single year.

A frequently used benchmark for health spending is total health spending expressed as a ratio of the

Table 3-1 National Health Expenditures by Type of Service, United States, 2017

Expenditure Category	Amount (Billions of Dollars)	Percent of Total
National health expenditures	3,492.1	100.0
Health consumption expenditures	3,324.5	95.2
Personal health care	2,961.0	84.8
Hospital care	1,142.6	32.7
Professional services	920.0	26.3
Physician and clinical services	694.3	19.9
Other professional services	96.6	2.8
Dental services	129.1	3.7
Other health, residential, and personal care	183.1	5.2
Home health care	97.0	2.8
Nursing care facilities & continuing care communities	166.3	4.8
Retail outlet sales of medical products	451.9	12.9
Prescription drugs	333.4	9.5
Durable medical equipment	54.4	1.6
Other non-durable medical products	64.1	1.8
Government administration	45.0	1.3
Net cost of health insurance	229.5	6.6
Government public health activities	88.9	2.5
Investment	167.6	4.8
Research	50.7	1.5
Structures and equipment	116.9	3.3

Data from Centers for Medicare & Medicaid Services, NHE60-10_Final.csv. Table 4. Retrieved from https://www.cms.gov/Research-Statistics-Data-and-Systems/Statistics-Trends-and-Reports/NationalHealthExpendData/NationalHealthAccountsHistorical.html.

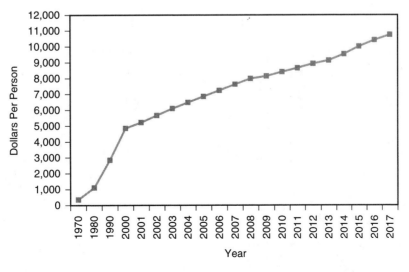

Figure 3-7 Per capita health expenditures, United States, 1970–2017.

Data from National Health Expenditures Tables, Table 1, CMS. Retrieved from http://WW W.CMS.gov/research-statistics-data-and-systems/statistics-trends-and-reports/national health expenditures data/downloads/tables.PDF.

total of all final goods and services produced in the economy during a year (the gross domestic product [GDP]). In 2017, the ratio for the United States was 17.9%. That is, of all final goods and services, 17.9% were healthcare goods and services. The ratio of national health expenditures to the GDP is generally considered a critical indicator of resource use in the healthcare sector. In fact, as seen in **Figure 3-8**, this ratio had been growing steadily and significantly over the past several decades (Centers for Medicare and Medicaid, 2018a). While there was a relatively stable period in the mid to late 1990s, when government spending was reduced, there was a rapid increase

in 2015 and 2016, reflecting the depressed economy, and a slight decrease in 2017. As seen in Figure 3-8, spending on healthcare goods and services as a percent of GDP was unabated. In fact, the national economy experienced tremendous growth during the 1990s, and this increase (which is the denominator in the ratio of health spending to GDP) helped reduce the ratio. In recent years, the ratio has increased again.

When compared with other developed countries, the United States has a very costly healthcare system. As can be seen in **Figure 3-9**, the health spending to GDP ratio is much lower for other countries (World Health Organization, 2018). In Germany, in 2015, for

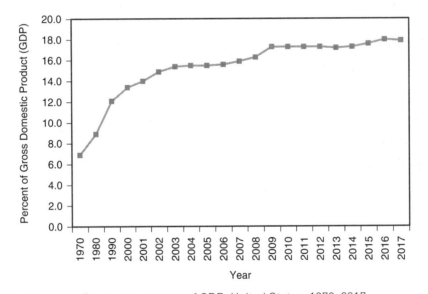

Figure 3-8 National health expenditures as a percent of GDP, United States, 1970–2017.

Modified from National Health Expenditures Tables, Table 1, CMS. Retrieved from http://WWW.CMS.gov/research-statistics-data-and-systems/statistics-trends-and-reports/national health expenditures data/downloads/tables.PDF.

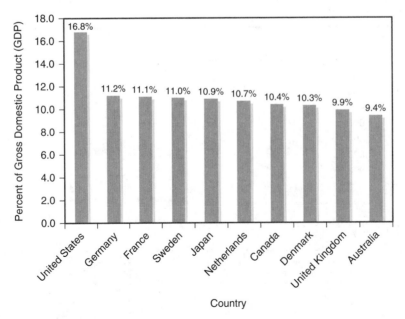

Figure 3-9 Current health expenditures as percent of GDP, selected countries, 2015.

Modified from World Health Organization. (2018). *Global health observatory data repository.* Geneva, Switzerland: Author.

example, the ratio was 11.2%, in the United Kingdom it was 9.9%, and in Australia, it was only 9.4%, compared to the United States at 16.8%. Investigators have focused on this statistic as an important indicator of the economic performance of the healthcare system (Anderson, 1997).

These data provide us with some idea of the direct costs of services provided. They do not, however, provide an indication of the total "burden" of costs—direct and indirect—that falls on all members of society as a result of illness. This total measure composes what are called the *social costs*.

Ideally, a cost-of-illness study will include all of the relevant resources that are influenced by the illness. The economic effects of illness can be experienced for years, and they can have a very broad impact in terms of the types of resources that are affected (Rice, Hodgson, & Kopstein, 1985).

An illness can be diagnosed years after it was acquired. For example, a person can be affected with the hepatitis C virus for many years before finally being diagnosed. It is only when he or she has been diagnosed that it is possible to measure the economic impact of the illness. Furthermore, the illness can generate economic costs for years after it has been diagnosed, even after the person has died. Chronic diseases last for years, and resources can be used as long as an illness lasts. If the person with the disease dies prematurely because of the disease, earnings that would have been experienced, but were not, are an indirect cost and part of the economic picture.

The following resource components might be affected by the illness: healthcare resources used in diagnosis and treatment (also called *direct care costs*); direct non-health resources, such as transportation, special diets, and household goods; patient loss of work time due to illness and injury (also called *indirect care costs*); and other related indirect costs, such as work time lost by unpaid caregivers. The collection of all of these data is expensive, and so most studies will not include all the components.

Cost-of-illness studies can be conducted on a prevalence or incidence basis. With a prevalence basis, the annual costs of all existing cases during a year (including newly and previously diagnosed) are included. The future mortality-related costs for all persons with the disease who died during the year are also included (Rice, 1990). In contrast, an incidence-based analysis includes all present and future costs *only for cases newly diagnosed during the year*. In theory, one can also conduct an incidence-based analysis for cases that were contracted during the year, although this is seldom done for chronic diseases because of a lack of data. The cost of a premature death would include the lost work time from future deaths.

The prevalence approach is useful for budgeting purposes. For many purposes, the incidence approach is preferred, although it is much easier to obtain prevalence data than incidence data. If we are conducting a study on the economic effects of preventing or detecting illness, we should obtain data on the costs of all downstream events of the illness. The incidence approach would provide that information. If we used the prevalence approach, we would be obtaining the cost of many of the cases in midstream.

Data on the cost of several of the more economically important illnesses are shown in **Figure 3-10**. The costliest condition is injuries, with direct costs of $145.1 billion and indirect costs of $556.8 billion. The disease with the highest direct medical costs is

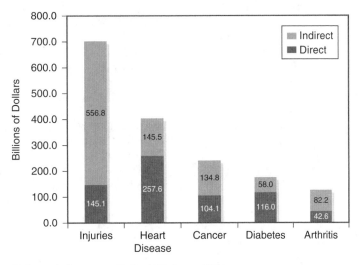

Figure 3-10 Cost of illness: Selected diseases, United States, c2006.

US Census Bureau, Income, Poverty, and Health Insurance Coverage in the United States: 2017. Dunlop D et al. The Costs of Arthritis. Arthritis Care Research 2003. Mensah and Brown. An overview of cardiovascular disease burden in the United States 2007. Kaiser Family Foundation. Retrieved from www.statehealthfacts.org

heart disease, with annual costs of $257.6 billion. However, persons who suffer from injuries are generally younger than those who suffer from heart disease, and so their indirect costs are higher. Diabetes and cancer have roughly the same total cost of illness, but diabetes generally occurs in older persons, and so the ratio of direct to indirect costs is greater for diabetes. Arthritis has low direct costs because the cost of treatment is much lower than for the other illnesses shown in the graph (Scitovsky & McCall, 1977).

Cost-of-illness studies can provide valuable information that can be used in budgeting decisions and in cost-effectiveness studies. Cost-of-illness studies focus on the economic component of trends in disease and consequently are useful for policymakers. It is important for policymakers to have a notion of the impact of disease changes on expenditures (Changik, 2014; Sheill, Gerard, & Donaldson, 1987). Much debate and misunderstanding has surrounded this topic. It should be understood that cost-of-illness studies are descriptive studies. One should not use the results of these studies by themselves to make policy recommendations. For these studies to be useful for evaluation purposes, the investigator must add additional information. Put another way, cost-of-illness studies describe what has happened. This can be very useful, but decision making requires more information—we must know why costs are what they are and what our objectives are.

Exercises

1. Describe the kinds of costs that insured individuals may be responsible for when they use healthcare services.
2. Through what mechanism do most people in the United States purchase private health insurance?
3. What population does the Medicare program cover?
4. What are the four parts of Medicare, and what does each cover?
5. What populations does Medicaid cover?
6. What distinguishes a preferred provider organization from a traditional health maintenance organization?
7. How does an accountable care organization differ from a health maintenance organization?
8. When would it be preferable to use opportunity costs rather than money costs?
9. What is a cost-of-illness study?
10. What is the difference between measuring the cost of illness using the prevalence and incidence approaches?

Bibliography

Anderson, G. F. (1997). In search of value: An international comparison of cost, access, and outcomes. *Health Affairs, 16*(6), 163–171.

Centers for Medicare and Medicaid Services. (2010). NHE60-10_Final.csv. Retrieved from http://www.cms.gov/Research-Statistics-Data-and-Systems/Statistics-Trends-and-Reports/NationalHealthExpendData/Downloads/tables.pdf

Centers for Medicare and Medicaid Services. (2018a). NHE60-10_Final.csv. Retrieved from https://www.cms.gov/Research-Statistics-Data-and-Systems/Statistics-Trends-and-Reports/NationalHealthExpendData/NationalHealthAccountsHistorical.html

Centers for Medicare and Medicaid Services. (2018b). Retrieved from https://www.medicare.gov/what-medicare-covers/what-part-a-covers

Centers for Medicare and Medicaid Services. (2018c). Retrieved from https://www.medicare.gov/what-medicare-covers/what-part-b-covers

Centers for Medicare and Medicaid Services. (2018d). Retrieved from https://www.medicare.gov/what-medicare-covers/what-medicare-health-plans-cover/

Centers for Medicare and Medicaid Services. (2018e). Retrieved from https://www.medicare.gov/drug-coverage-part-d/what-medicare-part-d-drug-plans-cover/

Changik, J. (2014). Cost-of-illness studies: Concepts, scopes, and methods. *Clinical and Molecular Hepatology, 20*, 327–337.

Gold, J. (2015). Accountable care organizations, explained. *Kaiser Health News*, September 14, 2015.

Higgins, A. M., & Harris, A. H. (2012). Health economic models: Cost-minimization, cost-effectiveness, cost-utility, and cost-benefit evaluations. *Critical Care Clinics, 28*, 11–24.

Kaiser Family Foundation. (2011). *Employer health benefits, 2011 annual survey*. Menlo Park, CA: Author.

Kaiser Family Foundation. (2018). *Employer health benefits, 2018 annual survey*. Menlo Park, CA: Author.

Kirschner, N. (n.d.). *Accountable care organization (ACO) 101, brief course*. American College of Physicians.

McLaughlin, C. G., Zellers, W. K., & Brown, L. D. (1989). Health care coalitions: characteristics, activities, and prospects. *Inquiry, 26*, 72–83.

Monheit, A. C. (2010). The free lunch society. *Inquiry, 47*(4), 272–277.

Reinhardt, U. E. (1993). Reorganizing the financial flows in American health care. *Health Affairs, 12*, 172–193.

Rice, D. P. (1990). Cost-of-illness studies: Fact or fiction? *Lancet, 344*, 1519–1520.

Rice, D. P., Hodgson, T. A., & Kopstein, A. N. (1985). The economic cost of illness. *Health Care Financing Review, 7*(Fall), 61–80.

Scitovksy, A. A., & McCall, N. (1977). *Changes in the cost of treatment of selected illness* (Publication no. HRA 77-3161). Hyattsville, MD: National Center for Health Services Research.

Sheill, A., Gerard, K., & Donaldson, C. (1987). Cost of illness studies: An aid to decision-making? *Health Policy, 8*, 317–323.

Sonofi-Aventis. (2018). *Payer digest, 2018.* Bridgewater, NJ: Managed Care Digest Series.

World Health Organization. (2018). *World health statistics, 2018.* Geneva, Switzerland: Author.

PART II

Explanatory Economics

CHAPTER 4

Demand for Health and Medical Care

OBJECTIVES

1. Explain the demand hypothesis and factors influencing demand and distinguish between the concepts of *demand* and *quantity demanded*.
2. Explain how an individual's demand curve and the market demand curve for medical services can be derived.
3. Define the concept of elasticity of demand and explain how to measure the concept using data on prices and utilization.
4. Identify the private, external, and social demand for health services.
5. Explain how time costs influence the demand for health services.
6. Explain the concept of discounting by which the consumer places lower valuations on future health benefits than on present benefits.

4.1 The Concept of Demand

The purpose of explanatory economics is to predict economic behavior. When analyzing demand behavior, attention is focused on the quantity demanded by consumers of a specific good or service. To perform the analysis, a demand model is used that serves two purposes: It categorizes the factors that might cause demand or quantity demanded to increase or decrease, and it hypothesizes how economic factors (e.g., price and income) influence demand or quantity demanded.

Models are devices used to obtain results. A model is a simplified representation of reality, not a complete description of it. The purpose of a model, however specified, is to present an "If . . . then . . ." type of explanation. In the case of the demand model, the reasoning is: "If factor *x* increases, then demand or quantity demanded will increase (or decrease, depending on what factor *x* is)." A good model screens essential causal factors and incorporates them into a logical, coherent system. Models enable simpler explanations of complex situations to be undertaken. Using these simpler models enables exploration of the actions and consequences of complex situations to be studied and understood. Using diagrams and equations, economic models attempt to explain events occurring in the world.

Even though every model is conjectural, it should explain something about movements in real phenomena (e.g., the quantity of medical care demanded). In assessing a model, it is therefore sufficient to examine whether its predictions concerning movements in selected phenomena are realized by comparing the predictions with actual movements in the phenomena as measured by data. In other words, accuracy of prediction is the test of an explanatory model.

This chapter introduces a simple model of the demand for a good or service. Section 4.2 sets forth the model, using an individual's demand for medical care as an example. Section 4.3 takes us behind the scenes and shows how the model of demand can be derived. Section 4.4 examines the factors influencing the market demand for a good or service. Section 4.5 develops the concept of *elasticity,* a tool used to measure the magnitude of the hypothesized movements, and Section 4.6 presents the demand analysis when insurance is present. Section 4.7 examines the characteristics of the market for healthcare services that differentiates it from the market for everyday goods and services. Finally, Section 4.8 presents some actual estimates of the demand relationship.

4.2 Individual Demand: The Price–Quantity Relation

4.2.1 Demand and Quantity Demanded

The exploration of the price–quantity relation begins with a specification of the terms of reference and definitions of the variables used. The unit of analysis is the individual consumer. Economic behavior involves attaining or attempting to attain goods and services. Because the focus is on health care, the service *physician care* is used as a major example. Physician care is defined as examinations and treatments administered by physicians to their patients. Physician care is only one of many goods and services in the healthcare sector, so the relations specified in this chapter can be applied to other health-related goods and services, including hospital services, pharmaceuticals, dental care, home care, preventive measures, nutritional services, nursing care, and the services of other health professionals.

As the model of physician care is developed, certain assumptions are made in order to simplify the complex healthcare market. In making assumptions, attention focuses on the major issues associated with a problem. Once the simpler model is understood, then the more complex world can be introduced. The assumptions made will vary with different situations or different questions to be studied. Assumptions will also vary with the length of time in which the situation occurs; assumptions involving short-run situations may be very different from those involving long-run situations.

Having identified the service in our analysis, a pervasive problem encountered in medical care organization analysis is defining and measuring quality differences among units of medical care. Examinations and treatments can vary in thoroughness, such as in the physician's technical competence or in the physician's bedside manner, or in other factors. When analyzing physician care as a service, these variations should be kept in mind.

Our service, physician care, is measured by the number of office visits to a physician by the typical consumer. Each visit is assumed to be identical with all others. Finally, we specify the time span as being 1 year. Given this time frame, our service measure becomes the number of physician office visits per year.

With this background, the demand hypothesis used to predict the effect of a change in direct per-unit price on the quantity demanded of a good or service can be presented. The hypothesis is that the lower the out-of-pocket price (the endogenous variable) offered to consumers (all other factors held constant), the greater the number of units of that good or service they will demand.

A number of conventions, or interpretations, are related to this hypothesis. "Quantity demanded" means the quantity demanded at any specific price, all other causal factors held constant. Quantity demanded is the amount that the consumer is *willing and able* to buy at the specified price. "Demand" means the set of quantities demanded at various prices, all other causal factors held constant. "Out-of-pocket price" means the price paid directly by consumers for a particular unit of the good or service. "All other factors" means those variables other than price that influence consumer demand behavior. The economic approach to consumer behavior is to specify an initial relation between out-of-pocket price and quantity demanded and then to introduce other causal factors to see how they affect the basic demand relation.

One such demand relation, assuming all other factors remain unchanged, is illustrated diagrammatically as line d_1 in **Figure 4-1**. The specific relation shown by this line, or curve, entails that at a price of $70 per visit, the consumer would be willing to visit the physician twice a year; at a price of $60 per visit, the consumer would be willing to make three visits; and so on. Assuming that the quantities demanded at all other prices trace out a straight-line relation, d_1 represents a particular demand curve at one specific level of demand. The lowercase letter d is used to indicate the behavior of a single individual.

The downward slope of the demand curve is explained by the possibility of substitution. Substitution occurs when goods and services can be used in place of each other to satisfy a desire or need to a similar level. This economic approach implies that very few, if any, goods or services are absolute musts.

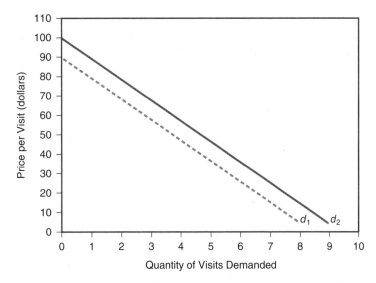

Figure 4-1 The demand relationship. Curves d_1 and d_2 show the quantity demanded increasing as the direct price decreases. Each curve represents a separate level of demand. With reference to curve d_1, curve d_2 represents an increase in demand, not just an increase in quantity demanded.

© Jones & Bartlett Learning.

The longer the time span during which the consumer adapts his or her behavior to any substitutes, the more relevant they become. A sore throat, for example, can be treated by a physician or by resorting to drugs or home remedies. Furthermore, even if the malady is treated by a physician, alternative types of broad-spectrum antibiotics can be used. In recent years, use of outpatient treatment instead of hospitalization has been suggested for many types of ailments. In the long term, health foods and other preventive services are substitutes for medical care in maintaining desired health levels. In these, as well as other instances, the hypothesized relation applies: the lower the price of any specific alternative, the more it will be demanded.

Other hypotheses than this demand relation might be put forward to explain consumer demand behavior. One alternative hypothesis that has received much attention in medical care literature is that at higher prices, individuals will still demand and pay for the same quantity of medical care. This alternative hypothesis would be represented by a vertical demand curve representing a perfectly inelastic demand curve. Similar vertical demand curves have also been hypothesized for other items considered necessities, such as housing, basic foods, and even alcohol.

Having two alternative hypotheses, we are faced with the problem of determining which is more useful for explaining actual behavior. Debating the issue by itself cannot resolve the controversy, however. The hypothesis chosen should be the one that most closely fits the actual data. The empirical testing of hypotheses is discussed in Section 4.8.

It should be emphasized that the focus here is solely on consumer behavior. Our hypothesis relates only to how much the consumer is willing and able to buy at any price. At this stage, we are not inquiring about whether the amount demanded will be supplied or even available.

4.2.2 Changes in Demand

The effects of factors other than the out-of-pocket price on the economic behavior of consumers are introduced by way of their influence on the basic price–quantity relation. These other exogenous factors can be placed into four broad categories: (1) income, (2) prices of other (related) goods and services, (3) tastes and preferences, and (4) expectations. Each category is considered in turn.

4.2.2.1 Income

The income of the consumer is generally assumed to be positively related to demand. That is, if income increases, the quantity demanded at each price will be greater if the good or service is a normal good. If the good or service is inferior, then the increase in income will result in a decrease in demand, other factors being equal. The basic relation between income and demand can be illustrated with the use of demand curves. Referring back to Figure 4-1, curve d_1 can now be interpreted as representing a level of demand at some initial level of income. Assume that, from this initial level, income increases. The hypothesized effect on demand is now at a price of $70, there will be three visits demanded instead of two; at a price of $60, there will be four visits demanded instead of three, and so on. The new demand level, corresponding to the higher income level, can be represented by the curve d_2. In the diagram, the relative position of the two curves summarizes the net influence of income on consumer behavior. A shift in demand from curve d_1 to curve d_2 is called an *increase* in demand, as opposed to a change in quantity demanded with a change in price, represented by movement along a static demand curve.

The same reasoning can be applied in reverse to a fall in income. This decline causes the consumer to demand less of the normal good or service at each price and can be represented by a shift from d_2 to d_1. This is called a *decrease* in demand, reflecting a reduction in quantity demanded at every price.

Income is frequently defined as an individual's earnings in a specific time period, and is used as an approximation to measure the ability of the individual to afford medical care. Another measure of ability to purchase medical care is the individual's level of wealth, including bonds, bank deposits, real estate, and other assets, minus any debt, such as bank loans and mortgages. A third measure is after-tax income. This measure is particularly important to take into account when considering changes in tax rates and their effects on purchasing power. Whatever measure is used should be a good approximation of the individual's ability to pay for medical care.

4.2.2.2 Prices of Related Goods and Services

The demand for a particular good or service is also influenced by the quantities of related goods and services consumed. The quantities of these related goods and services are, in turn, influenced by their prices. Two classes of good and service relations are of concern: complements and substitutes. A complementary good or service is one whose use is generally accompanied by the use of the good or service in question. Examples might include the services of a surgeon and the hospital's surgical services, or the services of a radiologist and radiograph film.

The hypothesis relating the demands of complementary goods and services is as follows: a fall in the price of a good or service increases the quantity demanded of that good or service, and it also leads to an increase in the demand for goods and services that are complements. Similar reasoning, in reverse, applies to an increase in the price of one good or service in a complementary set. For example, we can hypothesize that a fall in the out-of-pocket price of the surgical services involved in an elective procedure will lead to an increase in the quantity of services demanded; it will also increase the demand for hospital surgical services.

Complements play an important role in medical care demand. The close relation between radiology machines and radiologist services has frequently led to the assertion that much hospital demand is really determined by the quantity of physician services consumed.

The second type of good or service relation is a substitute, which is a good or service that can replace the original good or service. The hypothesis is that a fall in the price of a good or service increases the quantity demanded and leads to a reduced demand for substitute goods and services. For example, a rise in the price the patient pays for an additional day of hospital care decreases the quantity of hospital days demanded and, at the same time, increases the demand for home care, a substitute good.

Substitution is also the reason given for the downward slope of the demand curve for any good or service. For example, quantity of inpatient care demanded is negatively related to patient price, because inpatient care can be substituted for home care when the price of inpatient care falls and vice versa, assuming that the price of home care remains constant. A rise in the price of home care leads to additional substitution, resulting in an outward shift in the inpatient care demand curve. The slope of the demand curve of any good or service, as well as how much it shifts when substitute prices change, depends on how similar the patient perceives the substitutes to be.

4.2.2.3 Tastes and Preferences

Consumer tastes and preferences is a catchall category covering a large number of other factors that might influence demand. Tastes have sometimes been called *wants*, a term connoting the intensity of desire for particular goods and services. The elements that influence the intensity of an individual's desire for medical care include such things as health status, educational background, gender, age, race, and upbringing. Any of these can explain differences among individuals in the intensity of desire for medical care. That is, with other factors (incomes, prices of other goods and services, and so on) held constant, these differences can be used to explain why one individual's demand curve is d_1 (Figure 4-1) whereas another's is d_2.

Tastes and preferences are usually considered to be fixed from the standpoint of economic analysis, although some economic models recognize that advertising by firms can influence consumer tastes. Although tastes and preferences differ among individuals, they are hypothesized to be stable over fairly short periods of time. If they are stable, once the factors that underlie tastes are accounted for, differences in demand can be attributed to differences in incomes, prices of other goods and services, expectations, and factors influencing tastes and preferences. In addition to the dependence of tastes on health, which in itself transitory, physicians potentially can exert considerable influence over tastes for medical care. Changing tastes and preferences have played a large role in health economics.

4.2.2.4 Expectations

Consumers' expectations about the future may impact current demand for a good or service. For example, if consumers expect their incomes to be higher in the near future, then they may purchase more goods and services currently and save less. Another example of the impact of expectations is if consumers expect prices to increase, then they may purchase additional services at the current price.

4.3 Deriving the Demand Relationship

In Section 4.2, the demand for medical care was analyzed as if medical care were an ordinary good or service, like carrots or shoes. However, certain characteristics of medical care make it unlike many ordinary goods and services. Closer attention must be given to these characteristics to determine if and when standard demand analysis is appropriate for medical care. To do this, a theoretical model is presented focusing on the conditions that are required for the demand

relation to hold; special attention is paid to whether these conditions are likely to be met in the case of medical care.

The factors influencing a consumer's behavior with regard to the demand for a good or service can be placed under the categories of tastes and preferences, incomes, prices, and expectations. Assume that a typical individual has a choice of purchasing only two goods and services. These two goods and services are carrots and physician office visits. The assumptions underlying the model for the demand for these two products are examined.

4.3.1 Tastes and Preferences

Tastes are essentially desires for goods and services. These desires, or wants, are quantified using an index called *utility*. Utility reflects the level of satisfaction derived from the consumption of a good or service. The utility of carrots for an individual is shown in **Table 4-1**. The numbers in this table were devised to show an increasing total amount of utility (total utility) as more carrots are consumed, but more importantly, they were devised so that the increases gradually diminish.

The concept used to represent the increases in utility from successive quantities of a good or service is called *marginal utility*, which is the change in total utility resulting from a unit change in the consumption of the good or service. Thus, the marginal utility for the first carrot is 6; it is 5 for the second, and so on. This decrease in the size of the utility of successive quantities of a good or service is called *diminishing marginal utility*. Note that, in general, total satisfaction will still increase. This is a key assumption of demand analysis. The same assumption can be applied to medical care

Table 4-1 Relationship Between Quantity Consumed of Two Goods and Services and Utility of (Satisfaction Derived from) the Goods and Services

Medical Care			Carrots	
Quantity	Total Utility	Marginal Utility	Total Utility	Marginal Utility
1	22	22	6	6
2	42	20	11	5
3	60	18	15	4
4	76	16	18	3
5	90	14	20	2
6	102	12	21	1

as well, but the circumstances in which the relationship of diminishing marginal utility will hold needs to be explored in greater detail. We therefore list the conditions that must occur in medical care.

4.3.1.1 Health Status

The initial health status of the individual (H) is given and known by the individual. That is, the individual knows what medical condition exists.

4.3.1.2 Consumer Information

The relationship between medical care (MC) and health status (H) is also known by the individual; the individual knows how medical care will influence health status. Partly, this reflects that the individual has a good understanding of existing health problems.

4.3.1.3 Productivity of Medical Care

In general, it is assumed that the marginal productivity of medical care in influencing health is constant. As more units of medical care (visits) are consumed, equal additions to health status result. Obviously, there is a limit to how healthy an individual can become, and we will show what happens when this assumption is altered. For the moment, we will hold with the assumption of constant productivity.

4.3.1.4 Quality

The quality of medical care is also assumed to be constant. All visits provided by the physicians are of the same quality.

4.3.1.5 Other Taste-Influencing Variables

The utility function is dependent on a host of other variables, each of which may influence the individual's intensity of desire for medical care. These variables include the individual's education, upbringing or culture, marital status, and age, among others. For example, it is believed that higher levels of education increase an individual's desire for good health. Thus, it is important to know that in the back of any taste function lies a series of formative factors that cause the utility–quantity relation to be what it is. In this example, the assumption is that there are no other sources of utility except for medical care and carrots.

Given these assumptions, the type of relations between utility and medical care are shown in Table 4-1, the plausible hypothesis is that each added visit results in a smaller increment of additional utility.

4.3.2 Income

The second variable in the demand model is the individual's income. Assume the individual's income is $10 for the time period and that the individual lacks any accumulated wealth usable for purchasing care.

4.3.3 Prices of Other Goods and Services

Other variables include the prices charged for physician's office visits and carrots. Initially, the prices are set at $1 per carrot and $4 per physician's office visit. The purpose of the analysis is to predict what happens when the price of physician's office visits changes and, in the process, to make explicit what variables are initially being held constant in the analysis.

4.3.4 Behavioral Assumption: Utility Maximization

Finally, the behavioral assumption of utility maximization sets the model in motion. Assume the individual is a utility maximizer (i.e., the individual desires to gain the most satisfaction, or benefit, from his or her income).

4.3.5 Predictions

The model's conclusion stems from these assumptions together with assumptions about price changes. Let us first determine what quantities of medical care and carrots are demanded at the initial prices. In doing this, the focus is on the marginal utility (MU) per dollar of expenditure, or the ratio of marginal utility to price (P), which is expressed as MU/P. It is this variable that expresses the satisfaction per dollar of expense for each alternative use. At a price of $1 per carrot, buying a carrot will be the best bet for the first $1 of expenditure, because the first carrot yields 6 units of utility. The next item purchased will not be another carrot, because an additional expenditure here would yield 5 units of utility per $1, whereas a visit to the physician would yield 5.5 units (22 units/$4). Therefore, the individual visits the physician. The individual has now spent a total of $5 and has $5 left. The next items of expenditure will be a carrot and another visit to the physician (indeed, both have a MU/P ratio of 5). At this point, the individual has used all income and will have achieved an equal marginal utility per dollar for the last purchases of each good or service. The total utility (53) is the highest that can be attained with $10. This equality of MU/$P$ in each use indicates that the individual's income cannot be reallocated to a different mix of carrots and visits to obtain more utility.

To illustrate utility maximization, assume that, after the second carrot, the individual allocates the remaining $4 to the purchase of carrots instead of office visits. The marginal utility of the third, fourth, fifth, and sixth carrots would be 4, 3, 2, and 1, respectively. The individual would now be getting 1 unit of utility per $1 of expenditure instead of the 5 units obtainable by purchasing office visits. The total utility would be 43; and the individual would be better off with two carrots and two office visits than with this alternative set of purchases.

Having shown there is a utility-maximizing "equilibrium" quantity for each good or service, the assumption about price is changed to $3 per office visit. A carrot will still cost $1. This fall in the price of office visits results in an increase in the utility per dollar of office visits for all visits and makes them more valuable in dollar terms. Under this altered assumption, the individual will maximize utility by "consuming" three physician visits and consuming only one carrot.

The essential implication of this analysis is that when the price of office visits falls, the quantity demanded increases (assuming all other variables, including other prices as well as incomes, expectations, prices of related goods and services, and tastes and preferences, remain the same). This is a derivation of the demand relationship. This model holds only when other variables are held constant. Changing them will shift the demand relationship in one direction or the other, depending on the variable and the degree of change.

Next, we make a more realistic assumption that office visits have diminishing marginal productivity with respect to health. If additional units of health diminished in size with successive visits, then the marginal utility of office visits falls more quickly and reduces the relative desirability of additional units of office visits. There would still be a downward-sloping demand curve, but it would be shifted inward compared to the situation in which the productivity of office visits was constant.

4.4 Market Demand

The previous model provided a means of analyzing an individual's demand for office visits. To generalize the model to explain market (a network of buyers and sellers) demand, an additional assumption must be made. The assumption is that the more individuals there are who seek the product, the greater will be the market demand and the quantity demanded in the market at any price.

This is illustrated in **Figure 4-2**, which shows the demand curves of three individuals: d_b is Mr. B's demand curve, d_k is Ms. K's demand curve, and d_j is Mrs. J's demand curve. At a price of $20 per visit, Mr. B will demand three visits, Ms. K will demand two, and Mrs. J will demand none. At $15 per visit, Mr. B., Ms. K., and Mrs. J will demand five visits, four visits, and one visit, respectively. Using information on individual demand curves, and on the number of individuals, a market demand curve can be derived.

Given the three individual demand curves, the market quantity demanded at a given price will be the sum of the quantities demanded by all three individuals at that price. At a price of $20, the quantity demanded in the market will be five visits; at $15, the quantity will be 10. The market demand curve is

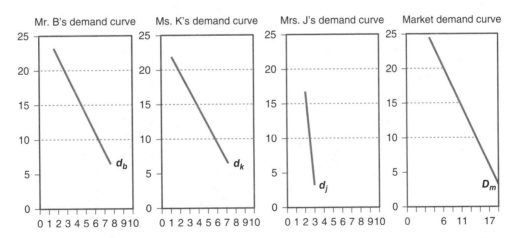

Figure 4-2 Individual and market demand curves. Derivation of the market demand curve from individual demand curves. The quantity demanded at each price by all consumers in the market is the sum of the individual quantity demanded. The market demand curve is the horizontal sum of all individual demand curves.

shown in Figure 4-2 as D_m and is the horizontal sum of the demands of the three individuals demanding visits.

The factors influencing market demand can be divided into two categories: (1) factors influencing individual demand only and (2) factors influencing market demand. The former includes prices, incomes, expectations, and tastes and preferences. If any of these change, individual demand, or the quantities demanded by individuals, will also change. If individual demand curves shift out, market curves will shift out as well. In addition to responding to changes in individual curves, market demand is influenced by changes in the number of participants in the market. For example, an influx of people into an area will cause market demand to increase. Also, possibly people who did not demand any medical care at higher prices will enter the market and become consumers of care as the price falls.

4.5 Measuring Quantity Responsiveness to Price Changes

Previously, a model was developed that enabled the prediction of how a particular factor affects quantity demanded or demand. Thus, when the out-of-pocket price falls, the quantity demanded will rise; that is, there is an inverse relationship between price and quantity demanded. The question now is by how much will the quantity demanded rise?

The concept used to measure quantity responsiveness to out-of-pocket price changes is the concept of *price elasticity of demand*. Price elasticity attempts to measure responsiveness when the only factor undergoing change, and thereby influencing the quantity demanded, is price.

The measure of elasticity is a measure of relative magnitudes and will not change if cents rather than dollars are used to measure price or single units rather than thousands are used to measure quantity. Elasticity is, thus, a pure measure of the magnitude of change. The formula used for small changes in price is the percentage change in quantity demanded divided by the percentage change in price. In symbolic terms, this is written

$$E_p = \frac{\Delta Q / Q}{\Delta P / P}$$

in which E_p is price elasticity, Q is the original quantity, P is the original price, and ΔQ and ΔP are changes in Q and P, respectively. This formula is known as a *point elasticity formula*, and point elasticity is appropriate for small changes along the demand curve. If the change in price is appreciable, an average elasticity measure over the range of the demand curve covered by the change is more appropriate. This measure, known as the *arc elasticity of demand,* is written as

$$E_p = \frac{(Q_2 - Q_1) / (Q_2 + Q_1)}{(P_2 - P_1) / (P_2 + P_1)}$$

in which Q_1 and P_1 refer to one price and quantity set and Q_2 and P_2 refer to a second set at another point on the same demand curve. In fact, both the price and quantity changes are expressed as ratios to average price and quantity levels, that is, as $(P_1 + P_2)/2$ and $(Q_1 + Q_2)/2$. The 2s would cancel out, leaving us with the formula as presented.

For example, assume the Richland County Health Department charges $3.00 per syphilis test in May and it performed 1200 tests. In June, the County Council raised the charges to $3.25 per test and only 1150 tests were performed in June. What is the price elasticity of demand?

The elasticity measure of a price change is a measure of responsiveness along a demand curve when all factors other than price remain constant. If other factors have changed, some adjustment must account for the extent to which these other factors influenced the quantity demanded. In our example, assume these other factors remained constant and only price influenced quantity. In this case, the price elasticity formula can be used directly:

$$E_p = \frac{(1150 - 1200) / (1150 + 1200)}{(3.25 - 3) / (3.25 + 3)} = -0.53$$

The elasticity of demand at that point is –0.53. The minus sign is frequently dropped from discussions, so price elasticity is quoted as the absolute value, for example, 0.53. This figure indicates the responsiveness of quantity to price.

Price elasticity is related to how total consumer expenditures respond to a change in the out-of-pocket price. For any elasticity measure whose absolute value is less than 1, total out-of-pocket expenditures will increase with a decrease in price; at such points on the demand curve, demand is said to be inelastic. When demand is relatively inelastic, the demand curve is steeper. In our example, total expenditures ($P \times Q$) were $3600.00 before the price change and $3737.50 after. Receipts from this source rose by $137.50 because of the nature of the responsiveness at that point on the demand curve.

An elasticity measure of –0.53 is thought of as relatively unresponsive; that is, a small relative price rise or fall will generate a smaller relative quantity change. If price increases by 1%, the quantity will decrease by only about 0.53%, and the total amount spent will increase. With an elasticity of –0.53, a reduction in price will lower total consumer expenditures because the relative increase in quantity purchased will not be sufficient to overcome the relatively greater price decrease. Thus, if the Richland County Health Department wants more revenue, and does not care about how many tests are performed, it should raise its price to $3.25.

Demand curves can also have unitary elastic and elastic portions. When the elasticity measures –1, demand responsiveness is said to be *unitary elastic*. In the case of a small change in price, total expenditures will remain constant. When the demand responsiveness is elastic (i.e., greater than 1 in absolute value), it means that the relative change in quantity consumed exceeds the relative change in price. If there is a small increase in price, the decrease in quantity will be relatively greater, and total expenditures will decline.

If there is a small decrease in price, total expenditures will rise. When demand is relatively elastic, the demand curve has a flatter slope.

These relations are shown in **Figure 4-3**. A straight-line demand curve for vaccinations is shown in Graph A. At a price of $10, no vaccinations are demanded, but as the price falls in $1 increments, vaccination demand increases by 100. Thus, at a price of $9, there will be 100 vaccinations demanded; at a price of $8, there will be 200 demanded; and so on. Graph B shows the total expenditures generated at each level of sales. Thus, if 100 vaccinations are sold, $900 in expenditures is generated, and so on (see **Table 4-2** for the actual values). Over a range, total expenditures increase, but eventually the increase levels off to a maximum, and beyond that point total expenditures begin to decline.

There is a connection between the elasticity along a specific segment of the demand curve and the total expenditures specific to relevant points on the curve. At relatively high prices and low quantities on a straight-line demand curve, only a relatively small

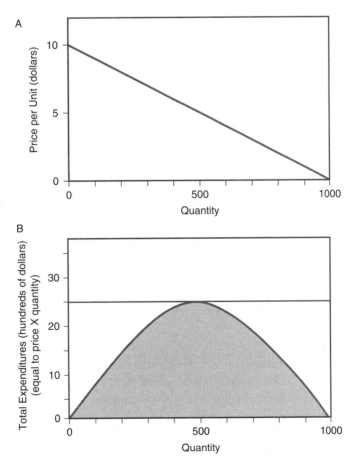

Figure 4-3 Relationship between price, quantity demanded, and total revenue. Graph A shows the basic relationship between quantity demanded and price. Graph B shows the relationship between total expenditures (which equals price times quantity) and quantity. Graph B is derived from Graph A.

Table 4-2 Price for Vaccinations, Quantity Demanded, and Total Expenditures

Price ($)	Quantity Demanded	Total Expenditures ($)
10	0	0
9	100	900
8	200	1600
7	300	2100
6	400	2400
5	500	2500
4	600	2400
3	700	2100
2	800	1600
1	900	900

© Jones & Bartlett Learning.

change in price (in terms of percentage) is needed to induce a relatively large change in the quantity demanded. The lower expenditures resulting from the fall in unit prices are therefore more than offset by the large increase in quantity demanded, and so total expenditures will increase. For example, in Table 4-2, for a reduction in price from $9 to $8, the arc elasticity of demand along that segment of the curve is −4.76. Demand is therefore said to be elastic, and if that reduction in price is instituted, total expenditures will increase (in this case, from $900 to $1600).

As we move down the demand curve, the relative price change becomes smaller in relation to the associated quantity change. Thus, the absolute value of elasticity falls. But as long as this value in absolute terms is greater than 1 (i.e., the elastic portion of the curve), total expenditures will increase, although not by as much as in higher-apriced segments. Eventually, the elasticity takes on a value of −1. At this point, price and quantity changes offset each other exactly, and total expenditures stay constant (the top of the total expenditures curve). As prices fall further, we move on to the inelastic portion of the demand curve. Price reductions offset quantity increases, and total expenditures fall. Thus, along any single straight-line demand curve, the elasticity of demand will decrease with successive reductions in price.

While elasticity is related to slope, it is not identical with the slope of the curve. For example, the slope of a linear curve is constant, but the elasticity varies

along the linear demand curve. Slope is defined as "rise over run," in which rise reflects the change in price and run reflects the change in quantity. As indicated, slope is the ratio of changes in two variables, and elasticity is the ratio of percentage changes in two variables.

For example, assume two demand curves in two different markets for physician visits cross at a price of $3 and 10,000 visits, as in **Figure 4-4**. The consumers in Market 2 are more responsive to price reductions than are those in Market 1. Let AD be the demand curve in Market 1 and BC be the demand curve in Market 2. Now let the price fall by 10 cents. Consumers in Market 1 demand 10,300 visits, whereas those in Market 2 demand 10,500. The arc elasticity in Market 1 is

$$E = \frac{300/20,300}{-0.10/5.90} = -0.87$$

The arc elasticity in Market 2 is

$$E = \frac{500/20,500}{-0.10/5.90} = -1.44$$

The demand curve BC is for a more responsive group of consumers, and the elasticity for a given quantity will be greater in absolute value than that of a less responsive group.

4.6 Insurance, Out-of-Pocket Price, and Quantity Demanded

A major factor in considering the demand for medical care is the role that insurance plays in influencing the out-of-pocket price of medical care. There are a number of different types of insurance arrangements that consumers can obtain, and these will affect the out-of-pocket price, and hence, the quantity demanded in different ways.

In analyzing the effect of alternative insurance arrangements, the initial demand curve reflects consumers having no insurance and paying the full price charged by the provider. This curve, in which full charge equals the out-of-pocket price, is labeled D_n in **Figure 4-5**.

Now, a coinsurance arrangement is introduced in which the patient pays a proportion of the charged price and the insurance company pays the remainder. For example, with a 20% coinsurance rate and a charged price of $20 per visit, the patient pays the provider 20% of the charged price, $4, and the insurance company pays the remaining $16. In this

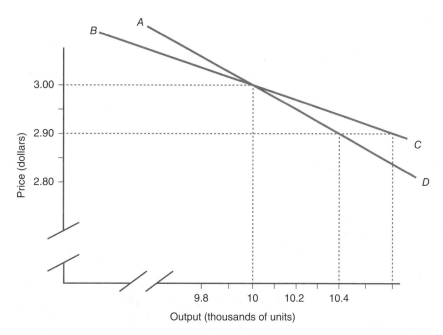

Figure 4-4 Responsiveness of quantity demanded to price for different sloped demand curves. Curve *BC* shows a greater responsiveness of quantity demanded to price than curve *AD*.

© Jones & Bartlett Learning.

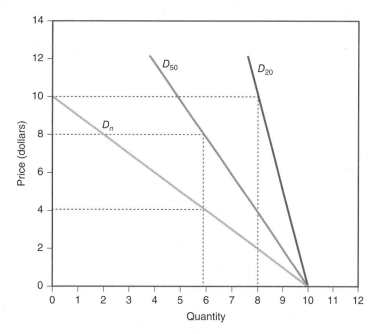

Figure 4-5 Demand curve with no insurance (D_n), with 50% coinsurance (D_{50}), and with 20% coinsurance (D_{20}). When there is a coinsurance rate, D_n also represents the relation between the quantity demanded and the out-of-pocket price.

© Jones & Bartlett Learning.

case, the out-of-pocket price and charged price now differ from one another. At any given charged price, the consumer faces a lower out-of-pocket price and hence, will move down the demand curve D_n.

If the coinsurance rate is 50%, the demand curve facing the provider is D_{50} (see Figure 4-5). Here, the out-of-pocket price is one-half the charged price, and the consumer demands a quantity determined by the

out-of-pocket price and the demand curve D_n. In fact, D_n becomes the demand curve relating quantity to out-of-pocket price. Thus, if the provider's charge were $8 per visit (in Figure 4-5), the consumer with a 50% coinsurance contract would pay a $4 out-of-pocket price and the quantity demanded would be six visits. If the coinsurance rate was 20%, the market demand curve facing the providers would be D_{20}. A charged price of $10 would mean an out-of-pocket price of $2 and a quantity demanded of eight. As the coinsurance rate falls, the market demand curve facing the providers shifts out, but the curve D_n continues to represent the relation between quantity demanded and out-of-pocket price.

Next, under an indemnity contract, a maximum fixed per-unit amount the insurer will pay for a service used is set. For example, an indemnity contract might specify that the insurer will pay up to $4 per visit. If the price is greater than $4, the consumer is responsible for the balance. In **Figure 4-6**, D_n is again the demand curve with no insurance coverage. Now, under an indemnity contract requiring the insurer to reimburse the provider up to $4 per visit, the demand curve facing the provider becomes D_{n+i}, which is the D_n curve raised by $4 at all points. The quantity demanded will reflect this lower out-of-pocket price. In Figure 4-6, a charged price of $8 means an out-of-pocket price of $4 and a quantity demanded of six. An increase in the amount by which the insurer indemnifies the consumer would shift D_{n+i} upward. The curve D_n would remain the same.

Finally, under a deductible, which is a fixed total amount that the insurer deducts from the bill, the consumer must spend up to this amount before coverage begins. Until the consumer spends this amount, the full price is paid for each additional unit consumed (the price paid for the next additional unit is called the *marginal out-of-pocket price*). The marginal out-of-pocket price before the deductible is reached is the charged price. If there is no coinsurance in addition to the deductible, the marginal out-of-pocket price after the deductible is met is zero.

To analyze the impact of a deductible on demand, assume that the curve shows the value to the consumer of each additional visit (the marginal value). If the patient consumes one visit, the value of the visit is $9. The second visit has a smaller marginal value, in this case $8. The two visits together would have a value of $17. These numbers, and the value of additional visits, are contained in **Table 4-3**. The table shows a declining marginal value for successive visits, consistent with the assumption in deriving the demand hypothesis.

Now assume a market price of $8 and a deductible of $32. At this market price, the out-of-pocket marginal price to the consumer will be $8 per visit until (and if) the deductible is met. Thereafter, it will be zero. In determining how many visits will be demanded, the consumer's valuation of visits in Table 4-3 is examined and compared with the marginal out-of-pocket price and the deductible level. At first the temptation might be to say that only the first two visits are worth at least the marginal out-of-pocket price and so only two will be demanded, concluding that, having spent $16 in total, the consumer did not meet the deductible, and so the visits will end at two.

But a logical "economic person" will realize that the purchase of the third and fourth units will use up the deductible of $32. Once the deductible is met, the rest of the visits demanded would be free!

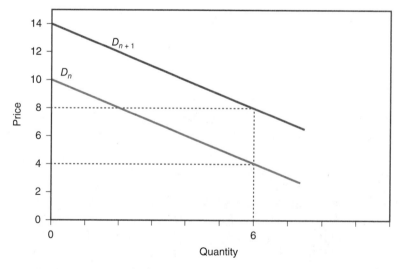

Figure 4-6 Demand curves with no insurance (D_n) and with an indemnity copayment amount (D_{n+1}). When there is a copayment, D_n also represents the relationship between the quantity demanded and the out-of-pocket price.

Table 4-3 Schedule of Value of Additional Medical Visits to Patient and Total (Summed) Value of All Units of Care

Quantity	Value of Additional Unit of Care to Consumer ($)	Total Value of All Care Received up to Given Quantity ($)
1	9	9
2	8	17
3	7	24
4	6	30
5	5	35
6	4	39
7	3	42
8	2	44
9	1	45
10	0	45

© Jones & Bartlett Learning.

Indeed, if the individual consumed nine units, the value would be $45, well in excess of the outlay of $32 for the first four units. In general, with a deductible, the amount demanded will be determined by the consumer's comparison of the additional value of all extra units with the additional out-of-pocket cost of all extra units. Even if the marginal value of the next visit (third, in this case) is less than its marginal out-of-pocket price, overall it will pay the individual to spend more in order to receive the benefits of the post-deductible units. If, however, the deductible was $100 and the charged price $8, the individual would stop consuming at two units because there would be no other quantity of consumption at which the total value to the individual exceeded what the individual had to pay.

Frequently, a deductible and a coinsurance are found together in the same policy. For example, the $32 deductible is combined with a 20% coinsurance (on units of care after the deductible has been reached). With a charged price of $8, the individual would then pay a marginal out-of-pocket price of $1.60 for each unit consumed after four. The individual would overspend the deductible in this case, but would demand only eight visits, because the ninth, costing $1.60, would have a marginal value of only $1.

4.7 Additional Factors Impacting Demand for Health Care

So far, the demand for medical care was introduced as if medical care were an ordinary everyday good or service. Some types of medical care *are* ordinary everyday goods and services. Pediatric well-child visits, the consumption of aspirin, and visits to a dentist are routine occurrences for many people. However, the circumstances surrounding many types of medical care are quite unlike the circumstances surrounding the use of everyday goods and services (Culyer, 1971). As a result, the traditional model must be modified to incorporate special factors. This section brings these factors into consideration by showing how they influence the demand relation.

4.7.1 Implications of Health Care for Life and Health

A widely cited characteristic of medical care is its ability to improve health. In some instances, timely medical care may prevent death or permanent disability. Where this condition holds (e.g., after a heart attack or a serious traffic accident), the question of substitutes, or price of services, has little importance. Presumably, the person would be willing to disburse all of his or her wealth to receive lifesaving medical care, and the demand curve would be vertical, reflecting absolute inelasticity of demand.

However, such instances are a very small portion of the total number of situations that cause individuals to seek medical care. In the vast majority of cases, alternative courses of action are available, and individuals have time to consider options. In fact, medical care should be viewed as a spectrum of services and goods rather than as a good or service only sought and consumed in an emergency. The less a situation calls for immediate action, and the greater the relevance of substitutes, the less steeply sloped the demand curve is for medical care. Substitutes are important even in emergency situations: individuals and planners have a wide variety of alternatives they can choose in advance of dire circumstances. Some of these choices are reflected in living wills and advanced directives, reflecting an individual's desires in cases of medical events.

Even though most medical problems are not emergencies, a reduction in medical care consumption can lead to a deterioration in health. In studying such a possibility, it may be desirable to analyze medical care demand from a multiperiod perspective. The imposition of a copayment on drugs or physician visits will generally lead to a reduction in the quantity demanded in Period 1. There is nothing in the theory of demand that says which units of medical care will no longer be demanded. Some units may have been unnecessary to begin with, but some may have been highly desirable given their effects on health status. When medical care is desirable, a reduction in its consumption in Period 1 may lead to a decline in health status in Periods 2, 3, or 4, and to possible increases in medical care demand in these subsequent periods.

This phenomenon was first examined following the imposition of a $1 copayment for each of the first two doctor's visits and $.50 for each of the first two prescriptions in the California Medicaid program. An original study (Roemer, Hopkins, Carr, & Gartside, 1975) stated that reductions in doctor's office visits and diagnostic tests after the copayment's introduction were accompanied by increases in hospitalization rates in subsequent periods. Although the data methods of the study were questioned, with no conclusive results (Chen, 1976a, b; Dyckman, 1976; Hopkins, Gartside, & Roemer, 1976), the study raised the issue of the importance of examining the wider effects of demand-reducing measures.

A subsequent study, based on the national Rand Health Insurance Experiment (Brook et al., 1983), examined the effects of reductions in use due to copayments on subsequent consumer health status and found that they were generally not adverse, except for certain groups. In particular, for poor individuals with hypertensive conditions, free care was associated with better blood pressure control and reductions in the risk of early death. There is a likelihood that, for selected groups, reductions in demand can have considerable impact on subsequent health status and medical care demand (Fein, 1981; Relman, 1983).

Research does indicate that price of healthcare services is relevant to the demand for many healthcare services, especially when viewed in terms of the impact of insurance on the utilization of healthcare services. For example, O'Neill and O'Neill (2009) reported that, in 2005, about 80% of insured women between the ages of 40 and 64 had received a mammogram during the past 2 years, but only 49% of uninsured women had received one. For the total population between the ages of 18 and 64, only 50% of those uninsured had received a routine physical during the past 2 years, compared to 78% of the insured population in that age cohort. While these are not direct measures of the impact of higher price on the demand for healthcare services, they can be used as proxies for determining the inverse relationship between price and quantity demanded in the market for selected healthcare services.

The consequences of being uninsured can be significant. An Urban Institute study (Dorn, 2008), estimated that applying the conservative increased risk of mortality associated with being uninsured of 15% to individuals between the ages of 25 and 64 resulted in over 101,000 excess deaths between 2000 and 2006, with 16,000 of them occurring in 2006.

For individuals with insurance, cost-sharing can still have a substantial impact on the demand for healthcare services. Zeber, Grazier, Valenstein, Blow, and Lantz (2007) found that increasing pharmacy copayments did result in a reduction in prescription utilization; however, following the reduction was a higher inpatient utilization resulting from cost-related nonadherence to treatment regimen. Similar impact findings were reported by Doshi, Zhu, Lee, Kimmel, and Volpp (2009), in which an increase in copayments for lipid-lowering medication adversely impacted medication adherence, including among those at high coronary heart disease risk.

4.7.2 External and Social Demand for Medical Care

Earlier, it was assumed that the sum of all individual's own demands for medical care was the same as the total societal demand for medical care. For certain social goods, such as medical care and education, however, it has been asserted that individuals would be willing to pay something to enable others to consume them. Many individuals would be willing to pay something to help ensure that a heart attack victim could reach a hospital in time; they would not be so generous if a person's car had broken down and $400 was "needed" for repairs. Furthermore, people's generosity probably extends only to certain types of medical care. The need for medical care with substantial health implications for the recipients (e.g., inoculations or care for the aged) elicits great concern; someone's desire to undergo cosmetic surgery does not.

To formalize the analysis of this phenomenon, the focus is on the consumption of a single individual, called A. The service whose demand is now analyzed is defined as individual A's consumption of medical care. A's own demand may be called *private* or *internal demand*.

Assume that the rest of society can be characterized as individuals B, who may also have a demand for A's consumption of medical care. Such a demand can be characterized in the same way as A's own demand;

as the price is lowered, B's demand for A's consumption of medical care will increase. This demand is in addition to A's own demand and can be called an *external demand*, because it comes from a force external to the consumer of the service. Examples of policies to influence the social demand for medical care are Medicare, Medicaid, and the Affordable Care Act. When society determined that the elderly and certain categories of low-income individuals weren't consuming sufficient medical care, policies were implemented to subsidize their purchase of additional services.

If society is defined as the sum total of A and B, then society's demand for A's consumption of medical care will depend on the private demand of A and the external demand of B. This total demand can be called *community* or *social* demand.

The effect of the external demand is to increase A's quantity demanded at any given price, assuming that the external demand is greater than zero at that price (see **Figure 4-7**). Society is the sum of all individuals, and the social demand for an individual's consumption of a given good or service is the sum of all private and external demands. The statement that "society wants everyone to have a decent level of medical care" can be interpreted to mean that, at the given price, there is a social demand for a "decent" level of care for each person.

There are a sufficiently large number of manifestations of external demands for medical care to impress on us how real this phenomenon is. The existence of philanthropic giving to such organizations as the American Heart Association, the United Way, the American Cancer Society, and the National Research Foundation provides evidence that donors are truly committed to enabling others to consume the services of these organizations, including health education and research. The majority of hospitals in the United States began as tax-exempt (not-for-profit) organizations with large charitable components. In recent years, these charitable components have decreased because of the growth of government health programs, such as Medicare and Medicaid, and private insurance. Such government programs themselves may be an expression of external demands expressed through the "political marketplace." Before the introduction of Medicare and Medicaid, physicians contended that a great deal of their medical services were provided as a form of charity.

4.7.3 Influence of Quality on the Demand for Medical Care

Earlier, the analysis of medical care demand was based on the assumption that each unit of medical care was like any other unit. Of course, this is not always the case. One of the more problematic tasks in analyzing resource allocation in medical care is coming to terms with quality differences.

Quality is not a single attribute, but rather a series of attributes, any of which can make the product appear better or worse to the consumer (Congress of the United States, 1988). Assuming the consumer is fully aware of how each of these attributes that determine the quality level of a product will affect him or her, and that quality is subjective in terms of how the consumer values these attributes of the good or service, their impact on demand can be evaluated.

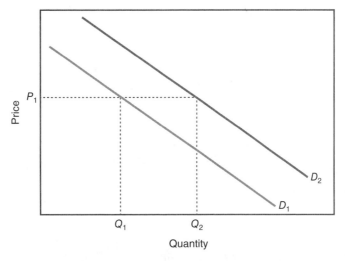

Figure 4-7 Social demand for medical care. At the price of P_1, individual A would purchase Q_1 units of medical care. But because society values A's use of medical services, society determines that at price P_1 individual A should consume Q_2 units of medical care. As a result, subsidies or other actions must be provided to increase A's demand for medical services to society's level of Q_2. Societies demand for aid, therefore, is the distance between Q_1 and Q_2.

There are three attributes of medical care that are used to identify quality (Donabedian, 1988): (1) the *structure* of the resources provided (e.g., the qualifications of the clinicians and the type of facilities); (2) the *process* of medical care (e.g., the thoroughness with which the diagnostic services are carried out or the comfort or luxury of the particular services provided); and (3) the *outcome,* or the level of medical excellence of the services. The latter attribute is associated with the accuracy of a diagnosis, the effectiveness of a treatment in restoring health, the effectiveness of a preventive course of action, and so on. Assuming that these aspects of quality can be accurately assessed, a consumer can make a personal evaluation of the overall quality levels associated with alternative units of medical care and can rank these alternative units according to their quality levels.

A reasonable hypothesis is that a higher quality level will increase the importance of medical care in relation to other goods and services at all levels of medical care consumption. This will result in an outward shift of the demand curve for medical care.

One qualification must be mentioned. If the quality of care is low, the demand may be less. But if low-quality care results in subsequent illness (e.g., if rheumatic fever develops from a failure to check for strep throat or if a patient with chicken pox contracts Reye's syndrome because aspirin was prescribed), it may lead to a greater demand for care in subsequent time periods (see **Figure 4-8**).

4.7.4 Time and Money Costs

Until now, the resource commitment necessary to obtain a unit of medical care has been measured by the per-unit out-of-pocket money price of that good or service. Thus, if a unit of medical care costs $5, then $5 was treated as an accurate measure of what a person had to give up (the opportunity cost) to obtain a unit of medical care. Yet the resources devoted to consuming a good or service include more than the money price of the good or service; when obtaining an office visit, people have to travel to and from the physician's office and wait to see the physician and be examined. The effort and time expended are personal resources and are part of the totality of resources committed to obtaining medical care.

The value of the time spent by a person traveling, waiting, and being examined is referred to as the time cost of obtaining medical care. The associated resource commitment is equivalent to the amount that could have been earned if the person had not visited the physician (assuming the person does forgo income in undertaking this action). If the person does not forgo income, valuable time is still given up. In this case, the opportunity cost of time would be taken to be equivalent to the value to the person of the activity given up. This latter magnitude is very difficult to measure, so for our purposes, we will assume that all time spent in obtaining health care can be measured in terms of the person's wage rate.

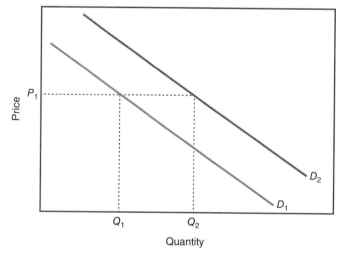

Figure 4-8 Increase in demand for medical care with improved quality of care. Demand curve D_1 reflects an individual's initial demand for medical care. When the quality of care is viewed as increasing, or improved, then the individual's demand for medical care will shift outwards to demand curve D_2, increasing the quantity demanded at each price of medical care. Notice that a change in quality shifts the entire demand curve, and doesn't cause just a movement along the original demand curve.

The total cost to, or total resource commitment made by, the person for each unit of health care can be expressed as $(w \times t) + p$, in which t is the amount of time involved in obtaining a unit of health care, w is the wage that would have been earned had the person worked during this time, and p is the money price of the health care.

Using the expression $(w \times t) + p$, the new hypothesis is this: as the total per-unit cost (time cost plus money price) falls, more medical care is demanded. For example, if the time required for a visit to the physician is 1 hour, the wage forgone is $20 per hour, and the money out-of-pocket price of a visit is $20, the total per-unit cost is $40. If the money price is set at zero by a government program or insurance, the total cost falls to $20 per visit. Medical care may still be too costly for some people, even at a zero out-of-pocket money price. If the government wishes to encourage consumption beyond this point, it might have to take steps that would lower waiting or travel time (e.g., by relocating a clinic to a more populous area).

Framing the analysis of demand in terms of total cost provides additional insight regarding issues of distribution. Even though money costs may be the same for all consumers, total costs may vary because of variations in w and t. For example, w may vary among consumers because some may have their wages docked if they take time off from work, whereas others may not. And t may vary because of variations in distances from care providers. When medical care is offered for "free," that is, at a zero money price, variations in quantity demanded will be determined by variations in time costs. In this circumstance, individuals who incur the lowest time cost will demand the greatest quantities, but may not be those with the most acute medical conditions. In this case, medical care would be rationed to those who are willing to wait and not to the most ill.

This problem arises when a program lowers the direct money price to zero while failing to increase supply sufficiently to meet the increased quantity demanded. An excess demand results, and queues may form. This raises the time cost, which becomes the mechanism by which medical care is rationed. Rationing, in and of itself, is not negative but simply a fact of life. Rationing is simply about making choices. If resources are limited, resulting in everyone not having everything they want, then choices will have to be made about how the limited resources will be used and who will be able to receive the resources. The issue becomes what is the best mechanism by which to ration the service to achieve the best or society-desired result.

4.7.5 The Demand for Health

In general, the output of the healthcare sector can be regarded either as health care or as health. An alternative formulation of consumer behavior in this area has been presented in terms of the demand for health (Grossman, 1972). Health can be regarded as an end in itself, something people want for its intrinsic characteristics or as a means to an end. For example, better health, by enabling a person to earn more income and purchase other goods and services, would function as a means for attaining a higher level of consumer consumption.

Assuming health to be an end in itself, it can be created or produced by the activities individuals undertake. These activities can include receiving medical care, engaging in self-care (exercise and proper diet), and so on. Such activities are substitutes because each contributes to achieving the desired end. The cost of each alternative activity can be expressed in terms of the resources an individual would have to commit in order to produce one healthy day. Because each activity will normally require time and purchased inputs on the part of the consumer, the cost of one healthy day can be expressed as follows:

$$c = (a \times w) + (b \times p)$$

In this equation, c is the unit cost (cost per one healthy day produced) of the activity; a is the amount of time required to produce one healthy day by engaging in the activity; b is the amount of purchased inputs required in conjunction with a to produce one healthy day; w is the opportunity cost of the individual's time and thus a measurement of the size of the resource commitment of one unit of time; and p is the price of one unit of purchased input. The cost of one healthy day (c) depends on a, b, w, and p. For each health-producing activity, there will be a different c.

If one activity, say self-care, is very productive (i.e., a and b are small), then the cost of producing an extra healthy day through self-care will be low. On the other hand, if self-care is not very effective in producing health, then a may be very high and c, in turn, will likely be high. Recall that, although the unit price of purchased inputs (p) may be high, the number of units required to produce a healthy day (b) may be low. Thus, purchased input-intensive activities, such as medical care, are not necessarily more costly than other health-producing activities. One prediction of this model is that, if the value of c of one type of health-producing activity rises relative to the value of c for another type, individuals will substitute in favor of the lower-cost alternative.

It is unlikely that a and b will remain constant across all levels of an activity. Instead, it is probable that the more an activity (e.g., physician care or self-care) is engaged in, the more a and b will increase. That is, it will take successively larger doses of personal effort and purchased inputs to yield a unit of health, reflecting diminishing marginal productivity. For this reason, the individual will probably demand both medical care and self-care. However, if a factor changes (e.g., there is an increase in the amount of waiting time necessary to obtain medical care), this will cause a shift in demand (e.g., more self-care and less medical care will be demanded).

Viewing the demand for health-related resources in this way allows us to incorporate the full resource commitment of alternative ways of producing health. In such a framework, medical care becomes one of several alternatives, and a broader picture of health-related resources can be obtained. However, while the picture is broader, it is also more complex, and for many purposes, such a broad and complex picture is not required.

4.7.6 Agency Theory and Supplier-Induced Demand

Many consumers do not know the effect of medical care on health, and physicians have been regarded as having two main roles: (1) To act in an advisory capacity and inform patients of their level of health and the activities and treatments that might improve their health; and (2) To undertake treatments upon which their patients have decided. When we introduce the physicians into the demand analysis, we widen the framework, for the patient's demand is now also dependent on the interaction with the physician.

A patient's perception of the level of his or her health and the probable effect of medical care on the patient's health can influence the patient's demand for medical care. Because the physician potentially has influence over both of these factors, the physician can conceivably change the patient's demand for medical care by providing pertinent information.

Assuming the physician knows the patient's health level and the effectiveness of medical care in producing health, and if the physician has an awareness of the patient's tastes and other circumstances (prices and income), then, assuming the physician behaves as a "perfect agent," he or she will provide a quantity of medical care that a fully informed patient would have chosen. However, principal–agent relationships are such that the agent (physician) may not behave in the best interests of the principal (patient). A deviation of the agent from the principal's own interests is called *supplier-induced demand*.

Supplier-induced demand will arise when there is a potential divergence of interest between the principal and the agent. Despite this divergence, there must still be a basis for the two to engage in a contractual relationship. However, when the principal uses the services of the agent, he or she, in effect, has entered into an agreement that the agent will meet the principal's needs. Problems with the relationship will arise when there is uncertainty and information asymmetry that makes it difficult for the two parties to agree on a fixed price, agree on a predetermined service that the agent will provide, and develop an adequate mechanism to monitor and enforce the agreement.

As an example of a principal–agent relationship that would not be plagued by agency problems, imagine a private home care nursing agency administering intravenous drugs on a daily basis to a bedridden client. The home care nurse will agree to show up at a specified time each day and administer the drugs. The client can clearly specify the contract with the agency. Also, the client can easily monitor the performance of the nursing agency, and if the nursing agency does not perform adequately, the client can terminate the contract.

When the patient interacts with a provider, there are four additional types of costs to the price, wait, travel, and examination costs:

1. *Search costs*, or the costs of determining specifications of the services needed and the prices of these services;
2. *Contract costs*, or the costs of reaching an agreement with the provider as to what services are to be provided;
3. *Monitoring costs*, or the costs of identifying the desired outcomes, collecting data on these outcomes, and determining whether the outcomes have been achieved; and
4. *Enforcement costs*, or the costs of ensuring that the provider meets the agreed criteria.

These costs are especially important in the present circumstances. The patient (principal), lacking relevant information, relies on the physician (agent) to provide advice on health status and alternative treatments and, in many instances, to provide the recommended therapy. In some circumstances, the physician's interests may diverge from those of the patient. The physician can then engage in supplier-induced demand by providing advice and therapies that are in his or her own interests rather than the interests of the patient. Despite the divergences of interests, the patient may still contract with the physician because, given the costs of engaging in the medical care process, what is provided by the physician may be the best alternative (Dranove & White, 1987).

Thus, supplier-induced demand is a phenomenon that has been linked to agency theory. Supplier-induced demand may be encouraged by certain payment mechanisms that provide incentives to physicians to deliver more services, such as fee-for-service. Under fee-for-service, the physician is paid for each unit of service performed, and so one of the conditions needed for principal–agent problems to arise—the divergence of interests—will be present. Monitoring and enforcement costs may be very high for the patient; therefore, the physician has both the incentive and the ability to engage in demand-inducing practices.

There are limits to supplier-induced demand. For one thing, with repeated events (e.g., common colds), the patient eventually gains information that can be used to evaluate health and medical productivity. In addition, information sharing between patients, between patients and other physicians (second opinions), or on the Internet, limits the degree to which a physician can sway the patient with incomplete or misinformation. That is, the patient's monitoring abilities are improved. Deliberate misrepresentation of information would be contrary to the physician's ethical codes. Finally, the assumption that the *physician* has perfect information about the patient's health status and the productivity of medical care is not always realistic. Diagnosis and treatment are often undertaken under conditions of uncertainty. Under such conditions, a physician experiments to obtain the best treatment, some argue this is why it is called the practice of medicine. Although the physician can still generate demand, it is impossible to say with certainty how much of the "experimentation" was intentional demand generation and how much was honest experimentation.

4.7.6.1 Demand Under Uncertainty: The Demand for Health Promotion

The simple analysis of demand for medical care was based on the assumption that the consumer knows with certainty what his or her state of health will be during the relevant time period. This underlying assumption is not plausible for many medical problems. In these cases, a consumer cannot be certain whether or not a problem will occur. The consumer does know, however, that he or she *might* be sick during a particular period and might have to visit a

healthcare provider and even be hospitalized. Issues related to the uncertain appearance of illness have a bearing on a number of health-related activities (Kenkel, 1991; Russell, 1984; Scheffler & Paringer, 1980). For example, people adopt healthy or unhealthy lifestyles; these lifestyles are often resource-intensive and will have an impact on the likelihood that the individuals will be sick.

The basic theory of the demand for health promotion activities presents a systematic view of how certain underlying variables—tastes, wealth, the cost of health promotion, the likelihood of an illness, and the loss resulting from the illness—can influence the decision to engage in these activities. The assumptions of the model are as follows:

1. *Time frame.* All activities and consequences occur in the current time period.
2. *Level of wealth.* Our individual initially has a level of wealth of $1000.
3. *Consumer tastes.* When an illness occurs, it leads to medical care expenses that constitute a loss of wealth. To specify what this loss means to the individual, a concept to characterize the individual's well-being at alternative levels of wealth—the concept of utility—must be included. Utility is a measure of consumer satisfaction and reflects the maximum amount of resources (money) an individual will exchange for a particular bundle of goods and services. One hypothetical individual's taste for wealth is presented in the form of an index of utility in **Table 4-4**. This index shows the level of utility that is associated with each specific level of wealth.

Thus, a level of wealth of $1000 is associated with a level of utility of 100, a level of wealth of $990 is associated with a level of utility of 99.8, and so on. The size of specific numbers in the utility index is arbitrary. What is important is that higher wealth gives higher utility (i.e., increased wealth makes the individual "better off"). Also, the function is characterized by diminishing marginal utility. That is, each additional $10 of wealth results in less additional utility than the previous $10. For example, at $850, an extra $10 will yield 3 extra units of utility; at $860, an extra $10 will yield 2.8 extra units; and so on.

If an individual has a diminishing marginal utility for wealth, he or she is said to be *risk-averse*. The basic idea is that, for a given wealth level, a loss of a given amount of wealth (e.g., $10) is of greater subjective importance (utility) to the person than would be a gain of an equal amount. Utility is the subjective index of the relative importance of wealth.

Table 4-4 Relationship Between Wealth and Utility

Wealth ($)	Total Utility	Marginal Utility
800	57.0	4.2
810	61.2	4.0
820	65.2	3.8
830	69.0	3.6
840	72.6	3.4
850	76.0	3.2
860	79.0	3.0
870	81.8	2.8
880	84.4	2.6
890	86.8	2.4
900	89.0	2.2
910	91.0	2.0
920	92.8	1.8
930	94.4	1.6
940	95.8	1.4
950	97.0	1.2
960	98.0	1.0
970	98.8	0.8
980	99.4	0.6
990	99.8	0.4
1000	100.0	0.2

© Jones & Bartlett Learning.

In this model, a utility function is unique to an individual. Thus, it does not imply that additional wealth means less to a rich person than it does to a poor person. This kind of comparison, called *interpersonal comparison*, would involve specifying different people's utilities on the same scale.

1. *Medical expenses in the event of illness.* If the individual becomes sick, he or she will face medical expenses of $150. This expenditure is assumed to restore the loss in health fully so that $150 is the full value of the loss when the individual is sick.
2. *The cost of health promotion activities.* The consumer uses up resources when engaging in health promotion, including time, professional services,

and supplies. In our example, we will assume that these costs total $20.

3. *Likelihood of illness.* The element of uncertainty assumes that probabilities can be assigned to the various possible health states the individual may experience. Without any health promotion activities, there is a 0.3 probability of illness (i.e., of 10 people in similar circumstances, 3 will become ill) and a 0.7 probability the individual will remain well and will not incur any medical costs. These are the only two possibilities in this illustration, so the sum of the probabilities equals 1. With health promotion activities, the probability of being healthy increases to 0.9 and the probability of being ill falls to 0.1.
4. *Behavioral assumption.* The individual wants to maximize the expected value of his or her utility. Thus, the individual will choose that course of action from which he or she can expect to receive the highest level of utility.

The model's conclusions are obtained by determining how, under these assumed conditions, the individual will behave so as to maximize expected utility. Under the option of not engaging in health promotion, the expected utility for the individual is 92.8 $[(0.7 \times 100) + (0.3 \times 76.0)]$. This is because when the individual is healthy, he or she has a utility of 100.0 (corresponding to a wealth of $1000), and when he or she is ill, the utility is 76.0 (corresponding to a wealth level of $850). If the individual engages in health promotion activities, the expected utility will be derived from the probabilities and utility levels when he or she is healthy or ill, but has spent $20 on health promotion activities (which occur whether the individual is healthy or not). Therefore, the expected utility is 95.3 $[(0.9 \times 99.4) + (0.1 \times 69.0)]$. The individual is better off when he or she engages in health promotion activities under these circumstances.

However, this will not always be the case. If any of our basic assumptions change, so may our conclusion. The individual will be less likely to engage in health promotion when any of the following occurs: the cost of health promotion increases, health promotion has a reduced impact on illness, or the individual experiences an increase in risk aversion.

4.7.6.2 Limitations of the Model

The theory of the demand for health care under conditions of uncertainty has the virtue of explicitly organizing some of the variables that are central to the decision to engage in activities that promote health. As presented, however, it has an important limitation.

The utility function, which is supposed to measure satisfaction, does not include health. This is a shortcoming of the model, because well-being can depend on health status as well as wealth. The model looks only at financial aspects of the situation, in effect assuming that the care consumed fully and instantly restores health, with no utility implications of either the illness or the process of getting care. Clearly, this is an unrealistic assumption. Including health status creates a much more complicated model that is more difficult to apply, and while it is important to understand that we have abstracted from reality, this should not detract from the value of the model. The present model has the virtue of focusing on the benefits of risk shifting, which is an economic good that is distinct from medical care.

4.7.6.3 Discounting Future Values

Another factor that affects health promotion behavior is the individual's valuation of benefits in different time periods. Health promotion activities, such as the use of condoms, smoking cessation, vaccinations, and clean needles (for drug users), and unhealthy activities, such as smoking, engaging in unsafe sex, and excessive drug use, generally do not have good or bad impacts on health immediately. It takes a long time, sometimes years, for individuals to experience adverse health effects. The timing of health benefits will have an influence on the demand for health-related activities that promote these benefits.

It is generally assumed that $1000 in current benefits will be worth more to an individual than $1000 in benefits 1 year from now. The value of the preference for earlier rather than later periods can be expressed in terms of a discount rate, called r. If an individual is asked how much money he or she would accept at the end of 2020 rather than have $1000 at the beginning of 2020, the person might take $1100 at the end of the period. In other words, $1000 on January 1, 2020, would be worth as much as $1100 one year later. The discount rate is 0.1, and the discounting equation is expressed as $1000 × (1 + 0.1) = $1100, or symbolically as $1000 × (1 + r) = $1100. This may be rewritten as $1000 = $1100/(1 + r). This equation says that, in the individual's eyes, $1100 one year hence will be equivalent to $1100/(1 + r), or $1000, now. The discount rate for an individual is derived largely from introspection—from an acceptance that a given future amount and a lesser current amount provide the same satisfaction *at the present moment.*

The same principle holds for comparisons between December 31, 2020, and December 31, 2021. That is, $1000 at the end of 2020 is equivalent to $1100 at the end of 2021 if the individual's discount rate is 0.1. By inference, then, $1000 at the end of 2021 would be worth $1000/[(1 + r) × (1 + r)] on January 1, 2020 [also expressible as $1000/(1 + r)^2$]. Similarly, $1000 on December 31, 2022, would be worth $1000/(1 + r)^3$ at the start of 2020, and so on. Generally, improved health, or added life, yields a stream of benefits. That is, a saved life on January 1, 2020 will yield benefits in 2020 (valued as of December 31, 2020), 2021 (valued as of December 31, 2021), 2022 (valued as of December 31, 2022), and so on. If the benefits are $2000 each year, the *present value* of future benefits can be expressed as $2000 + 2000/(1 + r) + 2000/(1 + r)^2$, and so on, for as long as benefits last. The letter usually used to symbolize the annual benefits is B, with subscripts 0, 1, 2, . . . for right now (0), 1 year hence (1), 2 years hence (2), and so on. In our current example, $B_0 = B_1 = B_2$, and the present value of benefits can be expressed symbolically as

$$B_0 + B_0 / (1+r) + B_0 / (1+r)^2$$

If the number of years that benefits will last is quite large, and the value of the benefits for every year is the same, the present value of the benefits can be expressed as B_0/r. If benefits of $10,000 a year will last forever, and if the discount rate is 0.1, the present value of these benefits will be 10,000/0.1, or $100,000. Benefits lasting for long periods can be approximated using this formula.

The discount factor can be quite substantial for benefits that will not be experienced for many years. For example, hepatitis C may not be recognized for 20 years. If hepatitis C imposes health-related costs of $1000 in 20 years and the discount rate is 10%, then the present value of these imposed costs is $148.64 [$1000 / (1 + 0.1)^{20}$].

Not everyone will have the same discount rate. An individual who has a very strong preference for current satisfaction rather than future benefits will have a high interest rate, perhaps 15% or 20%. On the other hand, a person who places very great importance on future satisfaction will have a very low discount rate, perhaps 2% or even 0%. In the latter case, there would be no discount rate, and present and future values would be the same.

Table 4-5 Calculation of Present Value of Benefits Under Alternative Discount Rates

Part A: Discounting Factors						
Discount rate	$(1 + r)$	$(1 + r)^2$	$(1 + r)^3$	$(1 + r)^4$	$(1 + r)^5$	
0.04	1.04	1.08	1.12	1.17	1.22	
0.08	1.08	1.17	1.26	1.36	1.47	
0.12	1.12	1.25	1.40	1.57	1.76	
Part B: Discounted Present Value of Benefits ($10,000)						
Discount rate	$B/(1 + r)$	$B/(1 + r)^2$	$B/(1 + r)^3$	$B/(1 + r)^4$	$B/(1 + r)^5$	Present value (row sum)
0.04	9,615	9,246	8,890	8,548	8,219	44,518
0.08	9,259	8,573	7,938	7,350	6,806	39,927
0.12	8,929	7,972	7,118	6,355	5,674	36,048

© Jones & Bartlett Learning.

Table 4-5 presents a series of discounted values, varying according to discount rates (4%, 8%, and 12%) and time periods (1–5 years). For example, in Part A, at a discount rate of 8% and a 4-year time horizon, the value of $(1 + r)^4$ is 1.36. The present value of a benefit of $10,000 that occurred in 4 years, discounted at a rate of 8%, would, therefore, be $7350.

Often, benefits will repeat themselves from year to year. For example, a $10,000 benefit may be experienced in each of the next 5 years. If the discount rate was 4%, then the present value of the benefits for each of the next 5 years would be $9615; then $9246; and so on for 5 years. The present value of $10,000 for all 5 years together, called the annuity value, is $44,518, as shown in Table 4-5 Part B. Annuity tables would contain present values summed over each time horizon.

4.8 Elasticity of Demand Estimates

Demand responsiveness can be measured by natural experiments and controlled trials. A natural experiment (in the demand context) occurs, for example, when a change in insurance coverage is implemented by an insurer. The results of such a policy action can be used to determine demand responsiveness by conducting before-and-after comparisons of the data. Assuming all else has remained the same (e.g., that an increase in a deductible has not driven the sicker insureds to buy more complete insurance elsewhere), we can use the data to measure the degree of responsiveness. Natural experiments, unfortunately, often do not provide sufficient information. The investigators have no control over insurer policy decisions and are therefore restricted to researching the changes in price and coverage introduced by the insurers.

A more flexible, but also more expensive, approach is to do a controlled experiment. In this approach, study groups are selected randomly (to avoid any bias due to self-selection, such as sicker individuals choosing more complete insurance coverage) and assigned to specific categories (e.g., 20% coinsurance, 40% coinsurance, etc.). Differences in utilization (which are assumed to be caused by differences in demand) can be measured, and thus, a measure of demand responsiveness can be obtained.

An example of a natural experiment in the demand field occurred in 1977, when the United Mine Workers introduced a $250 deductible for inpatient services and a 40% coinsurance for physician and outpatient visits up to a maximum family liability of $500. Prior to this, the insureds had no out-of-pocket expenses.

Scheffler (1984) conducted a study of the impact of this cost-sharing on hospital admissions, average length of hospital stays, the probability that an insured would have at least one physician visit, and the number of times an insured visited a physician. According to the analysis, in the 5 months prior to introduction of the hospital deductible (the comparison period), the hospital admission rate was 6.8 per 1000 enrollees, and the average length of stay per hospitalization was 5.42 days. The corresponding figures for the 5 months after introduction (the study period) were 4.8 per 1000 for admissions and 6.45 days per hospitalization. The longer average length of stay in the study period may have been due to the fact that only sicker cases were hospitalized, with individuals with typical short lengths of stay now not being admitted to the hospital at all. With regard to physician visits, the study's results indicated that the proportion of the population seeing a physician at least once fell from 44% in the comparison period to 28% in the study period, and the average number of visits of those who did see a physician at least once fell from 2.3 to 1.6.

The results of this experiment, like the results of other such studies, convincingly demonstrate the immediate impact of cost-sharing policies on utilization. But do the reductions in utilization last? Are there bad consequences farther down the line? One study (Scitovsky & McCall, 1977) verified that reductions in physician visits did last several years, but several others have raised doubts as to whether longer-term impacts occur.

By far, the best-known controlled experiment in this area is the six-site Health Insurance Experiment conducted by the Rand Corporation (Newhouse et al., 1981). In this study, 2756 families agreed to participate in an experiment in which each family was assigned to one of five groups with different coinsurance rates. The rates included free care (0 coinsurance), 25%, 50%, and 95% coinsurance, and a deductible with 95% coinsurance (all services, such as physician visits and hospitalization, were covered under the single rate). Those families with greater potential out-of-pocket expenses than their pre-experiment coverage were compensated accordingly. Upper limits were placed on each family's out-of-pocket expenses. The families participated for 3–5 years.

The results dramatically indicated the differential impact of higher out-of-pocket expenses. For example, those with free care incurred average expenses for all services of $401, whereas those with 25%, 50%, and 95% coinsurance incurred expenses of $346, $328, and $254, respectively. Furthermore, these differentials held up over several years. Because the experiment was designed to control for all other intervening factors (e.g., health status, income, etc.), the results have had a considerable impact in health policy circles. The fact is that such controlled results are seldom obtained.

Several questions have been raised concerning the applicability of the study's results. First, the experiments affected only a small portion of the entire healthcare market in each of the six communities studied. If coinsurance rates were raised for the entire market, or a substantial portion of the market, would providers (physicians) react and generate additional demand, thus changing the results? Furthermore, the

aged (and presumably the fragile) were omitted from the study. Would their responses be any different?

Despite the unanswered questions, such studies have moved us closer toward developing a quantitative measure of the impact of out-of-pocket price on demand. As seen previously, demand elasticity depends on the starting point on an individual's demand curve, which, in turn, is affected by the individual's level of insurance. A rough estimate of demand elasticity when consumers have 0%–25% coinsurance is –0.2 (Newhouse, Phelps, & Marquis, 1980).

Such an estimate can be used in the following way. If the price for a physician visit is $100, the coinsurance rate is 10%, and initially there are 120 visits, what would be the expected number of visits after the coinsurance rate is raised to 20%? The answer (assuming an elasticity of –0.2) is obtained by solving for Q_2 (visits in Period 2), in which

$$E = \frac{(Q_2 - Q_1)/(Q_2 + Q_1)}{(P_2 - P_1)/(P_2 + P_1)}$$

or

$$-0.2 = \frac{(Q_2 - 120)/(Q_2 + 120)}{(20 - 10)/(20 + 10)}$$

The result gives a value for Q_2 of 104 visits (rounded to the nearest integer). In this case, the total price did not change, although the coinsurance rate and therefore the out-of-pocket price did. A similar analysis could be done if the charged price and the copayment rate had both been changed.

A number of studies have been conducted analyzing demand in the nursing home market. Nursing home care is a healthcare service whose demand has distinct characteristics that have an impact on its elasticity of demand. First, there are a significant number of self-pay (uninsured) patients in this market; in 2009, out-of-pocket payments accounted for 29% of all nursing home expenditures. For those patients who are not covered by public insurance (primarily through Medicaid), the out-of-pocket price becomes an important variable, because private insurance for long-term care is still a minor factor. Second, there are close substitutes for nursing home care. Home health care is, in many instances, a viable alternative to nursing home care. Also, some patients who are hospitalized and could be moved to a skilled nursing care facility "economize" on skilled nursing home care by remaining in the hospital longer and transferring later or not at all. The existence of close substitutes increases the elasticity of demand for nursing home care.

Lamberton and colleagues (1986) conducted a cross-county study of nursing home demand in South Dakota. In analyzing the relationship between nursing home days and such variables as price, income, and home care visits, they estimated an elasticity of demand for private patients of –0.76. They also detected a significant negative relationship between home care visits and nursing home care, which substantiated the hypothesis that the two forms of care are substitutes. These results, which show that nursing home care has greater elasticity of demand than hospital care, were expected. Given the current interest in expanding long-term care insurance, an elasticity of this magnitude indicates that the demand for long-term care would increase substantially, if long-term care insurance were to increase (because the out-of-pocket price of long-term care would be lowered).

An original component of the Affordable Care Act was a requirement for the states to expand coverage to certain uninsured persons under Medicaid. However, courts found that states could not be mandated to expand Medicaid, but it had to be voluntary. As a result, only 33 states elected to expand Medicaid coverage. This difference in adoption of Medicaid expansion by states enables examination of the impact of Medicaid expansion on utilization of healthcare services.

A substantial number of research studies on the effects of Medicaid expansion under the Affordable Care Act on utilization of healthcare services has been conducted. Soni, Simon, Cawley, and Sabik (2018) found that Medicaid expansion resulted in significantly greater increases in cancer diagnosis rates, especially in diagnosis in the early stages of cancer. A GAO report (2017) demonstrated that Medicaid expansion states reported improved access to behavior and mental health services. Loehrer et al. (2018) found that patients admitted to academic medical centers or their affiliated hospitals with one of five common surgical conditions was associated with significantly greater probability of receiving optimal care in Medicaid expansion states. Yue, Rasmussen, and Ponce (2018) found Medicaid expansion was associated with gains in health insurance coverage, enrollees having personal physicians, and affordability among low-income, nonelderly adults. Results of the various studies highlight the impact that Medicaid expansion had on the utilization of healthcare services.

Exercises

1. Distinguish between demand and quantity demanded.
2. Indicate how each of the following factors will change the individual demand curve for aspirin tablets:
   a. an increase in income
   b. an increase in the price of Tylenol (a substitute)
   c. an increase in the price of bottled water (a complement)
   d. an increase in the number of people with headaches
   e. the discovery that aspirin, if taken regularly, reduces the severity of heart attacks
3. Determine how each of the following factors would shift the demand curve for chiropractic visits:
   a. an increase in the out-of-pocket price of chiropractic visits
   b. an increase in back problems
   c. a reduction in the out-of-pocket price for chiropractic visits
   d. an aging of the population
   e. an increase in the out-of-pocket price of back surgery (a substitute for chiropractic services)
   f. a reduction in the price of radiographs (a complement of chiropractic services)
   g. an advertising campaign that makes people more aware of the benefits of chiropractic care
4. In a small town in Florida, a food supplement sold for $2.00 a bottle in May. In total, 2000 bottles were sold. In June, nothing else changed but the price of the supplement, which was increased to $2.20. A total of 1900 bottles were sold. What is the arc elasticity of demand?
5. Determine how each of the following factors would shift the demand for home care:
   a. an increase of $10 in the price per day charged by nursing homes, with the government picking up the entire price increase

b. an increase, from $12 to $15, in the price paid out-of-pocket by users of home care

c. an increase in the number of people being discharged early from hospital

d. an increase in productivity among home care providers

e. an increase in the percentage of low-income people in a given population

6. The elasticity of demand for physician visits was determined to be –0.2. The president of the local health insurance company wants to add a copayment of $0.50 onto each physician visit. Currently, there is no copayment. The number of insured people is 3,000,000, and currently, the population uses 2.4 visits per capita. How many visits will they use after the introduction of the copayment?

7. Name three different ways of identifying quality. How would an increase in quality affect the demand for medical services?

8. Mrs. Smith earns $20 an hour. Normally, she has to drive into St. Cloud from her home (150 miles away) for a medical consultation. The drive is 2.5 hours each way. Mrs. Smith usually has a 1-hour wait, and the consultation takes about an hour. Mrs. Smith estimates that the cost of the transportation is 50 cents a mile. What are Mrs. Smith's travel and waiting costs for each visit?

9. What is information asymmetry and how does it result in a principal-agent problem?

10. What is supplier-induced demand? How is it related to a principal-agent problem?

Bibliography

Brook, R. H., Ware, J. E., Jr., Rogers, W. H., Keeler, E. B., Davies, A. R., Donald, C. A., Goldberg, G. A. … Newhouse, J. P. (1983). Does free care improve adults' health? *New England Journal of Medicine, 309*, 1426–1434.

Chen, M. K. (1976a). Penny-wise and pound foolish: Another look at the data. *Medical Care, 14*, 958–963.

Chen, M. K. (1976b). More about penny-wise and pound foolish: A statistical point of view. *Medical Care, 14*, 964–968.

Congress of the United States. (1988). *The quality of medical care*. Washington, DC: Congress of the United States, Office of Technology Assessment.

Culyer, A. J. (1971). The nature of the commodity "health care" and its efficient allocation. *Oxford Economic Papers, 23*, 189–211.

Donabedian, A. (1988). The quality of care. *JAMA, 260*, 1743–1748.

Dorn, S. (2008). *Uninsured and dying because of it: Updating the Institute of Medicine analysis on the impact of uninsurance on mortality*. Washington, DC: Urban Institute.

Doshi, J. A., Zhu, J., Lee, B. Y., Kimmel, S. E., & Volpp, K. G. (2009). Impact of a prescription copayment increase on lipid-lowering medication adherence in veterans. *Circulation, 119*, 390–397.

Dranove, D., & White, W. D. (1987). Agency and the organization of health care delivery. *Inquiry, 24*(4), 405–415.

Dyckman, Z. Y. (1976). Comment on "copayments for ambulatory care: Penny-wise and pound foolish." *Medical Care, 14*, 274–276.

Fein, R. (1981). Effects of cost sharing in health insurance. *New England Journal of Medicine, 305*, 1526–1528.

Grossman, M. (1972). *The demand for health*. New York, NY: National Bureau of Economic Research.

Hopkins, C. E., Gartside, F., & Roemer, M. I. (1976). Rebuttal to "comment on 'copayments for ambulatory care: Penny-wise and pound foolish.'" *Medical Care, 14*, 277.

Kenkel, D. S. (1991). Health behavior, health knowledge, and schooling. *Journal of Political Economy, 99*(2), 287–305.

Lamberton, C. E., Ellingson, W. D., & Spear, K. R. (1986). Factors determining the demand for nursing home services. *Quarterly Review of Economics and Business, 26*, 74–90.

Loehrer, A., Chang, D. C., Scott, J. W., Hutter, M. M., Patel, V. I., Lee, J. E., & Sommers, B. D. (2018). Association of the Affordable Care Act Medicaid expansion with access to and quality of care for surgical conditions. *JAMA Surgery, 153*(3), e175568.

Newhouse, J. P., Phelps, C. E., & Marquis, M. S. (1980). On having your cake and eating it too. *Journal of Econometrics, 13*, 365–390.

Newhouse, J. P., Manning, W. G., Morris, C. N., Orr, L. L., Keeler, E. B., Leibowitz, A., … Brock, R. H. (1981). Some interim results from a controlled trial of cost sharing in health insurance. *New England Journal of Medicine, 305*, 1501–1507.

O'Neill, J. E., & O'Neill, D. M. (2009). *Who are the uninsured? An analysis of America's uninsured population, their characteristics, and their health*. Washington, DC: Employment Policies Institute.

Relman, A. (1983). The Rand health insurance study: Is cost sharing dangerous to your health? *New England Journal of Medicine, 309*, 1453.

Roemer, M. I., Hopkins, C. E., Carr, L., & Gartside, F. (1975). Copayments for ambulatory care: Penny-wise and pound-foolish. *Medical Care, 13*(6), 457–466.

Roemer, M. I., & Hopkins, C. E. (1976). Response to M. K. Chen. *Medical Care, 14*(11), 963–964.

Russell, L. B. (1984). The economics of prevention. *Health Policy, 4*, 85–100.

Scheffler, R. M. (1984). The United Mine Worker's health plan. *Medical Care, 22*, 247–254.

Scheffler, R. M., & Paringer, L. (1980). A review of the economic evidence on prevention. *Medical Care, 18*, 473–484.

Scitovsky, A. A., & McCall, N. (1977, May). Coinsurance and the demand for physician services. *Social Security Bulletin, 40*, 19–27.

Soni, A., Simon, K., Cawley, J., & Sabik, L. (2018). Effect of Medicaid expansions of 2014 on overall and early-stage cancer diagnoses. *American Journal of Public Health, 108*(2), 216–218.

United States Government Accountability Office (GAO). (2017, June). *Medicaid expansion: Behavioral health treatment use in selected states in 2014*. Washington, DC: GAO Report to

Congressional Requesters. Retrieved from https://www.gao.gov/assets/690/685415.pdf

Yue, D., Rasmussen, P., & Ponce, N. (2018). Racial/ethnic differential effects of Medicaid expansion on health care access. *Health Services Research, 53*(5), 3656.

Zeber, J. E., Grazier, K. L., Valenstein, M., Blow, F. C., & Lantz, P. M. (2007). Effect of a medication copayment increase in veterans with schizophrenia. *The American Journal of Managed Care, 13*(6, Pt 2), 335–346.

CHAPTER 5

Healthcare Production and Costs

OBJECTIVES

1. Define fixed and variable inputs and distinguish between a short-run and a long-run time horizon in identifying whether inputs are fixed or variable.
2. Explain the concept of a production function for medical services in terms of inputs and outputs, and show how it can be used to understand the substitution among inputs and the effect of changes in the volume of inputs.
3. Explain the concepts of *total cost*, *average cost*, and *marginal cost* and the relationships among them and show how to derive them from basic assumptions.
4. Explain the concept of *economies of scope*.
5. Explain the concepts of *short-* and *long-run cost curves* and indicate a likely shape for these curves.
6. Identify the likely actual shapes of cost curves for nursing homes, hospitals, physician services, and health insurers.

5.1 Introduction

This chapter focuses on the economic behavior of healthcare providers in the production of healthcare services. Examined first is how the resource commitment made by individual providers varies with the amount of production undertaken by these providers. Here, the focus is on the individual unit of production. The measure used to weigh the magnitude of the resource commitment of each production unit is the cost to the unit of resources used. How these costs vary as the size of operations of the production unit varies is then examined.

Before embarking on the analysis of costs, Section 5.2 considers the relationship between inputs (resources) and outputs (the input–output or production relation). The presentation is in purely "physical" terms and is designed to provide a brief summary of the role of production in determining cost. In

Section 5.3, the basic cost–output relationship is explored and three alternative ways of looking at this relationship are examined. Using the cost–output relationship as the basic reference point, in Section 5.4 the various factors that affect this relationship are examined, such as changing technology, the quality of care given, the incentives offered to providers, and the size of the production unit.

In Section 5.5, the impact of one particular organizational factor on a unit's operating costs—the relatedness of the types of services produced together in the same unit—is examined. Producing services of different types in the same unit may give rise to economies and diseconomies of scope. In Section 5.6, the impact of operating scale on a unit's costs is examined. Finally, in Section 5.7, the empirical estimation of cost curves in relation to physician practices, hospitals, nursing homes, and health insurance companies is investigated.

5.2 Production: The Input–Output Relation

5.2.1 Basic Relationship

Production involves the creation or addition of utility, which is the want-satisfying capacity of a good or service. The economic analysis of production involves the specification of alternative combinations of inputs that yield varying levels of outputs. Typically, inputs consist of mental and physical labor, capital equipment, raw materials, intermediate goods and services, knowledge, and entrepreneurial abilities, all of which exist in limited quantities. The production process itself in health care, its organization, and the technology used lie in the realm of administrative practice and medicine. The production process has considerable impact on economic variables and can be influenced by economic factors as well.

The production process is partially determined by the technology used. Roughly defined, technology is a way of transforming inputs into outputs. Outputs consist of finished goods or services, or intermediate goods and services used by others in the production process. The production process in medical care is determined by what things are done to the patients as well as the way they are done. In this sense, there are many "technologies," even for the same illness. To bring out the essential characteristics of the production (input–output) relationship, we focus initially on one technology and then later there is the introduction of complicating factors and the determination of how they affect this relationship.

The simplest production process can be illustrated by the hypothetical case of a solo private practice physician with a nursing staff who treats patients all with the same disease—the common cold. Treatment involves an examination, diagnostic tests, and a prescription of two aspirins and a glass of water. Two simplifying assumptions should be noted. *First*, the patients' conditions are homogeneous (the patients have equally severe cases of a single disease). *Second*, the treatment provided is of the same quality (all patients receive the same examination and the same tests and listen to the same instructions from the physician).

The production process involves the use of various resources (inputs). These resources can be divided into two basic groups: fixed and variable inputs. Fixed inputs are those whose use is restricted to their current function for the time period under consideration and cannot be varied or changed in the current production period. Given their specialized nature, the high costs of transferring them to other uses, or contractual arrangements in force, fixed factors cannot be used elsewhere in the economy during the current period of production. Furthermore, the producer cannot increase the quantity of fixed resources during this time period, or production cycle, which is assumed in this illustration to be 1 month. In this illustration, the fixed factors of production include the physician's office space, test equipment, and the physician's time.

An assumption is that office space and equipment are rented annually, and so their use for a 1-year period is fixed. As for physician time, assume that the physician has, by choice, decided to remain in his or her present position for at least the next production cycle and will work 40 hours per week. Physician time is, therefore, a fixed factor in this instance.

Whether or not a factor is fixed depends on the time period under consideration. If the time period involved multiple production cycles, then office space, equipment, and even physician time might vary. The variable factor of production in this illustration is nursing time. This input can be purchased in varying quantities by the physician during the production cycle. It will be assumed that one or more nurses perform all tasks during the cycle that the physician does not.

The production process consists of three types of tasks performed using the available nursing and physician resources. The first is the administrative tasks of setting appointments, keeping records, moving patients through the office, and billing patients. The second type is technical tasks, such as the testing of blood with the rented equipment. These two tasks are performed by the nurses in this illustration. Finally, there is the examination itself, which is performed by the physician. For simplicity's sake, assume no patient can be processed without the involvement of a nurse, so at least one nurse must be employed. Generally, of course, the physician is able to process some patients with no help, but assume this is not the case. Also assume that, within the current ranges of resource use considered, the physician can treat all patients who ask for an appointment; his or her time limitations do not create a "capacity" or shortage problem.

Now, attention in this illustration turns to determining the number of patients who can be treated at different levels of the variable input. The specification of this production relationship will be made under the condition that whatever the level of the variable input used in conjunction with the fixed inputs, the maximum number of patients possible is being served. This condition, discussed further at the end of this section, will hold only if the human resources (nurses) have incentives to produce as much as possible. Under this condition, a production function that expresses how output will vary when inputs are changed in quantity can be specified. In specifying this function, use L to refer to the nurses' labor input, which is measured by hours worked. All other factors, which in this illustration are fixed, will be called F for fixed. Output, called Q, is measured by patient visits (each visit is assumed to be identical in nature). The production function can be written $Q = Q (L, F)$, which means that Q depends on, or is a function of, L and F.

The production function is a summary of what goes into the process—the inputs—and what comes out—the output. With F fixed, only L can vary. By varying L, we are in fact specifying different combinations of L and F. With few nursing hours, a single nurse will perform all the nonexamination tasks and consequently cannot afford to specialize. Few patients will thus be treated. In **Table 5-1**, this is presented by showing only one patient treated as a result of the first 8 hours of nursing input. When more patients are treated, the single nurse can begin to perform some tasks for several patients together. This concentration of tasks allows additional output to be produced with fewer additional resources. Indeed, in this illustration, only seven additional nursing hours are required to process a second patient.

The additional production yielded by the use of one extra unit of the variable input is called the *marginal product*. It can be calculated by dividing the change in quantity produced (Q) by the change in the variable inputs (in this case labor or L) and can be expressed symbolically as $\Delta Q/\Delta L$. As can be seen in Table 5-1, at the lowest level of output (one visit), an extra nursing hour adds one-eighth of a visit to the level of output. At a level of two visits, the additional output of an extra nursing hour is one-seventh of a visit. This fraction represents the marginal product. This tendency toward an increasing marginal product, created initially by the productivity gains that the concentration of tasks allows, is reinforced by productivity gains from the specialization of tasks as output continues to grow. As more patients are processed and more nursing hours and more nurses are used, some tasks can be divided among the nurses, resulting in productivity gains from specialization.

But such gains cannot be reaped forever. Eventually, a large number of routine activities will lead to boredom. It also becomes increasingly difficult to manage the activities being performed by nurses as the size of the operation increases. In addition, the fixed amount of equipment in the office becomes heavily taxed and nurses have to wait to perform lab tests. This changes the relationship between additional inputs and additional output; to produce successively

Table 5-1 Relations Between Cost and Output

(1) Total Nursing Hours (L)	(2) Total Visits (Q)	(3) Marginal Product (ΔQ/ΔL)	(4) Total Fixed Cost (TFC) ($)	(5) Total Variable Cost (TVC) ($)	(6) Total Cost (TC = TFC + TVC) ($)	(7) Average Fixed Cost (AFC = TFC/Q) ($)	(8) Average Variable Costs (AVC = TVC/Q) ($)	(9) Average Total Cost (ATC = TC/Q) ($)	(10) Marginal Cost MC = (ΔTC/ΔQ) ($)
8	1	1/8	1,000.00	160.00	1,160.00	1,000.00	160.00	1,160.00	160.00
15	2	1/7	1,000.00	300.00	1,300.00	500.00	150.00	650.00	140.00
20	3	1/5	1,000.00	400.00	1,400.00	333.33	133.33	466.67	100.00
24	4	1/4	1,000.00	480.00	1,480.00	250.00	120.00	370.00	80.00
30	5	1/6	1,000.00	600.00	1,600.00	200.00	120.00	320.00	120.00
38	6	1/8	1,000.00	760.00	1,760.00	166.67	126.67	293.33	160.00
50	7	1/12	1,000.00	1,000.00	2,000.00	142.86	142.86	285.71	240.00
64	8	1/14	1,000.00	1,280.00	2,280.00	125.00	160.00	285.00	280.00
100	9	1/36	1,000.00	2,000.00	3,000.00	111.11	222.22	333.33	720.00
140	10	1/40	1,000.00	2,800.00	3,800.00	100.00	280.00	380.00	800.00

more units of output at these higher levels requires increasingly larger doses of nursing hours. Putting the argument in terms of marginal productivity, at higher levels of output, the marginal productivity of nurses' efforts begins to decline; this property is referred to as *diminishing marginal product.* Thus, in our illustration, at a level of output of four visits, the marginal product of an additional nursing hour is one-fourth of a visit; at a level of output of five visits, the marginal product falls to one-sixth of a visit; and for six visits, the marginal product is lower still, at one-eighth of a visit. Production has reached the stage of diminishing marginal productivity. It should be noted, however, that total output is constantly rising; the assumed relation in our production function stipulates that additional increases in output are harder and harder to come by as the size of output rises.

In viewing **Figures 5-1** and **5-2**, notice that these two curves reflect opposite sides of the same coin. That is, the production function gets flatter as total production (output) increases; also notice that the total cost curve gets steeper as the total production (output) increases. These two changes in the slopes of the curve occur for the same reason: diminishing marginal productivity, reflected in column 3 in Table 5-1.

The numbers used in this illustration were created to illustrate the principle being hypothesized: that marginal productivity eventually diminishes as output increases. Other equally illuminating illustrations could have been chosen to explain this principle.

5.2.2 Shifts in the Relationship

We have now defined a production function and specified, in general terms, the most important property such a function is expected to possess: the marginal product will eventually decline as more units of a variable input are added. This relationship was specified on the basis of restrictive underlying conditions. An examination can now be made of how the productive relationship will be affected by changes in these underlying conditions. These changes will be examined using the basic production (input–output) relationship specified in Table 5-1 as a point of reference.

A change in any of these underlying conditions either increases or decreases the amount of output obtained from given amounts of input. Either result will be regarded as a shift in the production relationship. An upward shift means that at each level of input, more output can be produced; a downward shift means that less output can be produced. Looking at an upward shift in marginal terms, at any level of input more additional output can be produced with an additional unit of the variable input. Expressed in output terms, at any level of output, less additional input is required to produce one extra unit of output.

Stating the same thing in marginal terms, we would say that the marginal product is greater at any level of output. Thus, at a level of output of eight visits, the original production relationship was such that an extra nursing hour employed led to an increase in

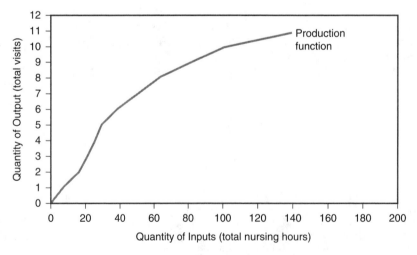

Figure 5-1 Production function. The production function illustrates the relationship between the number of nursing hours employed and the amount of total output produced in terms of the number of physician visits provided. The horizontal axis reflects the input *L* (nursing hours) in the first column of Table 5-1; the vertical axis reflects the output *Q* (total visits) in the second column of Table 5-1. Because of diminishing marginal product, the production function gets flatter as the number of nursing hours increases.

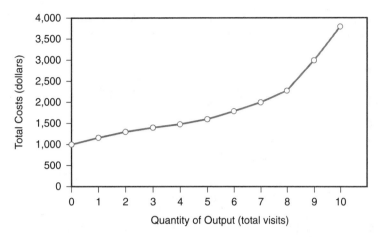

Figure 5-2 Total cost curve. The total cost curve illustrates the relationship between the quantity of output produced (*Q*) and the total costs of production. The horizontal axis reflects the number of physician visits produced (*Q*) in column 2 of Table 5-1; the vertical axis reflects the total costs (*TC* equals *TFC* + *TVC*) in column 6 of Table 5-1. As the quantity of output increases, the total cost curve gets steeper, reflecting the diminishing marginal product of the input.

© Jones & Bartlett Learning.

output of one-fourteenth of a visit. With an upward shift in the production function, an extra nursing hour might now produce one-tenth of a visit. Of course, the assumption that marginal productivity is diminishing still holds, but the entire relationship is such that now more can be obtained at any level of output.

Now, how changes in some of the underlying conditions affect the production relationship will be examined. The possible changes include a change in the case mix of patients seen by the physician and in the severity of illness of patients, in the quality of care provided to the patients, in the technology employed in the provision of care, in the amount of capital available that the physician uses, and in the underlying incentive structure that the physician faces in the provision of patient care.

First, a change in the case mix (type and/or severity of patients seen) would occur, for example, if the physician was confronted with a number of rheumatic fever cases in addition to patients presenting with common colds. More resources would need to be expended on each of these new type of cases, shifting the production relationship downward. The same type of downward shift would occur if the physician merely had to treat some patients with especially severe colds. These cases would require more resources and would thus shift the production relationship downward.

Second, the result of a change in the quality of care will depend on the precise meaning attached to *quality*. If greater thoroughness in performing an examination is an aspect of higher quality care, then the effect of providing higher quality care is to shift the production relationship downward,

because more resources would be required for each examination. Similarly, if more extensive patient education is an aspect of higher quality care, then the production relationship will again be pushed downward.

Third, high quality is frequently associated with high technology; in other words, highly trained specialists and sophisticated equipment. Offering the benefits of advances in technology thus usually entails an increase in capital, both human and physical. More input is required to produce a single unit of output (measured as a visit), and therefore the measured relationship between input and output will shift downward. However, note that more resource-intensive visits are qualitatively different than less resource-intensive ones. We cannot say that medical resources are less productive in any of these instances. Instead, a given amount of resources will produce a lower quantity of care, but this medical care is likely to be of a higher quality.

Of course, sometimes the introduction of a new piece of equipment can increase the quantity of output without changing the quality. As an example, if a computerized blood counter replaces a manually operated counter, more tests of the same quality can be processed with the same amount of variable input (technician time). The production relationship shifts upward in this case.

A final factor influencing the production relationship is the "management" incentive system. Our production relationship was derived using the assumption that the maximum output would be obtained at any given level of resource use. Incentives enter the picture when we consider the benefits that accrue to management (the physician, in our illustration) as a result of the way resources are used. If management is rewarded for keeping production costs low, then management will have an incentive to use as few resources as possible per unit of output. However, incentives can be structured in such a way as to encourage the use of more inputs. If, for example, the management receives a fixed rate of compensation that is positively related to its costs of production, then management will have an incentive to use more resources to perform each task. An example of this was the cost-based reimbursement system originally used to pay hospitals for services provided to patients. Even though the analysis of production lies in the realm of production management and medicine, the production relation cannot be analyzed in total isolation from the economic incentives that exist within the organization.

5.2.3 Substitution Among Inputs

The analysis of the previous section was based on the assumption that one variable input existed. In fact, there may be several variable inputs, and they may be substitutable for each other, at least to some degree. Let us suppose that there are two variable inputs, nursing time (N) and medical assistant time (A), in addition to the fixed inputs (F). The production function is now expressed as $Q = Q(N, A, F)$, where the output Q is a function of the variables N and A and the fixed inputs F.

Substitutability among inputs is often analyzed by assuming the level of output (Q) is held constant and then examining, for example, how much medical assistant time must be added to the process to offset a decrease in a unit of nursing time. This is called the *marginal rate of substitution* of medical assistants for nurses.

A number of areas have been identified in health care in which substitution makes sense. One study examined the use of paraprofessional surgical assistants as substitutes for physicians or surgeons in the role of assistant to the operating surgeon. The study found that trained assistants could replace physicians in this assisting role with no adverse effects on the operating surgeon's time, particularly in less complex operations (Lewit, Bentkover, Bentkover, Watkins, & Hughes, 1980). Increasingly, computer-assisted procedures are being substituted for physician-only procedures. One study (Iampreechakul, Chongchokdee, & Tirakotai, 2011) found that such substitution could decrease overall surgery time without decreasing accuracy. Another study by Patel, Youssef,

Vale, and Padhya (2011) found that the use of computer-guided endoscopic transsphenoidal surgery increased the procedure time available without additional personnel.

Another example of the substitutability of inputs is the use of drugs in the care of mental patients. To some extent, increased utilization of drugs reduces the amount of effort required of psychiatric hospital attendants. Also, physician assistants and nurse practitioners can perform many of the tasks that physicians traditionally perform (Kleinpell, Ely, & Grabenkort, 2008; Leski, Young, & Higham, 2010; Reinhardt, 1972), and dental technicians can perform simple tasks, such as cleaning teeth and doing easy repairs (Yee, Crawford, & Harber, 2005). Addesso, Nimmer, Visotcky, Fraser, and Brousseau (2019) found that the use of medical scribes increased efficiency in the emergency department of hospitals without decreasing patient satisfaction. A study involving eye care productivity found a significant positive correlation between the use of ophthalmology technicians and ophthalmologists' productivity in the Veterans Affairs Healthcare System (Lynch, Maa, Delaune, Chasan, & Cockerham, 2017).

Frequently, substitution is feasible and even economical, but barriers exist to limit it. For example, licensing laws may limit the degree to which nurse practitioners can substitute for physicians. In such cases, one must separate what is feasible from what is legally or institutionally permitted.

5.2.4 Volume–Outcome Relationship

The production function has been specified as a relationship between the volume of services provided and the quantity of inputs. As noted, there is also a relationship between the quality and volume of healthcare services. This relationship has often been demonstrated for specific surgical procedures.

Tsao et al. (2011) found that there were significantly higher quality and lower costs in high-volume kidney transplant hospitals in Taiwan than in low-volume hospitals. In a review of the literature, the authors Halm, Lee, and Chassin (2002) found that there was, in general, a positive association between higher volumes and better outcomes; however, the magnitude of the relationship varied widely among the studies, as did the methodological quality of the studies. Begg, Cramer, Hoskins, and Brennan (1998) found a significant association between volume and short-term outcomes in cancer care, which has been supported in more recent studies (Birkmeyer, Sun,

Wong, & Stukel, 2007; Joudi & Konety, 2005; Ward et al., 2004). Drews, Cooper, Onwuka, Minneci, and Aldrink (2019) found that morbidity following pediatric thyroidectomy was associated with surgery volume.

In discussing the relationship between volume and outcome, the focus can be on the volume of services that are provided by individual providers (surgeons or surgical teams) or the service volume of a healthcare organization (Garnick, Luft, McPhee, & Mark, 1989; Roukos, 2009; Tsao et al., 2011). Surgeons individually or as part of a team, can maintain their skills better when they perform more of the same types of procedures during a specified time period. If they do only a few operations of a given type within a given time frame, they may get out of practice, their team may lose its cohesiveness and skills, and the quality of their work may deteriorate. We would therefore expect a positive relationship between the volume of a given procedure for a given practitioner or team and outcomes of the care provided. Salemi et al. (2019) found patients undergoing a transfemoral transcatheter aortic valve replacement (TAVR) performed by a high-volume physician had significantly lower risks of death, stroke, or acute myocardial infarction.

A positive relationship between volume and outcome may also hold for an institution, but for different reasons. An institution with an especially large volume of certain procedures may hire specialized personnel and acquire specialized equipment. For example, in the area of rehabilitation, an institution with specialized personnel and equipment can return patients to normal functioning sooner. Thus, the relationship between volume and outcome can work separately for the surgical (or treatment) team and for the institution where the treatment occurs.

There is a confounding factor that can make it difficult to interpret an observed relationship between outcome and volume. If a surgical team is known to be more skilled, then the team will be sought out by patients. There could then be observed a positive relationship between outcomes and volume, but the high volume may not be the cause of the team's maintenance of its skills. Thus, a policy that encourages larger volumes for surgical teams regardless of their skill levels may not be successful in improving the overall levels of outcome. A further confounding factor may be that an especially skilled surgical team may attract the most difficult cases, which would tend to worsen outcomes irrespective of provider skills. In evaluating the outcomes of the providers and/or institutions, it is important to consider the case mix and severity of the patient population. Determining the causes of the observed relationship is important for policy reasons, although it may be difficult, in practice, to uncover the real causes.

5.3 Short-Run Cost–Output Relations

5.3.1 Production and Cost

Previously, the focus was on the relationship between output and alternative combinations of inputs. In specifying the production relation, the inputs were presented as separate entities that work together. The next step in our analysis is to present a measure of the overall commitment of resources by the provider in producing the output. One such measure, which places all inputs on a single scale measured in money terms, is cost. To a provider, cost means the value of inputs used in the production process. However, this value may not always be well approximated by money outlays.

Therefore, a broader view of cost—one that measures what the provider gives up by using all the resources committed to production, not just the ones paid for—is used in this section. Of central importance is the concept of opportunity cost, which is defined as the value that the provider gave up by not committing the resources to the next highest valued use. Another way of putting it is that the cost of resources is measured by the amount for which those resources could be sold in the market, or the market value of the resources used in the production process. This concept is particularly important when measuring the value of resources that are not paid to others (e.g., resources that the producer owns) and hence that appear to be free. If the owner of these unpaid resources is giving up some return on them, then there is a cost associated with them, and this cost must be estimated by calculating the probable market value of the resources. These resources are often considered to be implicit costs because they don't require an outlay of money.

Because we are concerned with the functioning of an organization, the cost of resource use will be considered from the organization's point of view. Any organization can undertake a resource commitment that does not appear in its paid-out costs. Nevertheless, if the organization commits its resources to a particular use, they are part of the organization's costs and should be counted as such. On the other hand, an economic unit outside the organization may make a resource commitment that allows the organization to function. For example, a person may give blood to a blood donor clinic, a benefactor may endow a hospital with an operating room, or a physician may volunteer teaching time at a medical school. In these instances, resources are used to undertake activities, but they are not part of the resource commitment of the institution. Rather, they are part of the total resource commitment required to undertake the activity. In this chapter, the concern is with the operations of healthcare organizations and so the focus is on the resource commitment made by these organizations in their activities. This leaves out the question of the total (or social) resource commitment made to perform any activity, including the commitment of donors, volunteers, benefactors, and government agencies.

In the analysis that follows, the definitions presented are placed in a time frame of 1 month, or a single production cycle. Given this time frame, the production costs can be separated into fixed costs and variable costs. Fixed costs are defined as those that do not change, or vary, with output within the relevant time frame of the production cycle. Variable costs, on the other hand, increase as output increases; they vary with output in the production cycle.

In the earlier physician's practice illustration, the fixed costs were those that did not vary during the month; they were the costs of the fixed factors, including space and equipment rental costs and the cost of physician time. Now, assume the space and equipment rental values to be $500 during the period. Also assume that the physician could have earned $500 working as an employee in a clinic rather than working in the private practice; this amount of $500 measures the *opportunity cost* the physician faced when making the decision whether to continue to practice privately. Given that the decision to practice privately has been made, the forgoing of other ways of using work time becomes a "sunk" cost, relevant more to the past than to the present. A *sunk cost* is one that has already been committed and cannot be recovered in the present (or even the future) time. Nevertheless, it is still a cost, and is classified as a fixed cost.

The total fixed costs thus, in this illustration, equal $1000. (The cost curve of a company incorporates the return that the owners could normally get on their assets, including their time, the buildings they own, and so on. This normal return is called *normal profit*, which is associated with the risk taken, not a specific percentage. Any return above normal profit is called *economic profit* and is typically viewed as excessive and not sustainable in the long run.)

Variable costs are costs of inputs that change as the firm alters the quantity of output produced during the production cycle. In our illustration, the only variable input is nursing hours. For illustrative purposes only, assume that the price of nursing services is $20 per hour. Thus, 8 hours of services cost $160. The relationship between the cost to the provider and the level of output can now be specified. This relationship depends on the quantities of resources used (determined by the production relationship) and the money paid for, or the opportunity cost imputed to, these resource services.

The relationship can be viewed in three different ways. *First*, costs can be examined from the point of view of the total resource commitment required to maintain production at any specific level of output. In this case, determination is made on how total costs vary with output. *Second*, the average value of resource commitment, that is, the total cost of the resource commitment required to produce the total output, or total costs divided by total output, can be determined. The value of this average resource commitment is called *average cost*. The *third* way of viewing costs is to examine the value of additional resources that must be committed to the production process to produce an additional unit of output. This value is called the *marginal cost*. The following sections discuss how each of these alternative measures varies as the level of output changes.

5.3.2 Total Cost

Total cost (*TC*) is the sum of all costs incurred in producing a given level of output; total variable cost (*TVC*) is the total cost of variable inputs for any level of output; total fixed cost (*TFC*) is the total cost of all fixed factors. Total cost is the sum of the total variable cost and the total fixed cost. Now, look at these types of cost with regard to the data contained in Table 5-1. The total fixed cost is $1000 whatever the level of output. Therefore, this cost, plotted on the graph in **Figure 5-3**, is represented by a straight horizontal line (*TFC*) at the $1000 level.

The behavior of the total variable cost depends on two factors: the relationship between output and variable inputs, specified in Section 5.2; and the unit cost of these variable resources. Figure 5-3 contains a total variable cost curve that reflects the data in our illustration.

The total cost curve (*TC*) is the vertical sum of the two curves *TVC* and *TFC* at each output level (see Table 5-1, column 6). The level of the *TC* curve is determined, in part, by the fixed cost; its shape is determined by the production function and the

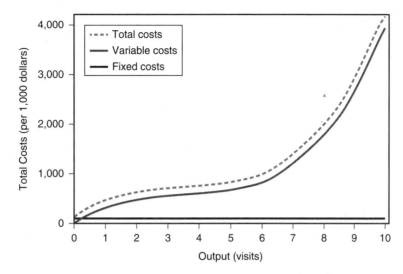

Figure 5-3 Relationship between total fixed costs, total variable costs, total costs, and level of output. At each production level, total costs can be divided between the fixed and variable costs. The fixed costs do not vary with output. This graph is based on data in Table 5-1.

© Jones & Bartlett Learning.

variation of output with variable inputs. Given the fixed per-unit price of the variable input ($20 an hour), the production function relation, translated into a cost–output relation, entails that the addition to total costs of the extra resource commitment levels off as output increases. Thus, the total variable cost is $160 at a scale of one visit, $300 at a scale of two visits, $400 at a scale of three visits, and $480 at a scale of four visits. This leveling off of cost is shown diagrammatically by the flattening of the section between 0 and 4 of curve *TVC* in Figure 5-3.

If additional resources had been increasingly more productive beyond this scale of input, the *TVC* curve would have continued leveling off. But beyond four units of output, diminishing marginal productivity begins to set in; and in terms of costs, this means that successively greater resource commitments are needed to attain successively higher levels of output. In Table 5-1, the total variable cost rises to $600, $760, $1000, $1280, $2000, and so on, and the total cost also rises rapidly. As seen on the curve, beyond a scale of 4, *TVC* is curving upward; at the extreme, it would become almost vertical. Thus, a considerable commitment in resources is required to move to a higher output level. The shape of *TC* is similar to that of *TVC*, except that *TC* is higher by $1000.

5.3.3 Marginal Cost

Implicit in the total variable cost–output relationship is the marginal cost–output relation. The marginal cost at any level of output is the additional cost required to move one unit higher on the output scale. It is thus

defined as the change in total costs divided by the change in the quantity of output $\Delta TC/\Delta Q$. Because *TFC* is constant over all levels of output, the marginal fixed cost would be zero at any value, because the additional fixed resource commitment is zero at all levels of output. Thus, the marginal cost is simply the addition to total variable cost needed to produce one extra unit of output. In Table 5-1, the marginal cost (*MC*) is shown in column 10. As can be seen, the extra cost of moving to one unit of output from zero is $160, to two units from one is $140, and so on. Until we reach four units of output, *MC* is falling.

However, because of the diminishing marginal productivity of variable inputs, coupled with the fact that the additional variable inputs used are all paid the same wage in this illustration, producing additional units of output eventually requires successively greater resource commitment. This is reflected in rising marginal cost after the fourth visit; the fifth visit costs $120 extra; the sixth, $160 extra; and so on. The marginal cost curve is shown in **Figure 5-4**. Note that beyond an output of 4, marginal costs cease falling and begin to rise in this illustration.

The concept of marginal cost is central to the analysis of most economic decisions. For the most part, the types of decisions that concern economists involve determining the consequences of employing additional (or fewer) resources for a particular purpose. For example, the concern might be with the implications of placing additional surgical services in either Boston or Boise, so the analysis might include determining the consequences of adding one or more paramedics to an existing medical practice in these two locations, or we

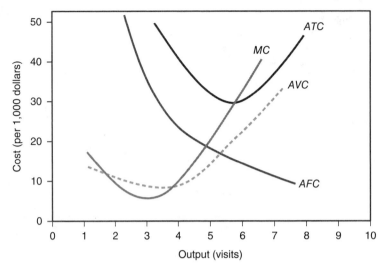

Figure 5-4 Relationship between costs and output. The average total cost is shown in total *ATC* and is separated into the two components of average fixed cost (*AFC*) and average variable costs (*AVC*). Marginal cost (*MC*) is the addition to total cost of the next unit produced. There is a unique relationship between *MC* and both *AVC* and *ATC*; when *MC* is above *ATC* (or *AVC*), the average cost is falling; when *MC* is greater than *ATC* (or *AVC*), the average cost is increasing; and when *MC* equals *ATC* (or *AVC*), the average cost is constant; that is, it has reached a minimum point.

might be interested in the consequences of decreasing the number of obstetric beds in a particular region of the country or a particular hospital. In these instances, as in most other cases of resource allocation, the allocation decision concerns whether to expand a particular facility or service or increase the available quantity of trained personnel. The concept used to measure the added resource commitment is the marginal cost.

5.3.4 Average Cost

The third way of looking at costs is to average the costs required to obtain a given level of output. The average total cost (*ATC*) is the total cost per unit of output and is defined for any level of output. It equals the total cost (*TC*) divided by the quantity of output (*Q*), or *TC/Q*. It measures the value of the average resource commitment required to sustain a given scale of output. However, because it is useful in making comparisons, this variable has been frequently used in empirical studies.

The behavior of the average total cost depends on the behavior of the average fixed cost (*TFC/Q*) and the average variable cost (*TVC/Q*). The average fixed cost is lower at successively higher levels of output in our illustration because the $1000 in fixed cost is spread out over more and more output. Thus, at one visit, the average fixed cost is $1000; at two visits, it is $500; and so on. The average variable cost initially falls at successively greater levels of output. At one unit of output, it is $160; at two, it is $150; at three, it is $133; and so on. The fall in average variable cost is

made possible by the increasing productivity of additional variable inputs at low output levels.

Another way of viewing this relationship is to consider that the marginal cost is initially below the average cost, which brings down the average cost as output increases. The marginal cost for the first visit is $160, and the average variable cost is $160. For the second visit, the marginal cost is $140. This brings down the average variable cost of the two visits to $150 (i.e., $300/2). The falling average variable and the average fixed cost, together, ensure that the average total cost (which is the sum of the two) will also fall as output expands. Eventually, after four visits, the marginal cost increases as output expands. Expanding output from four to five visits costs an extra $120, expanding to six visits costs another $160, and the marginal cost at seven is $240. However, as long as the marginal cost is lower than the average total cost, a further expansion of output will continue to reduce the average total cost.

For example, in Table 5-1 we can see that at five units of output, the total cost is $1600 and the average total cost is $320. An expansion of output by one unit to a level of output of six units would cost an additional $160. The *ATC* at six units of output decreases to $293.33 because the *MC* of the sixth unit of output is lower than the *ATC*, and so expanding output brings down the average. With a rising *MC*, this situation will not continue indefinitely. At some level of output, the *MC* will just equal the *ATC*, and at a still higher level, it will exceed it. The *ATC* must then begin to rise. In our illustration, the level at which the *MC* equals the

ATC is eight visits. As seen in Table 5-1, an expansion from seven to eight visits will cost an extra $280. With an *ATC* of $285.70 at the level of seven visits, expansion to eight visits leaves the *ATC* at about the same level. An expansion to nine visits has an *MC* of $720. This is above the *ATC* at eight visits. The *ATC* increases to $333.33 at nine visits.

The average cost curves are shown in Figure 5-4 in juxtaposition to the *MC* curve. These curves are based on the data presented in Table 5-1, but have been smoothed for convenience. The average fixed cost (*AFC*) curve declines over all levels of output. The average variable cost (*AVC*) curve declines until four visits. At five visits, the *MC* just equals the *AVC*, and so the *AVC* curve bottoms out. For output levels higher than five, the *MC* is above the *AVC*, and so the *AVC* increases with expansion of output. The *AVC* curve is thus U-shaped, indicating that at lower levels of output the *AVC* falls as output expands. The *AVC* curve then bottoms (where *MC = AVC*) and begins to rise. The *ATC* curve (remember, *ATC = AVC + AFC*) is also U-shaped. It is located above and slightly to the right of the *AVC* curve and also bottoms out where the rising *MC* cuts it.

The *ATC*, as already noted, has a fixed and a variable component. The relative sizes of these two components will determine at which level of output the *ATC* curve will begin to slope upward. The average fixed cost component (*AFC*) always falls as output increases, because the same fixed costs are spread over a greater output. The variable cost component (*AVC*) follows the rules of productivity and begins to rise, because eventually higher marginal costs will raise the average. The larger the fixed cost component, the greater the range over which the average total cost will fall. Hospitals have been identified as having large fixed cost components. If this is indeed true, then hospitals should experience a diminishing average total cost over a wide range of potential output levels.

The fixed cost component is related to the use of capital equipment. A heavy investment in capital equipment will create a large fixed cost. However, such equipment may permit additional procedures to be undertaken with a small additional commitment of resources up to high levels of output. In such a situation, although the fixed cost would be high, the marginal cost would be low, and the average total cost would fall over a wide range of output levels. In a related phenomenon, called *indivisibility*, expensive equipment, available in a large dose, cannot be divided into smaller units. It is operated at low levels of output at a high *ATC* and operated at high levels at a low *ATC*.

This section has identified three related cost–output measures: total cost, average cost, and marginal cost. Their shapes are dependent largely on the production relationship. As shown in Section 5.2, the production relation is subject to shifts caused by a variety of conditions. These same conditions can cause a cost curve to change its positions, as discussed next.

5.4 Cost Curve Position

The position of a cost curve is determined by the same factors that influence the production relationship. These factors in health care include the case mix and the severity of cases treated, the quality of care provided, the technology used, the volume of fixed factors employed in the production process, and the incentive system under which the provider is operating. In addition, change in input prices can affect the position of the cost curve. In the following discussion, each factor will be considered separately.

Given fixed inputs and fixed costs, a change in the case mix toward more complicated cases and an increase in the average severity level will increase the variable resources required per unit of output and will thus increase marginal and average costs at all output levels. The positions of both the *ATC* and *MC* curves will now be higher. The shifts in position are shown in **Figure 5-5**. Here, ATC_1 and MC_1 are the average total cost and marginal cost relationships before the change to a more complex case mix. This change in case mix results in a shift to ATC_2 and MC_2.

An increase in quality, if this entails more thorough examinations or treatments, will similarly shift the cost curves upward. The adoption of a technology that uses more resources per case will have a similar effect. Many recent technological innovations have been associated with a large capital investment for equipment as well as a larger flow of variable expenditures for the services of the highly trained personnel needed to operate this equipment. Examples of such technological innovations include open-heart surgery, a procedure that intrigued economists in the 1960s; coronary care units (CCUs) or intensive care units (ICUs), which are high-cost monitoring and life support units; computed tomography (CT) scanning; magnetic resonance imaging (MRI), a revolutionary and somewhat costly advance in radiology; and laparoscopic surgery, which allows a surgeon to perform an operation through a small incision. All these examples require a heavy investment in equipment, and the effect of introducing any of them would be to shift both the fixed and variable components of the *ATC* upward, thus increasing the *ATC* for all levels of output. However, it should be

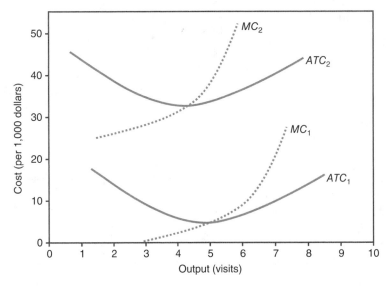

Figure 5-5 Shift in average and marginal cost curves. Curves ATC_1 and MC_1 indicate the initial relationship between costs and output. Curves ATC_2 and MC_2 represent the upward shift in costs at each level of output.
© Jones & Bartlett Learning.

remembered that an increase in the quality of services provided may accompany the introduction of new technology. One physician visit or one hospital stay is not always the same as another.

All technological innovations in medical care are not of this resource-using type, however. Innovations in pharmaceuticals have reduced the length of hospitalization required for some illnesses. Two notable examples are tuberculosis treatment and mental illness treatment. Furthermore, new laboratory equipment has allowed many tasks to be automated. This has led to falling average costs over broad ranges of output because of the low variable costs associated with the use of this equipment. Surgical interventions have also changed, with many surgical procedures becoming less invasive, thereby requiring fewer days in the hospital to recuperate and therefore leading to decreasing average costs.

The effect of incentives that encourage resource use is to raise the level of average cost associated with any single level of output. Assuming that a single least-cost position is associated with each output level, a least-cost average cost curve can be identified. Incentives to use resources will encourage the provider to choose a position above this curve. It has been questioned whether a cost curve that measures the cost–output relationship when given resources are not used to maximize output (i.e., a more-than-least-cost curve) is a meaningful concept. This is because more than one such average cost point may exist at any output level. There can be only one least-cost point, however, and in the least-cost case, a cost curve that supposedly represents a unique relation between cost and output can be uniquely determined. Once a provider chooses to use more than the least amount of resources to achieve

a given output level (with no change in quality), he or she can use these excessive resources to varying degrees. There is no longer a unique cost curve (Zuckerman, Hadley, & Iezzoni, 1994).

Another factor that might cause cost curves to shift is the price the provider pays for hired resources. In our illustration, if the physician had to pay $30 per nursing hour instead of $20, both the marginal and the average cost curves would shift upward. Conversely, if the price fell to $10, the curves would shift downward.

A final factor that can influence the position of the average cost curves appears when two or more types of variable inputs exist. When these inputs can be substituted for each other, at least to some degree, then a substitution of a less costly for a more costly input can lower the cost curves, although other factors may push them the other way. For example, if a paramedic is substituted for a physician but takes much longer to do the same task, the total or average cost may not shift downward as a result of the substitution. Also, keep in mind that the quality of the product may become lower (or higher) as a result of the substitution, and even though the output may cost less to produce, it might not be exactly comparable.

5.5 Economies of Scope

This discussion of costs has been presented as if a healthcare institution or provider had a single type of output. Although this assumption helps to clarify certain relationships between costs and output, it generally doesn't apply in the case of larger institutions, notably hospitals. Hospitals are multiproduct firms that offer a large number of separate product lines, such as clinical laboratory services, emergency department services, physical therapy, and intensive care (Berry, 1973; Goldfarb, Hornbrook, & Rafferty, 1980).

The product line dimension of output should be distinguished from the case-mix dimension. Case mix refers to the complexity of the types of diseases being treated. A hospital that treats a large number of different diseases has a different case mix than one that specializes in a few. If, as is sometimes done, severity is included as a dimension of case mix, then case-mix indexes can be developed (Hornbrook & Monheit, 1985). Each hospital also has a number of services or product lines. In fact, two hospitals can have very similar case-mix measures but very different service scopes. As a consequence, the relation between cost and scope offers itself as a possibly fruitful topic of investigation.

Economies of scope are savings derived from producing different products (output) jointly/simultaneously in the same production unit rather than producing them individually in separate production units. Let X_1 stand for one output (e.g., family planning services) and X_2 stand for a second output (e.g., pediatric services). Let $C(X_1)$ stand for the total cost of producing X_1, let $C(X_2)$ stand for the total cost of producing X_2 in a separate setting, and $C(X_1, X_2)$ stand for the cost of jointly producing X_1 and X_2 in the same production unit. Economies of scope arise when the cost of jointly producing specific quantities of the two services [$C(X_1, X_2)$] is less than the sum of the costs of producing each service separately [$C(X_1) + C(X_2)$]. In our example, economies of scope would exist if a clinic could jointly produce given quantities of family planning services and pediatric services more cheaply than the same quantities produced in sharply separated units or departments.

Economies of scope might arise when some of the tasks involved in providing two distinct services are complementary. For example, if family planning and pediatric services require a common core of testing capabilities, then providing the two types of services in separate units would cause duplication. Savings could be achieved by combining the two services into a single unit that caters to both groups of patients. Of course, it is also possible to have diseconomies of scope. This would occur when two types of output are best produced in separate units. For example, if psychiatric patients are treated with one regimen and home health service patients with a different one, combining the psychiatric and home health services in a single unit may be more costly than keeping them separate.

In one study of the economies of scope in health care, Cowing and Holtmann (1983) estimated economies of scale and scope for 138 short-term hospitals in New York State. They divided hospital output into five diagnostic categories (actually representing different case mixes rather than service scopes): medical-surgical, maternity, pediatric, other inpatient care, and emergency department care. For four of the services (pediatric care being the exception), marginal cost fell over low ranges of output and then became constant. These results indicate substantial economies of scale in these services and suggest that merging services produced on a small scale into larger units could yield considerable savings. However, with regard to the existence of economies of scope, the findings were generally negative. These findings, if they hold up in repeated trials, indicate that, on cost grounds alone, hospitals should specialize rather than become multiproduct organizations. One must be careful not to overgeneralize, because, even though economies of scope may not be widespread, specific services may have production conditions that, when combined, yield economies of scope.

Gonzales (1997) applied the economies of scope theory to the home health industry in Connecticut. In the study, costs initially decrease as the scope of services provided increases. However, as the scope of services continued to rise, the costs of providing the services increase even more, demonstrating diseconomies of scope. The provision of services under diseconomies of scope reflects the services being provided beyond the point at which they could be produced cost-effectively. Dunn, Sacher, Cohen, and Hsiao (1995) found that there were significant economies of scope in the provision of multiple surgeries. In Germany, McRae, Bruno, and Bard (2019) found considerable impact if similar services could be consolidated among different departments.

5.6 Long-Run Cost Curves

In deriving the cost curves in Section 5.4, the assumption was made that some of the inputs were fixed. Suppose a longer perspective is taken and enough time is allowed for the producing unit to change its "fixed" factors—to expand or contract its physical plant, to buy and sell equipment, and to hire and fire physicians. For planning periods of sufficient length, such changes are certainly possible. An analysis of relevant issues is called a *long-run analysis*.

Indeed, the factors that are considered fixed from the perspective of the short term are no longer fixed;

they too can vary. From the longer planning perspective, all resources are variable. Suppose a hospital board is planning to build a new facility from scratch. The board can choose either a 60-, 120-, or 250-bed facility, entailing a capital outlay of $20 million, $30 million, or $35 million, respectively. Associated with each size is the given annual capital cost of depreciation and the interest on the financial capital. During the planning period—up until the size decision is made—these capital costs can be varied (at three different levels) and thus are variable. That is, if the time horizon is sufficiently long, all costs in the production process become variable.

Associated with each facility under consideration is an average cost curve (either ATC_1, ATC_2, or ATC_3 in **Figure 5-6**), which includes capital costs (remember that, in the long run, there are no fixed costs). Now assume that each facility is least costly for a given range of output. For fewer than 1000 annual admissions, ATC_1 is the least costly; for over 3000 admissions, ATC_3 is the least costly. Depending on which level of output is chosen, one plant size will be the least costly. The dashed curve in Figure 5-6 represents the least cost that can be used to produce at any given output level (assuming we can choose the size of the facility). This is called the *long-run average cost (LRAC)* curve. It is made up of the minimum cost points at each output level. The *LRAC* is usually hypothesized, if it were represented in a smooth fashion, to be U-shaped. Such a shape would be generated by falling long-run average costs (economies of scale) at low levels of output, followed by constant and finally increasing costs (diseconomies of scale).

Before discussing such costs, it is necessary to specify whether the entity in question is a single operating unit (e.g., an individual hospital, nursing home, or ambulatory care clinic) or an entire system (e.g., a corporate chain). A single operating entity may be subject to eventual diseconomies, because the gains from specialization in certain tasks eventually run out. Also, a single hospital unit may be able to expand only by the addition of diverse units (e.g., a CT scanning unit or a physiotherapy department), and such units may be costly to manage in a single unit. For these reasons, the long-run cost curve of the single operating unit may exhibit diseconomies of scale.

A multi-plant system, such as a multi-hospital corporation, may exhibit economies of scale as it expands by acquiring additional distinct operating units. Certain functions, such as purchasing, may be run more efficiently on a scale that exceeds that of an individual operating unit. Furthermore, a multi-unit system can develop standardized procedures in patient records, accounting, and the like, and can make comparisons among units. For these reasons, as a system expands, it may exhibit economies of scale, at least up to a point.

5.7 Empirical Estimation of Cost Curves

5.7.1 Background

Average, or per-unit, cost is a convenient and accessible summary of a producer's performance. To obtain the average cost at any level of output, divide total cost by total quantity. Given the convenience of this measure

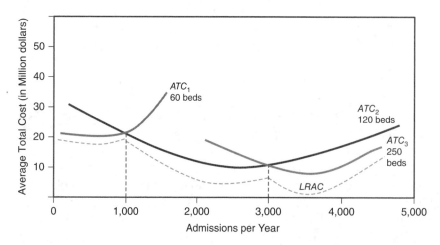

Figure 5-6 Relationship between short- and long-run average cost curves. Short-run curves (ATC_1, ATC_2, and ATC_3) are shown for three plant sizes (number of beds). The long-run average cost (*LRAC*) curve is derived from these curves (shown as a dashed line). The *LRAC* curve is the minimum cost point at each level of output. At 1000 admissions and 3000 admissions, the *LRAC* curve becomes associated with the different cost curves (different plant sizes), because it becomes more economical to produce successively greater output with larger sized plants.

of performance, it is natural that analysts would use it to compare providers who produce roughly the same product, but at different levels of output. Our simple, unqualified, short-run hypothesis would lead us to expect a U-shaped relation between average cost and output. However, inter-producer comparisons are fraught with complications.

Quality, case mix, and technology differences among producing units may make comparisons difficult. For this reason, as well as others cited in Section 5.4, producers may be operating on different cost curves, as shown in **Figure 5-7**, in which ATC_1, ATC_2, and ATC_3 are average short-run cost curves of three producers. As compared with Producer 1, Producer 2 is producing a higher quality product or serving patients with a more severe case mix, but is using the same amounts of fixed inputs. Therefore, Producer 2's cost curve (ATC_2) is above ATC_1 at all levels of output. To identify the shape of the short-run cost curve, one must control for factors that shift the curve. Assume, for example, that Producer 1's cost–output point is at x and Producer 2's is at v. Without knowing how the quality of services and other factors differed, it would not be possible to know if points x and v are on the same curve or on different curves.

In estimating long-run cost curves, even greater difficulties are encountered. Assume that Producer 3 has a more capital-intensive operation than Producers 1 or 2 because Producer 3 has invested more heavily in capital equipment to gain economies from automation. Also assume that the quality and case mix of Producer 3 are similar to those of Producer 1. The true long-run cost curve for the industry (assuming that these are the only two scales of operations available) is ATC_1 up to point t in Figure 5-7 and ATC_3 for scales of output above and beyond point t.

But when we start to estimate this curve, we do not know this. Among the data that are usually available for making such comparisons, only one observation for each producer is known. These observations tell us, for example, that Producer 1 is producing at 1000 units of output with an ATC of \$50, Producer 2 is producing at 1200 units with an ATC of \$80, and so on. (We may, of course, also have some information on some of the operating characteristics of each producer.) With this information, only one point on each producer's cost curve is known, which is not enough to tell us where on its cost curve each producer is operating.

If, for example, Producer 1 is producing at point T and Producer 3 at point Z, then both are on the long-run cost curve, and an estimation of a long-run cost curve with points such as these will give us a reasonably accurate picture of what the long-run cost curve looks like. But there is no reason why we should be so lucky. Producer 1 could well be producing at a high-capacity level, such as point Y, and Producer 3 could be at a low-capacity level, such as point S. While both are on their short-run curves, neither

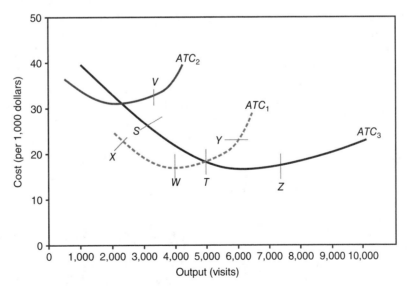

Figure 5-7 Identifying points on the average total cost curve. When data are gathered from producers on their average total cost and various output levels, care must be taken in interpreting these data points. Data points collected from different producers may be on similar *ATC* curves (such as *X*, *W*, *T*, and *Y*) or on different *ATC* curves (such as *V* and *Y*). The key to determining which is more likely is to identify extraneous circumstances (other than output) that might have caused producers to operate on different curves. These circumstances, if identified, would lead to the conclusion whether pairs such as *V* and *Y* are on different or similar curves. The circumstances that shift the cost curve (or lead to different cost curves) include differences in such things as input prices, quality of output, and capital equipment.

is on its long-run curve. There would be no way of knowing this, and if it was assumed that the estimate reflected a long-run curve, biased results would occur.

In fact, where on its cost curve each producer is producing depends on supply. It also depends on the producer's goals or objectives as well as the conditions underlying costs and revenues. Following are brief summaries of empirical evidence on producer cost curves for several health-related activities. When reviewing this material, keep in mind the difficulties in identifying actual cost–output relations.

5.7.2 Group Practices

Group medical practices have occasionally been held up as institutions that should yield considerable economies of scale and thus help raise output while moderating increases in total costs. Because a fairly large number of group practices are in operation, it might seem that the proposition that average costs are falling would be easy to test. However, because of the considerable variation in the types of group practices, difficulties in output measurements, and problems associated with gathering appropriate data, only tentative answers have been obtained.

The first statistical analysis was done using data collected on solo and group practices in the field of internal medicine (Bailey, 1968). Because the study compared practices in the same field, it circumvented problems associated with the inclusion of different production techniques used by different types of practices. The data collected showed that the average volume of services provided per physician, adjusted for the type of visit (e.g., routine visit, annual examination, or complete examination), was greater for solo practices than for group practices. Although the sample size was small, it cast some doubt on the existence of economies of scale.

There are several reasons why this finding may not be so surprising. First, the technology generally used in internal medicine is such that the gains from task specialization and the use of capital-intensive techniques may be achieved at a low level of output. For the tasks involved in operating an internal medicine practice, the *ATC* curve may reach a lower point at a scale of output supportable by one practitioner. Second, an incentive factor may be at work when several practitioners combine forces. This factor, which has a tendency to shift the *ATC* curve upward when the group is formed, is operative in situations in which members of the practice share revenues and costs. When this sharing occurs, the revenues that any single member of the group generates are shared, and the costs that he or she incurs are borne by all the members. Because

of reduced burden, the individual physician can make a heavier use of nurses' time and of equipment while feeling less impact than in a solo practice.

It is hypothesized that, under cost-sharing arrangements, each physician in the group will generate more costs than in a solo practice, pushing up the cost curve for the group. Furthermore, the larger the group, the higher will be the cost curve (assuming that offsetting factors do not exist; see Scheffler, 1975). A study that focused on physician practices found that a higher degree of specialization led to a decrease in costs, but that costs of group practices were higher than of solo practice. This finding could be explained by the indivisibility of expensive equipment—smaller practices lack the critical mass to invest in these expensive technologies (Kwietniewski, Heimeshoff, & Schreyogg, 2017).

Another study analyzed inter-practice variations in the relationship between staff salary costs and scale of output (measured by office visits) for a sample of single-specialty practices, although they were not all of the same specialty (Newhouse, 1973). The presence of cost-sharing was found to shift the cost curve upward for group practices. Furthermore, after adjusting for this incentive factor, the cost curve was found to exhibit economies of scale, indicating that such economies do exist among practices with no cost-sharing and also among practices with some cost-sharing. Because of the small sample, the inattention paid to case mix, and technology differences among practices due to specialty differences, the results are not conclusive.

Pauly (1996) investigated multispecialty group practices and found that the evidence does not suggest that such group practices will obtain economies of scope because of their diversity, but that they may be able to coordinate the process of care better. Engberg, Wholley, Feldman, and Christianson (2004) concluded that mergers among health maintenance organizations that produce Medicare and other products are likely to create diseconomies of scope that increase costs.

5.7.3 Hospital Marginal Costs

The importance of the topic of hospital marginal cost is related to the objective of reimbursing hospitals for the extra resource costs they incur when their volumes change. If a hospital is being reimbursed at the level of costs in 1995, and its admissions have increased by 5%, its additional costs may be greater than, equal to, or less than 5%. If the hospital is reimbursed an additional 5% (ignoring inflation) to cover the volume differential, and actual costs had gone up by 3%, the hospital would incur a windfall gain. On the other hand, the hospital would suffer a loss if its costs had increased by 10%.

Marginal cost variation is often measured using the ratio of marginal (*M*) to average (*A*) costs (*M/A*). Recall that if *M* is greater than *A* (or *M/A* > 1), then the average cost will increase (Section 5.3). For example, beginning from an initial output level of 1000 admissions and an average cost of $200 per case, if output expands by 5% (50 admissions) and *M* is $220, then *M/A* is 1.1. Expansion has raised the average cost, and if the hospital was reimbursed for the additional cases at $200 per case, it would incur a loss. If the hospital was reimbursed on the basis of its prior year's costs plus the marginal cost of its additional cases, it would be fully reimbursed for its costs.

This problem has arisen in a number of instances. During the early 1970s, when price controls were set on hospital revenues, allowable revenues were set at the previous year's revenue levels, plus an inflation factor, plus a volume adjustment based on estimates of *M/A* (Ozminkowski, Gaumer, Coit & Gabay, 1994). In the Finger Lakes region of New York State, a regional reimbursement experiment was set up: hospitals were reimbursed based on a base-year cost, plus an inflation factor, plus a volume adjustment that assumed that the value of *M/A* was 0.4 for inpatient care and 0.6 for outpatient care (Farnand, Jacobs, & Dickson, 1986). And currently, under Medicare regulations, hospitals are given extra reimbursement for cases in a particular diagnostic group whose length of stay or costs are outside diagnostic limits (outliers). The additional reimbursement is based on an *M/A* value of 0.6 for the extra days.

One way of estimating hospital marginal cost is to take short-term (e.g., monthly) values of operating costs and volume for a given hospital over a period (2–3 years) and find the average variation in costs with a given variation in output. Another way is to relate variation in costs and outputs across hospitals. The former method will probably give a more accurate estimate than the latter of short-run marginal cost, but there are difficulties even with it. Among these are that adjustments must be made for the cost levels of inputs (assuming they have changed) and that capital equipment and operating techniques must remain the same throughout the study period (otherwise the hospital will have moved from one short-run cost curve to another).

In addition, the marginal cost will depend on the measure of output (e.g., whether it is the length of stay or admissions). It will vary with the amount of the volume adjustment (e.g., 2% or 5%) and the relative permanence of the adjustment as estimated by the hospital administrator. For a volume increase that is small

or short-lived, the administrator may decide to tax existing resources for a time rather than immediately expand and thereby raise marginal cost. The estimate of *M* under these circumstances would appear to be lower than if the administrator responded more automatically.

For the preceding reasons, there is no accepted measure of the true short-run value of *M/A* (Lave & Lave, 1984). Estimates range from 0.2 to 0.6, but remember that the value will vary depending on a number of factors (Friedman & Pauly, 1983).

5.7.4 Hospital Economies of Scale

A large number of studies have investigated the possible existence of economies of scale in hospitals, with very mixed results (Berki, 1972; Frech & Mobley, 1995). Early studies identified economies of scale, but subsequent studies have uncovered no evidence (Lave & Lave, 1984) or conflicting evidence (Frech & Mobley, 1995). There is an explanation for the differences in findings.

As discussed earlier, the typical hospital is an organization with a complex case mix and a large number of different services. Each service has its own cost–output relation, which may exhibit economies of scale. The scope of services is greater for larger hospitals (Berry, 1973), but these hospitals may have more varied case types, so some services (e.g., cobalt therapy) that are devoted to specific case types may be operated at low capacity and high cost. A multi-product hospital can be quite large, yet have a number of services with considerable excess capacity (Finkler, 1979b). As a result, it might exhibit a higher average cost than many smaller hospitals.

One study (Hornbrook & Monheit, 1985) that incorporated both case-mix and service scope variables to investigate economies of scale found no such economies at the hospital level. But a number of studies of individual services, such as open-heart surgery facilities, CT scanner units, therapeutic radiology facilities, and hospital laundries, have found evidence of economies of scale (Finkler, 1979a; Gregory, 1976–1977; McGregor & Pelletier, 1978; Okunade, 1993; Schwartz & Joskow, 1980). This suggests that the economies of scale that do occur in some hospital departments are offset by diseconomies of scale in others.

Yatchak (2000) found that economies of scale had recently evolved for nonteaching and teaching hospitals, reflecting the pressure of market forces associated with decreased revenues. Valdmanis (2010) found that hospitals would benefit from decreasing costs by exploiting economies of scale. Burns and Lee (2006) found that hospital purchasing alliances represented an important source of economies of scale for hospitals.

A systematic research study by Giancotti, Guglielmo, and Mauro (2017) found consistent evidence of economies of scale for hospitals with 200–300 beds. They also found that diseconomies occurred in hospitals below 200 beds and in those above 600 beds.

5.7.5 Nursing Home Costs

A number of studies have been undertaken in the nursing home area with a view to determining the effect on costs of operating variables, such as volume of operations, product quality, case mix, and organizational characteristics (e.g., investor-owned or tax-exempt status and membership in a chain) (Bishop, 1980). The relevant variable for such studies is average cost, which is the most commonly available variable for a comparison of costs in different facilities. There is no agreement as to whether total costs (which include fixed costs, such as administrative costs, interest, and depreciation) or only variable costs should be used. Using just variable costs would be appropriate when focusing on short-term operations, whereas including capital and other fixed costs would be appropriate when dealing with long-term issues. For example, one might want to find out whether a large-scale plant is more efficient than a small-scale plant. Asking which is the most efficient implies that time would be allowed to develop a plant of the appropriate size.

Studies that have examined the relationship between average cost and various causal variables have uncovered some interesting relationships. There is disagreement as to the relationship between average cost and scale of operations (Bishop, 1980; McKay, 1988). The fact that a nursing home is a member of a chain does not appear to influence its costs (Ullman, 1986). On the other hand, investor-owned nursing homes have been identified as having a lower average cost than tax-exempt nursing homes (Ullman, 1984).

As with all cost studies in the healthcare area, such studies have had to deal with difficulties in measuring and netting out the impact of patient case mix and the level of quality, two factors that influence the level of care and hence nursing home costs. For example, it has proven extremely hard to identify patient characteristics associated with specific levels of care. Patients differ considerably with regard to health status, and their different needs should translate into differences in the level of care or resource intensity. Several case-mix classifications (for long-term care patients) that try to take into account resource-use differences have been developed. These measures are far from perfect, but even allowing for their shortcomings, their inclusion in the cost analysis may not be sufficient to account for differences in average cost that are related to level-of-care differences.

A nursing home that offers "high-quality" care as measured by resource-intensive processes (rehabilitation, nursing care) may provide more care to all patients regardless of their health status. Similarly, in a low-quality nursing home, all patients may receive fewer services than in the high-quality home, adjusting for health status. One must therefore find a quality measure that is independent of case mix or case severity in order to control for the influence of each factor on cost of care. Most measures of case mix do not adequately distinguish between case mix and severity, and so it has been very difficult to identify each factor's specific impact on cost.

Average cost is not the only relevant cost measure in nursing home analysis. Marginal cost is also important when forecasting resource use or when assessing nursing home profitability. A 1983 New York study (Nyman, 1988) analyzed the marginal cost of nursing homes, adjusting for variables, such as SNF/ICF days, average level of service in the institution, patient characteristics, input prices, and investor-owned or tax-exempt status. The marginal cost for the healthiest patients was $51 per patient day. For the least healthy patients, the marginal cost was $60. These rates can be compared with the reimbursement rate of $72, indicating a profit for patients at all levels.

5.7.6 Health Insurance Costs

Theoretically, health insurance administrative costs are potentially influenced by the scale of a firm's operations. Additionally, a very important factor affecting these costs is the ratio of group policies to all policies that an insurance company sells. Per policy, individual policies are more expensive to sell. Also, employers perform many of the functions for group policies that insurers perform for individual policies. This fact may influence public policy, because if individual and group policies have significantly different costs, the government may act to encourage holders of individual policies to obtain group policies.

One study examined health insurance administrative costs for a cross section of insurance companies that offer health insurance. The study found that both factors (scale of operations and type of policies) have a significant impact on these costs (Blair, Jackson, & Vogel, 1975). An unexpected finding of their study was that mutual (tax-exempt) companies had lower administrative costs than stock (investor-owned) companies, however, one might have expected the opposite to be true.

Exercises

1. Sweetgrass Radiology Labs has a fixed amount of radiology equipment. The laboratory can hire any number of radiology technicians per hour to produce radiographs, which are displayed on a screen. The relationship between the number of technicians hired per hour and the number of radiographs produced per hour is shown in the following table. Show the total and marginal products and indicate at each level of production whether the production function exhibits increasing, constant, or diminishing marginal productivity.

Radiograph Technicians per Hour	Radiographs Produced per Hour
1	10
2	26
3	50
4	74
5	94
6	100

2. St. Mary's Hospital owns a prime piece of real estate in the center of town. There is a small shopping center on this piece of land. Rents for each store are $8000 per month. The benefactor of this real estate, in her endowment to St. Mary's, stated that one of the stores should be operated as a clinic for the poor and be kept open 24 hours a day. St. Mary's has agreed to these conditions. It hires three nurses monthly at $6000 each. Furnishings are included in the estimate of the $8000 rent. Supplies are $20 per patient; there are 1600 patients a month, each of whom come in for one visit. What are the total monthly costs of operating the clinic?

3. City Home Care (CHC) hires a furnished office at $4000 per month, telephones at $400 a month, and a secretary at $4000 per month. These resources do not change, no matter how many clients are visited. Currently, CHC sees 900 patients a month, each three times (2700 visits in total). CHC uses 30 full-time nurses with their own cars, and they are paid $8000 per month each. There is a plentiful supply of additional nurses in town. These nurses can be hired almost on notice. Supplies are $40 per patient per month. What are the monthly money costs of operating CHC at its current level? Approximately how much would it cost to operate CHC at a level of 3150 visits per month assuming patients continued to be seen three times each month, and nurses were working at full capacity at the original level of patient visits?

4. The Jonesville Clinic is an inner-city clinic that provides primary care for indigent persons. Three physicians volunteer 5 hours a week each. Normally, physicians earn $450 per hour, but the clinic is lucky to get their services for free. The clinic hires two nurses annually at $54,000 each. Overhead, including secretarial time, is $45,000 a year. Ace Pharmaceuticals donates $6000 worth of drugs annually, and the First Street Mall donates a small office. The mall's owners could get $1200 monthly in rent for the office. What is the economic cost annually of operating the clinic?

5. The May Clinic rents a small office in Dubuque. May pays the building owner a rent of $6000 a month, which includes all utilities. It has signed a 3-year lease. May hires a general practice physician at $150 an hour, a nurse at $45 an hour, and a secretary at $30 an hour. May assumes that each patient uses $30 in supplies. In September, the clinic was open for 200 hours, during which all personnel were available at all times to staff the clinic. During that time, 3000 patients were seen. What were May's fixed and variable costs for the month?

6. Given the following monthly data for alternative operating levels at the St. Christopher's Ambulance, calculate the total fixed cost, average fixed cost, average variable cost, average total cost, and marginal cost for successive output levels. If St. Christopher's is operating at a level of three trips and it wants to determine the resources needed to make another trip, which statistic will it use?

Ambulance Runs	Total Variable Costs ($)	Total Costs ($)
0	0	1,200
1	1,300	2,500
2	1,400	2,600
3	1,500	2,700
4	1,800	3,000
5	2,400	3,900
6	3,600	4,800

Bibliography

Addesso, L. C., Nimmer, M., Visotcky, A., Fraser, R., & Brousseau, D. C. (2019). Impact of medical scribes on provider efficiency in the pediatric emergency department. *Academy of Emergency Medicine, 26*(2), 174–182.

Bailey, R. M. (1968). A comparison of internists in solo and fee-for-service group practice. *Bulletin of the New York Academy of Medicine, 44*(2nd series), 1293–1303.

Begg, C. B., Cramer, L. D., Hoskins, W. J., & Brennan, M. F. (1998). Impact of hospital volume on operative mortality for major cancer surgery. *JAMA, 280*(15), 1747–1751.

Berki, S. (1972). *Hospital economics.* Lexington, MA: D.C. Heath.

Berry, R. E. (1973). On grouping hospitals for economic analysis. *Inquiry, 10*, 5–12.

Birkmeyer, J. D., Sun, Y., Wong, S. L., & Stukel, T. A. (2007). Hospital volume and late survival after cancer surgery. *Annals of Surgery, 245*(5), 777–783.

Bishop, C. E. (1980). Nursing home cost studies and reimbursement issues. *Health Care Financing Review, 1*, 47–65.

Blair, R. D., Jackson, J. R., & Vogel, R. J. (1975). Economies of scale in the administration of health insurance. *Review of Economics and Statistics, 57*, 185–189.

Burns, L. R., & Lee, J. A. (2006). Hospital purchasing alliances: Utilization, services, and performance. *Health Care Management Review, 33*(3), 203–215.

Cowing, T. G., & Holtmann, A. G. (1983). Multiproduct short-run hospital cost functions. *Southern Economic Journal, 49*, 637–653.

Drews, J. D., Cooper, J. N., Onwuka, E. A., Minneci, P. C., & Aldrink, J. H. (2019). The relationships of surgeon volume and specialty with outcomes following pediatric thyroidectomy. *Journal of Pediatric Surgery, 54*(6), 1226–1232.

Dunn, D. L. Sacher, S. J., Cohen, W. S., & Hsiao, W. C. (1995). Economies of scope in physicians' work: The performance of multiple surgery. *Inquiry, 32*, 87–101.

Engberg, J., Wholey, D., Feldman, R., & Christianson, J. B. (2004). The effect of mergers on firms' costs: Evidence from the HMO industry. *The Quarterly Review of Economics and Finance, 44*(4), 574–600.

Farnand, L. J., Jacobs, P., & Dickson, W. M. (1986). An evaluation of the Finger Lakes Experimental Payment Program. *Inquiry, 23*(2), 200–208.

Finkler, S. A. (1979a). Cost effectiveness of regionalization: The heart surgery example. *Inquiry, 16*, 264–270.

Finkler, S. A. (1979b). On the shape of the hospital industry long run average cost function. *Health Services Research, 14*, 281–289.

Frech, H. E., & Mobley, L. E. (1995). Resolving the impasse on hospital scale economies. *Applied Economics, 27*, 286–296.

Friedman, B., & Pauly, M. V. (1983). A new approach to hospital cost functions and some issues in revenue regulation. *Health Care Financing Review, 4*, 105–114.

Garnick, D. W., Luft, H. S., McPhee, S. J., & Mark, D. H. (1989). Surgeon volume vs. hospital volume: Which matters more? *JAMA, 262*, 547–548.

Giancotti, M., Guglielmo, A., & Mauro, M. (2017). Efficiency and optimal size of hospitals: Results of a systematic search. *PLoS One, 12*(3), e0174533.

Goldfarb, M., Hornbrook, M., & Rafferty, J. (1980). Behavior of the multi-product firm. *Medical Care, 18*, 185–201.

Gonzales, T. I. (1997). An empirical study of economies of scope in home healthcare. *Health Services Research, 32*(3), 313–324.

Gregory, D. D. (1976–1977). Some evidence on the economic aspects of hospital cooperative ventures. *Journal of Economics and Business, 29*, 59–64.

Halm, E. A., Lee, C., & Chassin, M. R. (2002). Is volume related to outcome in health care? A systematic review and methodologic critique of the literature. *Annals of Internal Medicine, 137*, 511–520.

Hornbrook, M. C., & Monheit, A. C. (1985). The contribution of case mix severity to the hospital cost-output relation. *Inquiry, 22*, 259–271.

Iampreechakul, P., Chongchokdee, C., & Tirakotai, W. (2011). The accuracy of computer-assisted pedicle screw placement in degenerative lumbrosacral spine using single-time, paired point registration along technique combined with the surgeon's experience. *Journal of the Medical Association of Thailand, 94*(3), 337–345.

Joudi, F. N., & Konety, B. R. (2005). The impact of provider volume on outcomes from urological cancer therapy. *Journal of Urology, 174*(2), 432–438.

Kleinpell, R. M., Ely, E. W., & Grabenkort, R. (2008). Nurse practitioners and physician assistants in the intensive care unit: An evidence-based review. *Critical Care Medicine, 36*(10), 2888–2897.

Kwietniewski, L., Heimeshoff, M., & Schreyogg, J. (2017). Estimation of a physician practice cost function. *European Journal of Health Economics, 18*(4), 481–494.Lave, J., & Lave, L. B. (1984). Hospital cost functions. *Annual Review of Public Health, 5*, 193–213.

Leski, M., Young, M., & Higham, R. (2010). Managing inflammatory arthritides: Role of the nurse practitioner and physician assistant. *Journal of the American Academy of Nurse Practitioners, 22*(7), 382–392.

Lewit, E. M., Bentkover, J. D., Bentkover, S. H., Watkins, R. N., & Hughes, E. F. (1980). A comparison of surgical assisting in a prepaid group practice. *Medical Care, 18*, 916–929.

Lynch, M. G., Maa, A., Delaune, W., Chasan, J., & Cockerham, G. C. (2017). Eye care productivity and access in the Veterans Affairs Health Care System. *Military Medicine, 182*(1), e1631–e1635.

McGregor, M., & Pelletier, G. (1978). Planning of specialized health facilities: Size vs. cost and effectiveness in heart surgery. *New England Journal of Medicine, 299*, 179–181.

McKay, N. L. (1988). An econometric analysis of costs and scale economies in the nursing home industry. *Journal of Human Resources, 23*, 58–75.

McRae, S., Brunner, J. O., & Bard, J. F. (2019). Analyzing economies of scale and scope in hospitals by use of case mix planning. *Health Care Management Science.* doi:10.1007/s10729-019-09476-2

Newhouse, J. P. (1973). The economics of group practice. *Journal of Human Resources, 8*, 37–56.

Nyman, J. A. (1988). The marginal cost of nursing home care. *Journal of Health Economics, 7*, 393–412.

Okunade, A. A. (1993). Production cost structure of U.S. hospital pharmacies: Time series, cross sectional bed size evidence. *Journal of Applied Econometrics, 8*, 277–294.

Okunade, A., & Suraratdecha, C. (1998). Factor interchange and technical progress in U.S. specialized hospital pharmacies. *Health Economics, 7*, 363–372.

Ozminkowski, R. J., Gaumer, G., Coit, A. J., & Gabay, M. (1994). Hospital wage and price controls: Lessons from the Economic Stabilization Program. *Health Care Financing Review, 16*(2), 13–43.

Patel, S. N., Youssef, A. S., Vale, F. L., & Padhya, T. A. (2011). Re-evaluation of the role of image guidance in minimally invasive pituitary surgery: Benefits and outcomes. *Computer Aided Surgery, 16*(2), 45–53.

Pauly, M. V. (1996). Economics of multispecialty group practice. *Journal of Ambulatory Care Management, 19*(3), 26–33.

Reinhardt, U. (1972). A production function for physicians' services. *Review of Economics and Statistics, 54*, 55–66.

Roukos, D. H. (2009). Laparoscopic gastrectomy and personal genomics: High-volume surgeons and predictive biomedicine may govern the future for resectable gastric cancer. *Annals of Surgery, 250*(4), 650–651.

Salemi, A., Sedrakyan, A., Mao, J., Elmously, A., Wijeysundera, H., Tam, D.Y., ... Gaudino, M. (2019). Individual operator experience and outcomes in transcatheter aortic valve replacement. *JACC Cardiovascular Intervention, 12*(1), 90–97.

Scheffler, R. M. (1975). Further consideration of the economics of group practice. *Journal of Human Resources, 10*, 258–263.

Schwartz, W., & Joskow, P. (1980). Duplicated hospital facilities. *New England Journal of Medicine, 303*, 1449–1457.

Tsao, S. Y., Lee, W. C., Loong, C. C., Chen, T. J., Chiu, J. H., & Tai, L. C. (2011). High-surgical-volume hospitals associated with better quality and lower cost of kidney transplantation in Taiwan. *Journal of the Chinese Medical Association, 74*(1), 22–27.

Ullman, S. G. (1984). Cost analysis and facility reimbursement in the long-term health care industry. *Health Services Research, 19*, 83–102.

Ullman, S. G. (1986). Chain ownership and long-term health care facility performance. *Journal of Applied Gerontology, 5*, 51–63.

Valdmanis, V. G. (2010). Measuring economies of scale at the city market level. *Journal of Health Care Finance, 37*(1), 78–90.

Ward, M. M., Jaana, M., Wakefield, D. S., Ohsfeldt, R. L., Schneider, J. E., Miller, T., & Lei, Y. (2004). What would be the effect of referral to high-volume hospitals in a largely rural state? *Journal of Rural Health, 20*(4), 344–354.

Yatchak, R. (2000). A longitudinal study of economies of scale in the hospital industry. *Journal of Health Care Finance, 27*(1), 67–89.

Yee, T., Crawford, L., & Harber, P. (2005). Work environment of dental hygienists. *Journal of Occupational & Environmental Medicine, 46*(6), 633–639.

Zuckerman, S., Hadley, J., & Iezzoni, L. (1994). Measuring hospital efficiency with frontier cost functions. *Journal of Health Economics, 13*, 335–340.

CHAPTER 6

Behavior of Supply

OBJECTIVES

1. Define a supply curve in terms of the quantity of healthcare services supplied.
2. For a single investor-owned provider, describe a model that can be used to predict the quantity of healthcare services supplied.
3. Define a market, and describe and use a market model of healthcare supply.
4. For a single tax-exempt provider, describe an output-maximizing model to predict supplier behavior.
5. Describe the joint "quantity-quality" output-maximizing model to predict supplier behavior.
6. Describe the "administrator-as-agent" model to predict the effect of ownership status (investor-owned versus tax-exempt) on operating efficiency.

6.1 Introduction

This chapter is concerned with the determinants of the quantity and quality of output of various health-related products. The approach involves considering the behavior of organizations supplying these health-related products. In this chapter, hypotheses are provided regarding what causes suppliers to produce particular quantities and qualities of health-related goods and services. These hypotheses are formulated in terms of models of supplier behavior, and they incorporate the key causes of such behavior. The goal of the models is to isolate the direction in which individual factors cause supply to move, while keeping in mind other factors that may also be influencing supply movements. The emphasis is on understanding why the various quantities of healthcare goods and services are produced in the United States and what determines these quantities.

In presenting the hypotheses about supply behavior, a distinction is made between the supply of a single or individual producer and the supply of all producers in the market (i.e., individual versus market supply). It should be pointed out that, like in the analyses of demand, the focus is on the behavior of a group of market participants in isolation—in this case, the suppliers of the goods and services.

In this chapter, no single model of supplier behavior is presented as uniquely appropriate. The subject is complex, and the models presented offer suggestions rather than definitive answers. In particular, many healthcare providers differ with regard to the type of organization involved in the production of healthcare goods and services. Some healthcare organizations, such as investor-owned hospitals and nursing homes and physician practices, are profit-seeking institutions. Others, such as tax-exempt hospitals, the Red Cross, independent blood banks, and philanthropic organizations (e.g., the March of Dimes and the American Heart Association), operate under other legal and philosophical structures. This means that their "owners" (or, more appropriately, governors, boards, or trustees) can neither appropriate for themselves any profits that the organization might make nor sell the rights to the assets of the organization for personal gain. In this chapter, separate hypotheses are discussed for both types of organizations (investor-owned and tax-exempt).

Initially, in Section 6.2 a basic model of an individual profit-seeking supplier is developed, and then in Section 6.3 a model of the market supply behavior of a group of such investor-owned firms is presented. Because investor-owned and tax-exempt organizations can differ substantially, the following three sections focus on the effects that the tax-exempt organizational form has on the behavior of a tax-exempt organization. Much disagreement exists over the analysis of tax-exempt agency behavior. As a result, several alternative hypotheses about tax-exempt agency behavior are presented.

In Section 6.4, the tax-exempt agency hypothesis is examined as if it were an output-maximizing agency. In Section 6.5, this analysis is expanded to incorporate the behavior of the organization when quality in addition to quantity is incorporated into the output decisions of the organization. In addition, the organizational structure of the tax-exempt hospital, an unusual type of tax-exempt organization, is examined. In Section 6.6, a model is developed in which the tax-exempt agency is regarded as an instrument used to the benefit of its managers.

6.2 A Model of Supply Behavior: An Individual Investor-Owned Company

As a review of basic economic theory, please recall that supply reflects the quantity of a good or service that a producer is willing and able to provide in the market at a given price in a particular period of time. Note that this quantity supplied reflects the amount the supplier is willing to offer for sale, not the amount that was actually sold in the market. For a normal good or service, there is a direct relationship between price and quantity; that is, as price increases, the quantity a producer is willing and able to offer for sale in the market increases, other things being equal—ceteris paribus. This quantity offered for sale at various prices reflects the cost of resources required to produce the good or service and the profit required by the producer. Supply of a normal good or service is plotted graphically as an upward-sloping line, with the dependent variable quantity plotted on the horizontal axis and the independent variable price plotted on the vertical axis.

Price is the endogenous (internal) factor impacting the quantity offered in the market. A change in price will cause movement along a given supply curve,

reflecting a change in quantity supplied. An increase in price would cause an upward and to the right movement along the existing supply curve, while a decrease in price would cause a downward and to the left movement along the given supply curve.

Other factors impacting supply will cause a shift in the entire supply curve, reflecting that a different quantity of the good or service will be supplied at the original price as a result of the change in these exogenous (external) factors. This shift in the supply curve reflects a change in supply and not just a change in quantity supplied. In general, the exogenous factors impacting the supply of a good or service are:

1. *Costs of production resulting from changes in the price of inputs.* If the producer has to pay more for the inputs (resources) used in the production of the good or service, then the producer would need to receive a higher price for each unit produced, and so the supply curve would shift upward or leftward, reflecting a smaller quantity supplied at each of the original prices. The reverse is true if the price of the inputs decreased.

2. *Changes in the technologies used in the production of the good or service.* If the new technology results in greater efficiency in the production process, then the costs of production of the unit of output would decrease, resulting in a downward and rightward shift in the supply curve, reflecting a greater quantity supplied at each of the original prices.

3. *Changes in government taxes or subsidies associated with the production of the good or service.* If the government increases taxes, this would increase the cost to the producer and so the producer would need to receive a higher price for each unit produced, and so the supply curve would shift upward, reflecting a smaller quantity supplied at each of the original prices. The reverse is true if the producer receives a subsidy from the government for the goods or services produced.

4. *Changes in the prices of substitutes and/or complements.* If the number of substitutes for a good or service increases, then the producer will supply fewer units at the original prices, so the supply curve would shift upward and to the left to reflect this. If the number of complements increases, then the producer will supply more units at each of the original prices, so the supply curve will shift downward and to the right to reflect this.

5. *Changes in the general environment (economic and/or physical).* If the general environment improves, then the producer will be willing and able to

produce a greater amount of output and so the supply curve would shift downward and to the right.

6. *Changes in the goals of the firms.* If the goals of the firm change so that the new goal is to provide, for example, a higher quality of product, which can only be achieved by increasing the costs of production, then the supply curve will shift upward and to the left, reflecting a smaller quantity of output at each of the original prices.

7. *Changes in the opportunity costs of the alternative uses for the resources used by the supplier in the production process.* If the opportunity costs increase, this will increase the costs of production for the producer and so the supply curve will shift upward and to the left, reflecting a smaller quantity of output at each of the original prices. The reverse will occur if the opportunity cost of the alternatives decreases.

8. *Changes in price expectations.* If the producer expects prices to increase in the future, then the producer is likely to reduce the amount it is willing to supply currently, resulting in an upward or leftward shift in the current supply curve.

As discussed, a change in any of these exogenous factors will cause a shift, either outward to the right or inward to the left, of the entire supply curve. A shift outward in the supply curve reflects a greater quantity offered for sale at each price; an inward shift of the supply curve reflects a smaller quantity offered for sale at each price.

6.2.1 The Basic Model

The assumptions made in the initial supply model presented in this chapter fall into three categories: (1) revenue assumptions, (2) cost assumptions, and (3) assumptions about the objectives of the organization. In the following analysis, a laboratory (ABC Labs) that is owned by a pathologist and produces blood tests of a given level of quality will be used to illustrate the models and assumptions.

In this illustration, assume initially that the revenues of ABC Labs come from only two sources: payment received from the provision of patient services (termed *patient* or *earned revenues*); and a catch-all category called "other" sources (e.g., philanthropic or government grants, endowment funds, and other nonpatient-related sources). The assumption is that all revenues come from the payment for services provided (i.e., nonpatient-related revenues are zero). This assumption will be altered later in the analysis as the model presented becomes more complex.

With regard to patient revenues, the assumption is that ABC Labs is a "price taker"; that is, ABC Labs is a supplier that has no influence on the price it will receive for its output. The price-taker firm may occur because the price is set by an independent administrative agency (such as the government or an insurance agency) or because the lab is operating in a competitive situation in which the best price it can get for its product is the price prevailing in the market. The charging of higher prices by one supplier in a highly competitive market will simply drive consumers to the lower-priced competitors, preventing the higher priced supplier from selling the output produced. These lower prices will therefore prevent the higher priced supplier from achieving its goal of selling its product above the market price.

In this illustration, assume that ABC Labs receives $28 for each test performed. Its marginal revenue (*MR*), defined as the addition to total revenue (*TR*) for one additional unit of output produced and sold ($\Delta TR/\Delta Q$), is therefore also $28. The total and marginal revenues for output levels 0 through 10 are shown in **Table 6-1**, columns 9 and 10.

As for cost, the assumption is that ABC Labs has both fixed costs (costs that cannot be changed in a single production cycle) and variable costs (costs that change with changes in the quantity of output produced). The assumption regarding fixed costs is that the ABC Labs spends $14 monthly on equipment rental and mortgage payments. In addition, the assumption is that the pathologist-owner could earn a total of $10 if she worked elsewhere. This fixed cost sum is, at the same time, a monetary cost and an opportunity cost. That is, it incorporates a "normal" return on the investment of the owner's assets and efforts, reflected in the opportunity cost. The pathologist, once committed to work in the lab, gives up $10 per period that could have been earned with alternative activities. The total fixed costs are thus $24, and being fixed, they do not vary as the amount of output changes. The total fixed costs are shown in column 2 in Table 6-1; the associated average fixed costs (total fixed costs [*TFC*] divided by total quantity [*Q*] produced) are shown in Table 6-1, column 5.

Variable inputs are assumed to be employed in a least-costly manner (the total minimum variable cost for operating ABC Labs at different levels of output is shown in Table 6-1, column 3). The average variable cost (*AVC*) initially falls, and then subsequently rises (Table 6-1, column 6), and the marginal cost (*MC*) eventually rises (Table 6-1, column 8). The figures for the total cost (*TC*), the sum of the fixed (*TFC*) and variable (*TVC*) costs, are shown in Table 6-1, columns

Table 6-1 Illustrative Data on Relationships Among Revenue, Costs, Profit, and Output

(1) Quantity of Tests	(2) Total Fixed Costs (TFC)	(3) Total Variable Costs (TVC)	(4) Total Costs (TC)	(5) Average Fixed Costs (TFC/Q)	(6) Average Variable Costs (TVC/Q)	(7) Average Total Costs (TC/Q)	(8) Marginal Costs (ΔTC/ΔQ)	(9) Total Earned Revenue (TR = PXQ)	(10) Marginal Revenue (ΔTR/ΔQ)	(11) Profits (TR − TC)
0	24	0.00	24.00	0.00	0.00	0.00	0.00	0.00	0.00	−24.00
1	24	13.50	37.50	24.00	13.50	37.50	13.50	28.00	28.00	−9.50
2	24	21.00	45.00	12.00	10.50	22.50	7.50	56.00	28.00	11.00
3	24	26.30	50.50	8.00	8.83	16.83	5.50	84.00	28.00	33.50
4	24	34.00	58.00	6.00	8.50	14.50	7.50	112.00	28.00	54.00
5	24	47.50	71.50	4.80	9.50	14.30	13.50	140.00	28.00	68.50
6	24	71.00	95.00	4.00	11.83	15.83	23.50	168.00	28.00	73.00
7	24	108.50	132.50	3.43	15.50	18.93	37.50	196.00	28.00	63.50
8	24	164.00	188.00	3.00	20.50	23.50	55.50	224.00	28.00	36.00
9	24	241.50	265.50	2.67	26.83	29.50	77.50	252.00	28.00	−13.50
10	24	345.00	369.00	2.40	34.50	36.90	103.50	280.00	28.00	−89.00

4 and 7 (total and average values, respectively). Therefore, the cost curves are shaped as hypothesized in the chapter on healthcare production and costs (see **Figure 6-1**). Whereas in Table 6-1 the values jump in discrete steps, the curves are drawn as smooth functions for geometric convenience.

In graph A, the supplier produces where total profits, equal to the difference between total revenue (TR) and total costs (TC), are at a maximum. In graph B, the same conclusion can be derived in terms of marginal costs and revenues. Here the profit-maximizing point is where $MR = MC$. In the graph, since the price per unit is constant in this illustration, price (P), average revenue (AR), and MR are the same.

These dollar figures are approximated in graph A of Figure 6-1 for total values and in graph B for marginal revenue (MR), marginal cost (MC), average variable cost (AVC), and average total cost (ATC). Note that the TR curve rises at a rate of $28 per blood test and that MR is constant at $28. These are two different ways of saying the same thing: the revenue per unit of output sold is fixed at $28. This is a concrete expression of the initial assumption in the illustration that ABC Labs is a price taker, because ABC Labs can sell all desired products at that price but cannot sell any at a price above the market price of $28. Finally, because ABC Labs is an investor-owned company, it

seems reasonable to assume that its main objective is to maximize profits (total revenues [TR] minus total costs [TC]).

Now the conclusions regarding the basic model can be examined and the question underlying the analysis can be answered: What quantity of output will ABC Labs supply? The task is to present a hypothesis that will enable the prediction of which quantity will be chosen to be produced and offered in the market and how this quantity will vary when some of the underlying variables in the model—prices and costs—themselves vary.

Referring to Table 6-1, a specific quantity of output that achieves ABC Labs' profit-maximizing objective can now be derived from the model: profits are at a maximum at six units of output (here they amount to $73.00). The reasoning used to obtain this conclusion can best be presented in marginal terms. Assume that ABC Labs was initially supplying four units of output. Profits from four units, given the assumed revenue and cost conditions, equal $54.00. If ABC Labs produces and sells one more blood test, the additional or marginal revenue will be $28.00 (i.e., $MR = \$28.00$), and the additional costs of production (MC) will be $13.50. The additional profit obtained by expanding output from four to five tests will be $14.50, bringing total profits to a new level of

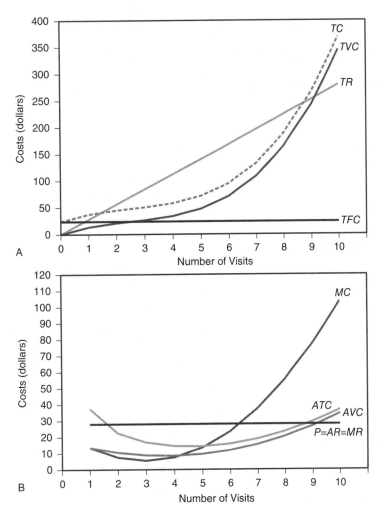

Figure 6-1 Supply relationship for a profit-maximizing firm in terms of total costs and revenues (graph A) and average and marginal costs and revenues (graph B).

$68.50. ABC Labs, being a profit maximizer, would expand production to at least five units.

In fact, ABC Labs will move beyond this amount of five units because profits can be further increased by doing so. The best ABC Labs can do, at the given price and cost conditions, is to produce six units of output. Expanding beyond six units still results in positive profits for a while, but these profits would be less than the profit at six units of output. According to this model, a profit-maximizing firm will continue to expand production as long as MR exceeds MC. If the model presented was dealing with smooth, continuous changes, the conclusion would be that a profit-maximizing firm will expand output up to the point at which MR = MC, as long as MC is rising with output. At this point, the firm is maximizing its profits, and so the quantity at which MC = MR is the supply position for which the firm should be aiming.

This conclusion is shown diagrammatically in Figure 6-1. In graph A, profits at each level of output

are shown as the vertical distance between total revenues and total costs at that level of output. Because profits are defined as total revenue minus total costs (TR – TC), then where this vertical distance is at a maximum (the greatest distance), profits are also at a maximum. In our illustration from the data in Table 6-1, this profit-maximizing point occurs at six units of output for a profit of $73.00 (allowing for small variations because the graph is drawn with continuous curves).

In graph B, the same profit-maximizing conclusion is shown, but is presented in terms of marginal costs and marginal revenues. Here, the point at which marginal revenue equals marginal cost (MR = MC) is the profit-maximizing quantity, that is, the quantity that will be supplied by a profit-maximizing producer. As the data in Table 6-1 show, a movement in quantity supplied in either direction from six units would detract from total profits and so would not be consistent with the profit-maximizing objective.

The first conclusion of this model, then, is that, given the stated revenue (i.e., price) and cost conditions, and given the profit-maximizing objective, a profit-maximizing firm will produce at the quantity at which $MR = MC$. Using this information, it is now possible to derive a supply curve, or a supply schedule, that shows what the quantity supplied will be at different prices. This analysis is shown graphically in **Figure 6-2**.

At each price above $8.50, the firm will maximize profits by supplying at the quantity where price equals MC. If the price is at $8.50, the firm will just be meeting its variable costs. At any price below this, the firm's variable production costs are greater than the revenue received and so production will result in larger losses than if the firm shuts down operations; therefore, the firm will not supply output at any price below $8.50. For price above $8.50, the firm's supply curve and its MC curve are the same.

If the price rises from $28 to $30, ABC Labs will add to its profits by expanding output to a seventh unit because, even though the cost of this unit is higher, the higher extra revenue will make it profitable to expand output. The same reasoning applies to additional price increases: higher prices will bring forth greater quantities supplied until marginal revenue equals marginal cost ($MR = MC$).

The same concept applies to price declines, with one major exception: eventually, the price could become so low that the owner of the firm would be better off, from the point of view of profits (or losses), to shut down operations and produce nothing. For all prices below this level of $8.50 (represented by point j in Figure 6-2), the quantity supplied by the firm would be zero, since the price below $8.50 would no longer be covering the variable costs incurred in the production of the output. Basically, the firm will continue to produce as long as the price covers variable costs and some of the fixed costs. If price falls below the variable costs, then the producer will stop production in order to minimize its losses.

The critical price below which the firm will shut down depends on the variable costs of the firm. Recall that fixed costs are the same thing as "already committed" costs that cannot be changed, while variable costs are those that can be avoided by not employing the variable factors in the production of goods and services; total costs are the sum of the two costs (fixed and variable) at each output level. If the price falls sufficiently, it is possible that even at its best level of output (from the profitability standpoint), the firm will be incurring a loss.

The criterion the firm would use in deciding whether to continue operating under such unfavorable circumstances is not whether the firm is incurring a loss, but whether it is minimizing its losses. The importance of variable costs in the decision-making process comes into play here. As long as the firm's total revenues (TR) are exceeding its total variable costs (TVC), the firm will be adding to a surplus of

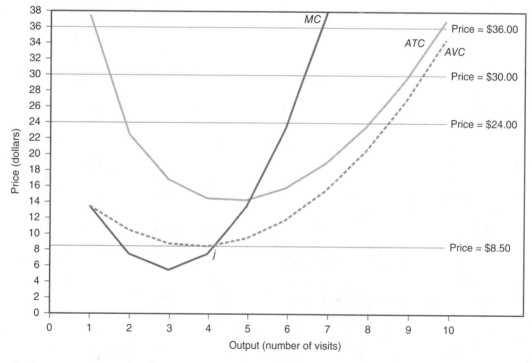

Figure 6-2 Profit-maximizing supply points at alternative prices.

revenue. In this case, total revenue minus total variable costs ($TR - TVC$) will be positive. Even though total profits may be negative, signifying a loss (total revenue minus the sum of total variable cost plus total fixed costs) [$TR - (TVC + TFC)$], the loss is less than it would be if the firm shut down entirely. For if the firm shuts down, both total revenue (TR) and total variable costs (TVC) are zero, and the losses would equal total fixed cost (TFC).

In sum, as long as the firm is meeting its variable costs and adding something to cover some or all of its fixed costs, the firm should continue to operate. In this case, its supply curve is traced out by the MC curve; that is, the costs of production shape the supply curve. In a profit-maximizing situation, the quantity supplied will be where price equals marginal cost. Should the price fall so low that at no level of output could the firm meet all its variable costs, then it should cease production and shut down.

A complete analysis of the firm's supply behavior can now be presented using the curves in Figure 6-2. If the price is equal to or greater than the lowest point on the average variable cost (AVC) curve (point j), then at some level of output, all variable costs will be covered and the firm will produce some output. If the price is lower than this critical minimum price, the firm will cease producing and shut down operations. If the price is above the critical minimum level, the firm will produce output at the quantity at which marginal revenue equals marginal cost ($MR = MC$) (i.e., when price = MC). The marginal cost (MC) curve of the firm then is its supply curve, relating price to output.

In the context of this analysis, it is possible to make some sense regarding the previous assumption that the costs incurred by an investor-owned firm are at a minimum. The producer has a choice of producing a given quantity of output at the lowest possible cost or above the lowest possible cost. (It was described in Chapter 5 on healthcare production and cost.) By choosing the lowest possible cost method of production, the firm can achieve its greatest profits because profits are defined as the difference between total revenues and total costs. If costs were above the minimum, they would cut into profits, which is contrary to the assumed goal of the investor-owned, profit-maximizing firm.

It should be noted that the supply relationship focuses on the behavior of suppliers in isolation. That is, the term *quantity supplied* refers to a distinct schedule of output the producer is willing and able to provide at various prices—that is of the supplier's responsiveness to price. In this chapter, the focus is on supplier behavior in isolation from demanders. Before

putting the separate forces, supply and demand, together, it is essential to understand how each operates on its own.

6.2.2 Nonpatient Revenues

The previous illustration assumed the only source of revenue for ABC Labs was revenue received for the provision of services to patients. Now a new element is introduced into our analysis: the receipt of nonpatient revenues. In this expanded illustration, the focus is on a particular form of unearned revenue, a grant or subsidy, that is unrelated to the amount of goods produced. Such a grant or subsidy might be received from a grateful donor, governments, or a foundation. While nonmarket-related revenue occurs in many different markets, these types of revenues are especially relevant for the healthcare industry. Many healthcare providers receive grants from different sources that are unrelated to the quantity of the goods or services produced by the providers. These grants can be viewed as supplemental revenue that is independent of the costs of producing a good or service. The analytical task here is to determine how this type of revenue might affect the provider's supply of a good or service.

The economic significance of a grant unrelated to output is that it provides a set amount of money regardless of whether the output of the supplier expands or contracts. Such a grant can be treated analytically in one of two ways, either as a fixed addition to revenue or as a fixed reduction from total costs (a negative fixed cost). While the rationale for the first option seems clear-cut, the rationale for the second requires some explanation. In a sense, a fixed subsidy reduces, by a fixed amount, the total costs that the provider must meet at each output level. Operationally, regardless of the way it is treated, it will have the same impact on profits. Therefore, in this illustration it will be treated as a reduction in total costs.

Assume that ABC Labs received a fixed subsidy of $10. This would increase revenues in Table 6-1 by $10 at each and every level of output. Profits would also increase by $10 at each level of output. In Figure 6-1, the increase would appear as an upward parallel shift in the total revenue (TR) curve.

What is important from a supply standpoint is that neither patient revenues (including marginal revenue – MR) nor variable costs (VC) are affected. Thus, while profits are higher by $10 at every output level, the maximum profitability level of output remains at six units. The fixed subsidy does not affect the most profitable level of output; it only affects the level of profits at that and every other level of output. In this case, the nonpatient revenue can be viewed similarly to the impact that fixed costs have on the production side. It is the marginal costs and marginal revenue that are considered in determining the level of output to supply in the market.

This conclusion would not hold if the subsidy was related to output, for example, if ABC Labs received a subsidy for each blood test performed. In that case, as output expanded, the marginal revenue would be the additional revenue from patient sources plus the additional (output-related) grant or subsidy revenues. When estimating the most profitable output level, the firm would then have to consider both sources of additional revenue and relate them to marginal cost.

The conclusion then is that a grant or subsidy that is not output related will not influence the supply decisions of a profit-maximizing firm; the firm's supply position will still be where marginal patient revenue equals marginal cost. The firm simply receives a greater profit at that point.

6.2.3 Shifts in the Supply Curve

In this section, consideration is given to what happens to the supply curve of the firm when factors that influence the position of the marginal cost (MC) curve change. These factors are referred to as exogenous (external) to the market and were reviewed at the beginning of this chapter. A supply schedule is simply a table, or listing, that provides varying values for the prices of a good or service and the corresponding

quantities that the producer/seller would be willing and able to offer for sale at each price during a particular period of time. The supply schedule can reflect either the behavior propensities of a single producer or the aggregation of producers across the market. The values listed in the supply schedule, when plotted in a graph, become the supply curve.

In general, as shown in **Figure 6-3**, any factor that causes the marginal cost (MC) curve to shift upward from MC_1 to MC_2 will amount to a leftward shift in the supply schedule of the firm (a decrease in supply). The quantity supplied at any price will be reduced from Q_1 to Q_2. Such shifts might occur because of higher input prices or a higher quality of product being produced, to cite two of the factors discussed in Section 6.2 that might cause the firm's cost curve to shift. In the case of the production of a higher quality product, for example, the net result is that a lower quantity will be produced by the firm at any given price when producing the higher quality costs more to produce. In the healthcare industry, it has been shown that higher quality care does not always increase costs (Rantz et al., 2010). There are other times when higher quality does cost more (Auerbach, Maselli, Carter, Pekow, & Lindenauer, 2010).

An upward shift in the MC curve of a profit-maximizing firm will mean a lower quantity supplied at any price. In this figure, a shift from MC_1 to MC_2 means a decrease in supply level indicated by the dotted line (the quantity supplied decreases from Q_1 to Q_2).

The same reasoning, in reverse, holds for downward (to the right) shifts in the marginal cost (MC)

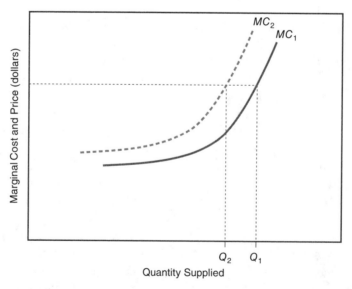

Figure 6-3 Shifts in the marginal cost curve for a profit-maximizing supplier. An upward shift in the MC curve of a profit-maximizing firm will mean a lowerquantity supplied at any price. In this figure, a shift from MC_1 to MC_2 means a decrease in supply level indicated by the dotted line (the quantity supplied decreases from Q_1 to Q_2).

curve. For example, an increase in the capacity of the firm to produce output, caused by a technological advancement, will cause the *MC*, and thus the supply curve, to shift to the right, indicating a willingness on the part of the firm to supply more output at any given price. Such expansion in output is likely when the firm is operating on the downward-sloping part of its long-run average cost curve. An expansion in output would allow it to move to a lower point on the long-run average cost (*LRAC*) curve (i.e., to a lower-cost short-run curve).

6.3 Market Supply

Now, it is easier to demonstrate how the analysis of individual supply movements can be extended to form a hypothesis about movements in product supply in a specific market. To do this, two new assumptions concerning individual supply behavior are introduced to the model:

1. There is a set number of suppliers in the market.
2. There are no agreements on the part of suppliers to restrict supply.

In the present model, two groups of factors influence market supply: the number of suppliers and the factors that influence individual supplier behavior.

In other words, the market supply schedule can be obtained once the number of suppliers and their individual supply schedules are known. Assume in this illustration that the market consists of three suppliers: ABC Labs, XYZ Labs, and GHI Labs (see **Figure 6-4**). Each lab has a given supply schedule. XYZ Labs supplies 5 tests at $1.00, a total of 10 tests at $1.50, a total of 15 at $2.00, and so on. GHI Labs supplies 3, 6, and 9 tests at these prices, respectively, and ABC Labs supplies 6, 9, and 12 tests. Given these schedules, and the fact that these three labs are the only ones in the market, the market supply curve is the sum of these individual supply curves at each price. At $1.00, the market supply of tests is 14 (5 + 3 + 6); at $1.50, a total of 25 tests are supplied; and at $2.00, a total of 36 tests are supplied. The market supply curve is shown as the horizontal sum of all individual supply curves in Figure 6-4. Given a particular price, the model predicts the quantity that will be supplied by all producers in the market.

The market supply shows the quantity supplied by all firms providing the product to the market at each price. It is obtained by simply summing individual suppliers' quantities at each price.

The market supply curve will shift outward (to the right) if, given the number of producers, any factors cause the individual supply curves to shift outward

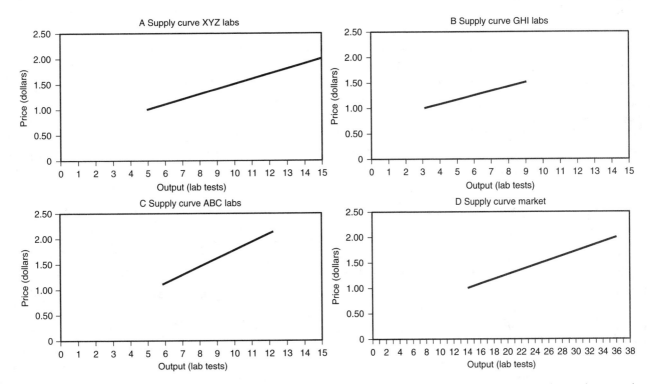

Figure 6-4 Derivation of the market supply curve from individual supply curves. The market supply shows the quantity supplied by all firms providing the product to the market at each price. It is obtained by simply summing individual suppliers' quantities at each price.

or if the number of suppliers increases. In either case, more will be supplied at any given price. Our model enables the classification of these influences and separates their effects on supply. The same type of analysis applies to reductions in supply, which would shift the supply curve upward or to the left.

With regard to the number of suppliers, just as profits are the motivating force behind the expansion (or contraction) of output by an individual firm, profits are a driving force behind the expansion of firms in the market—the entry of new firms into the market. At any particular time there are a number of prospective suppliers capable of acquiring the techniques and equipment needed to supply a product (e.g., blood tests in this illustration). If profits are high in the market, prospective suppliers will be motivated to enter the market and thus shifting the supply curve down and to the right. Of course, in real life, existing firms, protective of their high profits, may act to keep potential suppliers out, but this type of behavior is ruled out of the model discussed here.

6.4 Supply Behavior of Tax-Exempt Agencies: The Output Maximization Hypothesis

Tax-exempt (formerly known as not-for-profit) suppliers abound in the healthcare field. Tax-exempt designation indicates that these organizations do not pay taxes on the profits generated through the provision of goods and services or on the properties they own. As discussed earlier, members of the boards of directors and administrators cannot benefit personally from the operations of the tax-exempt organization. One reason for the tax-exempt status of healthcare providers appears to be the existence of external demands for healthcare products and services. These external demands may arise when people are concerned about, and willing to pay for, the health care others may need or utilize. To satisfy these external demands, individuals may form tax-exempt agencies whose purpose is to provide products and services to those perceived to be needy, usually on a less-than-cost basis. Health-related philanthropies, such as the American Heart Association, give away educational services that are financed by donors who want others to consume the services. The Red Cross blood program exists because there is sufficient concern on the part of blood donors about the health of those requiring transfusions.

Tax-exempt hospitals originally provided free and subsidized hospital care to the needy in substantial amounts; this care was financed largely through philanthropic donations, which can be regarded as payments to satisfy the donors' external demands for care to the needy. As the population grew, and the costs associated with hospital services increased, it became necessary for larger subsidies to be obtained for the hospital care provided to the needy. These subsidies tended to take the form of government-assistance programs supported through taxation. Public health departments attempt to satisfy external demands for health care through government-provided services.

There are, no doubt, other reasons for the formation of tax-exempt agencies. For example, these agencies may be formed as "captives" of other tax-exempt groups. During the 1930s and 1940s, Blue Cross plans began under the auspices of tax-exempt hospitals to ensure that hospitals were paid. The scope of the inquiry here does not encompass the conditions under which health service agencies become organized on a tax-exempt basis (see Culyer, 1971, for a more in-depth discussion). Rather, the existence of this type of organization is treated as a given and attention is restricted to the supply behavior of these agencies once they are formed.

To ensure that the services offered by a tax-exempt agency are provided in a reasonable manner, a governing board of trustees is formed. The members of a board of trustees cannot gain direct financial benefit from the organization, either in the form of profits or of proceeds from the sale of the enterprise. Furthermore, board members are frequently banned from garnering indirect gains, such as what might occur if a board member's law firm provided legal services to the organization. The board of trustees is primarily responsible for setting organizational policies, but many of their responsibilities are delegated to a full-time, salaried administrative (executive) staff. The actual responsibilities of each (the trustees and the staff), including the making of supply decisions, vary from organization to organization.

Several approaches can be taken in forming hypotheses about the supply behavior of tax-exempt agencies. One approach is to regard the trustees as being in charge of the day-to-day operations of the organization. Following this approach, the goals the trustees are likely to pursue would be hypothesized and then a model of the actions of the organization that incorporates these goals would be developed.

Another approach is to regard the salaried executives of the organization as the people who maintain control over decision making. In this case, hypotheses are made about their goals, and a model of organizational supply based on *these* goals is developed. No doubt the supply behavior of a real tax-exempt firm is influenced by both trustees and staff, but to keep the analysis simple, each approach is pursued separately. We begin with the trustee-dominance model. In this model, assume that the trustees' objective or goal is to maximize the output of the agency, that is, to carry out their mandate to the fullest extent possible by maximizing the quantity of services provided by the agency.

Now assume a tax-exempt lab is initially financed by a public-spirited benefactor. Cost and revenue conditions are the same as in the ABC Labs illustration, with the exception that the pathologist is under contract and receives an explicit payment of $10 per month for her services. From the point of view of the lab, once the contractual commitment with the pathologist is made, this becomes a fixed cost, and so the total fixed costs of the laboratory are $24 ($10 for the pathologist and $14 for the earlier rental obligations). The quality of the product is the same as in the previous illustration and is constant. Revenues are $28 per test, but now the reimbursement may be made by a third party. (Reimbursement or payment may be collected through individual donations or from a united agency.) The major difference between the two examples is that the tax-exempt lab seeks to maximize output rather than to maximize profits.

According to this model, because revenues come only from reimbursement for services, output will be expanded to the point at which the firm breaks even, that is, when total revenue equals total costs ($TR = TC$). In Table 6-1, given a price of $28, output will be expanded to eight units, because at nine units total cost equals $265.50, while total revenue is only $252.00. In graph A of Figure 6-1, the break-even point at eight units of output is shown in total terms. In graph B, the lab's operating point is where price per unit equals average total cost. The lab just covers costs for all units when it operates at this level.

Given the assumptions, output for an investor-owned profit-maximizing firm will be lower than that for a tax-exempt firm that behaves as hypothesized (i.e., maximizes output). The supply curve for an output-maximizing firm is its average total cost (*ATC*) curve for prices above the minimum point on the curve. If the revenues do not total at least this minimum amount, the firm runs a deficit and must raise the funds from nonpatient sources. For the moment, assume that nonpatient revenues are zero and that the firm has no reserves to meet a deficit. If it does not meet all its obligations, it will cease production and go out of business.

As long as the price is above the minimum point on the average total cost (*ATC*) curve, the supply curve of the tax-exempt agency that maximizes output is the *ATC* curve. As the price rises, so will the supply offered. Any factor that shifts the *ATC* curve downward (lower unit costs at any level of output) will cause the output to increase at any price.

The response of an output-maximizing tax-exempt firm to a fixed subsidy or grant is very different from that of a profit-maximizing firm. Recall that a fixed subsidy will not influence a profit-maximizer's supply, now assume that a donor gives the nonprofit lab a $25 subsidy unrelated to output. Analytically, this can be treated as an overall increase in total revenues or as an overall reduction in total costs (and a reduction in average fixed costs of $25.00/$Q$). In the former case, the analysis in Table 6-1 would be altered to show total revenue (*TR*) and profits higher at every level of output by $25. Whereas formerly, the output-maximizing output level was 8, with the subsidy, an output level of 9 will show an overall (operating and nonoperating) profit of $11.50 ($25.00 − $13.50). The lab would be losing money (in the red) at an output level of 10, but it could now meet all its costs at a level of 9, and this is where it would maximize output (subject to the fact that it must break even).

Graphically, if the fixed subsidy is treated as a reduction in fixed costs, it would appear as a downward shift in average fixed cost (*AFC*) and also average total cost (*ATC*) (because *AFC* is part of *ATC*). It will appear as an outward shift in the firm's supply curve, which is identical to the *ATC* curve. The conclusion in either case is the same: a nonoutput-related grant or subsidy will shift the supply curve of the output-maximizing firm and thus will lead to increased output. In this respect, the output-maximizing firm is very unlike the profit-maximizing investor-owned firm discussed earlier.

The market supply analysis in the case of tax-exempt organizations is somewhat more complicated than in the case of investor-owned organizations. If the assumption is made that each separate tax-exempt supplier has a vested interest in providing output to the needy, the market supply curve will be made up of the sum of what all the individual suppliers would be willing to supply at each price or reimbursement rate. That is, the market supply curve is the sum of the individual producers' supply curves for prices above the minimum *ATC*.

Individual tax-exempt suppliers might act competitively if the trustees developed some sense of identification with the organizations of which they were board members. However, if this sense of identification did not develop, trustees would not care which organization supplied the output to the needy as long as it was supplied by someone. In this situation, market supply would consist of a far more complicated set of arrangements, because trustees would pull their organizations out of the market when other organizations supplying the same product appeared. Assume that, in this illustration, organizational pride develops to the point that the standard market supply model is appropriate.

6.5 Supply Decisions Involving Quality

Until now, it has been assumed that quality of output was held constant and thus did not enter the supply decision. In fact, quality is an extremely important supply variable for suppliers, especially in the health-care system. In particular, it has frequently been asserted that hospitals seek to supply output of the highest quality. In this section, a model is developed to incorporate quality of care into the supply picture.

To understand the bias of tax-exempt hospitals toward high-quality supply, it is necessary to examine their unusual management structure. Like other tax-exempt firms, a tax-exempt hospital includes a board of trustees and a group of salaried administrators. However, physicians have a special relationship with the hospital: they are in charge of the medical activities of the hospital, and yet, for the most part, they are unsalaried staff members. Because their services are so crucial (indeed, the hospital's activities revolve around them), physicians have enormous influence over hospital supply decisions, and hospital supply policies are set by an informal arrangement among physicians, trustees, and administrators. This type of arrangement has been termed a "management triangle," depending on mutual accountability, interdependence, and responsibility for appropriate performance of their respective obligations. Hospital activities are the result of directives (sometimes conflicting) issued by three lines of authority: medical, trustee, and administrative. In particular, the medical influence in the decision-making process has been held to be responsible for the bias toward higher quality in hospital objectives, because physicians benefit considerably from high-quality inputs.

In most hospitals, the physicians form an organized medical staff, which is a self-governing entity that typically has the responsibility for determining the membership of the medical staff, performing credentialing of the members, granting privileges and peer-review activities, and providing timely oversight of the clinical quality of care provided and for patient safety. The medical staff seeks maximum physician autonomy with minimal interference in the practice of medicine from hospital procedures.

These goals of the medical staff may come in conflict with the hospital's goals of increasing efficiency in the production of medical services in order to improve the financial bottom line of the hospital, creating tension in the relationship. In many cases, the hospital has been viewed as a "free" workshop for physicians to perform their activities of delivering patient care, since the physicians do not have to pay for the equipment, supplies, or support personnel used in the provision of hospital care. In addition, because hospitals rely upon physicians for patients, and therefore financial resources, administration has attempted to create attractive practice environments for physicians. Because physicians are paid separately for their services from the hospital, the physicians have a financial interest in the facilities, technologies, and staff that can improve their personal productivity and increase ease of patient care, not necessarily what is best for the institution, as long as the hospital remains sufficiently financially viable to remain open.

A supply model that is based on the preceding analysis, but incorporates the bias toward quality, can be developed. Assume a given level of reimbursement, say $4000 per patient day (see **Figure 6-5**). Average total cost (*ATC*) curves are drawn for three different levels of quality of service; each higher level is produced with more resources. ATC_1 represents an *ATC* curve for a specific level of output and level of quality. ATC_2 and ATC_3 are similar curves for successively higher levels of quality.

The *ATC* curves represent relationships between *ATC* and output at various quality levels. ATC_3 represents the highest level, ATC_2 the intermediate level, and ATC_1 the lowest level. A tax-exempt producer who maximizes the quantity of output (given the quality level) will produce where the unit payment rate, or price, equals *ATC*. For the lowest quality level, the output will be 12. Higher-quality levels entail a reduction in the maximum output levels achievable given the payment rate.

An output-maximizing hospital will choose Q_1 (12,000) units of output at Quality Level 1; Q_2 (10,000) units at Quality Level 2; and Q_3 (9000) units at Quality Level 3. Indeed, a trade-off between quality and quantity of care typically occurs. Such a trade-off is shown in **Figure 6-6**, with quality of care represented on the vertical axis and the quantity on the horizontal axis. Curve *XY* shows the maximum output

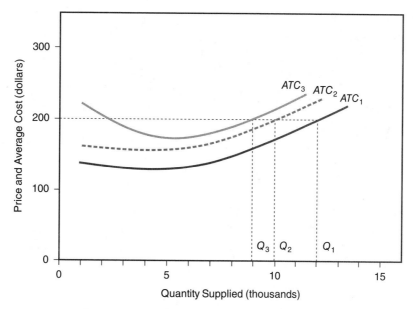

Figure 6-5 Alternative quantities and qualities supply by a tax-exempt supplier. The *ATC* curves represent relationships between *ATC* and output at various quality levels. ATC_3 represents the highest level, ATC_2 the intermediate level, and ATC_1 the lowest level. A tax-exempt producer who maximizes the quantity of output (given the quality level) will produce where the unit payment rate, or price, equals *ATC*. For the lowest quality level, the output will be 12. Higher-quality levels entail a reduction in the maximum output levels achievable given the payment rate.

© Jones & Bartlett Learning.

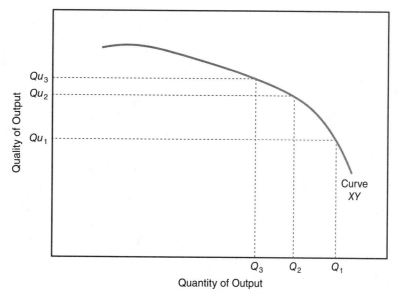

Figure 6-6 The tradeoff between quality and quantity. Based on Figure 6-5, for any given payment rate, a higher quality level can be achieved only with a lower quantity of output. The curve shows alternative levels of quantity and quality that can be achieved at a given payment rate (or price).

© Jones & Bartlett Learning.

that can be achieved for each level of quality given the reimbursement rate of $4000, and thus reflects the constraints or the choices facing the hospital. The actual combination of quality and quantity supplied will depend on the hospital's policies.

A highly quality-oriented hospital will choose a quality level close to Qu_3, whereas an output-oriented hospital will choose a level closer to Qu_1. If the assertion that hospitals are quality-oriented is correct, it might be expected that Qu_3 would be more frequently observed.

That is, of the various output combinations that a tax-exempt hospital can choose, it will tend to provide care of a higher quality level. By itself, however, this does not mean that such high-quality care in the market will be observed, for it must be remembered that currently only the supply side of the market is being examined. The quality of care actually produced will be determined by what the suppliers are willing to supply and what the consumers are willing and able to purchase. Determining what output actually is produced and utilized requires that the market in its entirety be examined.

Based on Figure 6-6 for any given payment rate, a higher quality level can be achieved only with a lower quantity of output. The curve shows alternative levels of quantity and quality that can be achieved at a given payment rate (or price).

6.6 Supply Behavior of Tax-Exempt Agencies: The Administrator-As-Agent Model

An alternative theory of resource allocation and product supply in tax-exempt agencies focuses on the behavior of the executive or administrator of the organization. The underlying assumption is that the administrator, even though just an agent of the trustees, has considerable control over the organization's resources. This seems a plausible assumption given that trustees of a tax-exempt agency typically can devote only a small portion of their time to trustee-related activities, whereas the administrator is usually a full-time employee. As part of this approach, a comparative analysis can be done that examines how the same administrator would behave if operating the same agency as an investor-owned enterprise or as a tax-exempt enterprise. The differences in behavior, which are due solely to the different incentive structures of the two types of organization, create differences in the use of the agency's resources and in the agency's output.

The theory can be viewed as simply an extension of the basic demand hypothesis. According to this hypothesis, the lower the direct cost of a good or service or other benefits to an individual, the more the good or service will be demanded. The extension of the hypothesis involves identifying the goods and services that are desired by the administrator of an agency, as well as their relative prices or costs under varying institutional circumstances. Because the focus is on the administrator's behavior, two types of benefits that can be obtained by the administrator in the context of the job are identified.

First, there are the pecuniary (monetary) benefits, especially the administrator's salary. In addition, if the administrator is a part or full owner of the agency, the pecuniary benefits will encompass the profits that accrue. Benefits of the second type, sometimes called *on-the-job* benefits, or amenities, are nonpecuniary. These include such things as high-grade office furniture, a relaxed work atmosphere, expenses-paid "business" trips to exotic places, and so on. Both types of benefits are desired by the administrator, but because their supply is limited, the administrator cannot have everything he or she would like. Recall that a fundamental assumption in economics is that resources are limited but wants and desires are unlimited.

Before developing the hypothesis about how much of each type of benefit will be demanded, the implications for the resource use of obtaining the two types of benefits are examined (Lee, 1971). First, when a smaller amount of resources is used to obtain a given output, an opportunity to increase profits is created. Nonpecuniary benefits also require the commitment of resources. Better office equipment, more liberal working conditions, better fringe benefits, and other on-the-job benefits are obtained from the expansion of the total resource commitment and result in an increase in costs and a reduction in profits. In a tax-exempt enterprise, this reduction in profits does not detract from the manager's pecuniary benefits, because he or she will not be rewarded on the basis of the profits the organization earns.

The hypothesis as to how the administrator will behave under these alternative incentive structures is based on the constraints facing the administrator in the two different environments. In a tax-exempt environment, because the administrator cannot convert profits into take-home pecuniary benefits (remember, the profits cannot be distributed to owners or stakeholders but must be reinvested in the organization), they must be converted into organizational resources if any benefit is to be obtained. On the other hand, the use of these extra resources in an investor-owned organization will detract from profits and hence potentially from take-home pecuniary benefits, assuming these are related. The personal costs of on-the-job benefits are lower for the administrator of the tax-exempt agency, and it is thus hypothesized that more of these nonpecuniary benefits will be demanded.

The implications of this hypothesis for tax-exempt resource allocation are considerable. The hypothesis implies that the tax-exempt agency will use more resources to get a given job done, and so its costs will be higher. The absence of incentives for efficiency has been the target of investigation, including its effect on tax-exempt agency operating costs, particularly in the case of tax-exempt health insurers (Frech, 1976), nursing homes (Borjas, Frech, & Ginsburg, 1983; Frech, 1985), and dialysis units (Lowrie & Hampers, 1981). Similar analyses comparing tax-exempt and investor-owned hospital behavior have not been as conclusive for several reasons.

First, to compare operating costs between tax-exempt and investor-owned hospitals, such variables as case mix, case severity, and quality must be used to adjust results. Assertions have been made that tax-exempt hospitals have a more complex case mix because investor-owned hospitals engage in "cream skimming" by encouraging the admission of low-cost cases. Evidence on this score seems mixed (Bays, 1979a, b; Renn, Schramm, Watt, & Derzon, 1985; Schweitzer & Rafferty, 1976). Even more difficult to determine is whether quality differentials exist by ownership category. Tax-exempt managers do have an incentive to produce quality care (which will show up in higher costs). The role of quality in pushing costs higher has yet to be fully explored.

Another difference that has been uncovered when comparing tax-exempt and investor-owned hospital behavior lies in the pricing area. Charges are the prices set by the hospital for its services. Two California studies found that investor-owned hospitals had higher charges (relative to costs) for ancillary (lab, radiology, pharmacy) services (Eskoz & Peddecord, 1985; Pattison & Katz, 1983). Generally, markups (charge-to-cost ratios) for ancillary services were found to be higher than basic room charges. Investor-owned hospitals also provided more (high-profit) ancillary services per patient than tax-exempts in the studies and were more profitable, although cost levels were similar. One possible explanation of this finding is that tax-exempt managers (or trustees) can gain nonpecuniary benefits from encouraging the use of hospital services by keeping patient charges low (which may result in lower profits) as well as by providing more free care to indigents.

A RAND report by Shugarman, Nicosia, and Schuster (2007) reviewed the literature between 1996 and 2006 regarding comparisons between tax-exempt and investor-owned healthcare organizations. This review provided conflicting evidence on the relationship between the type of hospital ownership and costs but provided consistent evidence that investor-owned nursing homes had lower costs. A study by Wheeler, Burkhardt, Alexander, and Magnus (1999) found that investor-owned hospitals offered less subacute care than did tax-exempt hospitals. When examining the amount of uncompensated care provided, Cram et al. (2010) found that the percentage of admissions that were classified as uninsured was lower in tax-exempt hospitals than in either investor-owned or government hospitals.

A study (Birmingham & Oglesby, 2018) found that tax-exempt hospitals had lower 30-day readmission rates than investor-owned hospitals in both 2010 and 2012, but both types of hospitals reduced their readmission rates after the implementation of the Hospital Readmission Reduction Program. Another study by Li et al. (2018) found that investor-owned inpatient rehabilitation facilities had significantly higher 30-day unplanned readmission rates than did tax-exempt inpatient rehabilitation facilities.

However, relying solely on the incentives identified in the administrator-as-agent model to explain cost and price differences between investor-owned and tax-exempt hospitals would be a mistake. The incentive differences are but one factor operating to influence costs (and possible cost differences) in the two types of organization. The reimbursement system is another major influence on cost and supply behavior. Indeed, the absence of cost differences between tax-exempt and investor-owned hospitals that was uncovered by investigators in California may have been partly due to the reimbursement system, which, at the time of the studies, encouraged cost inflation in all types of hospitals.

Exercises

1. Some 1000 patients called up Dr. Kalikorn and asked him to perform a new surgical procedure. Dr. Kalikorn booked all 1000 and told them that he could perform twice as many procedures if only he had more patients. What is his quantity supplied?

2. The state Medicaid agency sets the price for nursing home care. The unit price is $250 per day. This price is beyond the control of any nursing home. What is the marginal revenue for another patient day at Holly Head Nursing Home?

3. The following is a cost function for clinic visits in a small inner city clinic:

Quantity of Visits Supplied	Total Costs per Week ($)
0	20
1	30
2	60
3	90
4	150
5	230
6	330

a. Determine the marginal cost for each level of output.
b. If the price per visit is given to be $50, at what level of visits will the maximum profit position be? What are the profits at this level? What is the quantity supplied?
c. If the price per visit increases to $90, what will be the quantity supplied (assuming maximizing profits)?

4. Given the following data, answer questions (a) and (b). The total fixed cost for the Grand Forks Clinic is $60 per month. The total variable cost is given as follows:

Quantity of Visits Supplied	Total Variable Costs per Week
1	20
2	50
3	90
4	140
5	210
6	290

a. If the price per visit is $60, what is the quantity supplied?
b. If the total fixed cost increases to $80 and the price per visit is $60, what is the quantity supplied?

5. Given the following cost schedule for a regional hospital that seeks to maximize its profits, answer the following three questions:

Days of Hospital Care Supplied	Total Costs per Day of Care ($)
0	200
1	400
2	800
3	1400
4	2200
5	3200
6	4400

a. If the price per day is $440, what is the quantity supplied?
b. If the price per day increases to $640, what is the quantity supplied?
c. If the price per day is $900, what is the quantity supplied?

6. A clinic receives a per-visit payment of $40. It has an upward-sloping supply curve. Indicate the net effect on the quantity of visits supplied if the following occur:
a. The wage rates for the clinic nursing staff increase.
b. The fixed overhead costs (rent, electricity) increase.
c. The clinic's patients become sicker.
d. The clinic increases productivity.
e. The clinic decides to increase "quality" (defined as a more thorough examination for each patient).

7. Given an upward-sloping supply curve for radiographs by a radiology practice, predict how this curve will shift (supply will increase or decrease) if the following occur:
a. An increase in the wages of radiological technicians
b. A reduction in productivity
c. A decrease in the wages of technicians
d. An increase in the price of radiographs
e. An increase in the quality of services (radiologists spend more care in reading and interpreting radiographs)
f. An increase in the price of film
g. An increase in the number of patients with multiple and rare problems

Bibliography

Auerbach, A. D., Maselli, J., Carter, J., Pekow, P. S., & Lindenauer, P. K. (2010). The relationship between case volume, care quality, and outcomes of complex cancer surgery. *Journal of the American College of Surgeons, 211*(5), 601–608.

Bays, C. (1979a). Case-mix differences between nonprofit and for-profit hospitals. *Inquiry, 14*, 17–21.

Bays, C. (1979b). Cost comparisons of for-profit and nonprofit hospitals. *Social Science and Medicine, 13C*, 219–225.

Birmingham, L. E., & Oglesby, W. H. (2018). Readmission rates in not-for-profit vs. proprietary hospitals before and after the hospital readmission reduction program implementation. *BMC Health Services Research, 18*(1), 31.

Borjas, G. J., Frech, H. E., III, & Ginsburg, P. B. (1983). Property rights and wages: The case of nursing homes. *Journal of Human Resources, 17*, 231–246.

Cram, P., Bayman, L., Popescu, I., Vaughan-Sarrazin, M. S., Cai, X., & Rosenthal, G. E. (2010). Uncompensated care provided by for-profit, not-for-profit, and government-owned hospitals. *Health Services Research, 10*, 90.

Culyer, A. J. (1971). Medical care and the economics of giving. *Economica, 38*, 295–303.

Eskoz, R., & Peddecord, K. M. (1985). The relationship of hospital ownership and service composition to hospital charges. *Health Care Financing Review, 6*, 51–58.

Frech, H. E. (1976). The property rights theory of the firm: Empirical results from a natural experiment. *Journal of Political Economy, 84*, 143–152.

Frech, H. E. (1985). The property rights theory of the firm: Some evidence from the U.S. nursing home industry. *Zeitschrift fur die Gestamte Staatswissenschaft, 141*, 146–166.

Lee, M. L. (1971). A conspicuous production theory of hospital behavior. *Southern Economic Journal, 38*, 48–58.

Li, C. Y., Karmarkar, A., Lin, Y. L., Kuo, Y. F., Ottenbacher, K. J., & Graham, J. F. (2018). Is profit status of inpatient rehabilitation facilities independently associated with 30-day unplanned hospital readmission for Medicare beneficiaries? *Archives of Physical Medicine Rehabilitation, 99*(3), 598–602.

Lowrie, E. G., & Hampers, C. L. (1981). The success of Medicare's end-stage renal disease program. *New England Journal of Medicine, 305*, 434–438.

Pattison, R. V., & Katz, H. M. (1983). Investor-owned and not-for-profit hospitals. *New England Journal of Medicine, 309*, 347–353.

Rantz, M. J., Hicks, L., Petroski, G. F., Madsen, R. W., Alexander, G., Galambos, C., … Greenwald, L. (2010). Cost, staffing, and quality impact of bedside electronic medical record (EMR) in nursing homes. *Journal of the American Medical Directors Association, 11*(7), 485–493.

Renn, S. C., Schramm, C. J., Watt, J. M., & Derzon, R. A. (1985). The effects of ownership and system affiliation on the economic performance of hospitals. *Inquiry, 22*, 219–236.

Schweitzer, S. O., & Rafferty, J. (1976). Variations in hospital product: A comparative analysis of proprietary and voluntary hospitals. *Inquiry, 13*, 158–166.

Shugarman, I. R., Nicosia, N., & Schuster, C. R. (2007). *Comparing for-profit and not-for-profit health care providers: A review of the literature*. Santa Monica, CA: RAND.

Wheeler, J. R., Burkhardt, J., Alexander, J. A., & Magnus, S. A. (1999). Financial and organizational determinants of hospital diversification into subacute care. *Health Services Research, 34*(1, Pt 1), 61–81.

CHAPTER 7

Provider Payment

OBJECTIVES

1. Identify the major types of physician payment and compare their incentives using the principal–agent framework.
2. Explain the Resource-Based Relative Value Scale as a fee-for-service funding instrument.
3. Using the principal–agent framework, explain the incentives associated with each of the major types of hospital payment.
4. Explain the Medicare Severity-Diagnosis-Related Group (MS-DRG) payment system for Medicare.
5. Identify the major methods for paying long-term care facilities.
6. Explain the traditional method by which capitation rates were set by Medicare for health maintenance organizations.
7. Examine the impact of alternative provider payment methods on HMO performance.

7.1 Introduction

In the healthcare field, there is a wide variety of services; the major healthcare services are hospital, physician, pharmaceutical, long-term care facility, and home care and hospice services. In addition, there are a number of combined service units, such as health maintenance organizations, preferred provider organizations, medical homes, and accountable care organizations. For each of these types of services, there are alternative ways of paying the providers for their services. For example, physicians can be paid on a fee-for-service basis, by capitation, per case or episode, or by salary, and hospitals can be paid on the basis of a global budget, on a per-case basis, capitated, on a per diem basis, or for costs already incurred (retrospectively). Earlier, there was a movement toward prospective payment (i.e., payment by predetermined rates) for hospitals and away from retrospective payment, because of the adverse incentives created under retrospective reimbursement.

In recent years, Critical Access Hospitals, however, have had retrospective payment reinstated by Medicare.

Critical Access Hospitals (CAHs) are acute care hospitals that have converted from the original full-service hospital to a more limited service hospital and have received certification from the Centers for Medicare and Medicaid (CMS) as a CAH. They are eligible to receive cost-based payments plus 1% from Medicare, and to include capital improvement costs in the allowable costs for determining Medicare reimbursement. The rationale was this conversion had the potential for increasing revenue and reducing the risk of closure. However, CAHs continue to close at an alarming rate.

CAHs are limited to 25 or fewer acute care beds and must maintain an annual average length of stay of 96 hours or less for their acute care patients. CAHs must also be located more than 35 miles from another hospital, although exceptions are granted based on types of roads, weather, and other extenuating circumstances. In addition, CAHs must provide 24-hour emergency services with medical staff on-site or on-call available on-site within 30 minutes (the limit is 60 minutes if certain frontier area criteria are met).

It has been shown that the rate of payment may influence supplier behavior. In addition, payment bases are not neutral with respect to their impacts; that is, the basis of payment can have an impact on both the quantity and quality of services provided. The theory of agency can be used to shed light on the effects of the different types of payment on provider and consumer behavior. In this chapter, a description of the key forms of provider payment in the health-care field is provided.

7.2 Principal–Agent Relationships Among Payers and Providers

A principal–agent relationship or arrangement exists when one entity or individual (called the agent) acts on behalf of another individual or entity (called the principal). When the agent is an expert at making the necessary decisions that are in the best interest of the principal, and coincide with what the principal would do if he/she possessed sufficient information, knowledge, and expertise, the arrangement usually works well. However, if the interests of the agent and the principal differ or diverge substantially, or there is a conflict of interest between the agent and principal in carrying out the conditions of the arrangement, then the arrangement will usually not work well. For example, a conflict of interest may occur if the benefits to the agent (e.g., more income) from an action differ from the benefits to the principal (e.g., unnecessary care).

In the area of provider payment, the provider, acting as an agent, typically faces at least two principals: the patients being served and, when there is public or private health insurance, the insurers (Blomqvist, 1991). The primary focus in this chapter is on the relationship between payers (insurers) and providers (physicians, hospitals, and long-term care facilities) and the potential implications and impacts of the interactions between payers and providers.

Insurers must pay providers an agreed-upon amount when the providers bill them for services rendered to the members of the insurance plan. The payments for the services provided are designed to cover the average costs incurred by the providers for that service, including a reasonable profit (excess of income over expenses) for the provider. In addition, as will be seen presently, some payment types impose higher risks on the providers than others. Providers, in turn, may demand a risk premium (additional payment) to compensate them for incurring these risks, and if the providers are risk-averse, these risk premiums can be considerable, thus adding substantially to the insurer's costs.

In addition to the payment to providers, insurers and other payers also incur costs of interacting with the providers. These transaction costs include such things as the costs of searching for product availability, characteristics of the products, and prices; costs of negotiating and preparing contracts; costs of monitoring the providers' performance; and costs of enforcing the terms of the contracts. These transaction costs will vary according to the basis of payment. For example, if a particular payment basis encourages the provision of low-quality care or of the provision of excessive services, then additional monitoring and enforcement costs will be imposed on the insurer. In turn, the costs to the insurer are passed on to the consumers in the form of higher premiums. The higher the insurer's cost, the higher the premium the consumer (individually or through an employer) will have to pay. In this chapter, the economic implications of different payment systems in light of these concepts are examined.

7.3 Physician Payment

There are four major types of physician payment: fee-for-service, per case, per capita, and salary payment, as well as hybrid types, in which combinations of these major types are used. Oftentimes, the stated fee-for-service amount quoted is discounted to physicians, so the amount the physician receives is different from the amount charged.

7.3.1 Fee-for-Service Payment

The fee-for-service method of payment is similar to a piece-rate method. Under the fee-for-service method, the physician is paid a specific, predetermined amount for each individual service he or she provides to the patient. The services are broken down into types of units of service, such as a complete physical exam, a new patient visit, a follow-up patient visit, a tonsillectomy, and so on. Typically, the fee to be paid to the provider is set in advance (prospectively) to the service being delivered.

There are several ways in which the fees can be set by the third party. One, which most closely corresponds to the assumption of an absence of control by the provider over the fee, is the relative value scale used by Medicare and other payers (Carroll, 2011; Havighurst & Kissam, 1979; Hsiao & Stason, 1979; Malay, 2011). In this method, each category of service is assigned a relative value in accordance with some criterion (e.g., the number of minutes required to perform the procedure, the cost of supplies involved, the expertise required, the stress the provider incurs in the provision of the service, etc.). For example, in the frequently used earlier surgical component of the California Relative Value Scale, a single coronary bypass operation would have an index number of, for example, 25. This relative value could then be converted to fees by applying a conversion factor, or set dollar amount per unit. This conversion factor is applied to the relative unit values assigned to all services. If the conversion factor was, for example, $500 per point on the relative value scale, the surgeon would be paid $12,500 for the bypass operation.

While Medi-Cal, the California Medicaid program, has developed its own system now, the underlying principles are the same: a relative unit value is determined and a conversion factor is applied to the relative value of the healthcare services. A recent version of this mode of payment is discussed in the next paragraph. In this instance, the physician is viewed as a price taker. The physician can determine the amount of services to provide at that price but cannot influence the price received for the service once it has been set. The amount of services provided to patients then depends upon the provider's marginal cost of production.

A second type of fee setting does not really correspond to the assumption that fees are beyond the control of the individual provider. This method is referred to as the UCR (usual, customary, and reasonable) form of payment. *Usual* refers to the usual or typical fee charged by the billing physician, *customary* refers to fees charged by all physicians in the community, and *reasonable* refers to allowances for particular extenuating circumstances (Epstein & Blumenthal, 1993). Under this system, suppose Dr. Welby performed 100 varicose vein injections and charged an average of $200 per injection. Dr. Welby's usual fee for the procedure would then be $200. The customary fee would be derived from the frequency distribution of the fees charged by all physicians in the community for the procedure (e.g., the physicians in the 10th percentile might charge an average of $110, those in the 20th percentile might charge $126, and so on). The insurer then decides which percentile to use to set an allowable maximum fee. If the payer used the 70th percentile, then the associated charge might be $175. Dr. Welby would then be paid her usual fee or the customary fee, whichever was lower (in her case, the customary fee of $175, because her usual fee is $200).

The reason why the provider is not a pure price taker in this approach is that the provider's fee partly determines the customary fee prevailing in the market. If all physicians (or even some) raise their fees, the customary fee will increase as well. Each physician thus exerts some degree of influence over the market's fees. When there are many physicians in the market, the degree of influence may be small, and for analytical purposes, the physicians might take the customary fee as a given fee. (Note that the fee, in this case, is also beyond the control of the insurer.)

The use of the UCR payment method has often been viewed as inflationary (Miller, 2009; Simoens & Giuffrida, 2004). Because providers know that increasing fees charged in 1 year will impact the amount of the customary rate of fees charged the following year, the incentive provided is to increase the rate charged, creating a spiraling inflationary result. Even though the higher rate charged will not impact the current customary fee in the market, it does influence future customary rates.

The profit-maximizing model is useful for analyzing the effects of the level of rates in a fee-for-service payment system. Because the physician is paid a fixed rate per unit of service provided, the number of units produced will depend on what the payment rate is and on the physician's marginal costs for the specific service. If the marginal cost schedule slopes upward steeply, only a slight addition to supply will result from an increase in the fee (Chernew, Mechanic, Landon, & Safran, 2004; Miller, 2009; Phelps, 1976). Another important factor is the composition of fees. If surgical fees are high relative to general checkup fees, that is, if surgical operations yield considerably more profits relative to checkups, then surgeons will have an incentive to operate more. On the other hand, nonsurgical physicians will not have an incentive to perform more checkups, especially if the fee is set low, so that performing checkups might be only marginally profitable, if at all.

Indeed, fee-for-service payment is believed to encourage physicians to provide more medical care or increase the volume of care provided. As just seen, however, the degree of encouragement, if any, will depend on the relation between the fee and the service's marginal cost. Some analysts have taken the argument one step further and claimed that fee-for-service payment encourages many medically unnecessary practices (Goodwin, Singh, Reddy, Riall, & Yong-Fang, 2011; Klarman, 1963; Swensen et al., 2011). In the context of the present analysis, it is only possible to say whether additional services are likely to be offered; it is not possible to determine whether they would be medically unnecessary.

The fee schedule is a potentially powerful tool that third parties can use to influence both the type of services performed and where they are performed. For example, tonsillectomies are thought to be unnecessary in many instances. If a third party wanted to discourage the provision of this procedure, it could lower the amount of payment to the physician. On the other hand, if a third party wanted to encourage certain procedures to be performed on an outpatient rather than an inpatient basis, it could pay physicians differentially for the same procedure. For example, an insurance company could pay a provider $5000 for a colonoscopy performed in an outpatient setting and only $3000 for the same procedure performed in a hospital.

The profit-maximizing hypothesis can be altered to take into account alternative possible behavior patterns of the physician-owners of medical practices. These behavior patterns are influenced by the payment method. When price is fixed externally, then the provider can impact the quantity of services provided, and that quantity is influenced by the marginal cost of production. Marginal costs to providers include not only the direct costs of supplies, labor, overhead, and such but also the mental (psychological) costs associated with their behavior. How responsive physicians are to payment incentives may be influenced by the physicians' values and community standards.

7.3.2 Per-Case Payment

The second type of physician payment is on a per-case basis. Under this type of payment, the physician is paid a fixed amount for each type of case treated, much like the hospital-based diagnosis-related group (DRG) system. In fact, the DRG system is among the systems considered as a basis for per-case payment (Mitchell, 1985). In per-case payment, the physician bears the cost of any services he or she provides and is paid a sum for the entire case. For example, an obstetrician may be paid a sum for all prenatal care provided during the pregnancy as well as the delivery, regardless of the number of visits provided. If the physician reduces the number of services provided per case, more money will be left over as profit. Concern has been expressed that this payment method may lead to the underservice of patients.

Per-case payment for physicians is not widely being considered for all physicians at this time, in part because studies have indicated that there are wide variations in services for a single case type. This variation would result in difficulties in establishing rates, or fees, and would give providers greater leeway to select cases with potentially low costs and to refer potentially high-cost cases to other providers.

In many cases, it is difficult to determine when an outpatient case begins and when it ends. For example,

how would a beginning point be established for diabetes, especially if preventive interventions are undertaken prior to the onset of diagnosed diabetes? The same concerns arise in the care of most chronic health diseases or conditions; it is very difficult to establish the beginning and ending point of a chronic condition. Per-case payment has been used for obstetrical care by many insurers, in which a set fee is established for prenatal care and delivery. Per-case basis has also been applied to a number of surgical cases for physicians.

The Patient Protection and Affordable Care Act in 2010 has become a catalyst for developing innovative models for delivering and paying for health care in an effort to improve the efficiency and effectiveness of health care. One program, the Medicare Shared Savings Program, establishes financial incentives for Accountable Care Organizations (ACOs) to provide coordinated, well-integrated care across all types of providers. Emphasis in this program is placed on moving away from the fee-for-service chassis that rewarded volume and, instead, reward value and outcome by placing the provider at financial risk for the care required by a specific patient population. The goal of the shared savings program is to achieve better health for individuals, better health for the population, and to lower the rate of growth of healthcare expenditures.

Limitations currently faced by providers, however, include lack of integrated health information systems necessary to provide the clinical and financial data required to coordinate care among providers at different levels efficiently or effectively. ACOs intensify the incentives to improve quality and reduce costs in health care, allowing providers to receive a portion (share) of the savings generated. However, if providers only participated in the savings inside and were not also held accountable for rising costs, then anticipated reductions in the rate of increase were not achieved. While a number of different financial models have been adopted by these early ACOs, increasing emphasis is being placed on bundled payments.

A bundled payment, also known as an episode-based payment, case rate, package pricing, or global payment, is simply a single payment made for all healthcare services that a patient requires related to a specific course of treatment or condition over a period of time; the provider is not paid for each discrete service, interaction, or procedure. The single payment amount covers all providers and services performed for a clinically defined episode of care for a single patient, and that amount is then allocated among all the providers involved in the care of the patients. This bundled payment system is expected to create financial incentives to provide better coordinated care across providers to achieve high-quality outcomes because each provider in the chain of care does not receive a separate payment for every service. Bundled payments are designed to provide incentives for providers to coordinate care provided to patients, improving quality and containing costs.

Medicare's original shared savings program has been overhauled with the program called Pathways to Success. The Pathways to Success program sped up the process of requiring ACOs to take on real risk, but also offered ACOs the flexibility needed to coordinate care and innovate. One feature of the new program included increased access to telehealth services, including services provided to a patient in their place of residence. Also, ACOs were provided the ability to offer new incentive payments to Medicare beneficiaries if the beneficiary undertook actions to achieve good health, such as obtaining primary care services and any necessary follow-up care to improve outcomes. Many ACOs participating in the new program are taking on risk for spending increases above the cost targets in exchange for higher levels of shared savings and greater regulatory flexibility. If ACOs accept a sufficient level of risk, they can qualify as an advanced alternative payment model (APM). These advanced APM ACOs are exempt from the merit-based incentive payment system (MIPS) program and may qualify for additional incentive payments (Verma, 2019).

The merit-based incentive program adjusts payment to the group of providers based on their performance in four categories: quality, cost, promoting interoperability, and improvement activities. The performance categories are given different weights and used to calculate a final score (0–100), and these weights will change over time. For example, in 2019, the quality performance category accounts for 45% of the final score, but by 2021, quality performance will account for only 35% of the total score. A group's final score is compared to a performance threshold to determine payment adjustments. In 2019, the total performance threshold is 30 points. If a group's final score is above the threshold, then the group will receive a positive payment adjustment. If the final score of the group is below the threshold, the group will receive a negative payment adjustment. If the group's final score is equal to the threshold, then the group will receive a neutral payment adjustment. Groups in the lowest quartile will receive the maximum payment adjustment for a performance period (Staheli, 2016).

7.3.3 Per Capita and Salary Payment

The incentives for physicians who are paid on a per capita or a salary basis are decidedly different than the incentives in fee-for-service payment. In both cases, there is some incentive for physicians to provide no more than the basic minimum level of services. However, a physician who intends to remain in practice a long time could not afford to allow the quality of services to fall to too low a level.

Considerable evidence exists regarding the impact that the payment system has on physician practices. Reference has been made to the large difference in surgical operations in the United States and England, and the difference in general payment patterns is considered one underlying factor. In England, surgeons were, traditionally, paid on a salary basis, while in the United States, the usual payment basis is fee-for-service (Aaron & Schwartz, 1984; Chung et al., 2010), although the fee schedule has been changed considerably since the introduction of the Resource-Based Relative Value Scale (RBRVS) by Medicare.

In the United States, several physician payment experiments have been undertaken (Eisenberg & Williams, 1981; Myers & Schroeder, 1981; Rudmik, Wranik, & Rudisill-Michaelsen, 2014). In one, primary care physicians were given financial responsibility for the entire healthcare expenditures of their patients (a global capitation system); they shared in any surpluses of premiums over total medical care costs (including hospitalization costs, specialists' fees, laboratory fees, radiology fees, etc.), as well as in any deficits. The incentive was for them to reduce the expenditures paid out so that the surpluses they retained would be greater.

This global capitation experiment was based on a view of the physician as "gatekeeper" to the healthcare system, someone who has the ability to control a good deal of the patient's cost. The results showed a considerable reduction in overall expenses relative to a fee-for-service comparison group (Moore, 1979). Another study examined how physician prescribing behavior was affected by an ambulatory care center's introduction of monetary incentives to generate additional business. The findings showed there was a substantial increase in radiographs ordered by the physicians (Hemenway, Killen, Cashman, Parks, & Bicknell, 1990).

Briefly, capitation is a payment method by which a healthcare provider is paid a fixed amount of money for each individual enrolled in his/her member panel, usually on a monthly basis, regardless of whether or not the individual uses any services. The provider is placed at financial risk for all members in his/her panel. If the cost of services provided to the members of the panel is less than the fixed amount, then the provider retains the difference as additional income; if the costs are greater, then the provider suffers a loss in income. Capitation creates an incentive for providers to be efficient and effective in the provision of care in order to contain costs. A concern raised by capitation is that providers may in fact have an incentive to provide too few services to panel members or to limit members' access to services.

Salaried physicians, on the other hand, are paid a fixed amount (weekly or monthly usually), and the amount of the payment is not tied to the number of enrollees or the amount of services rendered, either in terms of services performed during each visit or the number of visits the member has. With a salary, the physician does not have a direct financial incentive to change treatment patterns because he/she does not face a financial risk, other than possible future salary increases. Under a salaried system, however, the physician does not have an incentive to increase the number of patients seen during office hours.

7.3.4 Agency Theory and Physician Payment

Many investigators have linked the fee-for-service payment system with the generation of a high volume of services and consequently with high expenditure levels. Usually, fee-for-service is compared with capitation funding in these investigations.

Under any payment system, the physician has the ability to generate additional services because of the information asymmetry between physician and patient. Information asymmetry occurs when at least some relevant information for the transaction is known to some, but not all, of the parties involved. This creates an imbalance of power in the decision-making process, potentially resulting in inefficiencies in market transactions. When acquiring information is expensive, such as a patient obtaining complete information regarding the symptoms and diagnosis of medical conditions and the treatment options available, then decisions may be delegated to the "expert" physician. In health care, this delegation removes the independence between demand and supply because the physician is also the supplier of the services demanded.

Under fee-for-service, the physician has the incentive to generate more services, especially if the fee exceeds the marginal cost of the service. By comparison, the physician will not have such an incentive under capitation. If the physician is not concerned about repeat visits, then he or she will have an incentive to reduce the volume of visits. However, if the physician has a desire to encourage repeat visits and continued enrollment by patients in his panel, then he or she will not want to reduce services to the point at which quality of care is compromised.

The capitation payment system imposes risks on the provider; the provider must incur the costs of all services for all patients enrolled in his/her panel, including the very high-cost ones. In determining his or her capitation rates, the provider will add a risk premium that will vary with his or her degree of risk aversion. This will be very high if the provider is risk-averse. A risk-averse provider is cautious, and desires to minimize exposure to risk, even when the potential benefit of the activity is rather large. The risk-averse provider, if given a choice, will select a guaranteed payoff rather than gamble that a payoff might be substantially larger. For example, if offered 50 cents guaranteed or offered a chance to receive a dollar or nothing depending on the results of the flip of a coin (which, technically, has a 50–50 chance of winning or losing), the risk-averse individual will select the guaranteed 50 cents.

A third-party payer (insurer) will incur contract costs under both fee-for-service and capitation funding. Under fee-for-service funding, the insurer must monitor the provider for excessive provision of services, while under capitation funding, the insurer must monitor the provider for low quality of care due to insufficient provision of services. There is no predetermined answer as to which funding system is more costly once societal costs are included, although most commentators would say that fee-for-service costs more.

7.3.5 A Resource-Based Relative Value Scale

Although Medicare had regulated fees since 1984, in 1989, Medicare adopted a variant of the UCR (usual, customary, and reasonable) system called *customary, prevailing,* and *reasonable* (CPR), where reasonable incorporates extenuating circumstances. In 1992, a new fee schedule was adopted to replace the old fee system. The new schedule has fixed fees that were based on resource-use measures. This system, called the resource-based relative value scale (RBRVS), attempts to classify the costs that would be incurred by physicians operating in a competitive environment. Based on the current procedural terminology (CPT) classification of conditions and interventions, a questionnaire was developed to capture the costs incurred in the classification scheme. The questionnaire was applied to national samples of physicians in 18 different specialties to develop a relative cost schedule for physician procedures or services. The cost categories include costs related to actual work done by a physician, costs of operating practices, and practice liability (malpractice) insurance.

The national survey interviewed a sample of physicians about the physicians' time required, mental effort and judgment, physical effort and technical skill, and psychological stress associated with each procedure (Hsiao et al., 1988). These elements were combined into the physician work component. For example, an office visit for internal medicine might have had a work index of 100, whereas a resection for rectal carcinoma might have had an index value of 445. To these work indexes were added practice cost factors and the professional liability insurance costs. Practice costs were determined by specialty based on a survey of costs and revenues by physicians in each specialty. Beginning in 1998, some CPT codes were assigned two RVUs: a lower unit value for procedures performed in a facility and a greater one for procedures or services performed at a nonfacility site (e.g., a physician's office or a patient's home). On average, the physician work component accounts for 51% of the total relative value for each service, the practice expense component accounts for 45%, and the professional liability component accounts for 4%.

In 2000, CMS replaced the cost-based professional liability of relative values with resource-based professional liability insurance RVUs. In addition, each CPT code is assigned a "global period" value that incorporates the following: (1) preoperative visits after the decision is made to operate beginning with the day before the day of surgery for major procedures and the day of surgery for minor procedures; (2) intraoperative services that are normally a usual and necessary part of a surgical procedure; and (3) all additional medical or surgical services required of the surgeon during the postoperative period of the surgery because of complications which do not require additional trips to the operating room.

Since costs vary by geographic location, CMS also establishes three geographic practice cost indices (GPCIs). The cost of living GPCI is applied to the physician work relative values, the practice cost GPCI is applied to practice expense relative values, and the professional liability insurance costs GPCI is applied to professional liability relative values.

The results of the calculations indicate the value of the services relative to each other, not their value in dollars. The relative valuations must then be assigned a dollar value, the conversion rate, in order to be translated into a fee schedule. For example, if the dollar value assigned to the schedule was $1 per index point, then the physician would receive $445 for a resection for rectal carcinoma (which was given an index value of 445 points).

The relative value of each service is multiplied by Geographic Practice Cost Indices (GPCIs) to adjust for locality cost differences. Differences are also paid based on facility or nonfacility practice type. Because the physician work relative values are based on the CPT (Current Procedural Terminology) codes, new and revised codes necessitate annual revisions in the RBRVS. The CPT codes reflect tasks and services performed by a medical practitioner in the provision of medical, surgical, and diagnostic care. In 2019, there were over 10,000 CPT codes in use. Medicare actually uses HCPCS codes (Healthcare Common Procedure Coding System); their Level I HCPCS codes are identical to CPT codes, and their Level II codes are additional codes typically associated with services provided outside the physician's office.

CMS publishes information on RVUs for CPT codes in the Federal Register. The CY 2019 conversion factor was $36.0391 (Federal Register, 2018). The effects of such changes can be analyzed in terms of the supply analysis presented in this chapter. An increase in the fee for a procedure should increase the quantity supplied of that procedure, and a reduction should reduce the quantity supplied. Thus, for those procedures whose fees are increased, the quantity supplied will increase.

This is shown in **Figure 7-1**, in which S_1 is a supply curve for a single profit-maximizing physician (ignore S_2 for the moment). Initially, the fee for an office visit is $40, and at this level the physician will be willing to supply 240 office visits. An increase in the fee to $100 will result in a willingness to supply 650 visits. According to this analysis, a fee increase will increase the quantity of procedures and a fee reduction will reduce the quantity. It should be noted that this discussion is restricted to the issue of supply. The number of services actually provided will depend on the quantity of services *demanded*.

Curve S_1 shows a situation where higher fees result in more labor (and less leisure). Curve S_2 shows the case where higher fees result in physicians taking more leisure time and cutting back on work. The behaviors in the two cases are the same up to where the fee per visit is $40.

There are some other qualifications that should be kept in mind. The first is the appropriateness of this analysis for dealing with labor supply issues. After all,

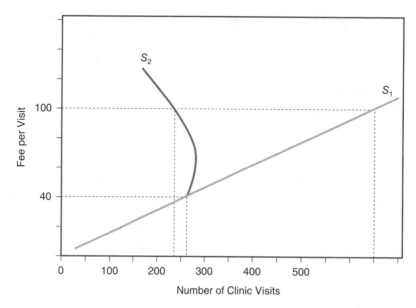

Figure 7-1 Supply curves for physician services under two sets of assumptions. Curve S_1 shows a situation where higher fees result in more labor (and less leisure). Curve S_2 to show the case were higher fees result in physicians taking more leisure time and cutting back on work. The behaviors in the two cases are the same up to where the fee per visit is $40.

© Jones & Bartlett Learning.

the physician's labor (work effort) is a key factor in the supply of physician visits. Individual physicians have limitations on their work time, and the supply model needs to be modified to take this into account.

At lower income and wage levels, the propensity to substitute work for leisure may be strong enough to more than offset the income effect. As the wage rate rises, the physician can work more hours to earn even more income—in other words, shift leisure hours to work hours, and the substitution effect dominates. An upward-sloping supply curve would result. However, at higher wage levels, the physician may work fewer hours and spend more hours in leisure activities, in which case the income effect may more than offset the substitution effect, and a backward-bending supply curve would result. In this case, the supply curve would slope upward and to the left. Recall that the income effect reflects the change in the described hours of work resulting from a change in income when the wage is held constant. The substitution effect reflects the change in desired hours of work resulting from a change in the wage rate, holding income constant. Leisure is a normal good and so higher income implies a desire for more leisure and fewer hours of work (income effect), but a higher wage raises the relative price of leisure, implying a desire for more hours of work (substitution effect). The net effect will depend upon which of the two effects is stronger.

In this example, in Figure 7-1 where S_1 and S_2 diverge, S_1 shows the substitution effect dominating

and S_2 shows the income effect dominating. Up to this point, where it begins to bend backward, the supply curve of S_2 is the same as the supply curve of S_1. The supply curve of S_2 begins to bend back just before 300 office visits. Up to the fee of $40, the physician behaves as in curve S_1. If the fee rises above $40 per visit, the physician's supply will increase in smaller amounts and eventually begin to decrease. If this is the way physicians behave, then raising fees above the maximum point will cause physicians to cut back on the number of services they are willing to provide. An increase in primary care fees, then, may not necessarily cause an increase in the quantity of primary care supplied. However, there is little evidence to support the notion of a backward-sloping supply curve of labor in the physician market.

7.4 Hospital Payment

7.4.1 Alternative Bases of Payment

Until the early 1980s, hospitals were paid on a retrospective cost basis. That is, a third-party insurer would pay a hospital for the expenses it had already incurred in the provision of services (if payment was on a cost basis) or the charges it had already billed (if payment was on a charge basis). There are numerous variations of retrospective payment. The third party can pay on a cost-plus basis, which means it can pay the hospital for its allowable operating costs plus a specified amount (say, 2% of costs) for capital equipment. In another method of payment, the third party pays the hospital whichever is lower, costs or charges. There is also considerable variation in how costs are defined. Allowable costs could exclude costs not directly related to patient care (e.g., indirect educational costs). Whatever the arrangement, retrospective payment has one overriding effect on supply and costs: it encourages an organization to expand. Increases in both the scope and quality of services tend to occur, and if the provider is a maximizer of anything (e.g., profits or perquisites), retrospective payment can lead to higher costs, more services, and higher quality services.

In response to this recognized bias in retrospective payment, a number of prospective payment plans have been introduced. Prospective payment involves setting the basis of payment before the payment period in which the services are provided. As a result, this sort of payment schema puts the provider "at risk" for any excess of cost over revenue. There are many different bases for setting the rate of prospective payments and an infinite number of rate levels. In this section, several of the alternatives are examined and their hypothesized effects on cost and quantity discussed.

To help classify the effects of different types of payment to hospitals, the following formula will be used to break out the components of total cost: Total Cost = Cost per service × Services per Day × Days of Stay per Admission × Number of Admissions. Now the likely effect of three types of prospective payment—per service, per diem (per day), and per admission—on an output-maximizing hospital will be explored.

In per-service payment, the hospital will receive a fixed prespecified amount for each service performed (e.g., an operation, a radiograph, or kidney dialysis). The amount for each service is set in advance (e.g., $90 for a specific lab test, $3275 for a complete full-body CT scan, etc.). The second method of payment is per diem, or per day, payment. Under this method, an amount to be paid for a hospitalization is arrived at by multiplying the payment amount per day by the number of days of care provided. The third prospective payment method, per-admission payment, rewards the hospital only for adding more patients. Under the per-admission method, payers usually adjust the payment by a case-mix or severity index because cases differ considerably by diagnosis and severity. For a discussion of a diagnosis-adjusted per-admission payment system, see Section 7.5. Even cases within a diagnosis group may differ from one another; in such circumstances, the per-admission and per diem bases of payment may be combined. This will be discussed next.

7.4.2 Agency Theory and Hospital Payment

The agency framework can be used to analyze the effects of the different hospital payment schema. As usual, the key issues include uncertainty, information asymmetry, and monitoring and other transaction costs.

7.4.2.1 Retrospective Payments

Retrospective payment is the funding of allowable costs that were actually incurred in the provision of services. Under retrospective funding, the payer incurs all the financial risks. Under retrospective payment, the provider has an incentive to increase the quality and volume of services, as it will receive payment for these; the hospital bears no financial risks. In order to protect itself financially, the payer must incur substantial expenses to set standards and monitor and enforce them. These transaction costs can be quite high because of the technical nature of medical care, including the wide variety of diagnoses and treatments; the complexity of the product leads to information asymmetries such that the provider may have considerably more technical and detailed knowledge of the patient than does the payer. These factors increase the monitoring and regulatory cost to the payer.

7.4.2.2 Prospective Fee-for-Service System

Prospective payment means setting the rate in advance of the provision of the service. Fee-for-service means that a fee for each service is set before the services are provided. Under this type of payment, almost all of the financial risk is still imposed on the payer. This is because all services provided by the hospital will be paid for by the payer. As long as the per-service rate exceeds the hospital's marginal cost, the hospital will have an incentive to add additional services. The payer would have to set standards and monitor and enforce them, thus incurring costs. The detailed knowledge possessed by the hospitals would create considerable information asymmetries. Information asymmetries would add considerably to the costs incurred by the payers.

7.4.2.3 Per Diem Fees

Under a flat per diem fee (e.g., $4000 per day in 2019), there will be a sharing of financial risks between the payer and the hospital. The longer the hospital keeps the patient, the more it will be paid. Because the latter part of most hospital stays is less costly to the hospital than the earlier portion, since most tests and procedures occur in the first few days, the per diem rates are likely to exceed the marginal costs of the latter part of a stay. This provides an incentive for the hospital to extend the patient's stay.

The actual rates paid in relation to cost will create very important incentives. The per diem cost of a case depends on the diagnosis. For example, a liver transplant case will have daily costs that are well above the average; in 2019, the average cost of a liver transplant was $500,000. A hospital that performs transplants could lose money on such operations if the same rate was applied to each day of stay regardless of diagnosis or procedure. The provider would require a risk premium if a flat per diem payment system were implemented because the hospital might demand additional compensation if it admits and treats high-cost cases.

In addition, the payer would incur the cost of monitoring the stays. The hospital will have considerable leeway in extending stays; because the hospital has considerably more information on the patients and their conditions than the payers, information asymmetries will arise. One factor that must be kept in mind is that it is the physician who controls admission to and discharge from the hospital, not the hospital administrators. While hospitals can influence physicians, they do not control the final decisions. The payer would have to develop standards, write contracts, monitor these, and enforce them. These costs could be substantial to the payer.

7.4.2.4 Per-Case Payment

Because of the wide range of diagnoses and treatments, almost all per-case payment systems make use of case-mix groups. Each group contains cases that use roughly the same amount of resources, and payers pay the hospitals the same sum of money for all cases within each group. Under such a system, the risk to the payer is reduced considerably. However, there is still a wide range of costs within each diagnosis group; sometimes, the within-group variation in resource use is said to be due to "severity." Hospitals that attract higher severity cases, either because they are referral centers or inner-city hospitals, may lose money due to the higher costs. They may, therefore, refuse to accept such cases without some kind of severity adjustment. In addition to these additional costs, a case-mix system contains considerable informational asymmetries. The providing hospitals have considerable discretion in assigning patients to diagnosis groups. In order to counteract this tendency, the payer will have to develop an adequate reporting system and ensure that

it is being followed. The development and maintenance of such a system will impose considerable costs on the payer.

7.4.2.5 Per-Case Payment with Adjustment for Outliers

In order to reduce the costs imposed on providers who accept more severe cases under a flat per-case payment system, many payers have developed a two-part system. Cases within each diagnosis group are divided into two groups, typical cases and outliers. Using the distribution of stays within each diagnosis group, a trim point is established that separates long-stay outliers from typical cases. The actual setting of the trim point is arbitrary and depends on how much pressure the payer wants to impose on the provider to reduce its stays. Outliers are paid in two parts: a per-case portion to cover those days inside of the trim and an additional per diem payment to cover the additional days. Thus, the risk of very high-cost cases due to very long stays will be borne, in a large part, by the payer. Outliers can also be established for cases that result in abnormally high cost for the diagnosis for reasons other than length of stay. Again, the risk is shifted to the payer for these cases.

7.4.3 Other Hospital Payment Issues

When evaluating types of hospital payment, several things have to be kept in mind. First, a distinction must be made between an all-payer system and a multipayer system. In an all-payer system, each payer pays the same rate for each service. For example, assume that Medicare, Blue Cross, and commercial insurers each have one-third of the overall caseload of 300 cases in a hospital, and that the case mixes and severities of the patient groups are identical (so there is no objective basis for differential payments among the three payers). Assume further that the regulatory authority in the state has determined that the hospital's allowable revenues should be $900,000 for these 300 cases. This means that each insurer "should" pay $300,000, and this is what each insurer would pay in an all-payer system.

A multipayer system is more like a free-for-all, with each payer setting up its payment rules unilaterally or based on market principles. For example, assume in the preceding example that the regulatory agency regulates only Medicare and Blue Cross rates and that it allows each to pay $270,000 instead of the original $300,000. The commercial group rates, however, are unregulated. In this instance, the hospital must charge the commercials more to cover its deficit, since Medicare and Blue Cross only pay $540,000 of the $900,000 revenues required. Whether or not it collects all its bills is another issue. What is significant here is that the hospital is no longer simply a price taker, and so a more complex model that can incorporate the reaction by the hospital to the unregulated rate is needed.

A second important factor to keep in mind is that other parts of the healthcare system may be affected by the hospital payment type and level. For example, if a system penalizes a hospital for keeping patients hospitalized for more than a specified time, this will most certainly reduce length of stay in the hospital. It may have other effects as well. For instance, if home health care or long-term care facility care is paid separately, the hospital may open up a long-term care facility or begin a home healthcare program to which it could discharge its patients, especially if there is not a sufficient supply of the services available to handle the increased demand as patients are discharged sooner.

A considerable number of experiments with prospective payment have also been conducted at the state level (Alderwick, Hood-Ronick, & Gottlieb, 2019; Bauer, 1977; Carter, Jacobson, Kominski, & Perry, 1994; McConnell et al., 2017; Simoens & Giuffrida, 2004). Most of these have occurred in multipayer systems, and so their effects are harder to identify than they would be in an all-payer system. One such experiment, conducted by the New York State legislature, set rates on a per diem basis for Medicare- and Blue Cross-paid patients according to a preestablished formula beginning in 1970. This had the effect of rewarding hospitals for longer stays. In testing for the effect of this type of payment, a comparison was made between length of stay and occupancy rates after 1970 in New York State and those in several comparison states, where prospective per diem rates were not in force (Ohio and the New England states). Between 1970 and 1974, New York showed a slight increase in the average length of stay and no net change in the occupancy rate (i.e., the average percentage of beds filled). Both of these indicators of hospital supply decreased considerably in the control states during the same period of time. This suggests that the payment mechanism had its expected effect (Berry, 1976).

A 2019 study by Frank and Fry examines the impact of Medicaid expansion on access to Naloxone, a drug that can reduce deaths due to opioid overdose. The Affordable Care Act (ACA) included a provision that gave states the option of expanding their Medicaid program to cover low-income, childless adults,

with the federal government assuming a higher majority of these additional costs (100% of the costs in the early implementation years and 90% in subsequent years). As of 2018, 37 states had expanded their Medicaid program, and 14 states had not. In this study, the amount of Medicaid-covered Naloxone used between 2009 and 2016 was examined in terms of participation in Medicaid expansion or not. The authors found that before Medicaid expansion, the number of Naloxone prescriptions per Medicaid enrollee were similar in expansion and nonexpansion states. On average, the states that participated in the Medicaid expansion program had 78.2 more prescriptions for Naloxone per year compared to states that did not expand Medicaid (a nearly 10-fold increase over the preexpansion years. The conclusion was that Medicaid expansion contributed to the growth in Medicaid-covered Naloxone more than state-level Naloxone policies, reflecting the impact of reduced cost on increased demand.

7.5 Diagnosis-Related Groups

In 1983, the federal government introduced a new prospective payment system (PPS) for Medicare Part A hospital patients. In this system, payment for all Medicare discharges is on a per-diagnosis basis. The following discussion reviews how diagnoses are grouped into separate diagnosis-related groups (DRGs) and how rates are set for each DRG.

The DRG system is one of many possible ways of classifying patients according to common elements (Hornbrook, 1982). There is the presumption that, if the classification system is to be used for payment purposes, all cases in each group must be similar with regard to resource use. Based on several patient characteristics (the major diagnostic group, the presence of comorbid diagnoses, the presence of a surgical procedure, and discharge status), an algorithm was developed to assign individual cases to groupings that exhibit common resource-use tendencies (as measured by length of stay) (Fetter, Youngsoo, Freeman, Averill, & Thompson, 1980).

In 2007, the DRG system was substantially revised, and the newly restructured DRGs are now known as MS-DRGs (Medicare Severity-Diagnosis Related Groups), and the numbering goes through 999, although gaps have been left throughout the sequence of numbers to allow for modifications and new MS-DRGs in the same body system to be located more closely in the numerical sequence. One additional modification in 2008 involved hospital-acquired conditions; these conditions are no longer considered to be complications if they were not present on admission, which results in reduced payment from Medicare for conditions apparently caused by the hospital. **Figure 7-2** provides the logic used in the development of Medicare Severity-Diagnosis Related Groups.

Once a major diagnostic category has been determined, then the first branch involves the performance of an operation procedure. If surgery was performed, then the type of surgery is determined. If no surgery, then the principal diagnosis is determined. For either surgery or no surgery, if applicable, then whether or not a complication or comorbid condition occurred is determined.

In the MS-DRG system, there were a total of 761 DRGs in 2019; CMS implemented 18 new MS-DRGs for FY 2019 and deleted 11 MS-DRGs. Under the new system, the age 0–17 category has been dropped. The main patient characteristics now incorporated in the determination of the classification of the patient are the principal diagnosis, up to 25 additional diagnoses, and up to 25 procedures performed during the stay. In a small number of cases, classification is also based on the age, sex, and discharge status of the patient.

There are now three levels of severity: MCC—Major Complication/Comorbidity, which reflects the highest level of severity; CC—Complication/Comorbidity, which is the next level of severity; and Non-CC—Non-Complication/Comorbidity, which does not significantly affect severity of illness and resource use.

MS-DRGs were developed based on the major diagnostic groups the disorders fell into and on such factors as the need for surgery and the presence of complicating diagnoses. The criteria were selected so that cases in each category would use similar amounts of resources and thus could be paid with a single rate. There were 538 categories in the 2006 DRG classification system and 761 in the 2019 MS-DRG system.

Based on cross-hospital studies, an average cost for each DRG was estimated. Factors in the calculation included the lengths of stay (within the DRG) in routine and special care, per diem costs in routine and special care, and the estimated per-case cost of ancillary services (laboratory, radiology, drugs, medical supplies, anesthesia, and other services) (Pettengill & Vertrees, 1982). Each DRG was then assigned a relative weight intended to approximate the relative amount of resources used by an average case in the group.

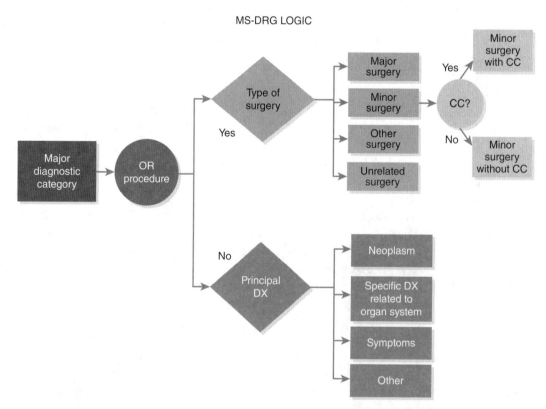

MS-DRG LOGIC

Figure 7-2 Logic used in the determination of MS-DRGs. Once a major diagnostic category has been determined, then the first branch involves the performance of an operation procedure. If surgery was performed, then the type of surgery is determined. If no surgery, then the principal diagnosis is determined. For either surgery or no surgery, if applicable, then whether or not a complication or comorbid condition occurred is determined.

For example, in 2019, a rectal resection without an MCC (DRG 332) had an assigned weight of 3.3982, and a digestive malignancy with percutaneous transluminal coronary angioplasty (PTCA) without CC/MCC (DRG 376) had an assigned weight of 0.9157. This means that, in comparison to an "average" diagnostic group (with a weight set equal to 1), a typical case of DRG 332 uses 3.3982 times the average amount of resources, and a case of DRG 376 uses fewer than average resources at 0.9157 times the average amount.

Using these weights and the frequency of types of cases, a hospital can develop a case-mix-adjusted admissions measure. This measure would presumably be a better approximation of the resources required to serve the hospital's patient population than mere admissions or patient days (which have traditionally been used).

For example, assume that both Aiken and Bethesda General Hospitals treated 200 patients in 2019, with an average length of stay of 5 days. Both would have a measured output of 1000 patient days. Assume, however, that of Aiken's 200 cases, half were heart failure and shock without CC/MCC (MS-DRG 293, with a weight equal to 0.6553) and half were heart failure and shock with MCC (MS-DRG 291, with a weight equal to 1.3458). Then Aiken's case-mix-adjusted measure of admissions would be equal to 200.11 [(0.6553 × 100) + (1.3458 × 100)]. Bethesda's case mix included 100 cases of coronary bypass with PTCA with MCC (MS-DRG 231), with a weight equal to 8.2115 and 100 cases of coronary bypass without cardiac catheterization without MCC (MS-DRG 236), with a weight equal to 4.0291). Bethesda's adjusted output would be equal to 1224.06 [(8.2115 × 100) + (4.0291 × 100)].

With the hospital's output being measured in terms of case-weighted admissions, a payment rate (called a standardized payment amount or conversion factor) must be set for each single point (relative weight = 1.00). Originally, this rate had national-, regional-, and hospital-specific components. Currently, the standardized amount includes a labor-related share and a nonlabor-related share. The labor-related share is adjusted by a wage index to reflect area differences in the cost of labor. The wage-adjusted standardized amount is multiplied by a relative weight for the MS-DRG. In 2020, the national operating standardized amount was $5654.12.

If the wage index of the region in which the hospital is located is greater than 1, then the labor share of the national adjusted operating standardized amount for 2020 was 68.3% and a nonlabor share was 31.7%. If the wage index is less than or equal to 1, then the labor share of the national adjusted operating standardized amount for 2020 was 62% and the nonlabor-related share was 38%. In addition, these rates were further adjusted for the following in 2020: (1) if the hospital submitted quality data and was a meaningful electronic health record (EHR) user an additional 2.6% was added to the labor and nonlabor-related rates; (2) if the hospital submitted quality data but was not a meaningful EHR user then only 0.35% was added to the rates; (3) if the hospital did not submit quality data but was a meaningful EHR user, then an additional 1.85% was added to the rates; or (4) if the hospital did not submit quality data and was not a meaningful EHR user, then 0.4% was deducted from the labor-related and nonlabor-related rates.

In 2020, the capital standard federal payment rate that was awarded to eligible hospitals was $462.61 (FY2020 FR Tables 1A–1E). To qualify for a capital payment adjustment based on new technology or new medical services, hospitals must demonstrate that the new technology or service is a substantial clinical improvement over technologies or services otherwise available, and that, absent the add-on payment, the hospital would be inadequately paid under the regular MS DRG system.

Under the Hospital-acquired Condition Reduction program, hospitals will incur a 1% payment reduction if they rank in the worst-performing quartile (25%) of all applicable hospitals, relative to the national average, of conditions acquired during the applicable period and on all the hospital's discharges for the specified fiscal year. The goal is to create an incentive to improve quality of care by reducing issues leading to hospital infections.

If a hospital treats a high percentage of certain low-income patients, it receives a percentage add-on payment applied to the MS-DRG adjusted-base payment rate. This add-on payment is known as the disproportionate share hospital (DSH) adjustment. If a hospital is training residents in approved residency programs, it receives a percentage add-on payment for each case paid, which is known as the indirect medical education (IME) adjustment. The percentage the hospital receives for IME depends on the ratio of residents to patients.

In addition, hospitals receive a reduction to their base operating payment if they are found to have excess readmissions based on the hospital's risk-adjusted readmission rate for acute myocardial infarction (AMI), heart failure (HF), pneumonia, chronic obstructive pulmonary disease (COPD), elective primary total hip arthroplasty/total knee arthroplasty

Table 7-1 Relative Weights for Selected MS-DRGs, 2019

MS-DRG	MDC	Type	MS-DRG Title (Description)	Relative Weight
332	06	Surg	Rectal resection W MCC	3.3982
333	06	Surg	Rectal resection W CC	1.9278
334	06	Surg	Rectal resection W/O CC/MCC	1.3062
374	06	Med	Digestive malignancy W MCC	2.0650
375	06	Med	Digestive malignancy W CC	1.2067
376	06	Med	Digestive malignancy W/O CC/MCC	0.9157

Table developed from information on CMS website, FY_2019 NPRM: Table 5. https://www.cms.gov/Medicare/Medicare-Fee-for-Service-Payment/AcuteInpatientPPS/FY-2012-IPPS-Final-Rule-Home-Page-Items/CMS1250520.html

(THA, TKA), and coronary artery bypass graft (CABG) surgery (**Table 7-1**).

Medicare also pays the hospitals for certain additional costs that fall outside of the basic case-mix formula known as outlier-related costs. An *outlier* is a case whose cost is sufficiently high that it falls outside certain predetermined limits. Outlier rules were developed to pay hospitals for cases that used an unusually high amount of resources. Rates for paying hospitals for outlying portions of cases are set by Congress. Originally, there were two kinds of outliers: day and cost outliers. A day outlier for a specific DRG was a case whose length of stay exceeded a preset number of days (e.g., 24 days if the DRG had an average length of stay of 6 days); all days in excess of this trim point (e.g., 24 days) were called *outlying days*. For example, if the trim point for DRG 103 is 24 and a case has a stay of 32 days, then 8 of these days will be deemed outlying days and additional payment made to the hospital for these 8 days. The hospital had to absorb the costs of the days between the DRG specified days and the trim point.

In 1997, Medicare stopped paying for long-stay outliers and provided extra funding only on the basis of high-cost cases. A high-cost outlier is one whose adjusted charges exceed the fixed loss threshold ($27,545 in FY 2019). For these cases, charges submitted by the hospital are adjusted using the cost-to-charge ratio of the hospital. The cost-to-charge ratio is the ratio between a hospital's expenses and what it charges. A hospital-specific cost-to-charge ratio is applied to the covered charges for a case to determine whether the costs of the case exceed the fixed-loss outlier threshold. Payments for eligible cases are then made based on a marginal cost factor, which is a percentage of the costs above the threshold. In 2019, the percentage was 80%. Outlier payments cover about 5.1% of total per-case payment, and their importance will vary depending on the degree of complexity of the hospital's cases.

7.6 Long-Term Care Facility Payment

Because there is such wide variability in long-term care facility (nursing home) lengths of stay, it is not feasible to pay long-term care facilities on a per-case basis. They are, therefore, typically funded on a per diem basis. Medicaid state agencies, being the largest third-party payers of long-term care facilities, have traditionally paid long-term care facilities in two different ways: with a flat per diem (per day) rate or with a facility-specific per diem rate. Facility-specific rates are largely retrospective and consequently can result in high costs. In flat-rate payment, a single rate is paid to all long-term care facilities, regardless of patient characteristics, quality levels, and so on. Often, a separate rate will be paid by level of facility—skilled nursing facility (SNF) or intermediate care facility (ICF).

One feature of the flat rate is that, at least in the case of investor-owned long-term care facilities, the facilities have an incentive to minimize costs. This may lead to some problems, however. Long-term care facilities might seek to attract patients who are healthier or who need less care (and hence cost less to treat), or they might compromise on quality (which would also lower costs and increase profits). As long as long-term care facilities seek profits to some degree (they might also have other objectives), they will tend to lower costs when such a payment mechanism is in place. It is primarily to balance the incentive to select patients with fewer needs that case-mix measures have been introduced (Schlenker,

1986). The primary purpose of case-mix payment in long-term care is to relate payment rates to required levels of care and help ensure that patients receive appropriate care.

One case-mix measure that has been developed is called *Resource Utilization Groups* (RUGs) (Fries & Cooney, 1985). This measure has now been superseded by RUGs II (Micheletti & Shlala, 1986), RUGs III (Fries et al., 1994), and RUGs IV (Urban Institute, 2007). The RUGs case-mix measure is based on a set of hierarchical groups related to levels and types of services (rehabilitation, extensive services, special care, clinically complex cases, impaired cognition, behavioral problems, and reduced physical functioning) and, within these hierarchical groups, scores on the activities of daily living (ADL) scale. The ADL scale assigns numerical scores according to the degree of physical functioning an individual can attain in each of six categories: bathing, dressing, toileting, feeding, transferring between locations, and continence (Katz, Ford, Moskowitz, Jackson, & Jaffe, 1963). RUGs III used four of these categories: eating, transferring, bed mobility, and toileting. Based on the points assigned to each of these, in combination with the hierarchical groups, the patient was assigned to 1 of 44 RUGs III categories. The RUGs IV system contains 53 categories. The categories are assigned weights according to their relative costs (see, e.g., Schlenker, Shaughnessy, & Yslas, 1985), and payment is made in accordance with these relative weights.

Such a system overcomes the first disadvantage mentioned: that case-mix selection creates a bias in favor of light-care patients. Indeed, if the weights of each category are in line with the relative costs of treating patients, then the selection bias should be removed. This does not mean that other selection biases do not exist. Indeed, three other types of biases that result from a RUGs type of payment system have been identified (Butler & Schlenker, 1989). The first of these is a bias against patient rehabilitation. If a patient improves, he or she moves into another payment category and the long-term care facility loses revenue. If the case-mix-payment system is oriented toward patient condition rather than services, then the long-term care facility will incur higher costs by rehabilitating patients. An incentive not to rehabilitate would therefore be present (Smits, 1984).

To counteract this, a payment program might pay long-term care facilities on the basis of outcomes or pay at the higher payment level for a limited period of time even when the patient improves. A second bias in such a system involves the provision of unnecessary care. If the payment system pays more for certain services (e.g., rehabilitation), then this might give the long-term care facility an incentive to provide such services, sometimes unnecessarily. As for the third bias, the long-term care facility has a motive to misreport patient status, thus acquiring a higher payment rate.

The best way to eliminate these biases may be to adopt regulations and institute a monitoring system. New York State, which adopted the RUGs II system, had a regulatory system to monitor the quality of care in long-term care facilities (Micheletti & Shlala, 1986). Such a monitoring system was developed because the payment system was not sufficient to achieve all of the public policy goals of the long-term care facility system.

RUGs IV was implemented in 2009, with the design such that the overall payment would be the same as under RUGs III. However, the distribution of the overall payment did change, with the payments for complex medical groups increasing substantially. There are now 66 RUGs, compared to the original 53 used by RUGs IV. The RUGs system uses the Minimum Data Set (MDS) to calculate the group to which the resident is assigned.

The MDS is a standardized primary screening and clinical assessment tool for facilitating care management in nursing homes because the assessment involves a comprehensive evaluation of the functional capabilities of the resident and enables staff to identify health problems. All residents in Medicare- or Medicaid-certified homes are assessed regardless of the payment source of the individual. The MDS 3.0 contains 15 categories, designed to capture the physical, psychological, and psychosocial functioning capacity of residents and the rehabilitation and restorative services needed by the residents. The MDS plays an important role in monitoring the quality of care provided to nursing facility residents

On October 1, 2019, Medicare implemented the Patient-Driven Payment Method (PDPM), a case-mix classification almost exclusively based on verifiable resident characteristics, not volumes of services provided. This system adjusts five different case-mix components reflecting the varied needs and characteristics of a resident's care, which is then combined with the noncase-mix components, resulting in the full skilled nursing facility prospective payment system (SNF PPS) per diem rate for the resident.

While the RUG IV system determined therapy payments based on the amount of therapy provided, PDPM classifies residents based on a clinical category and function score into one of 16 physical therapy (PT) and occupational therapy (OT) case-mix groups for each of the two components. The PT and OT components are variable rates and reduced by 2% every 7 days after the first 20 days of the SNF stay.

The speech-language pathology (SLP) case-mix groups contain 12 classifications based on clinical reasons for the SNF stay, the presence of a swallowing disorder or mechanically altered diet, and the presence of a SLP-related comorbidity or cognitive impairment. The existing RUG-IV methodology for classifying residents into nonrehabilitation RUGS was included in order to assist in the development of a nursing classification that explains nursing utilization, rather than therapy utilization. The nontherapy ancillary (NTA) component is based on the presence of comorbidities and extensive services received by the resident and residents are classified into one of six NTA case-mix groups. The NTA component is also a variable rate and is reduced by the length of stay.

The PDPM classifies each resident into these five components and provides a single payment based on the sum of these individual classifications. The payment for each component is calculated by multiplying the case mix index for the resident's group first by the component federal base payment rate, then by the specific day in the variable per diem adjustment schedule. These payments are then adjusted to the noncase-mix component payment rate to create a resident's total SNF PPS per diem rate under the PDPM. The goal of the system is to improve services provided to the residents and to reward the facility for providing the appropriate level of care.

7.7 Health Maintenance Organizations

The major characteristics of a health maintenance organization (HMO) from a supply standpoint are that it is simultaneously responsible for two types of services: health insurance and health care. Health insurance coverage is sold to customers on a per capita basis. The medical care itself is provided, or contracted for, by the HMO directly. The HMO assumes all the financial risk for providing this care. At the same time, its physicians act as gatekeepers and therefore have some degree of control over the patients' utilization of care.

In discussing the supply incentives inherent in such an organization, it must be recognized that an HMO can make a number of different types of arrangements with the physicians with which it contracts and with the hospitals to which it sends its patients. The arrangement made impacts the relative risks of the HMO and the provider.

The per capita funding formula provides an incentive for any investor-owned HMO to minimize costs (all other factors being held constant). An HMO can reduce its costs by lowering the use of services by existing patients, encouraging the enrollment of members who are at low risk, and disenrolling high-risk patients. Lower cost enrollees would include such groups as younger members, nonsmokers, individuals who exercise, and so on. In order to encourage healthy enrollees to select it, the HMO can design a product with this end in mind. It might, for example, have more pediatricians and fewer gerontologists on staff, specialize in sports medicine, and open more branches in the suburbs and have few or no branches in the inner city (Enthoven, 1988; Hellinger, 1995; Luft, 1986). Indeed, the likelihood of an HMO encouraging self-selection and thus having an enrollee mix that does not reflect the demographics of the general population has resulted in the development of adjustment formulas to compensate payers for potential differences in enrollee risk and the cost of utilization (Anderson, Steinberg, Holloway, & Canton, 1986). These formulas are used to calculate higher payment rates for higher risk individuals, thus inducing HMOs to enroll these individuals.

One such adjustment formula, Medicare's former average adjusted per capita cost (AAPCC) formula, was used to determine the rates at which Medicare paid HMOs. The rates were based on Medicare's own current payment rates for hospital and physician services in the fee-for-service system. AAPCCs were calculated for separate groups of patients (factors used in constructing the groups included gender, age bracket, county, welfare status, and institutionalization). For example, the monthly AAPCC for noninstitutionalized females aged 70–74 who were not on welfare in Washington County, Oregon, was $62 for hospital services and $30 for medical services. The Medicare rate to be paid to the HMOs for these individuals was 95% of the AAPCC of $92. The rationale behind this payment rate was that, for those individuals who did shift from fee-for-service coverage to HMO coverage, Medicare would save 5% of its average cost. The HMO would benefit if it could provide coverage at a cost lower than this.

One criticism of this payment system was that it did not pinpoint risk categories accurately enough and that HMO cream skimming was a distinct possibility, even with the AAPCC adjustments. For example, the AAPCC did not take into account the amount of prior health services used, which is a good indicator of future utilization of services. If an HMO could use this information to supply a product with characteristics that appeal to low-risk individuals, then it could obtain a large share of low-cost users, even allowing for AAPCC adjustments. The result could be costly to Medicare, whose 95% rule was designed to achieve savings for the program.

In the following illustration, assume that there are 100 individuals in County A who are enrolled in Medicare and who have the following characteristics: the individuals are 70–74 years old, female, noninstitutionalized, and nonwelfare. If these 100 individuals were in the fee-for-service program, Medicare would pay, on average, $92.00 a month for each. For each such individual attracted by an HMO, the HMO will receive 95% of the AAPCC, or $87.40 monthly. If the HMO is successful, through careful design of product characteristics, in drawing 10 very healthy, low-risk females from this group of 100, its average costs for these members will likely be below the $87.40 rate. The total cost to Medicare for these HMO members will be $87.40 times 10, or $870.40. The fee-for-service sector will now be left with a higher cost pool, having lost 10 lower-than-average-cost members, and its costs will rise. It is thus possible that this payment scheme could end up costing Medicare more money.

A second problem with this system was that it created a wide regional variation in rates. Medicare paid low rates for residents who lived in counties where costs were low, and as a result HMOs tended not to offer their plan in counties with low AAPCC rates.

In order to address these problems, Medicare instituted a new risk-premium-setting mechanism in 2000. This system was called "Medicare + Choice" and was instituted under a new Part C of Medicare. The risk-adjustment factors included prior hospitalization and demographic factors. The demographic factors included age, gender, disability status, Medicaid eligibility, and institutional status. In this illustration, for example, an HMO that newly enrolled a male aged 66 would receive a payment of $3720 annually, an average of $310 per month. If the person was also Medicaid eligible, the HMO would receive an additional amount, bringing the payment up to $4185 per year for that individual.

Continuing with the illustration, if the individual had been hospitalized in the previous year, and if his or her diagnosis fell into a serious category, the HMO would receive an additional payment to cover a higher risk status. There were 15 illness categories that were based on reason for hospitalization. The new categorization system is called Principal Inpatient-Diagnostic Cost Group (PIP-DCG). As an example, PIP-DCG 8 is asthma, and if a person has been hospitalized for asthma in the previous year, Medicare would add an

additional amount annually onto its rate, bringing it to $5230 per year (Health Care Financing Administration, 1999).

In developing a single rate, Congress hoped that HMOs would increase supply in areas currently underserved by HMOs because of low rates. The new system appears to better address certain risk factors associated with the HMO enrollees, but HMOs may continue to overserve low-cost areas and underserve areas where costs are high.

7.8 Provider Supply Under Managed Care

7.8.1 Agency Theory and Incentive Contracts

The quantity and quality of services that an HMO supplies to its members are determined, to a large extent, by the healthcare providers with whom the HMO contracts. The HMO is reliant on these providers to assess the HMO members' conditions and to provide appropriate levels of care. The manner in which the HMO compensates these providers will affect their supply behavior (Coller, 2011).

The HMO management does not usually know its members' health status or what and how many treatments are appropriate. The providers have the best information about these matters, and so there is an "information asymmetry" between the two groups. Consequently, it is possible, within limits, for the providers to act strictly in their own interest and not in the interest of the HMO or its members. In order to encourage the providers to act in the interest of the HMO, the HMO management can design a compensation scheme for the providers. Agency models can be used to analyze such compensation schemes. The two contracting bodies in such models are the *principals* (HMOs) and their *agents* (providers). A model in this section is presented to examine how alternative compensation schemes influence the supply behavior of providers.

The principal, or HMO, contracts with its members (on a per capita payment basis) to provide them with care.

- *HMO objectives.* In this illustration, assume that the HMO's objectives are to maximize profits. However, also assume that there is a minimum profit level that is acceptable to the HMO; in this illustration, assume this minimum profit is $1 million. Profits are equal to total revenue minus total cost.

- *HMO revenues.* The HMO's revenues depend on the capitation rate applied to its members and the number of members who join the HMO. In this illustration, the capitation rate is held constant.
- *HMO costs.* The HMO's costs include those that are incurred in treating the HMO members who become patients.
- *HMO–provider interaction.* In many respects, the HMO is dependent on its agents, the providers of care (physicians, physical therapists, hospitals, etc.), for the achievement of its profit targets. Providers can influence HMO profits by varying their levels of effort. If providers function at very low effort levels, patients will be dissatisfied with the health care they receive and will switch to other health plans. As a result, HMO profits will be low. As physician efforts increase, quality of care will improve and more members will join. However, additional physician effort means more lab tests, more procedures, and so on. While this will bring in more members to the HMO, it will also increase costs. Eventually, the additional effort will work against profitability, and profits will fall. Graph

A of **Figure 7-3** shows the relationship between the HMO's profits and the effort of the agents. At some effort level (E_3), profits will be at a maximum level. At other effort levels (E_1 and E_4), profits will be at minimally acceptable levels. HMO profits, then, are directly tied to the efforts of its contracting physicians. The physicians know how much effort they are providing and how much is required to treat their patients. The HMO cannot directly observe this effort. This is another way of saying that there is an information asymmetry between the principal and its agents. While the HMO cannot directly observe physician efforts, it can observe its profits. This performance indicator will come in useful when the HMO sets compensation policies for the physicians.

Graph A, the top diagram, shows the relationship between providers' average effort and the HMO's profit. The HMO's minimum acceptable profit level is $1,000,000. Graph B indicates the provider level of effort under alternative payment schemes. The marginal cost (*MC*) of additional effort is the same under

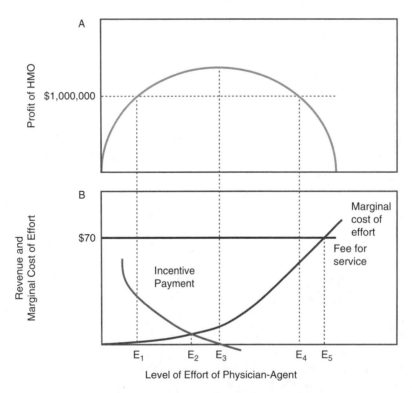

Figure 7-3 Optimal compensation of healthcare providers by an HMO. Graph A, the top diagram, shows relationship between providers' average effort and the HMO's profit. The HMO's minimum acceptable profit level is $1,000,000. Graph B indicates provider level of effort under alternative payment schemes. The marginal cost (MC) of additional effort is the same under all schemes. Under a straight salary, the provider will supply the minimum level of effort acceptable to the HMO E_1. Under fee-for-service, at assumed wage of $70, the provider will supply up to E_5, but only E_4 is acceptable to the HMO. Under a profit incentive E_2 is provided, slightly less than the HMOs maximum profit, because the incentive system is not "perfect."

all schemes. Under a straight salary, the provider will supply the minimum level of effort acceptable to the HMO E_1. Under fee-for-service, at an assumed wage of $70, the provider will supply up to E_5, but only E_4 is acceptable to the HMO. Under a profit incentive E_2 is provided, slightly less than the HMOs maximum profit, because the incentive system is not "perfect."

- *Physician objectives.* Now the assumptions about the behavior of the physicians are examined. In this illustration, assume that the objective of each physician is to maximize net income (profits), which is equal to revenues from the HMO minus the personal costs of supplying care (or exerting effort). With a rising marginal cost curve for effort, the maximization point (which indicates what level of effort will be chosen by the physician) occurs where the marginal revenue (MR) equals the marginal cost (MC) for the physician. Recall that profits are maximized when $MR = MC$.
- *Physician costs.* Assume in this illustration that all provider revenues come from the HMO (i.e., that each provider has no additional source of revenue). The relationship between alternative payment schemes that the HMO can institute and physician revenues will be discussed later. The physician costs in this illustration are the opportunity costs to the physician of engaging in productive practices. The physician places a value on his or her time, and this value is based on alternative uses of the time spent in providing care. Assume that the marginal cost to the physician of time spent on patient care increases as more time is spent. Put another way, as more time is taken away from leisure activities, the value of the last unit of time increases. This rising marginal cost curve of effort is shown in graph B of Figure 7-3.
- *Physician revenues.* The proposition being established in this section is that the level of effort selected by the physician will be influenced by the basis and level of payment. Three alternative forms of compensation are now examined: salary, fee-for-service payment, and incentive compensation based on the HMO's profits.

If the physician is paid a straight salary, any additional effort by the physician results in costs but yields no extra revenue. There is a minimum acceptable level of effort that the physician must put in—the level that corresponds to the minimum profit target of the HMO (level E_1). The physician will provide this level of services but no more under a salary system.

Assume now that the physician is paid a fee of $70 per service provided to an HMO member. Extra effort on the part of the physician will result in extra services provided. These extra services result in marginal revenues of $70 per service (see the straight horizontal line at $70 in Figure 7-3). The physician would maximize net income at a level of effort of E_5. However, because the HMO's profits are below those that are acceptable to the HMO, the physician will be required to reduce his or her effort level to E_4. If the fee falls below $70, then the physician will choose an effort level below E_5. If the fee level increases, then the effort level will also increase. It is quite possible therefore to have a low effort level under fee-for-service payment if the fee levels are low enough.

The HMO can also develop a contract for physicians that provides specific incentives. Recall that the HMO does not know how much effort is provided by the physician. The HMO only has a proxy for this based primarily on the HMO's financial performance (in this illustration, HMO profits). As an incentive, the HMO can pay the physician a fixed percentage of HMO profits. Under this incentive system, the marginal revenue (MR) curve for the physician will appear like that in any demand situation—it will decline to a level of zero as profits increase to their maximum. Beyond this point, the MR to the physician will be negative because HMO profits are falling. However, in these circumstances, the physician will not choose the level of effort that corresponds to maximum HMO profits but will choose instead level E_2, where the marginal revenue and marginal cost curves intersect. This will provide the HMO with lower than maximum profits but more profits than under a salary compensation scheme. There are numerous other compensation schemes involving incentives that can be selected, some of which are more complicated, but may motivate the physician to supply an effort close to the optimal level from the point of view of the HMO.

7.8.2 Management of Provider Behavior

In addition to setting contracts, insurers can engage in the direct management of provider supply behavior with the objective of influencing utilization patterns. The direct management of providers is an activity that is most closely associated with HMOs because of their close association with physicians. However, in recent years, the management of care has become widespread under all types of payment arrangements. Most of these practices have been focused on the use of hospital inpatient care, primarily because of the expense of this mode of care.

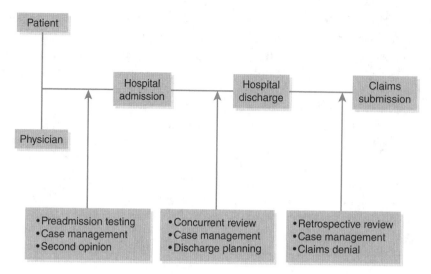

Figure 7-4 Techniques for managing provider behavior. Provider behavior can be regulated before, during, or after hospital admission, or acombination of these three time periods. Prior to hospitalization, insurers can requireproviders to seek permission (pre-authorization); during hospitalization, insurers canmonitor length of stay or use of procedures (concurrent review); and followinghospitalization, insurers can conduct reviews and deny claims (retrospective review).
© Jones & Bartlett Learning.

There are a number of different measures that insurers can use to influence providers' supply of hospital care (Korenstein, Falk, Howell, Bishop, & Keyhani, 2012; Scheffler, Sullivan, & Ko, 1991; Wallack & Tompkins, 2003). They include overall case management, preadmission management (e.g., second opinions and preadmission testing), concurrent management (e.g., concurrent review and discharge planning), and posthospital review (e.g., retrospective review and claims denials). **Figure 7-4** indicates where the measures are applied. Each measure involves the setting of standards and the review of patients in accordance with these standards.

Provider behavior can be regulated before, during, or after hospital admission, or a combination of these three time periods. Prior to hospitalization, insurers can require providers to seek permission (preauthorization); during hospitalization, insurers can monitor length of stay or use of procedures (concurrent review); and following hospitalization, insurers can conduct reviews and deny claims (retrospective review).

Many of the regulations set by HMOs carry substantial financial penalties, such as nonpayment for a claim. For example, if a second opinion is required before surgery, payment might be denied if the surgeon operated without a confirming opinion. Probably for this reason, the private regulation of providers has impacted utilization and costs. Earlier studies have indicated savings of about 7% overall (Feldstein, Wickizer, & Wheeler, 1988; Wickizer, Wheeler, & Feldstein, 1989), although the savings achieved depended on the type of program and types of penalties imposed (Keyhani, Falk, Howell, Bishop, & Korenstein, 2013; Scheffler et al., 1991). A more recent study by Stevenson, Ayanian, Zaslavsky, Newhouse, and Landon (2013) found that Medicare patients being cared for by managed care were in a better position to be promoted recommended services and discouraged from receiving burdensome procedures with little clinical value at end of life relative to traditional fee-for-service Medicare.

Exercises

1. What are four different methods for reimbursing physicians? How will each of these methods of paying physicians influence the volume of services supplied?

2. What "perverse" incentives must an insurer guard against in fee-for-service and per capita funding?

3. What is the Resource-Based Relative Value System, and how were fees set in order to influence the volume of surgical and medical services?

4. What is retrospective hospital payment, and what incentives are created by this type of payment?

5. What is prospective payment? List three alternative bases of prospective hospital payment.

6. How will each of the following bases for hospital payment affect the number of admissions, the average length of stay, the volume of services per day, and the unit cost of services (cost per service):
   a. Fee-for-service payment
   b. Per diem payment
   c. Fixed-fee per admission

7. Indicate the effect of each of the following hospital payment systems on the relative risks of the insurer and the hospital:
   a. Retrospective payment
   b. Prospective fee-for-service payment
   c. Per diem fees

8. What is the benefit of a diagnosis-related grouping system over a flat per diem payment system?

9. What methods can be used to fund a long-term care facility on a prospective basis?

10. What incentives do HMOs have with regard to
    a. Recruiting members
    b. Providing services to its members

Bibliography

Aaron, H., & Schwartz, W. B. (1984). *The painful prescription*. Washington, DC: Brookings Institution.

Alderwick, H., Hood-Ronick, C. M., & Gottlieb, L. M. (2019). Medicaid investments to address social needs in Oregon and California. *Health Affairs, 38*(5), 774–781.

Anderson, G., Steinberg, E. P., Holloway, J., & Canton, J. C. (1986). Paying for HMO care: Issues and options in setting capitation rates. *Milbank Quarterly, 64,* 548–565.

Angier, H., O'Malley, J. P., Marino, M., McConnell, K. J., Cottrell, E., Jacob, R. L., … DeVoe, J. E. (2017). Evaluating community health centers' adoption of a new global capitation payment (eCHANGE) study protocol. *Contemporary Clinical Trials, 52,* 35–38.

Bauer, K. (1977). Hospital rate setting—This way to salvation? *Milbank Quarterly, 55,* 117–118.

Berry, R. E. (1976). Prospective reimbursement and cost containment. *Inquiry, 13,* 288–301.

Blomqvist, A. (1991). The doctor as double agent: Information asymmetry, health insurance, and medical care. *Journal of Health Economics, 10,* 411–432.

Butler, P. A., & Schlenker, R. E. (1989). Case-mix reimbursement for nursing homes. *Milbank Quarterly, 67,* 103–136.

Carroll, J. (2011). Changing payment methodologies force physicians into larger groups. *Managed Care, 20*(2), 14–16.

Carter, G. M., Jacobson, P. D., Kominski, G. F., & Perry, M. J. (1994, Winter). Use of diagnosis-related groups by non-Medicare payers. *Health Care Financing Review, 16,* 127–158.

Chernew, M. E., Mechanic, R. E., Landon, B. E., & Safran, D. G. (2011). Private-payer innovation in Massachusetts: The "alternative quality contract." *Health Affairs, 30*(1), 51–61.

Chung, K. C., Kotsis, S. V., Fox, D. A., Regan, M., Burke, F. D., Wilgis, E. F. S., & Kim, H. M. (2010). Differences between the United States and the United Kingdom in the treatment of rheumatoid arthritis: Analyses from a hand arthroplasty trial. *Clinical Rheumatology, 29*(4), 363–367.

CMS. Critical access hospitals. Retrieved from https://www.cms.gov/Medicare/Provider-Enrollment-and-Certification/CertificationandComplianc/CAHs.html

CMS. Details for title: FY 2020 final rule and correction notice tables. Retrieved from https://www.cms.gov/Medicare/Medicare-Fee-for-Service-Payment/AcuteInpatientPPS/FY2020-IPPS-Final-Rule-Home-Page-Items/FY2020-IPPS-Final-Rule-Tables.html?DLPage=1&DLEntries=10&DLSort=0&DLSortDir=ascending

Coller, B. S. (2011). Realigning incentives to achieve health care reform. *JAMA, 306,* 204–205.

Eisenberg, J. M., & Williams, S. V. (1981). Cost containment and changing physicians' practice behavior. *JAMA, 246,* 2195–2201.

Enthoven, A. (1988). *Theory and practice of managed competition in health care finance.* Amsterdam, The Netherlands: North-Holland.

Epstein, A. M., & Blumenthal, D. (1993). Physician payment reform: Past and future. *Milbank Quarterly, 71,* 193–215.

Federal Register. (2018, November 23). Retrieved from http:\\federalregister.gov/d/2018-24170

Feldstein, P. J., Wickizer, T. M., & Wheeler, J. R. (1988). Private cost containment. The effects of utilization review programs on health care use and expenditures. *New England Journal of Medicine, 318,* 1310–1314.

Fetter, R. B., Youngsoo, S., Freeman, J. L., Averill, R. F., & Thompson, J. D. (1980). Case mix definition by diagnosis-related groups. *Medical Care, 18*(Suppl 2), 1–53.

Frank, R. G., & Fry, C. E. (2019). The impact of expanded Medicaid eligibility on access to Naloxone. *Addiction, 114*(9), 1567–1574.

Fries, B. E., & Cooney, L. M. (1985). Resource utilization groups. *Medical Care, 23,* 110–122.

Fries, B. E., Schneider, D. P., Foley, W. J., Gavazzi, M., Burke, R., & Cornelius, E. (1994). Refining a case mix measure for nursing homes: Resource utilization groups (RUG-III). *Medical Care, 32,* 668–685.

Goodwin, J. S., Singh, A., Reddy. N., Riall, T. S., & Yong-Fang, K. (2011). Overuse of screening colonoscopy in the Medicare population. *Archives of Internal Medicine, 171*(15), 1335–1343.

Havighurst, C. C., & Kissam, P. (1979). The antitrust implications of relative value studies in medicine. *Journal of Health Politics, Policy and Law, 4,* 48.

Health Care Financing Administration. (1999). *Medicare + Choice rates—45 day notice.* Baltimore, MD: Health Care Financing Administration. Retrieved from http://www.hcfa.gov/stats/hmorates/45d02.htm

Hellinger, F. J. (1995). Selection bias in HMOs and PPOs: A review of the evidence. *Inquiry, 32,* 135–142.

Hemenway, D., Killen, A., Cashman, S. B., Parks, C. L., & Bicknell, W. J. (1990). Physicians' responses to financial incentives. *New England Journal of Medicine, 322,* 1059–1063.

Hornbrook, M. (1982). Hospital case mix: Its definition, measurement, and use. Parts 1, 2. *Medical Care Review, 39,* 1–43, 73–123.

Hsiao, W. C., Braun, P., Dunn, D., Becker, E. R., DeNicola, M., & Ketcham, T. R. (1988). Results and policy implications of the resource based relative value study. *New England Journal of Medicine, 319,* 881–888.

Hsiao, W. C., & Stason, W. B. (1979). Toward developing a relative value scale for medical and surgical services. *Health Care Financing Review, 1,* 23–39.

Katz, S., Ford, A. B., Moskowitz, R. W., Jackson, B. A., & Jaffe, M. W. (1963). Studies of illness in the aged. *JAMA, 185,* 914–919.

Keyhani, S., Falk, R., Howell, E. A., Bishop, T., & Korenstein, D. (2013). Overuse and systems of care: A systematic review. *Medical Care, 51*(6), 503–508.

Klarman, H. E. (1963). The effect of prepaid group practice on hospital use. *Public Health Reports, 78,* 955–965.

Korenstein, D., Falk, R., Howell, E. A., Bishop, T., & Keyhani, S. (2012). Overuse of health services in the United States: An understudied problem. *Archives of Internal Medicine, 172,* 171–178.

Lave, J. R. (1984). Hospital reimbursement under Medicare. *Milbank Quarterly, 62,* 251–268.

Luft, H. S. (1986). Compensating for biased selection in health insurance. *Milbank Quarterly, 64,* 566–591.

Malay, D. S. (2011). Payments for surgical services and the medical inflation rate. *Journal of Foot & Ankle Surgery, 50*(1), 74–76.

McConnell, J. M., Renfro, S., Chan, B. K., Meath, T. H., Mendelson, A., Cohen, D., ... Lindrooth, R. C. (2017). Early performance in Medicaid accountable care organizations: A comparison of Oregon and Colorado. *JAMA Internal Medicine, 177*(4), 538–545.

Micheletti, J., & Shlala, T. J. (1986). RUGs II: Implications for management and quality in long-term care. *Quality Review Bulletin, 12,* 236–242.

Miller, H. D. (2009). From volume to value: Better ways to pay for health care. *Health Affairs, 28*(5), 1418–1428.

Mitchell, J. B. (1985). Physician DRG's. *New England Journal of Medicine, 313,* 670–675.

Moore, S. (1979). Cost containment through risk sharing of primary-care physicians. *New England Journal of Medicine, 300,* 1359–1362.

Myers, L. P., & Schroeder, S. A. (1981). Physician use of services for the hospitalized patient. *Milbank Quarterly, 59,* 481–507.

Pettengill, J., & Vertrees, J. (1982, December). Reliability and validity in hospital case-mix measurement. *Health Care Financing Review, 4,* 101–128.

Phelps, C. E. (1976). Public sector medicine. In C. M. Lindsay (Ed.), *New directions in public health care* (pp. 129–166). San Francisco, CA: Institute for Contemporary Studies.

Rudmik, L., Wranik, D., & Rudisill-Michaelsen, C. (2014). Physician payment methods: A focus on quality and cost control. *Journal of Otolaryngology-Head and Neck Surgery, 43,* 34.

Scheffler, R. M., Sullivan, S. D., & Ko, T. H. (1991). The impact of Blue Cross and Blue Shield plan utilization management programs, 1980–1988. *Inquiry, 28,* 276–287.

Schlenker, R. E. (1986). Case-mix reimbursement for nursing homes. *Journal of Health Politics, Policy and Law, 11,* 445–461.

Schlenker, R. E., Shaughnessy, P. W., & Yslas, I. (1985). Estimating patient level nursing home costs. *Health Services Research, 20,* 103–128.

Simoens, S., & Giuffrida, A. (2004). The impact of physician payment methods on raising the efficiency of the healthcare system: An international comparison. *Applied Health Economics and Health Policy, 3*(1), 39–46.

Smits, H. L. (1984, Winter). Incentives in case-mix measures for long-term care. *Health Care Financing Review, 6,* 53–59.

Staheli, W. (2016, January 29). What is MIPS? *Find-A-Code.* Retrieved from https://www.findacode.com/medicare/mips/

Stevenson, D. G., Ayanian, J. Z., Zaslavsky, A. M., Newhouse, J. P., & Landon, B. E. (2013). Service use at the end-of-life in Medicare advantage versus traditional Medicare. *Medical Care, 51,* 931–937.

Swensen, S. J., Kaplan, G. S., Meyer, G. S., Nelson, E. E., Hunt, G. C., Pryor, D. B., ... Chassin, M. R. (2011). Controlling healthcare costs by removing waste: What American doctors can do now. *BMJ Quality & Safety, 20*(6), 534–537.

Urban Institute. (2007). *Final report to CMS options for improving Medicare payment for SNFs.* Washington, DC: Author.

Verma, S. (2019, July 17). More ACOs taking accountability under MSSP through pathways to success. *Health Affairs Blog.* doi:10.1377/hblog 20190717.

Wallack, S. S., & Tompkins, C. P. (2003). Realigning incentives in fee-for-service medicine. *Health Affairs, 22*(4), 59–70.

Wickizer, T. M., Wheeler, J. R. C., & Feldstein, P. J. (1989). Does utilization review reduce unnecessary hospital care and contain costs? *Medical Care, 27,* 632–647.

CHAPTER 8

Competitive Markets

OBJECTIVES

1. Specify the assumptions of a competitive market model.
2. Use the competitive model to predict movements in price and utilization due to changes in factors that influence supply and demand for health services.
3. Use the supply–demand framework to predict the factors that influence shortages and surpluses in health care.
4. Identify the evidence for and against the competitive model.
5. Describe the factors that influence how the competitive bidder sets the price for a contract.
6. Define the concept of supplier-induced demand and describe the influence of supply on price in a market in which supplier-induced demand exists.

8.1 Introduction

A number of hypotheses about the behavior of entities demanding and supplying goods and services in the marketplace have been developed in previous chapters. The hypotheses deal with the demand behavior and supply behavior of entities in isolation; that is, demand and supply behaviors are examined individually. As a result, although a way of predicting what quantity would be demanded (supplied) at any price was developed, the basic model did not incorporate simultaneous consideration of the behavior of the supplying and demanding entities and, thus, could not indicate whether the same quantity would be both demanded and supplied. The model up to this point could not indicate if the behaviors would result in market equilibrium.

The focus now shifts to models in which entities demanding and entities supplying goods and services in the market interact. The setting in which this interaction between buyers and sellers occurs is called a *market*. A market in economics is a set of arrangements that brings buyers (demanders) and sellers (suppliers) together, although especially in today's environment, a market should not be thought of as a physical

location. Rather, the term *market* denotes the web of interactions among those who have commercial relationships or the potential to have such relationships with other buyers and sellers of similar goods and services. For example, a market for psychiatric services can be thought of as consisting of a group of consumers and a group of mental health providers who have the potential to enter into business relations with all members of the other group. Central to the analysis of the functioning of a market is the price that the buyer pays and the seller receives for the goods and services. In previous explanations, the price at which the exchange took place was assumed to be given for both groups; variations in price were beyond the control of any one buyer or seller. Yet, as a consequence of the related interactions of these groups, prices are set; as a result of some change in demand or supply behavior, prices change.

The market analyses that are now examined involve two categories of concepts:

1. *Phenomena to be explained.* These are objective events, such as changes in the price or the quantity of medical care utilized. The phenomenon of interest might be a rise in prices, and the models

here would be used to explain why the phenomenon occurred.

2. *Behavioral relationships.* The economic "forces" influencing these phenomena have been referred to as *demand* and *supply*. The strength of these forces can be increased or decreased by individual factors, such as incomes and tastes on the demand side, and input prices and productivity on the supply side. Demand can be increased, for example, by higher consumer incomes, and supply can be decreased by higher input costs. As a consequence of changes in causal factors, demand or supply will change, as will price and quantity. The economic models developed and utilized should be able to predict such causal chains of events.

In this chapter, one particular market model is developed and used to explain the outcome of price and quantity in the medical care market. This is the competitive market model, which treats the market as an interactive mechanism with many suppliers competing for consumer business. Such a model is helpful in explaining a broad range of phenomena. It offers hypotheses to explain rising prices; increasing or decreasing utilization; shortages in such goods and services as physicians' services, nursing services, and blood; and surpluses in such goods and services as hospital beds. Thus, it is a valuable starting point for any analysis of markets.

The competitive market model is presented in Section 8.2, and the predictions of the model are discussed in Section 8.3. Although the competitive model is able to generate a large number of predictions, not all the predictions are borne out by actual events. Indeed, several events are either at odds with, or fail to corroborate, the predictions of the competitive model. Since accurate prediction is the bottom line of explanatory economics, Section 8.4 is devoted to a discussion of corroborating evidence relating to the competitive hypothesis. Section 8.5 discusses a recent application of the competitive hypothesis in the healthcare field, in particular, the use of the model to explain selective contracting. Section 8.6 concerns a deviation from the competitive market that involves the notion of supplier-induced demand in health care.

8.2 The Competitive Model: Assumptions

In this discussion of the competitive model, a market for physician services will be used to illustrate the concepts. The product in this discussion is physician visits, which is assumed to have constant quality, with each physician visit characterized by the same accuracy of diagnosis, effectiveness of treatment, and personal attentiveness (bedside manners).

- *Individual demand.* The initial demand assumption is that each consumer has a normal demand curve for physician visits (recall that a demand curve for a normal good or service slopes downward and to the right). This includes the stipulation that consumers are fully informed about the nature of the services they require and the benefits that they can obtain with the purchase of physician visits. This stipulation implies that physicians cannot *directly* influence consumer demand for physician visits.

- *Market demand.* A further assumption is that there are many consumers in the market, and that these consumers (buyers) are competing for physician services. This assumption rules out the possibility that buyers are large enough, or can join together through unions, associations, or other entities into a purchasing group, to have any influence over the price at which physician services are supplied. The market demand curve (*D*) in this illustration is shown in **Figure 8-1**. Here conditions are assumed to be such that, at a price of $45 per visit, the quantity demanded is 600 visits: at $40, the quantity demanded is 700 units; at $25, the quantity demanded is 1000 units; and so on. Curve *D* traces out this relationship. Any change in the underlying causal factors (e.g., tastes and preferences) will shift demand. These causal factors are listed in the diagram for the purpose of reminding the reader of the underlying assumptions of the model. For further review, refer to Chapter 4.

- *Individual supply.* The supply assumptions can similarly be separated into assumptions about individual suppliers and about the supplier group or market supply. Individually, each supplier of a normal good or service has an upward-sloping marginal cost curve. Assuming supplier profit maximization and no supplier influence over price (a competitive market assumption), the marginal cost curve is the supply curve in a competitive market.

- *Market supply.* With regard to the group of suppliers, the assumptions are that there are a large number of suppliers, the suppliers do not collude with each other in order to influence price, and none of the suppliers is large enough by itself to influence the price of the good or service in the market.

Consumers are assumed to have knowledge of the price offers of alternative suppliers and so can

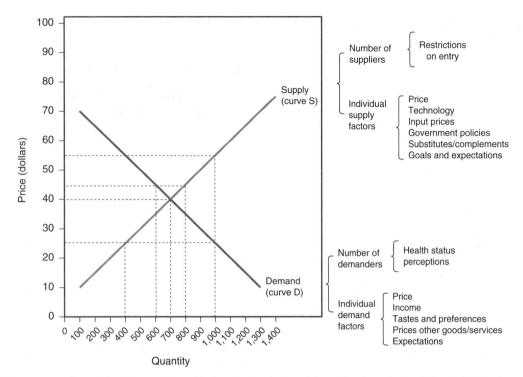

Figure 8-1 Representation of the interaction of behavioral relationships. The description is included in the text. My understanding is that the descriptive statements are not being included as a legend in the figure, but rather in the text.

compare the suppliers' prices when making purchase decisions. Because of consumer knowledge of market prices, any supplier charging a higher price than the lowest price that would prevail in a competitive situation would not be able to sell any units. Charging a lower price would simply mean forgoing some profits, since the supplier is able to sell its total output at the higher price. And so, in such a market, each supplier will take the price as given and supply the quantity at which price (P) equals its marginal cost of production (MC). The market supply will be the summed individual suppliers' marginal cost curves, which is the same as the sum of the individual supply curves. Market supply is shown in Figure 8-1 as curve S, and as illustrated there would only be 400 units supplied at $25, 700 units supplied at $40, 800 at $45, 1000 at $55, and so on. The factors influencing the position of the supply curve are also shown in Figure 8-1. For further review, refer to Chapter 6.

The phenomena, price and quantity, are influenced by supply and demand. These, in turn, are affected by a number of individual causal factors (listed in the diagram). The positions of the supply and demand curves have been set based on the assumption that supply and demand are at given levels. Changes in the magnitude of any of the underlying factors will cause a shift in supply or demand (or both).

Under these conditions of supply and demand, bargaining occurs between consumers (demanders) and producers (suppliers). An equilibrium in the market is reached when the quantity demanded by consumers equals the quantity supplied by producers. In Figure 8-1, this occurs at the intersection of the demand curve and supply curve, at the price of $40 and at the quantity of 700 units. The next section is devoted to the predictions of the model. That is, it presents what the market outcome would be expected to be (in terms of prices and quantities), if such assumptions and conditions were approximated in reality.

8.3 The Competitive Model: Predictions

8.3.1 Overview

Several important groups of conclusions can be drawn from the competitive model regarding how resources are allocated in any sector of the economy, including the healthcare sector. These conclusions are presented next. As you read the subsequent sections, it is important to keep in mind that these conclusions are presented as possible explanations for events, and whose usefulness is determined by how well the explanations conform to actual experience observed.

8.3.2 Market Price

In a competitive market, a single price will emerge that clears the market; that is, this price will enable suppliers to sell all they are willing and able to sell, and enable consumers to purchase all they are willing and able to buy. Competitive bidding in the market will lower the price, if a surplus of output exists (i.e., if there is unsold output or excess capacity) and will raise the price in the case of a shortage. Only when buyers are satisfied with the quantities they purchase at the established price and sellers are satisfied with the quantities they sell at the established price and are making the maximum profits will market equilibrium be established (i.e., quantity supplied equals quantity demanded). In our illustration in Figure 8-1, equilibrium will be reached at a price of $40 and a supply of 700 visits.

If the price is higher, say, $45, then only 600 units of service (physician visits) will be demanded, whereas the suppliers will be willing and able to supply 800 visits at $45. To eliminate this excess supply capacity, physicians will lower both their prices and the number of visits supplied. The quantity demanded will increase at the same time as the price is lowered. The process of price and quantity adjustment goes on until both groups are simultaneously satisfied with the price and quantity. The quantity supplied will just equal the quantity that consumers demand. The same process will occur in reverse if the price is below $40, in which case prices will be driven up and quantity adjusted to the equilibrium point.

It can be shown that the end result of this process is a single price charged by all producers in a competitive market. If any single physician charged more than the equilibrium price per visit, then his or her patients, given the assumption that consumers possess full knowledge of prices charged by other physicians, would obtain medical care elsewhere. The physician would be forced to bring his or her price down to the price other physicians are charging in order to be able to provide any visits to consumers. On the other hand, if a physician sets fees below the equilibrium level, patients will flock to this physician, creating an overload of work. Given a rising marginal cost (*MC*) schedule for this physician, if services are provided to the additional patients, the profits gained from the sale of each additional visit will, in fact, be negative. The physician with such an *MC* schedule would have been better off profit-wise to accept the highest price, which is the market price. That a single market-clearing price will emerge over time is, thus, one conclusion, given the assumptions inherent in the competitive model.

8.3.3 Price and Quantity Movements Caused by Demand Shifts

Additional conclusions based on the competitive model can be drawn regarding price and quantity movements when there is a change in any of the factors that influence demand. This set of conclusions is illustrated in **Figure 8-2**. Assume D_1 to be the demand curve consistent with the given initial values of underlying causal factors of demand (income, tastes and preferences, prices of other goods and services, expectations, and health status). Let S be the supply curve, which remains stable in this illustration because all supply shift factors (technology, input prices, governmental policies, substitutes and complements, and goals and expectations) are assumed to remain constant. The equilibrium price for these conditions is P_1 ($40), and the equilibrium quantity for the market is Q_1 (700 visits). If any of the initial conditions that influence demand change, causing an increase in demand to D_2, for example, there will be a new equilibrium price ($45) and a new equilibrium quantity (800 units).

The willingness of consumers to buy more at each higher price allows the producers to increase profits by producing more output (up to 800 units). Such a shift in demand can be caused by higher consumer incomes or a greater degree of illness in the population. Or, it can be caused by an increase in the amount of health insurance purchased, which also causes demand to shift out (see Section 3.6). In any case, with a change in a demand factor that shifts the demand curve upward and to the right the result is the same—higher prices and greater quantities. The opposite situation, lower prices and fewer quantities, would be the consequence of a change in demand factors shifting demand downward and to the left.

If the quantity utilized is to increase, additional quantity must be available and suppliers willing to provide the units. *Utilization* refers to the actual quantity exchanged or traded in the market. Utilization should not be confused with the amount demanded, because when there is disequilibrium, more (or less) might be demanded than is supplied. Nor should utilization be confused with the quantity offered by the supplier, because at any one price more (or less) might be supplied than consumers are willing to purchase at that price. Disequilibrium situations occur when the price does not adjust to allow the quantity demanded and the quantity supplied to equalize. Disequilibrium

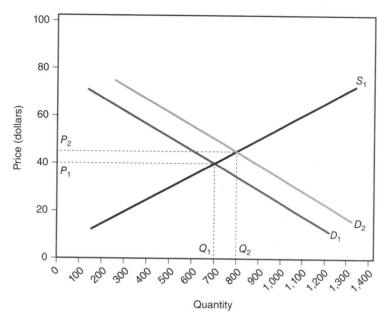

Figure 8-2 Representation of shift in demand with stable supply. An initial set of supply and demand forces, characterized by D_1 and S, will produce given price and output levels. An increase in demand to D_2, with a stable S, will cause price and output to increase.

© Jones & Bartlett Learning.

can be dynamic—the market has not had time to adjust to the change—or it can be static—something (e.g., government policies or market power) in the market is preventing it from making the appropriate adjustments to reach equilibrium

8.3.4 Price and Quantity Movements Caused by Supply Shifts

Another set of conclusions based on the model concern changes in factors (technology, input prices, government policies, substitutes or complements, or goals and expectations) that cause the supply to shift. What occurs if there is an increase in supply is shown in **Figure 8-3**. In this illustration, the good or service becomes less scarce (more abundant) and the supply shifts from S_1 to S_2. Given an assumption that the demand remains the same (constant), then the supply increases relative to the demand and the price decreases. As a result, a new lower price ($35) and a higher level of utilization (800 units) are predicted. Of course, a change in a factor that causes a reduction in supply will have the opposite effect on the price and the quantity utilized.

Changes in supply can occur because of changes in circumstances that are beyond the control of supplying firms (and to which they then react), or because of changes that the present or potential suppliers themselves initiate in the provision of the good

or service. For example, if hospitals or public health departments decide to hire medical technicians (an input in the production of physician visits), they will enter the market and bid for the existing supply of technicians. This will raise the price of technicians that all market participants have to pay, because the supply will initially remain relatively stable while the demand will increase. An increase in the price of technician services (or for that matter of any input) will shift the supply curve of all producers who use this input upward and to the left. Thus, the market supply curve will shift upward and leftward as well, and the price of physician services will increase.

Under the assumption in the competitive model that suppliers are profit maximizers, provider-initiated changes in supply will be undertaken by suppliers when these changes have the potential to add to profits. Three types of situations that will result in changes in supply are discussed in the following paragraphs:

1. a change in input combinations used to produce output brought about by existing suppliers
2. an increase in the capital stock (output capabilities) of existing suppliers
3. entry into the market by new suppliers

An example of the first situation, a change in input combinations, might occur if physicians were to hire nurse practitioners to perform, at a lower cost, services previously performed by the physicians themselves. Such a change might be the result of the

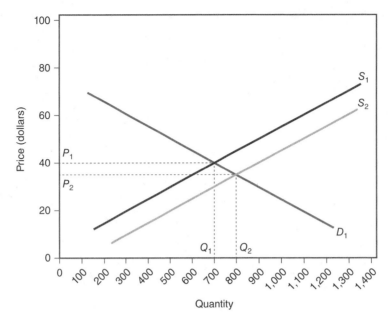

Figure 8-3 Representation of shifting supply with stable demand. Beginning with an initial demand and supply levels D_1 and S_1 and resulting price and output levels, an increase in supply to S_1 will cause output to increase and price to fall.
© Jones & Bartlett Learning.

passage of legislation allowing such substitution to occur in the provision of physician visits. The effect would be to shift the average total cost (ATC) curve downward and the marginal cost (MC) curve to the right. In a competitive market, one supplier making such a change would not cause a large shift in the market supply curve. Prices would remain about the same, and that one supplier would reap an increase in profits. However, if all suppliers made a change, the market supply curve would shift downward and to the right considerably, and the price of medical care would then decrease. Consumers would reap the benefits from such actions, assuming quality remains constant.

The net profit position of each provider after all suppliers have acted may not be any greater than before, because the price of output has decreased, but it is important to note that the providers make their decisions to undertake cost-reducing activities based on current or existing prices. In the competitive model, providers do not collude with their fellow suppliers, and they do not always anticipate that prices will fall as a consequence of their concerted actions. The end result of their actions in the market, however, is lower prices and greater utilization.

The same process occurs, for example, in the second situation when existing suppliers invest in the expansion of plant and equipment (capital). Additions to capital are often made in anticipation of additions to profits because of lower unit production costs. If these investments cut costs, and if they are sufficiently widespread in the industry, the net effect will be to lower prices and raise utilization. As a result, after these effects have worked themselves out in the market, profits may be no greater than before (they may even be less).

These effects have been presented here in a before–after manner (price and utilization before the change in price and utilization after the market has had time to adjust to the changes). In actuality, the change typically takes a considerable amount of time to occur. The potential for profits must first be realized, then planning for the additions and financing the changes must occur, and the additional capital equipment and plant capacity must then be constructed and put into use. As a result, the increase in supply and the fall in price may take months or even years to occur. For this reason, the analysis of provider behavior involving capital additions, with resulting shifts in average and marginal cost curves, has been referred to as *long-run analysis*. (It is generally difficult to decide when a change in supply conditions is long run and when it is short run. Short-run changes are usually assumed to be changes in quantity supplied that occur without changes in capital equipment.)

The third type of variation in supply occurs when new (profit-seeking) suppliers enter an industry or a market in response to high profits in the current market situation. Such a movement of resources into a market results in an increase in supply and a consequent fall in price and an increase in utilization. In this instance, since the cost conditions of existing suppliers remain the same, the profit levels must fall for all existing suppliers.

The conditions that determine how easily potential providers can actually enter the industry and place their products on the market are referred to as *conditions of entry*. These conditions depend on existing productive techniques, as well as on legal impediments. In some industries (for example, hospitals), extensive capital requirements preclude many firms from entering because of the large financial commitment necessary to undertake the capital investment and commence production. Such requirements may exist for some types of medical care, such as invasive specialized surgery, although the financial impediments are not nearly as great as they are, for example, in the automobile industry. For many types of medical care, financial impediments are not the most relevant barriers to entry. More relevant are the legal impediments, such as the licensing requirements for medical personnel and facilities. Licensing regulations frequently amount to restrictions placed on potential entrants into an industry.

8.3.5 Simultaneous Demand and Supply Shifts

In addition to creating movements in either demand or supply alone, where the effects are readily predictable, underlying factors may cause shifts in both the demand for and the supply of a good or service at the same time. At this stage of the analysis, it is critical to specify that the reference is to separate factors causing changes in demand and in supply. That is, for example, an increase in the number of people with a medical condition occurring at the same time as an influx of physicians into the market will cause both demand and supply curves to shift; the increase in the illness level will cause demand for physician visits to increase, and the increase in the number of physicians will cause the supply of physician visits to increase. In **Figure 8-4**, this is shown as an upward and to the right shift in demand from D_1 to D_2 and, at the same time, a downward and to the left shift in supply from S_1 to S_2.

Although quantity increases in this illustration, the net effect on price is ambiguous and will depend on how much each curve shifts, that is, on the changes in the values of the causal variables and the degree to which they cause demand and supply to shift. In the specific case illustrated in Figure 8-4, price will remain constant at P_1. But, if the extent to which both curves have shifted is not known, the model fails as a predictive device for price.

A second type of simultaneous shift may occur when the same factor that causes demand to shift independently causes supply also to shift. An increase in quality of physician visits, for example, will cause supply to decrease (given the assumption that increasing quality causes an increase in production costs) and demand to increase. When demand increases

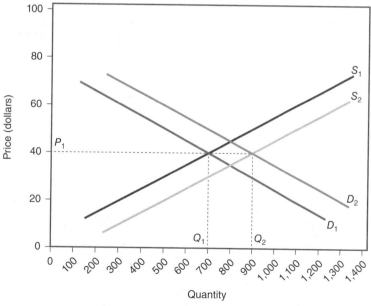

Figure 8-4 Representation of the simultaneous shifting of demand and supply curves. Beginning with initial demand and supply levels D_1 and S_1 and resulting price and output levels, a simultaneous shift in demand and supply curves (to D_2 and S_1) will have an ambiguous effect on price and will increase output. The extent of both shifts determines the effects on price and quantity. Some directional shifts, such as a decrease in demand and a simultaneous increase in supply, will lower the price but have an ambiguous effect on quantity traded.

and supply decreases, price will increase, but quantity will increase, fall, or remain the same depending on the extent of the shifts. (Another type of simultaneous shift that does *not* belong in this category is when the factors affecting supply and demand are not independent, such as when physicians can induce consumer demand. This phenomenon is discussed in Section 8.6.)

8.3.6 Shortages

The predictions provided so far have been concerned with what happens to the equilibrium price when one or several factors change. Not all situations are such that the quantity demanded is the same as the quantity supplied. The medical care market, for example, often experiences shortages in services available. A shortage occurs when the quantity demanded exceeds the quantity supplied at the current price. The model discussed so far shows that in a competitive market with free bidding, a shortage will cause the price to rise. Then, the suppliers will offer more services and the consumers will reduce their demand, making the shortage disappear. That is the theory, although persistent shortages have been observed in the blood market, the market for nurses, the physician services market, and, in some countries, the hospital market. A slight modification of the competitive model allows us to predict why these shortages occur and how they can be eliminated.

Refer to the illustration in Figure 8-1. Assume that, because of a government regulation that has been implemented, the price is prevented from rising above $25 per visit. Perhaps the regulation was passed and enforced to increase access to medical care for low-income consumers, who otherwise may go without needed medical services if the price is $40. The consequences of the passage of the regulation can be determined using the competitive model. At $25, consumers will be more willing and able to visit their physicians, and according to the illustration in Figure 8-1, 1000 consumers will call for appointments and visit their physicians. But at this price, it would be unprofitable for physicians to see 1000 patients. Indeed, the physicians will reduce the quantity of visits supplied in the market and will see only 400 patients. A queue or waiting list will form of untreated patients; in this case, 600 patients who want treatment will be unable to see a physician. Some shortages observed in the market are the result of such price ceilings. In a competitive market, a shortage can only persist if the price is somehow restricted and forced to remain below the market-clearing price (in this illustration, the market-clearing price is $40). This will usually be done by an official or semiofficial agency that can overrule the price that market forces set.

A shortage can also occur, for example, when health insurance is purchased, or when a government program "guaranteeing" access to medical care is instituted. In such situations, the consumers may face a zero out-of-pocket money price, which will result in a high quantity demanded (e.g., 1200 units, as shown in **Figure 8-5**). The reimbursed price to the provider may be only $20 per unit, and at this price only 700 units are provided. In our illustration, it would take a price of $70 per visit to bring forth a

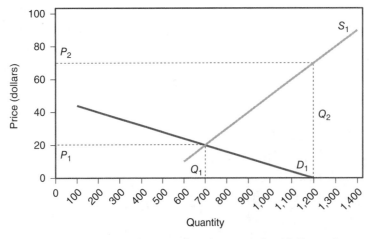

Figure 8-5 Representation of supply and demand forces using the example of full-service coverage by a third-party. Beginning with initial demand and supply levels D_1 and S_1 and resulting price and output levels, a simultaneous shift in demand and supply curves (to D_2 and S_1) will have an ambiguous effect on price and will increase output. The extent of both shifts determines the effects on price and quantity. Some directional shifts, such as a decrease in demand and a simultaneous increase in supply, will lower the price but have an ambiguous effect on quantity traded.

supply of 1200 units. At the administered reimbursement rate of $20, there is a shortage of 500 units.

Full-service (zero out-of-pocket price) coverage with a reimbursement rate of $20 will lead to a quantity demanded of 1200 and a quantity supplied of 700. To reach a quantity supplied of 1200, the payment rate would have to be $70 (curve S_1).

The situation just described requires some type of mechanism to ration the 700 available units, assuming that the quality produced remains the same. One tactic is to make the prospective patients wait in line; those who are willing to pay the "time costs" will receive the service (Buchanan, 1965; Culyer & Cullis, 1976; Drumm, Arkins, & Dayan, 2010; Sloan & Lorant, 1976; Tikkahen & Osborn, 2019). Another possibility is for the providers to lower the quality of their product, for example, by reducing the time devoted to providing the service to each individual. This action would reduce demand, since the physician visits would not have the same value as before, and it would increase supply, since more visits could be provided. As a result, the shortage would be reduced and perhaps even eliminated.

8.3.7 Surpluses

The usual definition of a surplus is that there is an excess of quantity supplied over quantity demanded at a given price in the market. For a surplus to persist over time, some factor in the market must keep quantity supplied above quantity demanded. If the price in the market was kept permanently above the equilibrium price, a surplus would persist: in this case, suppliers would be willing to provide more units of the good or service than consumers would be willing to purchase. In Figure 8-1, if the suppliers' reimbursed price and the consumers' out-of-pocket price were both $45 and could not be lowered because of regulations, a surplus would exist. In this case, suppliers would be willing to supply more units at that price (800) than demanders would want (600), and the suppliers would find themselves with excess capacity (200 units).

For a surplus to persist, something must prevent the market price from falling in response to pressures in the market, because in a normal competitive situation an excess supply would induce suppliers to lower their prices to induce demanders to purchase more. If the government pegged or supported an above-equilibrium price in the market, a surplus would occur. In the case of health care, where insurance exists, a surplus can occur if the reimbursement rate suppliers receive induces a greater quantity

supplied than the quantity demanded by consumers at the price they have to pay out of pocket for health care. In Figure 8-1, if the total reimbursement physicians received was $55 but the out-of-pocket price consumers paid was $40, a surplus of 300 visits would exist (1000 visits supplied but only 700 visits demanded).

In the early 1990s there was much talk of a "physician surplus" (Burns, 2009; Otari et al., 2009; Schwartz & Mendelson, 1990). In discussions of this topic, one heard talk of falling physicians' fees and incomes (although this was not always borne out by the data). To the extent that the fees and incomes of physicians were falling during that period, this situation was not a surplus in the technical sense. Falling fees are characteristic of prices responding to a shift in supply on the way to a new equilibrium point. For a surplus to develop and remain, the market is not allowed to move to a new equilibrium; it must remain in *dis*equilibrium.

The surplus in hospital beds is more likely a case of permanent disequilibrium than is the physician market. High hospital reimbursement rates have induced a large quantity supplied; at given out-of-pocket prices, there has not been enough quantity demanded to clear the market. This is reflected in an average occupancy rate of 65.9% in acute care hospitals in the United States in 2017 (Elflein, 2019). This 65.9% occupancy rate means that out of every 100 beds available, on average, only 65.9 beds were occupied by a patient.

8.3.8 Multi-Market Analyses

The competitive model is also well suited to making predictions about the effect of supply and/or demand changes in one market on the price and quantity of goods and services in a related market. To illustrate, assume there are two substitute services available, inpatient and outpatient surgical care for tonsillectomies. Because of the development of quicker acting anesthetics and less invasive techniques, outpatient surgery has become more feasible for a number of conditions. Further, the total cost of outpatient surgery is much less than inpatient surgery for most cases, and outpatient surgery, for many procedures, is now covered by almost all insurance carriers.

Analytically, the impact of moving from no outpatient coverage for a procedure (e.g., tonsillectomy) to outpatient coverage by insurance is shown in **Figure 8-6**. The pre-outpatient insurance coverage market for inpatient tonsillectomy procedures

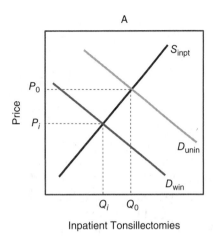
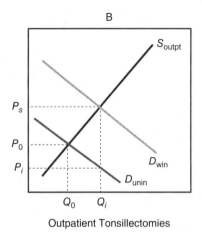

Figure 8-6 Representation of multimarket analysis. Demand curves in inpatient and outpatient markets are related (the services are substitutes). When the out-of-pocket price in the outpatient market falls (because of an implementation of insurance coverage), the demand curve in the inpatient market shifts inward and price and quantity fall and the demand curve in the outpatient market shifts outward and price to the patient falls and quantity increases, while price to the outpatient provider increases to a subsidized price of P_s meet the increased demand of Q_i.

© Jones & Bartlett Learning.

is characterized in Graph A. Here S_{inpt} is the inpatient supply curve of tonsillectomies and D_{unin} is the original inpatient demand curve without insurance. Without health insurance coverage of outpatient tonsillectomies, the inpatient equilibrium point is reached at a price of P_0 and quantity of Q_0 In graph B, reflecting the outpatient tonsillectomy market, D_{unin} is the original demand curve for outpatient tonsillectomies (without insurance) and S_{outpt} is the supply curve for outpatient tonsillectomies. Note that in this illustration the demand function for *inpatient* care is dependent on the out-of-pocket price for *outpatient* tonsillectomy surgery, because the two are substitutes in many cases.

Initially, there is no insurance coverage for outpatient tonsillectomies and P_0 is the prevailing price and Q_0 outpatient tonsillectomies are demanded. An implementation of insurance for outpatient tonsillectomies will shift the market demand curve for outpatient tonsillectomies outward (from the D_{unin} to D_{win} in graph B) and simultaneously lower the out-of-pocket price of outpatient care from P_0 to a point such as P_i, with quantity increasing to Q_i. In order for supply of outpatient tonsillectomies to increase to meet demand, the subsidized price paid to the providers will need to increase to P_s. This will result in graph A in an inward shift in the D_{unin} curve for inpatient care to D_{win}. The inpatient price for tonsillectomies will fall to P_i and the quantity of inpatient tonsillectomy procedures will be reduced to Q_i.

Similar types of analyses can be conducted for other types of substitute procedures. It can also be

conducted for complements, such as film and radiologist services. In some cases, it is not clear whether two services are substitutes or complements. For example, it is not clear whether nursing home care replaces hospital care or is used in conjunction with it. The same holds for home health care and hospital care. In these instances, the model cannot provide unambiguous conclusions.

8.4 Evidence for and Against the Competitive Model

8.4.1 Overview

There has been some use of the competitive model in explaining resource allocation trends in medical care markets. In the physician services market, for example, the phenomenon of rapidly rising physician fees, both before and after the watershed year of 1966, when Medicare and Medicaid were instituted (see Chapter 14), was explained using the competitive model by hypothesizing that the rapid increase in medical care insurance caused demand shifts and consequent rising prices. In the physician services market, the length of time required to train new physicians means a slow supply response to changing market conditions, even in a competitive market, and prices would be expected to rise to balance the market (Garbarino, 1959; Ginsburg, 2010; Newhouse, Phelps, & Schwartz, 1977).

In the hospital care market, the same type of explanation can be made for rising hospital costs, with one modification. Although insurance was increasing during this time period, hospital input prices, notably employee wages, were also rapidly rising. This latter phenomenon would shift the supply curve inward as costs of production increased. Couple this with a rapidly outward shifting demand curve for hospital care because of increased insurance coverage, the net effect would be a larger price increase. Whether utilization would increase or decrease would depend on the magnitude of both shifts. As seen in Chapter 3, hospital utilization increased. An "after the fact" explanation would state that the supply and demand shifts were such that the increase in utilization was likely to occur. (An application of the competitive model to the hospital field is found in Ro [1977].)

The competitive model has also been used to explain the persisting queues and unmet demands that have resulted from the institution of the National Health Service (NHS) in Great Britain in 1946. The initial NHS program was characterized by a zero money price paid by consumers at point of service, per capita remuneration for general practitioners, and salaried remuneration for surgeons and other hospital-based physicians. The competitive model applied to this type of healthcare system would predict large increases in quantity demanded following the lowering of the price to consumers to zero. Supply decisions were passed into the hands of the central government under the NHS, and large increases in the supply of physicians did not materialize. As a result, persistent shortages occurred, particularly in hospital care (Culyer & Cullis, 1976; Yeginsu, 2018).

Although the competitive model is a useful device for explaining price and quantity movements and uncovering the causes of shortages or surpluses of medical care, much attention has been focused on the shortcomings of the model. Evidence of the existence of shortcomings in the competitive market model might be obtained in three ways. First, data on market outcomes, such as profits and prices could be examined. If profit and price outcomes are not what would be expected in a competitive market (i.e., not what the competitive model predicts would happen), it could be inferred that the model does not explain what has been observed and so alternative models to better explain the data would be sought.

Second, some conditions and characteristics of a market, such as consumer ignorance or product quality level differences, might be observed. If the observed characteristics are at odds with the competitive model's assumptions, then a different model that incorporates realistic assumptions should be considered.

Third, direct actions on the part of providers that suggest the prevalence of noncompetitive practices might be observed. These observations might include constraints on certain activities usually thought of as competitive, such as easy entry into the market. Now, the discussion turns to examining some of the evidence that suggests the competitive model has serious flaws as a model of the healthcare market. The flaws do not necessarily mean the competitive model should be abandoned, but that modifications are necessary to incorporate the conditions interfering with its efficient functioning.

8.4.2 Excessive Profits

Studies made of the profits accruing from medical practice have shown these profits to be persistent and considerable. These profits, which are the net incomes (revenues minus expenses) of the physicians operating the practices, must be adjusted for the relative costs incurred in medical training, including fees paid and earnings forgone during medical school and residency. Even after adjusting for these costs, the net present value of medical practice indicates the existence of persistently high profits (i.e., earnings in excess of normal returns) (Cooper, 2011; Lindsay, 1976; Murphy, 2016; Popa, 2019; Sloan, 1976).

Generally, the competitive model predicts that such excess profits would eventually be bid away by new providers entering the industry to take advantage of the high returns. This has not occurred in medical practice. Although the number of physicians and the ratio of physicians per capita have been increasing, there has not been a noticeable decrease in physician incomes. As a result, it becomes necessary to examine what is keeping the competitive market from operating efficiently and to modify the model to enable more accurate predictions to occur.

8.4.3 Fee Differences Among Patients

The competitive model predicts that one price will prevail in the market for all suppliers and demanders. That is, the market-clearing price is the same for all producers and all consumers. Before the spread of health insurance, physician pricing was characterized by a sliding scale of fees, with high-income patients paying higher prices than low-income patients. The stated objective of the sliding fee scale was to enable all patients to have access to needed medical care. While the spread of health insurance coverage has reduced the need for physicians to use a sliding fee scale, there are still substantial variations in the prices paid by different insurance carriers for the same or similar service, continuing to limit the allocative role of a single price in the physician market. This phenomenon has led many economists to reject the competitive model as inappropriate for the physician services market and to substitute a monopoly model (De Jaegher & Jegers, 2001; Kessell, 1958; Leonard, Stordeur, & Roberfroid, 2009; Newhouse, 1970; Ruffin & Leigh, 1973; Wu & Masson, 1974; see Chapter 9). The monopoly model was believed to be more applicable because it enables producers to segment the market and charge different prices to each segment instead of a uniform price to all consumers.

8.4.4 Quality of Care

The competitive model assumes that a homogeneous service is being bought and sold and that competition for the good or service is based on price. Yet, product quality is a major element of the output of physicians and hospitals, and health insurance companies often offer different types of policies in terms of coverage (viewed as differences in the quality of the health insurance policy as well as differences in service).

When a supplier can vary its quality, it can attract consumers on the basis of its quality rather than just on price. It follows that some "brand loyalty" may ensue because of the real or perceived quality, and buyers will not switch brands easily (because of a slight increase in price or deferential in price, for example). This phenomenon is called *product differentiation*, and it implies that each supplier then faces a downward-sloping demand curve, not a horizontal one (as is the case in perfect competition) since the producer can sell as much of its output as it is willing to sell at the prevailing market price, and can now choose to compete with other providers on the basis of price or product quality. The competitive model is not equipped to handle this feature of the healthcare market, which requires a somewhat more complex model. The violation of the homogeneous product assumption in the competitive model means additional modifications to the model are required in order to enhance its predictive ability.

8.4.5 Restricting Competitive Behavior

Additional evidence of anticompetitive control mechanisms in the healthcare market is found by examining the behavior of physicians when they are confronted with potentially competitive colleagues. Historically, two restrictive practices have been used by physician-organized associations: the prohibition of advertising of physician fees and limiting the participation by physicians in prepayment group practices if the physicians wished to retain their membership in good standing in the association. In a competitive world, such as that set out in the model in Section 8.2, advertising is unnecessary because consumers possess complete information and so know all about physician fees. But in the real world, considerable consumer ignorance exists, allowing different prices to exist, and so advertising by certain physicians would reduce ignorance about alternative physician prices (and perhaps qualifications). Coupled with fee cutting (price reductions), advertising would result not only in more business for the fee-cutting advertiser, but, generally, would result in lower prices and reduced profits in the industry.

Advertising bans had been enforced by state medical societies (Kessell, 1958), and although such bans are no longer legally enforceable, their existence in the past was considered evidence that physicians were able to intervene in the market on behalf of themselves and eliminate some degree of competition in the market. Bans on advertising (and other competitive practices) have been used as evidence of the availability of mechanisms to restrict competition in the market for physician services. While advertising currently exists, most of the advertisements do not focus on the price of physician services, and so consumers are still not able to shop easily for the lowest cost providers.

8.4.6 Consumer Ignorance and Supplier-Induced Demand

The competitive model operates under the assumption that consumers possess a considerable degree of information about their medical condition, the healthcare products they need, and the outcomes associated with the use of the products. In fact, consumers appear to operate under a considerable degree of ignorance in the area of health and healthcare services, which has led some commentators to view physicians as essentially agents acting on behalf of consumers (Calcott, 1999; Carlsen & Grytten, 2000; Feldstein, 1974). If physicians do behave as agents for their patients, the implicit assumption that suppliers and demanders are acting independently must be rejected. Under the condition that patients lack complete information and so physicians act as their agents in making decisions to consume healthcare services, then demand is subject to direct supplier influence.

Nor can the assumption be made that, if physicians do act as agents for their patients, physicians always behave in the patients' best interests. Because of information asymmetry, the possibility exists that physicians can use their knowledge and influence to further their own interests, rather than the interest of their patients. Consumer demands can be shifted by the suppliers through the provision of incomplete or biased information.

Demand shifting can be detected in market outcome statistics in some circumstances. According to the competitive theory, an increase in the per capita supply of physicians results in an increase in market supply of services. With everything else held constant, this increase in supply should bring down the price of health care. Yet, it has been alleged that the relationship between physician per capita supply and price is exactly opposite to that predicted by the model; that is, the more physicians per capita in an area, the higher the observed price of physician services (Evans, 1974; Fuchs & Kramer, 1972; Pelech, 2018). The reason why this phenomenon is not considered proven is that a number of intervening factors also exist that may cause demand to rise at the same time as physician supply increases.

In the following illustration, a simple comparison of two hypothetical medical markets is analyzed, one in a small town and one in a large metropolitan center with several medical schools. The large city may have more physicians per capita than the small town, and yet the price for a visit to a physician in the larger city may be greater. This "raw" relationship by itself does not mean that the higher supply has caused the higher price in the market.

Many other intervening variables must also be taken into account, among them the amount and type of health insurance coverage, the health status of the two populations, and the type and quality of care provided in the two locations. The third factor, the quality of care, is especially important in making comparisons between the two communities, mainly because it is such a difficult variable to measure and, thus, may be ignored in many analyses. It may well be that the quality of care in the larger city is higher than in the smaller town. If all factors other than the quality of care were adjusted for, a positive relationship between physician density and price might still be observed. Until quality has been adjusted for, however, we cannot be certain that the higher price is not due to the fact that better quality service is being provided.

There is still evidence that the cost of health care varies substantially across the United States for comparable populations. For example, a report by the Network for Regional Healthcare Improvement (2018) found that the Maryland region had cost 20% below the benchmark average, while the Colorado region had cost 19% above the benchmark average. These variations have continued over time.

Another factor to take into consideration when comparing urban and rural physician-to-population ratios is the role of specialists and the critical mass of population required to support specialists. Since, for example, fewer people require the services of an oncologist than a general internist, the population base required to support the oncologist is larger, making direct comparison of physician-to-population ratios in urban and rural areas difficult and even misleading (Hicks & Glenn, 1991; Stensland & Stinson, 2002).

These types of confounding relationship have caused controversy regarding the observed relationship between price and physician density (Sloan & Feldman, 1978). Some commentators have proceeded as if the relationship were true and have constructed alternative supplier-induced demand models as explanations for the observed results.

8.5 Competitive Bidding

The competitive market has often been held up as an ideal system for allocative efficiency, a standard against which other allocative arrangements might be judged. One mechanism that has been put forward as potentially providing a competitive-style outcome for public programs is the use of competitive bidding. Competitive bidding occurs when a purchaser (e.g., a government agency) requests bids from alternative competing providers and then allocates the right to treat patients based on the bids. The object of this practice is to have the patients treated for the least cost to the public agency.

One approach to developing a model of the competitive bidding process is to examine the behavior of an individual supplier who is facing a single paying agency and who is competing with other providers for the right to provide the services. In constructing such a model, it is essential to recognize that the bids by providers are made under conditions of uncertainty and risk. When the providers submit their bids to the agency, the bidders do not know for certain whether or not they will be selected as providers. The behavior of the providers in this situation can be modeled in a manner similar to that of consumers who are faced with the risk of incurring major/catastrophic medical expenses.

The bidder faces one of two possible outcomes: (1) the bid submitted is accepted and then the bidder must provide services to the designated population for that price, or (2) the bid is rejected and the bidder will not have access to that population. To simplify matters, assume that no losses to the provider are associated with an unsuccessful bid (i.e., the bidder is no worse off if the bid is not accepted than if he or she had not bid). What the bidder must do in deciding whether or not to bid, and if making a bid at what level, is to compare the outcomes of the various bids being considered in order to assess which bid will prove the most satisfactory.

A simplified model is presented in numerical form in **Table 8-1**. In this model the following assumptions are made. *First*, a request is put out by the public agency calling for providers to bid for the right to serve a given number of patients in a public program. The bids submitted by the providers are to be expressed in per capita terms for a certain defined set of services (physician care, hospital care, and pharmaceuticals). *Second*, five options (labeled A through E) are being considered by the bidder: bids of $100, $95, $90, $85, and $80 per person in the program. *Third*, the bidder knows that as he or she lowers his or her bid, the probability of having the bid accepted by the agency increases.

As illustrated in the table, at a bid of $100, there is a 20% chance the bid will be accepted. This chance of the bid being accepted rises to 90% with a bid of $80. *Fourth*, the bidder's profits, if the bid is accepted, are equal to the revenues less the costs of serving the designated number of patients. Given the number of patients (Q) and the costs per patient (C), the higher the accepted bid (B), the higher will be the profits [equal to $(B \times Q) - (C \times Q)$]. *Fifth*, the profitability situation of the bidder is then translated into a wealth level for the provider. Assume also that, without a contract, the bidder's wealth would be $200, since the bidder will not have access to the program's population base. A successful bid, thus, adds to the successful bidder's wealth level by the level of the bidder's profits.

The bidder is, thus, faced with a trade-off between profits (and hence wealth) and the probability of a successful bid. The individual bidder can increase the likelihood of a successful bid, but only by lowering the price of the bid and, thus, lowering the profits that can be achieved. Given the range of alternatives, the decision is to determine which bid to submit. As set up now, the model is very basic, because it does not incorporate the objectives of the bidders or the bidding rules set up by the contracting agency.

With regard to bidder's objectives, assume first that the bidder is extremely risk averse—the bidder does not like uncertainty or risk. He or she puts a high personal value on small gains and successively lower additional values on potential larger gains (i.e., wealth), for the bidder has a diminishing marginal utility). Under this assumption, reflected in column 6 of Table 8-1, the bidder will choose the option that maximizes his or her *expected* utility, measured as the product of the probability of success (column 3) and the utility associated (column 6 or column 7) with the wealth level of that option. In the illustration provided, the risk-averse bidder will choose Option E, which yields an expected utility of 90 (0.9 × 100). Option D, for example, would yield an expected utility of 88 (0.8 × 110) for the risk-averse bidder. Although the profits for Option D are greater, the bidder prefers to select a very safe but relatively unprofitable option.

Table 8-1 Hypothetical Bidding Data

Utility Levels						
Option	Bid Price ($)	Probability of Acceptance	Profits (If Bid Accepted) ($)	Wealth Level (If Bid Accepted) ($)	Risk Averter	Risk-Taker
A	100	0.2	800	1,000	126	2,000
B	95	0.4	400	600	122	800
C	90	0.6	200	400	118	400
D	85	0.8	100	300	110	200
E	80	0.9	50	250	100	100

Alternatively, a risk-taker, whose tastes might be like those summarized in column 7 in Table 8-1, considers high levels of wealth to be most important, which is shown by the sharply increasing utilities of wealth in column 7. To a risk-taking bidder, substantial profits are so important that they overshadow the very small chances of attaining them. To the risk-taker, Option E has an expected utility of 90 (0.9 × 100) (the same as for the risk-averse bidder), whereas Option A has an expected utility of 400 (2000 × 0.2) for the risk-taking bidder. Option A is the one that would be selected by the risk-taking bidder.

Competitive bidding does not automatically lead to a low-price bid. Much of the outcome depends on the bidders' costs and goals. But, there are several other factors as well that impact the decision making in the bidding process. *First*, an increase in the number of bidders will reduce the probability of any single bidder being successful. Depending on the bidders' utility schedules, a larger number of competitive bidders may cause each bidder to reduce his or her bid, trying to improve the chances of submitting the winning bid.

Second, there are a number of different selection and reimbursement methods to which a contracting agency can resort. These methods may influence the bidding strategies of the bidders (Christianson, Smith, & Hillman, 1984; Miller, Rossiter, & Nuttall, 2002; Town, Feldman, & Kralewski, 2011). One such method is to reimburse each winning bidder (more than one provider in an area may be chosen as a winner) at the level of the bid he or she submitted. Thus, if Bidder 1 submitted a bid of $95, Bidder 2, $90, and Bidder 3, $85, and if Bidders 2 and 3 are selected as providers, then Bidder 2 would be reimbursed at $90 and Bidder 3 at $85. This method tends to encourage bidding providers to gamble and seek a higher price, since there is a potential reward to them for doing so (they are reimbursed at the price they bid if their bid is accepted). An alternative method will increase this tendency to gamble. If the set of rules specified that all winning bidders would be reimbursed at the amount submitted by the lowest winning bidder, there would be no benefit to a winner making a higher bid if the bidder believes that some other winner will bid lower. Indeed, submitting a higher bid merely reduces the chances of being a successful bidder.

Competitive bidding rules may lead to a competitive market-type outcome. Whether or not it does will depend on a number of factors, including the number of bidders, their attitudes toward risk, and the bidding rules set up by the agency. In 1982, the California legislative assembly passed a law allowing selective contracting by third-party payers with hospitals and physicians. Previously, third-party payers in California could not exclude any providers from the group they were obligated to reimburse for services provided.

In the 1990s, managed care grew rapidly as a tool for reducing the rate of increase in healthcare costs. One mechanism used by managed care companies to restrain costs was to limit the providers included in the plan, selecting the lowest cost providers. However, opponents were successful, in many states, in getting "any willing provider" laws passed, which required plans to accept any provider into the plan that was willing to accept the terms of the plan. This effectively removed the ability of managed care plans to limit provider participation and control costs. Currently, most willing provider statutes have been eliminated as governments and private insurers have moved toward accountable care organizations (ACOs) and efforts to reduce costs and improve outcomes for the population. ACOs are selected in the enrollment of providers to serve their members.

8.6 Supplier-Induced Demand

8.6.1 A Pedagogic Model

In Chapter 3, the focus was on the asymmetry of information between consumers and providers in the medical care market. The possibility was presented that consumers may not have good information about their health status, the treatment options available, or the probable effect of medical care on their health. Although consumers are not likely to be completely ignorant regarding their health and health care, they do often rely on physicians to act as their agents and inform them about these variables. Physicians can, in many instances, provide information that will allow patients to formulate a reasonable demand curve. However, this information provided may not be fully complete. Physicians can affect the demand curve for medical care by providing information that is biased or incomplete. If physicians do induce demand unnecessarily, perhaps in response to the excess capacities of their practices, then where the ratio of physicians to population is high, demand will be shifted out more. Ultimately, the extent of unnecessary inducement of demand is an empirical question—and a difficult one to answer.

A large number of studies have been developed that attempt to incorporate supplier-induced demand into the framework of medical markets to explain the wide variation in services to treat the same diagnosis in patients. Many of these models focus on the provider (physician) and assume implicitly that the ability to shift demand is unlimited. Because consumers have access to information about the quality of advice they receive from their physicians, it is more realistic to recognize that limitations to demand generation may exist. The following presents a simple model of medical care markets that brings out some of their more important features (Cooper, 2011; Leonard et al., 2009; Mohammadshahi et al., 2019; Mulley, 2009; Pauly, 1980; Peacock & Richardson, 2006; van Dijk et al., 2013).

In this model, assume that consumers' "taste" for medical care depends on information about initial health status (H_0); the effect of medical care on health ($\Delta H/\Delta M$, where M stands for medical care); and the impact of health on utility, incomes, and prices. It also depends on the number of physicians in the market. In particular, a lower physician (DOC) to population ratio (shortened to *DOCPOP*) will lead to a higher demand for each physician in the market.

For each patient in this illustration, assume there is a "true" level of H and $\Delta H/\Delta M$ that can be determined by the patient's physician. If the physician is fully truthful with the patient, a demand curve for the patient can be derived (D_{true} in **Figure 8-7**). This demand curve is downward sloping, which means that, for any given level of belief about H and

$\Delta H/\Delta M$, the quantity demanded will be responsive to the out-of-pocket price of the patient.

Assume, however, that the physician has the ability to tell the patient that H and $\Delta H/\Delta M$ have values higher than the actual ones. If the patient believes the physician, the patient's demand curve will shift upward into the right (i.e., at any price, the quantity demanded will be greater than under the actual values). However, the physician is only one source of information, and the patient can get information elsewhere if he or she questions the physician's assessment. It is, therefore, likely that there is an upper limit to the physician's ability to generate demand that is not grounded in reality. In this model, the demand curve at this upper limit is called D_{limit} in Figure 8-7.

8.6.2 Supply

Having specified the demand characteristics of the model, the supply side of the market is now examined. With regard to physician behavior, the following assumptions are made in this illustration:

- Each physician has an upward-sloping marginal cost (MC) curve (i.e., as more services are provided, marginal costs increase), resulting in an upward-sloping supply curve (S).
- The price of services is fixed by a fee schedule, and so fees are beyond physician control.

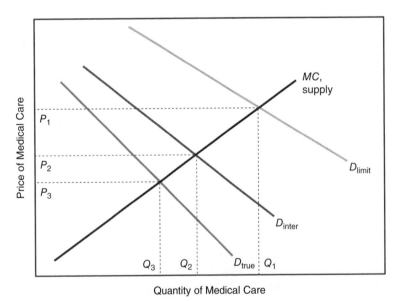

Figure 8-7 Representation of supplier-induced demand. The three demand curves, D_{true}, D_{inter}, and D_{limit}, represent the demand of three successive levels of supplier inducement; no unnecessary inducement (D_{true}), an intermediate level of inducement (D_{inter}), and the maximum level of inducement possible (D_{limit}). The physician's marginal cost is MC. Three alternative fee levels, P_1, P_2, and P_3, are shown. The quantity of medical care "induced" will depend on the fee level, the degree of inducement, and the physician's MC. However, at high fee levels, patient-influenced limitations may be a factor in determining utilization.

8.6.3 Objectives

A number of studies have identified a number of different possible physician objectives, ranging from healing patients to maximizing profits. In this illustration, assume each physician's goal is profit maximization for the sake of convenience, not because it is necessarily the most realistic assumption. It also elucidates the "worst case" scenario, and shows how the most selfish physicians will behave under specified conditions without restraint or remorse. This worst case scenario ignores factors that may limit a physician's demand inducement, including guilt for misleading patients, ethical norms, a strong sense of professionalism, competition, and increasing regulatory oversight and the reporting of comparative data on physicians.

The model presented in Figure 8-7 has been designed to predict the quantity of medical care provided in the market. In the illustration, it is shown that the quantity of medical care provided will depend on the specific price received by the physician. Assume initially that there is a high price for physician services, such as P_1 in Figure 8-7. At this price, the physician will generate demand up to the limit and provide services at level Q_1. At this point, marginal revenue (*MR*) is greater than *MC*, and the physician would be able to earn additional profits if demand could be generated beyond D_{limit}. However, the patient cannot be pushed further, and so this is the best the physician can do.

If the price were lower, for example at P_2, the physician would generate demand up to some intermediate point D_{int} and would provide Q_2 units of service. Beyond this point, *MC* would exceed *MR*, and the physician would have reduced profits with the inducement of further demand. At an even lower price, for example P_3, the physician would not generate any unnecessary demand and would provide Q_3 units of service. The conclusions of even this simple model are that, with the most selfish of physicians, the quantity demanded—and the degree of demand generation—will depend on the given price in the market.

Next, assume that there is an increase in the supply of physicians in this illustration (i.e., an increase in the *DOCPOP*). From the viewpoint of the individual physician currently in the market, such an increase would lead to a reduction in each demand curve (D_{true}, D_{int}, and D_{limit}), because these curves are the individual physician's demand curves and each physician will have a smaller share of the market. In these circumstances, each physician's quantity of services supplied will be reduced. Overall demand

cannot be generated beyond the maximum, and, at a price such as P_3, there is not likely to be any change in overall services.

As pointed out above, there are a number of reasons why consumers might not be totally gullible and vulnerable to demand-generating tactics. *First*, consumers can obtain information from sources other than their physicians, especially given access to the internet today. *Second*, a number of studies have suggested that there is a limit to the willingness of physicians to generate demand (Rossiter & Wilensky, 1983; Stano, 1987a, b; Xirasagar & Lin, 2006), although the nature of this reticence has not been spelled out. Analysts have alternatively modeled the generation of ungrounded demand as a cost to physicians and as a cause of disutility (perhaps as a result of feelings of guilt). In either case, generating too much unnecessary demand will make the physicians (as well as the patients) worse off.

As has been hypothesized in this illustration, the generation of ungrounded demand will result in higher marginal costs to the physician and, depending on revenues, may yield more profits. But what if the physician's objectives included patient well-being? The impact of this goal will be to reduce the degree to which the physician would be willing to generate demand.

The above-illustrated model has dealt with demand generation and patient utilization at given prices. It presents a pedagogic treatment of the issue of demand generation and its likely degree of restriction. However, it ignores the fact that, contrary to what might be expected, higher physician fees have been associated with an increase in *DOCPOP*. The following discussion focuses on possible explanations of this surprising relationship between fees and supply.

8.6.4 DOCPOP and Physician Fees: A Positive Relationship?

One hypothesis concerning price formation in the physician services market is that when supply increases (the supply curve shifts downward and to the right), price increases (Evans, 1974). This prediction is contrary to that of the competitive model, which predicts that price will fall when supply increases. The standard competitive model discussed in this chapter is represented graphically in **Figure 8-8**. In this figure, D_1 represents an initial demand level and S_1 an initial supply level. The initial supply level corresponds to an initial supply of physicians (an initial level of *DOCPOP*). Now, assume there is an increase in the level of *DOCPOP* to the point where

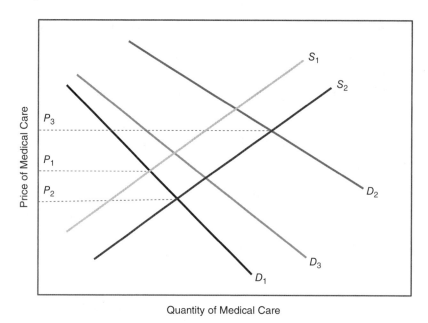

Quantity of Medical Care

Figure 8-8 Difficulties in identifying supplier-induced demand based on actual market data. An increase in the physician population will result in an increase in supply from S_1 to S_2. Absence of supplier-induced demand, this will cause a fall in price from P_1 to P_2, a result of a movement along demand curve D_1. However, supplier-induced demand is consistent with both an increase in price (if demand shifts to D_2) and a reduction in price (if demand shifts, but only to D_3).

© Jones & Bartlett Learning.

the supply shifts downward and to the right to S_2. Physicians, according to this theory, will offer more services, and, as supply shifts out, prices will fall and utilization will increase. This prediction does not square with the alleged empirical fact that increases in price accompany increases in physician supply (*DOCPOP*).

In order to fit the theory to the facts observed, a number of researchers have contended that suppliers can shift demand through supplier-induced demand. For example, assume the suppliers in this illustration could push the demand curve out to D_2. Even if the supply was to increase from S_1 to S_2, the equilibrium price would increase to P_3. Of course, supplier-induced demand can also occur when prices *fall* after an outward shift in supply. If, following an increase in supply to S_2, suppliers were only successful in shifting the demand to D_3, the price would fall, even though suppliers had been successful in shifting the demand. Thus, a fall in price when supply increases is consistent with both the competitive and the supplier-induced demand theories! This makes it impossible to distinguish between them. Only when prices are observed to rise following an increase in *DOCPOP* and all else stays the same can the supplier-induced demand model be assumed to be the appropriate model.

The major problem in verifying the existence of supplier-induced demand lies in the fact that

other demand- and supply-influencing variables are changing along with *DOCPOP*. For example, assume that supply shifts from S_1 to S_2 and a price increase from P_1 to P_3 is observed. In order to be sure that supplier-induced demand is actually being observed, then control of all other variables that could affect demand and supply has been achieved. If, for example, S_1 represents supply conditions in Salt Lake City and S_2 conditions in San Antonio, the demand differences between the two markets may have occurred because of supplier-induced demand or a myriad other demand-influencing factors, such as health status, quality of care, insurance coverage, and so on. Further, even if differences in *DOCPOP* between the two markets have been controlled for, there must be no other intervening supply variables that could have resulted in greater increases (or decreases).

A number of statistical studies have been undertaken to estimate the extent of supplier-induced demand. The majority of these have focused their attention on *utilization* of medical care and how it has been influenced by *DOCPOP*. For example, Rossiter and Wilensky (1983) studied data obtained from a national sample survey of families (known as the National Medical Care Cost and Expenditure Survey) to determine the effect of a number of variables, such as direct price, travel time, health status, and the physician-to-population ratio, on the number of physician-initiated visits. Physician-initiated visits, although suggested by physicians, are not the same as physician-induced visits, since the term *inducement* connotes lack of necessity. There is no way of telling from a data set such as that used by the authors the degree to which physician-initiated visits were unnecessary and induced by physicians for their own benefit. The results of the study indicated a very small effect of *DOCPOP* on ambulatory care utilization: An increase in the ratio by one physician per 100,000 population resulted in an increase in expenditures on physician-initiated visits of only seven cents. However, the authors did not directly test the supplier-induced demand hypothesis.

Cromwell and Mitchell (1986) and Fuchs (1978), on the other hand, did directly test for the effect of supplier-induced demand in the market for surgery by examining the effect of surgeon population ratios on surgery utilization and surgeons' fees. The data set in the Cromwell–Mitchell study consisted of metropolitan area statistics on families' characteristics and surgical utilization obtained from the Health Interview Survey of the National Center for Health Statistics coupled with Medicare surgical fee data. The authors studied how both surgical fees and surgery utilization rates differed among markets (metropolitan areas)

when variables, such as age distribution, education level, average coinsurance rate, the number of general practitioners per 1000 population, and the number of surgeons per 1000 population varied. They also controlled for the supply effect of higher fees causing more surgeons to locate in the area.

Their results indicated a price elasticity for surgical operations of -0.15, when all identified demand-shifting variables were held constant. With regard to the variable *DOCPOP* for surgeons, they identified a considerable effect of this variable on surgical utilization and on surgical fees. In the case of utilization, the magnitude of the relationship was such that a 10% increase in surgeons in the population resulted in a 9% increase in surgical operations. With regard to fee increases, a 1% increase in surgeons in the population resulted in a .9% increase in surgeons' fees. The authors presented these results as indicative of a significant supplier-induced demand effect in the market for surgery. However, because of the many variables influencing supply and demand and the difficulty of controlling for these in statistical tests, there is controversy surrounding any results in this area (Cooper, 2011; Dranove & Wehner, 1994; Feldman & Sloan, 1988; Mohammadshahi et al., 2019; Mulley, 2009; Peacock & Richardson, 2007; van Dijk et al., 2013).

Exercises

1. Predict the effect of the following changes in the market price and quantity utilized of eye examinations conducted by ophthalmologists:
   a. an increase in the degree of insurance coverage for eye exams (i.e., lower insurance copayments by the patients)
   b. an increase in the number of ophthalmologists
   c. an increase in the average age of the population
   d. a reduction in the price of optometry services (which are substitute services)
   e. an increase in the price of eyeglasses, which are complementary goods

2. Given an initial equilibrium in the market for clinical care, predict the effect of the following changes in equilibrium price and quantity:
   a. an increase in nurses' wages in the clinic market
   b. an increase in the number of clinics
   c. an increase in clinic productivity
   d. a reduction in supply costs for clinics

3. For-Profit Labs, Inc. (FPL) is a private laboratory that does only routine blood counts. With total assets of $8,000,000 last year, FPL took in $3 million in revenues and had expenses of $200,000. The average firms in other industries make a return of 10% on their assets. The market for lab services is potentially competitive, but right now there are only a few firms in the industry. However, lab technicians are free to enter the industry if they wish. Firms in the industry charge $300 for blood counts, and their costs are $20. What do you expect will happen in the long run?

4. The market for physiotherapist visits is shown in the accompanying diagram. The current equilibrium price is $30 and the equilibrium quantity is 150 visits. The healthcare authorities are concerned that the price is too high and so have proposed lowering the price to $10 per visit. They contend that at a lower price more people will get to use these services. Predict the

effect on quantities demanded and supplied and on quantity of services actually utilized as a result of such an intervention.

5. The demand and supply for hospital care in the Garden State is given in the following diagram. Currently, the state legislature has mandated that all hospital care must be free and that providers will be reimbursed at a rate of $450 per day. The Hospital Association has expressed its concern that at this reimbursement rate there will not be enough hospital care to "go around" and meet all the demands. It is proposed that the reimbursement rate be increased to $600 a day. What is the quantity demanded and supplied and the quantity utilized at the two rates? What is the total amount funded at the two rates?

6. The state healthcare commission is planning to put out bids for care. Physician Group A is considering making a bid but is unsure how much to bid. Group A's actuary has developed four options: bid a price per capita of $1000, $800, $600, or $400. Group A currently has a

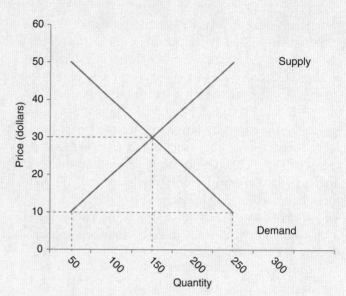

wealth level of $1000. Added profits associated with each level are provided in the accompanying table. Also provided in this table are the estimated probabilities of each of the four bids being accepted and Group A's utility of each wealth level. Given that Group A is a risk-averse, utility-maximizing entity, what bid should it make?

Option	Bid Price ($)	Probability of Bid Being Accepted	Added Profits If Bid Is Accepted ($)	Wealth Level If Bid Is Accepted ($)	Utility of a Given Level of Wealth
A	1000	0.2	4000	5000	380
B	800	0.4	3000	4000	400
C	600	0.6	2000	3000	280
D	400	0.8	1000	2000	200
No bid				1000	100

Bibliography

Buchanan, J. M. (1965). *The inconsistencies of the National Health Service*. Occasional paper 7. London: Institute of Economic Affairs.

Burns, J. (2009). Is the doctor in? Proven strategies for physician recruitment and retention. *Journal of Medical Practice Management, 24*(6), 344–346.

Calcott, P. (1999). Demand inducement as cheap talk. *Health Economics, 8*(8), 721–733.

Carlsen, F., & Grytten, J. (2000). Consumer satisfaction and supplier-induced demand. *Journal of Health Economics, 19*(5), 731–753.

Christianson, J. B., Smith, K. R., & Hillman, D. G. (1984). A comparison of existing and alternative competitive bidding systems for indigent medical care. *Social Science and Medicine, 18*, 599–604.

Cooper, R. A. (2011). Geographic variation in health care and affluence-poverty nexus. *Advances in Surgery, 45*, 63–82.

Cromwell, J., & Mitchell, J. B. (1986). Physician induced demand for surgery. *Journal of Health Economics, 5*, 293–313.

Culyer, A. J., & Cullis, J. G. (1976). Some economics of hospital waiting lists in the NHS. *Social Policy, 5*, 239–264.

De Jaegher, K., & Jegers, M. (2001). The physician-patient relationship as a game of strategic information transmission. *Health Economics, 10*(7), 651–668.

Dranove, D., & Wehner, P. (1994). Physician-induced demand for childbirths. *Journal of Health Economics, 13*, 61–73.

Drumm, T. L., Arkins, J. P., & Dayan, S. H. (2010). Retailicine, somewhere between retail and medicine. *Facial Plastic Surgery Clinics of North America, 18*(4), 491–498.

Elflein, J. (2019, March 18). Hospital occupancy rate in the U.S. from 1975 to 2017. *Statista* (data from AHA and USDHHS). Retrieved August 17, 2019, from https://www.statista.com/statistics/185904/hospital-occupancy-rate-in-the-us-since-2001/

Evans, R. G. (1974). Supplier induced demand: Some empirical evidence and implications. In M. Pearlman (Ed.), *The economics of health and medical care* (pp. 162–173). London, England: MacMillan.

Feldman, R., & Sloan, F. (1988). Competition among physicians. *Journal of Health Politics, Policy, and Law, 13*, 239–264.

Feldstein, M. S. (1974). Econometric studies in health economics. In M. Intriligator & S. Kendrick (Eds.), *Frontiers in quantitative economics, 2*, 377–437. Amsterdam, The Netherlands: North-Holland.

Fuchs, V. R. (1978). The supply of surgeons and the demand for operations. *Journal of Human Resources, 13*(suppl.), 35–55.

Fuchs, V. R., & Kramer, M. (1972). *Determinants of expenditures for physicians' services in the United States, 1948–1968* (Publication no. HSM 73–3013). Washington, DC: National Center for Health Services Research.

Garbarino, J. W. (1959). Price behavior and productivity in the medical market. *Industrial and Labor Relations Review, 13*, 3–15.

Ginsburg, P. B. (2010). Wide variation in hospital and physician payment rates evidence of provider market power. *Research Briefs, 16*, 1–11.

Hicks, L. L., & Glenn, J. K. (1991). Rural populations and rural physicians: Estimates of critical mass ratios. *Journal of Rural Health, 7*(4), 357–371.

Kessell, R. (1958). Price discrimination in medicine. *Journal of Law and Economics, 1*, 20–53.

Leonard, C., Stordeur, S., & Roberfroid, D. (2009). Association between physician density and health care consumption: A systematic review of the evidence. *Health Policy, 91*(2), 121–134.

Lindsay, C. M. (1976). More real returns to medical education. *Journal of Human Resources, 11*, 127–129.

Miller, P., Rossiter, P., & Nuttall, D. (2002). Demonstrating the economic value of occupational health services. *Occupational Medicine, 52*(8), 477–483.

Mohammadshahi, M., Yazdani, S., Olyaeemanesh, A., Sari, A. A., Yaseri, M., & Sefiddashi, S. E. (2019). A scoping review of components of physician-induced demand for designing a conceptual framework. *Journal of Preventive Medicine and Public Health, 52*(2), 72–81.

Mulley, A. G. (2009). Inconvenient truths about supplier induced demand and unwarranted variation in medical practice. *BMJ, 339*, b4073.

Murphy, B. (2016, April 12). Which physicians generate the most revenue for hospitals. *Hospital CFO Report.* Retrieved August 15, 2019, from https://www.beckershospitalreview.com /finance/which-physicians-generate-the-most-revenue-for -hospitals.html

Network of Regional Healthcare Improvement. (2018). *Healthcare affordability: Data is the spark, collaboration is the fuel.* South Portland, ME: Author.

Newhouse, J. P. (1970). A model of physician pricing. *Southern Economic Journal, 37*, 147–183.

Newhouse, J. P., Phelps, C. E., & Schwartz, W. B. (1977). Policy options and the impact of national health insurance revisited. *International Journal of Health Services, 7*, 503–509.

Otari K., Waterman, B., Faulkner, K. M., Boslaugh, S., Burroughs, T. E., & Dunagan, W. C. (2009). Patient satisfaction: Focusing on "excellent". *Journal of Healthcare Management 54*(2), 93–102.

Pauly, M. V. (1980). *Doctors and their workshops.* Chicago, IL: University of Chicago Press.

Peacock, S. J., & Richardson, J. R. (2007). Supplier-induced demand: Re-examining identification and misspecification in cross-sectional analysis. *European Journal of Health Economics, 8*(3), 267–277.

Pelech, D. (2018). *An analysis of private-sector prices and physician services.* Washington, DC: Congressional Budget Office.

Popa, R. (2019, July 19). How did independent physician practice profits change in the past year. *Becker's ASC Review.* Retrieved August 05, 2019, from https://www.beckersasc.com /benchmarking/how-did-independent-physician-practice -profits-change-in-the-past-year.html

Ro, K. K. (1977). Anatomy of hospital cost inflation. *Hospitals and Health Services Administration, 22*, 78–88.

Rossiter, L. F., & Wilensky, G. R. (1983). A reexamination of the use of physician services. *Inquiry, 20*, 162–172.

Ruffin, R. J., & Leigh, D. E. (1973). Charity, competition, and the pricing of doctors' services. *The Journal of Human Resources, 8*(2), 212–222.

Schwartz, W. B., & Mendelson, D. N. (1990). No evidence of an emerging physician surplus. *JAMA, 263*, 557–560.

Sloan, F. A. (1976). Real returns to medical education. *Journal of Human Resources, 11*, 118–126.

Sloan, F. A., & Feldman, R. (1978). Competition among physicians. In W. Greenberg (Ed.), *Competition in the health care sector* (pp. 57–131). Washington, DC: Federal Trade Commission, Bureau of Economics.

Sloan, F. A., & Lorant, J. H. (1976). The allocation of physicians' services. *Quarterly Review of Economics and Business, 16*, 86–103.

Stano, M. C. (1987a). A further analysis of the physician inducement controversy. *Journal of Health Economics, 6*(3), 228–237.

Stano, M. C. (1987b). A further analysis of the "variation in practice styles" phenomenon. *Inquiry, 23*(2), 176–182.

Stensland, J., & Stinson, T. (2002). Successful physician-hospital integration in rural areas. *Medical Care, 40*(10), 908–917.

Tikkahen, R., & Osborn, R. (2019). *Does the United States ration health care.* New York, NY: The Commonwealth Fund.

Town, R., Feldman, R., & Kralewski, J. (2011). Market power and contract form: Evidence from physician group practices. *International Journal of Health Care Finance & Economics, 11*(2), 115–132.

Van Dijk, C. E., Van den Bert, B., Verhey, R. A., Spreeuwenberg, P., Groenewegen, P. P., & de Baker, D. H. (2013). Moral hazard and supplier induced demand: Empirical evidence in general practice. *Health Economics, 22*(3), 340–352.

Wu, W. S., & Masson, R. (1974). Price discrimination for physicians' services. *Journal of Human Resources, 9*, 63–79.

Xirasagar, S., & Lin, H. C. (2006). Physician supply, supplier-induced demand, and competition: Empirical evidence from a single-payer system. *International Journal of Health Planning & Management, 21*(2), 117–131.

Yeginsu, C. (2018, January 3). N.H.S. overwhelmed in Britain, leaving patients to wait. *The New York Times.* Retrieved August 17, 2019, https://www.nytimes.com/2018/01/03/world/europe /uk-national-health-service.html

CHAPTER 9

Market Power in Health Care

OBJECTIVES

1. Use the monopoly model to predict the price charged or quantity of services utilized.
2. Use the monopoly model to explain how providers are able to charge different groups of patients different prices.
3. Describe the functioning of a market in which the buyers have market power.
4. Describe a measure of market power and demonstrate how it can be applied in a market situation.
5. Describe the determinants of market power.
6. Explain the concept of nonprice competition and describe a model with market power and nonprice competition.
7. Demonstrate how the monopoly model can be used to predict resource allocation in markets with preferred provider organizations.

9.1 Introduction

The previous chapters have focused on the characteristics and functioning of the competitive market. The competitive market is considered to be the most efficient type of market, although it does not necessarily consider the issue of equity or equality in terms of the allocation of resources. And, while the competitive market is efficient, some features have been identified in the healthcare system that violate the conditions of a competitive market, and so attention now turns to focus on other types of markets in order to improve analysis and understanding of the functioning of the healthcare system.

Recall from the earlier discussion that under competition, market conditions are such that no single buyer or seller can influence the price at which the exchange of goods and services take place. *Market power* refers to the ability of one participant in a market to influence the terms and conditions by which exchanges occur in the market. Market power can be wielded by either buyers or sellers. For example, a heart surgeon can be in a position to influence the fee that patients or insurers pay, if he or she is the only heart surgeon in the region. Similarly, an insurance company, or government health insurance program, can be in a position to influence the rate or price at which it pays providers for supplying services to its members. If an insurer, public or private, has sufficient power that it has the ability to set the price unilaterally, providers have to accept that price if they are to provide services to the insured population.

Essential ingredients of market power are the limited availability of viable substitutes for the service and the ease with which buyers and sellers can weigh the alternatives available. A hospital may be the only hospital for hundreds of miles, in which case, it possesses some degree of market power (i.e., it has some leeway in setting prices and other terms for the services it provides). On the other hand, a large number of health maintenance organizations (HMOs) or accountable care organizations (ACOs) may be vying to become providers for a firm's employees; in this case, the HMOs have little or no market power, although the firm may possess some market power if it employs a large enough number of individuals from the community.

The examination of the existence of market power is important because, if possessed by either buyers or sellers, it might allow them to wield undue influence over the use of resources to their benefit and to the detriment of the other bargaining parties in the market. In this chapter, an analysis of how market power influences market outcomes (i.e., prices, quantities, and quality) is presented. The analysis is "explanatory," in the sense that the question being asked here is how one set of factors (related to market power) influences specific phenomena or outcome. Discussion of the desirability (or undesirability) of market power must wait until measures with which to gauge actual market conduct are available.

Several models are examined in this chapter that explain resource allocation when either buyers or sellers possess some degree of market power. In Section 9.2, two models of the behavior of the ultimate wielder of market power—the monopolist—are examined that offer predictions about how monopolistic suppliers and/or demanders set price and quantity in the market. All suppliers and demanders would benefit if they possessed substantial market power, and so a pertinent question is, how is market power obtained?

In Section 9.3, the determinants of market power are considered. This section includes a general discussion of market power, as well as an account of how providers in one market possessing many of the preconditions of a competitive market, e.g., the physician services market, were nevertheless able to develop and maintain a considerable degree of market power and use that power to bolster their incomes.

The monopoly model and the competitive model are two polar extremes of models of market power. In many (perhaps most) markets, market power and competition are mixed to varying degrees. In Section 9.4, several models of incomplete market power are discussed that describe how product quality can be an important outcome in provider competition. Just as in the competitive market model, it is very difficult to find a pure monopoly industry in the real world. Most sellers in the market face some level of competition, but the existence of even limited market power leads to the potential for abuse in the market.

9.2 Monopolistic Markets

9.2.1 Simple Monopoly

A monopoly is defined as a single firm having sufficient market power, possibly because it is selling a unique good or service, to have complete control over the quantity produced and its price in the market. Monopoly literally means one seller. A supplier has monopoly in a market when it is the sole source of supply in that market. In a monopolistic market, the demanders do not have any close substitutes for the good or service, and there are restrictive barriers to the entry of new sellers into the market. Of course, some degree of substitutability for the good or service usually exists. For example, in health care, an alternative to specific treatment for a defined illness or injury usually exists, even if that alternative is to do nothing to treat the condition.

The monopoly model will be illustrated in the context of a supposed monopolistic market, the market for pediatric ambulatory services. In this illustration to develop the monopolistic model, it is assumed that, in this market, there is a single group practice of pediatricians. The product the market exchanges is defined as quality-constant pediatric visits. The simple monopoly model illustrated here consists of demand, cost, and behavioral assumptions.

9.2.2 Demand

With regard to demand in this illustration of a monopoly market, it is assumed that the pediatric group faces a single market demand curve (see **Table 9-1**). The demand curve of a monopolist is downward (negative) sloping, since the monopolist, unlike in a competitive market, faces trade-off between price and quantity. The only way the monopolist can increase quantity sold in the market is to lower the price of a good or service. In a competitive market, remember that the producer can sell any quantity it is willing and able to sell at the market price. To increase the quantity of the good or service sold, the monopolist must lower price. Likewise, if price is increased, then quantity sold will be reduced.

Notice that in this illustration there is a price ($100) at which patients will abstain from making any visits to the pediatric group. As movement occurs down the slope demand curve presented, movement occurs through elastic, unit elastic, and inelastic portions of the demand curve, and correspondingly the total revenue (TR) will first increase, then level off, and finally decrease with this downward movement. The marginal revenue (MR) of the group is falling throughout the movement in this illustration, although it is

Table 9-1 Revenue and Cost in a Hypothetical Monopolistic Market

(1) Price ($)	(2) Units of Output	(3) Total Revenue (TR) ($)	(4) Marginal Revenue (MR) ($)	(5) Total Cost (TC) ($)	(6) Marginal Cost (MC) ($)	(7) Profits (TR – TC) ($)
100	0	0	–	30	–	–30
90	1	90	90	40	10	50
80	2	160	70	60	20	100
70	3	210	50	90	30	120
60	4	240	30	130	40	110
50	5	250	10	180	50	70
40	6	240	–10	240	60	0
30	7	210	–30	310	70	–100

© Jones & Bartlett Learning.

positive when it is associated with the elastic portion of the demand curve and zero at the unit elastic point on the demand curve.

For the provider, the *MR* represents the additional total revenue (*TR*) that will be received by lowering the price enough to sell one more pediatric visit. It is important to note that as the provider lowers its price of a pediatric visit, it sells more units, but all of the visits have to be sold at the new, lower price, not just the last unit sold. The *MR* of the monopolist is the net change in *TR* and is equal to the difference in the two *TR*s at the two quantity levels.

The monopolist has the ability to set prices at any level in the market it wishes. This ability to set price unilaterally represents the ultimate degree in market power. Of course, it is important to remember that the price it sets will influence the quantity demanded by the buyer, something the monopolist will need to keep in mind when setting the price to offer its products in the market.

9.2.3 Cost

In this illustration, assume that the total fixed cost (*TFC*) is $30 and that the total variable cost (*TVC*) is increasing in such a way that marginal cost (*MC*) increases as output expands (see Table 9-1, column 6). The total cost (*TC*) is the sum of *TVC* and *TFC*. Recall that short-run cost curves reflect the law of diminishing returns and so most monopolist will also have a U-shaped cost curve, similar in shape to those in a competitive market. It is also important to remember that a monopolist's demand curve is identical to the market demand curve since it is the only supplier in the market.

9.2.4 Objectives

Profits (column 7 in Table 9-1) are equal to total revenue (*TR*) minus total cost (*TC*), and profits will initially increase and then decrease as output expands. The price that will be charged and the output (and profit) levels that will be attained cannot be determined until the objectives the provider is pursuing are known. It is initially assumed in this illustration that the provider's objective is to maximize profits.

The analysis of the monopolistic model is as follows. First, the price the monopolist sets will be the point on the demand curve at which *MR* comes closest to (or equals) *MC* (without *MC* exceeding *MR*). In this illustration, assume that the monopolist initially set its price at $100 per visit. At the $100 price it would have no buyers of its good or service (see Table 9-1), and its losses would be confined to its fixed costs of $30 because it would have no variable costs at zero output. If price in this illustration was lowered to $90, one visit would be sold and the *MR* would be $90. One additional visit would cost only $10 extra (*MC* = $10 as total cost increases from $30 to $40) and would add $80 to the previous output level's profits (from –$30 to + $50). Total profit would therefore be $50.

This is certainly better than not operating at all, but not as good in this illustration as lowering the price to $80, selling two units in total and deriving an additional $70 in revenue in the process (*MR* $160 – $90 *or* = $70). At the level of two visits, it would cost the pediatricians only $20 more to provide this added visit, and another $50 (MR – MC) would be added to the previous profit level, making the profits $100 in total. Indeed, the pediatric practice would continue to lower its price to $70, selling three pediatric visits. The pediatric group would stop supplying visits there because beyond this level of output, TC increases more than TR increases, and as a result MR – MC becomes negative. In this illustration with data in Table 9-1, any further increase in output would detract from the total profits of the pediatric group.

This analysis of the data in Table 9-1 is shown graphically in **Figure 9-1**. The revenue and cost function curves in Figure 9-1 have been smoothed-out to better illustrate their relationships. Here it is seen that the MR and MC curves intersect (meaning MR = MC) at a quantity of between 3 and 4 (because of our smoothed-out values). This corresponds to a price on the demand curve of between $60 and $70. Profitability cannot be increased by raising or lowering the price from that point.

The demand curve of the monopolist slopes downward and to the right since its demand curve is the market demand curve. The degree of elasticity determines the steepness of the demand curve—the more elastic the demand, the more gentle is the slope of the demand curve. The demand curve of the monopolist is also the average revenue curve for the monopolist. When the monopolist lowers price

in order to increase quantity sold, all units sold in the market will be sold at the new lower price, not just the last unit sold. The MR curve is always below the monopolist's demand curve because the monopolist's demand curve is the same as the average revenue curve. For the monopolist, both average revenue and marginal revenue decrease as quantity increases.

The following material discusses the implications of the monopolist model. *First*, the monopolist will set the price at that point on the demand curve above where the MR and MC curves intersect. Because MC is positive, MR must also be positive (because MR = MC at the profit-maximizing point). It is important to note that MR is positive only at those quantities that correspond to the *elastic* portion of the demand curve. Therefore, a monopolist will set the price only on the elastic portion of its demand curve. Indeed, if the price was set on the inelastic portion of the curve, say at $30, MR would be negative, meaning that a reduction in output coming from a price increase would decrease total revenues. At the same time, a reduction in output would reduce TC. Profits would therefore always be greater at a higher price when the monopolist is producing on the elastic portion of the demand curve. See **Table 9-2** for a further explanation of the relationship between price elasticity and total revenue.

In addition, because the most profitable level of output is determined by MR and MC alone,

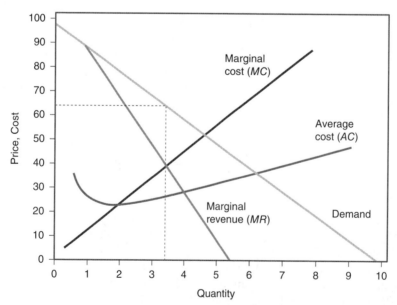

Figure 9-1 Equilibrium price (P) and output (Q) in a monopolistic (single seller) market. The monopolist faces a given demand curve for the service, and from this curve is derived its marginal revenue (MR) curve. The monopolist's cost conditions are presented in marginal (MC) and average (AC) terms. The profit maximizing monopolist will set price and quantity such that MR = MC. Equilibrium price is between $60–$70, and equilibrium quantity is between 3-4 units. (This graph is based on data in table 9-1).

Table 9-2 Total Revenue (*TR*) Resulting from Elasticity

(1)	(2)	(3)
Elasticity	**Price Increase**	**Price Decrease**
Inelastic (<1)	*TR* increases	*TR* decreases
Elastic (>1)	*TR* decreases	*TR* decreases
Unitary (=1)	*TR* the same	*TR* the same

© Jones & Bartlett Learning.

and because *MC* is unaffected by fixed costs, the profit-maximizing price will similarly be unaffected by changes in fixed costs. Continuing the previous illustration, assume that fixed costs increase to $50. Profits would be lower by $20 at every level of output. But the maximum profit level of output would still be the same (at *Q* = 3), only now the provider would be earning less profit. This important result implies that if the provider's fixed costs increase (e.g., because of an increase in mortgage rates), it cannot do anything about it. If it tries to pass on these added fixed costs to the consumer by raising the price, it will only be moving away from the profit-maximizing position; in raising the price, it will sell less, and total revenue will decrease more than total cost. This, of course, is not true for an increase in variable costs since these costs are associated with quantity produced (i.e., *MC*).

In a similar vein, if the profit-maximizing monopolist received a fixed subsidy from the government (i.e., one unrelated to output produced) of $20 to treat low-income patients, *TR* would be increased at every level of output by $20, but *MR* would not be affected. The monopolist's profit-maximizing price will not change. That is, the profit-maximizing monopolist will not lower the price to induce people to demand more.

One outcome of the monopoly model is that the firm could be persistently earning excess economic profits. Excess economic profits are defined as profits greater than the amount required to cover the opportunity costs of the resources invested in the firm. Firms require a normal profit to entice investors and owners to put their resources into the firm. Because the average cost (*AC*) curve incorporates all the monopolist's costs, including opportunity costs, the monopolist's profits in this analysis are equal to *TR* – *TC* or, using average terms, the product of the unit margin (*P* – *AC*) times output (*Q*), where *P* is price. These excess profits are true economic profits. That is, they are profits

over and above all the costs required to operate the enterprise, including a normal rate of return for the owner's efforts and capital.

Furthermore, nothing in the model will allow the monopolist's profits to be bid away. There are no potential entrants into the market who can charge a lower price. As a result, the monopolist can earn above-normal profits that persist over time. Note the contrast with the competitive market model, in which entry is inexpensive and any excess profits will attract new entrants who will expand supply and lower price and profits.

9.2.5 Price Discrimination

Under some conditions, a monopolist can further increase its profits by charging different prices for the same product to different buyers. This is called *price discrimination*, which can be practiced only when there is market segmentation and the product or service in the lower price market cannot be resold (a secondary exchange) in the higher price market. In addition, the demand elasticities in the two markets have to be different to make the practice worthwhile.

Now, assume that a pediatric practice can separate its patients into two distinct markets according to patient income. Assume further that demand elasticity is influenced by income so that each market will have a different demand curve. Thus, one of the preconditions for price discrimination is met. The product sold is patient visits. These can hardly be purchased in one market and resold in the other, so the other precondition is met as well. The demand curves for the two separate markets, "high income" and "low income," are shown in **Figure 9-2**, graphs A and B. The cost assumption is that the *MC* eventually rises, as shown in graph C. Note that there is one *MC* for the entire operation; production is not separated. The behavioral assumption is that the pediatric practice seeks to maximize its profits.

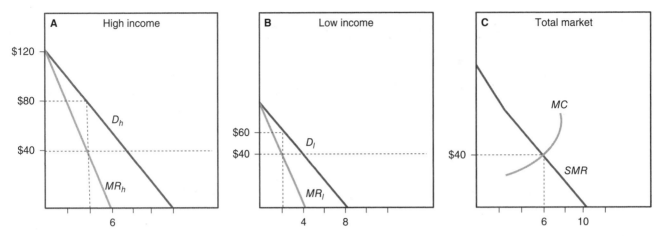

Figure 9-2 Price setting by discriminating monopolist. If the monopolist can separate its market into two submarkets, "high income (h)" and "low income (l)," the price charged in each submarket will be derived from firm level conditions, and will occur where the marginal revenue (MR) in the submarket equals the overall marginal cost (MC) to the firm. The curve SMR in Graph C shows the total quantity in all submarkets at each level of MR. Note that the equilibrium occurs in each market at the same value of MR.

© Jones & Bartlett Learning.

If the monopolist can separate its market into two submarkets, "high income (h)" and "low income (l)," the price charged in each submarket will be derived from firm-level conditions, and will occur where the marginal revenue (MR) in the submarket equals the overall marginal cost (MC) to the firm. The curve SMR in graph C shows the total quantity in all submarkets at each level of MR. Note that the equilibrium occurs in each market at the same value of MR.

Given these assumptions, the monopolistic model can be used to explain the monopolist's pricing policy. In doing so, the equi-marginal principle of maximization must be used. To maximize profits, the provider will set the price (and therefore the quantity) in each market, so that (1) the MR earned by lowering (raising) the price in all markets is the same; and (2) overall, the MR in each market is equal to the MC of producing that total level of output.

The derivation of the profit-maximizing prices is shown in Figure 9-2. The curve MC shows the provider's marginal cost for all units provided (it does not have a separate cost for each market), and the curve SMR (sum of marginal revenue) shows the quantity that would be supplied overall, when the firm allocated output to each market according to the specific level of MR. SMR is thus the sum of quantities in both markets at a given level of MR. Given the MR curves for the low-income and high-income markets (MR_l and MR_h) at an MR level in both markets of $40, the corresponding quantities in the markets are 2 and 4, respectively. The SMR curve for those quantities will be at a quantity of 6, in which $Q_m = Q_l + Q_h$.

The firm's maximum profit position will be determined by equating MC with the MR in each market. Overall, this occurs when MC = SMR (at quantity 6 in this illustration). The corresponding outputs in each market are 4 and 2, and the prices in the two markets that equate the MRs are $80 and $60, respectively. Profits, which are equal to the sum of TR in each market less TC, will be greater than if the same price was set in all markets.

Price discrimination such as this cannot exist in a competitive market, and this is one reason why physician pricing has been characterized as monopolistic. In a competitive market, if two submarkets had different prices, "traders" would buy goods in the low-price market and resell them (at a higher price, but below the market price) in the second market. For many years, physicians, particularly specialists, resorted to a sliding scale of fees when setting prices, charging the higher-income patients more than the lower-income ones (Kessell, 1958). By the 1970s, physician services became more highly insured, and the sliding scale all but disappeared at that time (Filler, 2007; Gattuso, 1997; Greenberg, Peiser, Peterburg, & Pliskin, 2001; Newhouse, 1970). However, different insurance plans still pay different prices for the same service in many instances.

9.2.6 Physician Pricing and Supply in Public Programs

A variant of the price monopoly model outlined in Section 9.2.5 has been used to explain physician pricing and supply in relation to the payment policies of Blue Shield (Sloan & Steinwald, 1978), Medicare

(Paringer, 1980; Rice, 1984), and Medicaid (Cromwell & Mitchell, 1984; Hadley, 1979; Kushman, 1977) and the 1972–1975 price limitations set by the Economic Stabilization Program (Hadley & Lee, 1978/1979).

The Medicare studies examined the effect of Medicare payment levels (80% of the reasonable charges) on the assignment decision—the decision of physicians to accept the Medicare-determined fee as full payment for their services in addition to the 20% copayment the patient pays of the allowable costs. On an individual-case basis, physicians were originally allowed to accept Medicare assignment of their patients. A physician who accepted the reasonable fee in full (i.e., who accepted assignment) for a specific patient receives 80% of the fee directly from Medicare and can bill the patient for the 20% copayment. If the physician did not accept assignment for that patient, the patient could be billed whatever fee the physician chose. In this case, Medicare would reimburse the patient directly for 80% of its reasonable fee, and the physician would collect the entire charge from the patient at the time of service.

The acceptance by physicians of assignment relieves patients from the financial risks associated with higher physician fees. Currently, physicians can no longer decide to accept assignment on a case-by-case basis. Instead, the physician must choose to accept the Medicare-approved amount as payment in full on all claims or not participate in the Medicare program. When the physician agrees to accept assignment, then the patient may only be billed for the deductible and coinsurance amounts.

The analysis is set out graphically in **Figure 9-3**. The physician is assumed to be a monopolist facing two submarkets: one with private patients and one with patients in a public program. (The extra billing is ignored in this illustration in order to simplify the model.) The output is defined as patients served. D_p is the demand curve for private patients, and MR_p is the related MR curve for private patients. The public agency reimburses the physicians for its patients at a fee level of F_m; because the fee level is fixed, F_m is a horizontal line and is also the physician's MR for public patients. Assume in this illustration that the physician's MC curve is at MC_1. Finally, assume that the physician is a profit maximizer.

With an MC such as MC_2, the monopolist would not supply any output to the public patients; the price and output levels in the private market would be P_n and Q_2.

According to the equi-marginal principle, the physician will supply services to Q private and $(Q_3 - Q_1)$ public patients because at this output $MR_p = F_m$ and both are equal to MC_1. The private patients will be charged a price of P_m. To attract any additional private patients, the physician would have to lower the price to private patients below P_m, which would imply an MR for private patients below that for public patients.

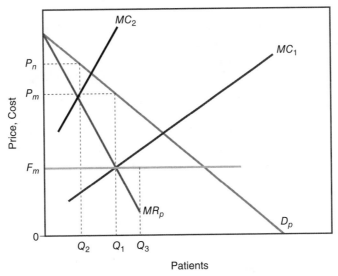

Figure 9-3 Price setting by a monopolist facing private market and a publicly financed market. In this market, demand is represented by D_p, marginal revenue by MR_p, and with the publicly financed market having a set fee, marginal revenue is represented by F_m. With a marginal cost of MC_1, the monopolist will set the price to equate the MR in both markets. In this case, the price in the private market is set at P_m. The marginal revenue for public and private patients will be the same, MR_p. Total output supplied is Q_3, with $Q_3 - Q_1$ going to the public patients. With an MC such as MC_2, the monopolist would not supply any output to the public patients; the price and output levels in the private market would be P_n and Q_2.

A profit-maximizing physician will thus prefer to serve additional public patients for which the MR is constant at a level F_m rather than lower price and have a marginal revenue below F_m.

A lower public fee would lower the supply to the public patients (it would also cause the physician to lower his or her private fee because the physician will now move down the MR_p curve). A physician facing the same demand curve, but with a higher MC (say, MC_2), will not supply any services to public patients and will set a private fee of P_n. This analysis demonstrates that the public and private sectors are interdependent. A public program that lowers fees will reduce the supply to the public market and will also affect the private market.

A model similar to the one discussed in the previous section has been used to explain hospital cost shifting, a tactic purportedly used by hospitals to raise fees on self-pay and commercially insured patients in response to low payment levels by Medicare, Medicaid, and in some instances, Blue Cross (Danzon, 1982; Dobson, Davanzo, & Sen, 2006; Dowless, 2007; Frakt, 2011; Sloan & Becker, 1984; Sloan & Ginsburg, 1984; Zimmerman, 2011).

9.2.7 Nursing Home Markets and Public Rates

The two-payer monopoly model is also suited to analyzing economic behavior in the nursing home market. Care provided in nursing homes generally enhances quality of life rather than curing a particular health problem. The demand for long-term care reflects a basic demand rather than a derived demand for health. Generally in this market, there are two major groups of payers: self-pay (relatively uninsured) resident and state Medicaid agencies. Many Medicaid agencies typically pay nursing homes a flat rate, whereas self-pay residents are typically charged according to market conditions. With Medicaid agencies having limited budgets and having the power to set rates, one option available in pursuing the goal of budget containment is to set low rates. In doing so, the Medicaid agencies must recognize the tradeoffs involved.

Because the nursing homes can differentiate their products, they can develop some form of "brand loyalty" on the part of residents and prospective residents. When they have residents with some degree of preference, nursing homes will face demand curves that have some elasticity (i.e., are downward sloping). The more loyal their residents are, the more inelastic their demand curves will be.

Figure 9-3 can therefore also be interpreted as pertaining to nursing home markets. In this diagram, assume that F_m is the rate that Medicaid pays to nursing homes, D_p is the demand of private-pay residents, and MC_1 is a nursing home's marginal cost. At the fee level (and marginal revenue) of F_m, the nursing home will equate its marginal cost so that it is equal to the MR for each class of residents. It will therefore serve Q_3 residents, with Q_1 of these being private and $Q_3 - Q_1$ being Medicaid. If the Medicaid agency lowered its rates below F_m, fewer Medicaid residents (and more private-pay residents) would be served. Shortages of Medicaid resident nursing home beds would therefore appear (Grabowski, 2002; Gulley & Santerre, 2007; Paringer 1980).

From a structural perspective, nursing home markets may resemble a monopolistically competitive industry. The nursing home provider basically faces three market segments. One segment reflects the private-pay market for residents paying more than the state-set Medicaid rate. This segment faces a downward-sloping demand curve. The second segment is the Medicaid-eligible people in the market, and because Medicaid pays a single rate, the demand curve is horizontal. The nursing home cannot impact the price received for these residents. The remaining third segment supply is provided to private-pay residents who pay less than the Medicaid rate. As long as the nursing home has excess capacity and the price received covers variable costs and some fixed costs, nursing homes will sell services to this third downward-sloping demand segment.

9.3 Monopsony—Buyers' Market Power

A large buyer that faces many small sellers may be in a position to exert market power. Market power possessed by buyers is referred to as *monopsony*, as opposed to monopoly for sellers. In the healthcare sector, the monopsony model has been applied to situations as diverse as the labor market for nurses, the purchase of hospital services by such big insurers as Blue Cross plans (Foreman, Wilson, & Scheffler, 1996; Staten, Dunkelberg, & Umbeck, 1987), the purchase of specialized medical services by managed care plans (Pauly, 1998), and the procurement of organs for transplantation (Barnett, Beard, & Kaserman, 1993).

The basic monopsony model can be illustrated by the example of a large hospital chain that is a purchaser of aspirin. The supply curve faced by the monopsonist is the result of many small sellers' willingness

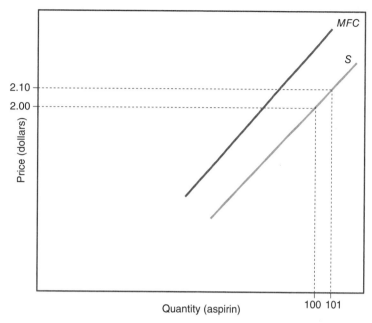

Figure 9-4 Supply and marginal factor costs (*MFC*) for buyer with market power. The *MFC* curve is derived from the supply curve (*S*) when the buyer has market power.
© Jones & Bartlett Learning.

to produce and sell aspirin at any given price. Higher prices result in a greater quantity supplied, so the supply curve looks like *S* in **Figure 9-4**.

For the monopsonist, however, the supply price associated with any quantity of aspirin does not give a true indication of the cost to it of expanding its purchases. In order to induce suppliers to sell added quantities, it must offer a higher price. Of course, it must pay this higher price, not just on the added purchases, but on all its purchases. This means that for the monopsonist, the marginal cost of an additional unit of aspirin is higher than its price. This is illustrated in Figure 9-4. Initially, the buyer is purchasing 100 units at a price of $2, spending a total of $200. To induce sellers to supply 101 units, the price offered must rise to $2.10. The new total spending on aspirin is thus $2.10 × 101 = $212.10. So the added expense is not just the $2.10 price for the 101st unit, but also the additional $10 paid on the initial 100 units. The expense of adding another unit of an input for a monopsonist is called the *marginal factor cost (MFC)*, and it will be higher than the supply price, as shown by the *MFC* curve.

Because there are many substitutes for a single aspirin product, the hospital chain will have a somewhat elastic demand curve, indicating the marginal benefit for any quantity (based on increased revenue the input will enable it to earn). In making a purchase decision, it will weigh this marginal benefit against the *MFC* and buy the quantity at which these two are equal. At any quantity less than this, there would be increased profit as a result of expanding purchases. At any higher quantity, profit would be enhanced by a reduction in quantity purchased.

The result is shown in **Figure 9-5**. A total of Q_0 units will be purchased at a price of P_0 per unit. The contrast of this result with the result that would occur in perfect competition is noteworthy. If the demand curve had represented the total demand of many small buyers, equilibrium would have been at P_cQ_c. So the effect of monopsony is to decrease price and quantity compared to what would occur in perfect competition.

9.4 Market Structure and Its Determinants

9.4.1 Measuring Market Concentration

Market structure has a major influence on market power. The structure of a market is usually presented in terms of an index, or percentage, representing the size of the largest firm (or four or eight firms) relative to the overall market's total output. Another method is measuring the distribution of firm size in the market. A four-firm concentration ratio shows the percentage of the total market (in terms of sales, assets, or some other selected indicator of firm size) represented by the largest four firms. For example, a completely monopolized market has a concentration ratio of 100%; a market with 20 firms, total sales of $1 billion, and combined

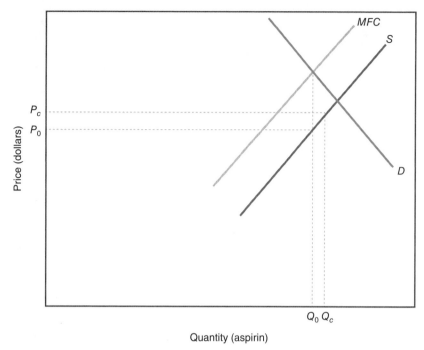

Figure 9-5 Price setting with buying power. *D* is the monopsonist's demand curve and indicates marginal benefit to the monopsonist of an additional unit purchased. To maximize profit, the monopsonist would purchase the quantity at which marginal benefit (*MB* or *D*) equals *MFC* (Q_0 in this case). The price paid for this amount is P_0. Under monopsony, price and quantity (P_0, Q_0) are lower than they would be under perfect competition (P_c, Q_c).
© Jones & Bartlett Learning.

sales for the largest four firms of $500 million would have a four-firm concentration ratio of 50%. The choice of four or eight firms is arbitrary and does not indicate the concentration of the remainder of the market.

A more general measure of concentration, which includes the output of all firms in the market, is the Herfindahl-Hirschman Index (*HHI*). According to this index, concentration is measured as the sum of the squared market share of all firms, where market share is an individual firm's output divided by the total output in the market.

$$HHI = \sum_{n=i} (S_i)^2$$

in which S_i is the market share of firm *i*. The summation sign (Σ) indicates summation over all firms. The largest *HHI* possible is one, indicating one firm controls the entire market. To illustrate, if a monopolist with sales of $300 million is the only firm in the market, its *HHI* is ($300/$300 million) or 1. If there were three hospitals in the market, each with sales of $100 million, the *HHI* for that market would be 0.3333 [(100/300)² + (100/300)² + (100/300)²], or 1/9 + 1/9 + 1/9 = 3/9 = 1/3 or 0.3333.

There is no true cutoff point for a concentrated versus a nonconcentrated market, although a figure of

about 0.1800 is sometimes used by the U.S. Department of Justice and the Federal Trade Commission to indicate a market is concentrated and a value of 0.2500 to indicate the market is highly concentrated (Cerullo, Lee, & Offodile II, 2018; Gaynor & Town, 2013; Wilder & Jacobs, 1986). Generally, it is thought that the greater the degree of concentration, the greater will be the ability of the leading firms to influence price, quantity, and other characteristics of output.

9.4.2 Determinants of Market Structure

Market structure can be thought of as having market and governmentally imposed (regulatory) determinants. The implications of two determinants can be illustrated with the health insurance market. In the United States, the health insurance market is largely a localized market; in part because each state requires operating licenses for any insurance company operating within the state and also because of unique historic relationships between local providers and some insurers (primarily the Blues). Aside from government insurance, health insurance has typically been broken down into two categories of operators: the Blues and the commercial insurance companies.

The Blues comprise Blue Cross (BC) (for hospitalization insurance) and Blue Shield (BS) (for medical and other insurance). In some states, the two plans are combined.

Originally, the Blues were tax exempt in terms of organization. Commercial insurers included a large number of mutual (member-owned) and commercial (investor-owned) firms, none of which had a substantial share of the healthcare market. Blue Cross and Blue Shield collect about one-quarter of the total health insurance premiums nationally, although their share of the private insurance market varies considerably by state. Currently, the Blues have been converted from tax-exempt organizations to investor-owned organizations. In 2015, there were 36 independent BC/BS companies in 50 states, the District of Columbia, and U.S. territories and they accounted for 41% of the total health insurance market.

9.4.3 Economies of Scale

Among the most important market determinants of market power are economies of scale, which reflect an increase in efficiency of production as the quantity of a good or service produced increases. Usually, the average cost per unit of output decreases when economies of scale are achieved because fixed costs are shared over an increased number of units of output,

and usage level of inputs increases more slowly than usage level of outputs.

Now assume in this illustration that the market demand for private health insurance is D_m in **Figure 9-6**, and that the long-run average cost curve for a state-of-the-art insurance company is *LAC*. Two things should be noted in the illustration. First, the long-run average cost incorporates capital and other fixed setup costs, as well as current operating costs; if there are high start-up costs for the industry, the *LAC* at low output levels will be quite high. Second, the *LAC*, in the illustration, includes insurance administration and transaction costs and the amount the insurance company reimburses the providers. In the example, the shape of the *LAC* curve is such that the minimum cost is reached at a large scale of output (e.g., about 13 million subscribers).

9.4.4 Pricing Policies

Given certain cost conditions, one firm could capture a considerable portion of the market. To do so, however, it must resort to a second, and related, market share determinant: pricing policy. If the insurance company sets a very low price relative to costs of other insurers (represented by the curve LAC_2), say, $80 per subscriber per month, market demand would be quite large (13 million subscribers). In this case,

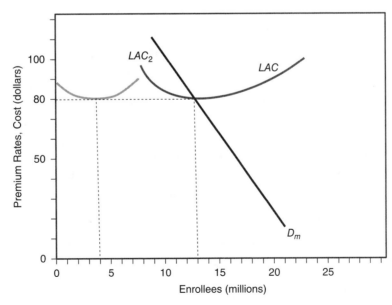

Figure 9-6 Output in an insurance market under alternative cost conditions. D_m represents market demand for insurance coverage. If the cost conditions are represented by cost curve *LAC*, one firm can capture a substantial portion of the market by virtue of its economies of scale and pricing policies. A producer with the cost conditions represented by *LAC* could set a price of $80; if it did so and chose to supply 13 million policies (as shown by the dashed lines), another producer with the same cost conditions could not reach a large enough scale of output to match the first producer's cost (and price).

the insurance company would have considerable discretion in choosing its own output level; the level chosen would depend, of course, on its objectives. If it provided services for 10 million subscribers at this price, there would be an excess demand of 3 million potential subscribers. If the technology of insurance provision was known to other potential entrants, a second firm could provide insurance on a cost basis like that represented by the LAC_2 curve. However, to reach a unit cost of $80, it would need to operate at a scale of 4 million subscribers. Because the potential entrant could not obtain such a volume with only 3 million customers not being served by the large firm, it might simply produce at a higher cost, charge a higher price, and obtain a smaller share of the residual market.

The final distribution of market shares will thus depend on the size of potential economies of scale relative to the potential market and also on the pricing policies of the larger firms. As seen in Figure 9-6, if the initial insurance company charged a higher price, say, $90 or $100, potential entrants would have less problem gaining an entry to the market.

On the other hand, if the state-of-the-art cost curve was like LAC_2 (with no substantial economies of scale), no firm could obtain a substantial share of the market, and a concentration of firms would be unlikely. There is some evidence economies of scale exist in health insurance operations, but these economies are not of the magnitude that would permit a single firm to dominate the health insurance market (Beaulieu, 2004; Blair, Jackson, & Vogel, 1975; Carroll, 2011; Town, Feldman, & Kralewski, 2011).

9.4.5 Input Prices and Taxes

A third cause of market concentration relates not to the cost–scale relation, but to the potentially different levels of cost curves for different providers. If, for example, one provider could obtain its inputs (workers, materials, etc.) at a lower cost than a second provider, its cost curve would be lower at all scales of output than the cost curve of the second provider. The first firm could capture a larger share of the market by turning its cost advantage into a price differential.

One such input price differential is the discount that many Blue Cross plans receive from hospitals (Feldman & Greenberg, 1981a, b; Goldberg & Greenberg, 1985), which is perhaps partly due to the special traditional relationship between Blue Cross and hospitals (Blue Cross was founded by hospitals).

Whereas commercial insurance companies typically have paid hospitals closer to full charges, about half of the Blue Cross plans have received discounts ranging from 2% to 30% and averaging from 8% to 15%. These discounts have the effect of lowering the LAC curves of the Blue Cross plans relative to the commercial ones, allowing Blue Cross to gain an increased market share by charging lower premium rates. One estimate attributed 7% of Blue Cross's market share to this cost differential (Feldman & Greenberg, 1981a, b).

9.4.6 Regulation

There might also be regulatory causes of market concentration. Like the Blue Cross discount, discriminatory regulations can give one firm, or type of firm, a cost advantage that allows it to lower price and increase market share. One such regulation was the tax on health insurance premiums, which was imposed on commercial insurance companies in all states; in some states, the Blue plans were exempt from such a tax, which was about 2% of premiums. In addition, the Blue plans, being nonprofit, were exempt from paying income taxes and, in some states, from property taxes. Such exemptions lowered the Blues' total costs of production, giving them a cost advantage in the insurance market. This last cost advantage was lost when the Blues lost their tax-exempt status and were forced to convert to investor-owned status.

However, these cost advantages need not always result in a larger market share for the firm. Firms can incur additional costs providing on-the-job benefits for the administrators, such as fancy offices, club memberships, etc. This is particularly true for tax-exempt firms, whose profits cannot be directly shared by the administrators. Thus, any cost advantage possessed by a tax-exempt firm can be appropriated by the managers rather than be passed on to consumers in the form of lower premiums. On-the-job amenities have been hypothesized to be a factor in the behavior of Blue Shield plans that were not "controlled" by physicians. Blue Shield plans deemed to be physician controlled were found to have lower operating costs. One possible explanation is that the physician-controlled plans passed on surpluses to the physicians in the form of payments. Nonphysician-controlled plans could appropriate potential surpluses and in the process, generate higher operating costs (Clark & Thurston, 2000; Einav & Finkelstein, 2011; Eisenstadt & Kennedy, 1981; Enders, 1995).

9.4.7 Market Power in the Market for Physicians' Services

Market structure and market power are not always equivalent. In the physician services market, there are a number of manifestations of market power, and yet the market structure does not have a high degree of provider concentration. For instance, for many years, physicians were able to maintain a sliding scale of fees (charging different prices for the same services), indicating price discrimination. Also, their incomes have been well above normal, even allowing for the high cost of medical training. Yet significant economies of scale in medical practice are not present, and there is a very low degree of market concentration, conditions that normally accompany monopolistic pricing and profit levels.

The explanation for this paradox is that the medical profession developed a mechanism of control to police its members and prevent them from engaging in such competitive practices as price-cutting (Kessell, 1958; Rayack, 1970). This control mechanism was basically in the hands of organized medical associations at the county, state, and national levels.

The key players in this control mechanism were the teaching hospitals, the American Medical Association (AMA), the local medical associations, and practicing physicians, especially surgeons and specialists (see Figure 9-7). The operation of the mechanism depended on the fact that it benefitted several of the key groups: (1) residents were an important (and low-cost) input in the operation of teaching hospitals, and (2) physicians, especially surgeons and specialists, needed membership on hospital medical staffs to have adequate access to patients to make a good, secure living.

The basis of the mechanism was a convention developed by the AMA regarding the certification of teaching hospitals. According to this convention, known as the Mundt Resolution, hospitals that were certified as teaching hospitals were "advised" that their medical staffs should be composed only of physicians who were members in good standing in local medical societies. Because the AMA certified teaching hospitals, the resolution carried substantial weight.

The following is an illustration of how the resolution helped to limit competitive behavior on the part of physicians. County medical association members generally disapproved of price-cutting and other competitive practices. One target of their disapproval was prepaid group practice medicine. Prepaid group practices (proto-HMOs) charged a single fee for all members, thus undermining the price discrimination system that had become prevalent in the fee-for-service world. The expulsion of physicians who joined prepaid group practice staffs from county medical societies occurred in several instances (Kessell,

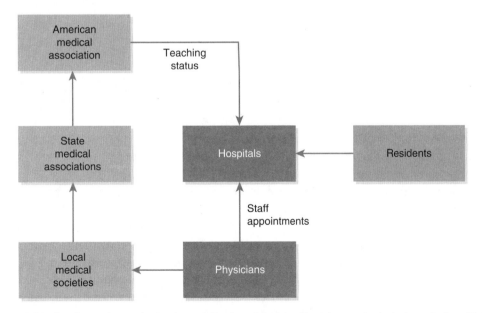

Figure 9-7 Control mechanisms that exist in the medical profession. Key players include hospitals with teaching programs that require accreditation from the Council on Teaching Hospitals (AMA associated) and physicians (who benefit from staff appointments in hospitals). Membership in local medical societies was required for staff appointment to a hospital, a regulation enforced by the AMA through its control over hospital accreditation. Local medical societies could enforce regulations (regarding pricing policies, for example) due to their control over membership.

1958), and the threat of expulsion was sufficient to make physician recruitment difficult for these practices. In addition, other competitive activities, such as advertising, were also discouraged by the organized medical profession.

The control of competitive practices by the medical profession at-large has not relied solely on such formal mechanisms. With the growth of specialization, physicians have become increasingly dependent on referrals from their colleagues, especially from primary care physicians. Physicians who engaged in competitive practices could be "controlled" to some degree by the threat of losing referrals from their colleagues (Baker, Bundorf, Royalty, & Levin, 2014; Cooper & Kramer, 2010; Havighurst, 1978; Trunkey, 2011).

In recent years, there has been a considerable amount of regulatory activity, especially on the part of the federal government, to contain anticompetitive practices on the part of physicians and other healthcare providers. One such activity is the Stark Law, which prohibits referring patients to an entity in which the physician or a family member has a financial relationship. This law provides significant civil penalties, but not criminal penalties, substantially affecting costs of providing services.

Mergers and acquisitions in health care also receive careful scrutiny to ensure that the resulting entity does not have sufficient market power to provide fewer choices for consumers, charge higher prices, and/or provide worse service. In addition, attention is given to ensure healthcare providers do not establish "destroyer prices" (prices set below the actual cost of production) to prevent entry into the market or bankrupt existing providers to reduce competition in the area.

The number of acquisitions in the healthcare industry, especially among hospitals and hospital systems, has been intense in recent years. While these activities are often presented as enabling the resulting organization to improve efficiency in the delivery of care, reduce the amount of excess capacity in the market, increase the ability of the organization to accept risk-based payment because of increased volume, and to reduce transaction costs in the market, these activities are being carefully evaluated to ensure the market is not becoming so concentrated that the resulting organization has sufficient market power to prevent efforts to contain costs and to enable the organization to increase the price of services in the market.

Most antitrust evaluations consider horizontal consolidation (e.g., hospitals merging with or acquiring another hospital) in measuring the concentration of market share and its potential impact on market prices. In determining the acceptability of proposed mergers, courts are increasingly considering the balance between the enhanced consumer welfare by the consolidation and the increased potential ability of the organization to control price. This consideration of social welfare has allowed some mergers to occur that did give an organization a majority of the market share in an area when the court determined that the reduction in costs to the consumer or the improvement in quality outweighed the costs of increased market power of the organization in the community.

In addition to the horizontal consolidation of organizations, there has also been an increase in activity in the vertical consolidation of organizations. In a vertical consolidation, there is an increase in the amount of factors of production and distribution under the control of a single organization. As an illustration, in health care, hospitals have been acquiring physician practices as a way of gaining more control over the referral of patients to their hospital, or they have acquired nursing homes and/or home health agencies as a way of gaining more control over the placement of patients once the need for the acute care services provided in the hospital has been met. The hospital may also acquire other suppliers of inputs into the production process, such as laundry services, pharmacies, medical supplies and equipment, and so on.

There has been some speculation that as large healthcare systems form Accountable Care Organizations (ACOs), they will also absorb the financing component or insurance functions as well. Accountable Care Organizations, or similar organizational structures, are viewed as having the potential to improve the quality of health care and slow the rate of growth in healthcare expenditures.

The foundation of ACOs is the reorganization of healthcare services around a team of providers, technology, and knowledge that is focused on the needs of the patient population in an area. The ACO expands the patient-centered medical home concept beyond just the primary care relationships to include the entire continuum of health care. This horizontal consolidation of the healthcare system is being viewed as allowing better cost control and the provision of higher quality of care because it enables better overall cost management, less variation within the population served, and an improved ability to track quality because the system is not so fragmented and data are available in a single location for the patient.

In an Accountable Care Organization, not only do providers—primary care physicians, specialists, hospitals, home health agencies—work collaboratively, they also accept collective accountability for the cost and quality of care delivered and the outcomes achieved by the patients in a defined population. For ACOs to achieve these anticipated results, there must be clinical and financial alignment as well as systematic consistency of quality. Efforts to align the goals and incentives of all participants in the healthcare system face many barriers and challenges. In the current healthcare system, there are wide disparities in the incomes of the different specialties and in the methods by which the providers are paid. Given the current fragmented system, it is difficult to determine the size of the patient population that will be necessary to enable the ACO to operate efficiently and to have sufficient data available to produce meaningful outcome results.

There are also inconsistencies currently in how outcomes are measured, making it difficult to arrive at consensus on a single, consistent set of measures for accountability. If these large, integrated organizations are formed, issues involving antitrust laws, antikickback laws, and the physician self-referral Stark Laws will also need to be considered. The integration of clinical and financial processes will also require significant amounts of resources to ensure sufficient capacity is available to the ACO.

The ACO model is also viewed as having a potential to reduce the number and consequences of medical errors in the United States. Because the foundation of the ACOs is the coordination of care through collaboration among healthcare providers, the expectation is that the team approach inherent in the ACO will decrease the errors occurring in the system. Because many current errors occur during the handoff of the patients among providers in different settings, the reduction in the fragmentation in the system is expected to reduce errors and duplication of care, which can also result in fewer errors and better outcomes.

In addition to the direct costs associated with medical errors, because they typically result in additional services being provided and longer lengths of stay in hospitals, in admissions and readmissions to hospitals, and therefore higher costs, errors also result in indirect or social costs to patients and the economy. The value of the lost lives due to medical errors and the disabilities caused by these errors adds substantially to the cost of the healthcare system. One study (Van Den Bos et al., 2011) put the annual cost of measurable medical errors that harm patients at $17.1 billion in 2008. A second study (Goodman, Villarreal, & Jones, 2011) found that in addition to the direct costs of medical errors, the social costs ranged from $393 to $958 billion due to premature deaths and disabilities in 2008. Improvements in the quality of care that reduce the occurrence of adverse events could have a significant impact on controlling the rate of increase in healthcare costs.

While ACOs and other regulatory programs were directed at improving quality and increasing focus on patient-centered care, there is still a substantial amount of fragmented care being provided in the healthcare system. The reality is healthcare professionals still possess a significant amount of monopoly power in the healthcare delivery system, and paternalistic approaches are still prevalent. Increasingly, however, attention is focusing on approaches that will more fully respect the preferences of patients, their values, and their personal experiences when interacting with the healthcare system.

To reduce the monopoly role of the healthcare professionals in the delivery of care, the patient-as-partner approach is being advanced. In this approach, the idea is to make the patient a true member of the healthcare team. Since the patients live with the medical condition, the information and expertise they usually possess could make valuable contributions to care. In addition, because of the knowledge the patient has, he or she can make valuable contributions to research and the training of future healthcare professionals. This focus on the patient-as-partner approach could reduce the asymmetrical power relationship between provider and patient in the healthcare system, bringing about a better balance of power and improving the healthcare delivery system (Karazivan et al., 2015).

9.5 Nonprice Competition and Market Power

9.5.1 Overview

The vast majority of healthcare markets are neither perfectly competitive nor completely monopolistic. Consumers develop some loyalty, or attachment, to specific providers, but this loyalty is not total. Furthermore, product quality or attributes other than price play a key role in the output of most healthcare providers; therefore quality has a key role to play in the competitive process as well. In this section, we discuss market power and the role of nonprice competition is discussed.

In addition to price, there are many product attributes that have the potential to attract patients. Providers can increase convenience by adding office hours in order to reduce their patients' waiting time. They can build satellite facilities and clinics to cut down on their patients' travel time. Pharmacists can initiate delivery services, emergency services, family prescription-monitoring records, and prescription waiting areas. Insurance companies and health maintenance organizations (HMOs) and other types of managed care organizations have a wide variety of services that might be covered, and they can also vary the degree to which these services can be covered (e.g., through the use of copayments, deductibles, and treatment limitations). Note, however, that in all such instances, additional quality is expensive to provide.

In the market there are three relevant varieties of price–quality competition to be discussed: (1) price competition alone, (2) quality competition alone, and (3) joint price and quality competition. Price competition simply involves the direct use of monetary incentives/disincentives to allocate goods and services in the market. Quality competition uses nonmonetary incentives/disincentives to allocate goods and services, while the price–quality joint model uses a combination of both price and quality to allocate resources.

9.5.2 Monopolistic Competition

Since neither the pure competition model nor the pure monopolistic model explains behavior observed in the healthcare market, a different model is necessary. One model that has been developed to handle product differentiation resulting from the establishment of brand names and advertising in the market is monopolistic competition. Since the producers sell products that are somewhat different, each producer has some power over the price of its own product. The monopolist's part of the model reflects the ability of a firm to raise its price, even if other producers of similar products do not, and not lose all of its sales. The monopoly power is limited, however, since there are a number of similar products being sold in the market. This competitive part of the model results in a single firm's demand curve being much flatter than the industry's demand curve.

In the healthcare system, competition in both price and quality results in the *monopolistic competition model* being used to analyze results and implications. In a monopolistic competition model, the fundamental conditions include the assumption that there are many competitors and potential competitors in the market (i.e., there is low-cost and freedom of entry into the market). Each firm can vary its product quality (e.g., location of facilities, operating hours, etc.), and in the process will develop some consumer loyalty (and hence market power). That is, consumers will not be as willing to change suppliers at the small decrease in price as in the quality-constant perfect competition case.

The model of monopolistic competition can be developed using the illustration of an HMO. Assume that Palmedico HMO is one among a number of alternative providers (some of which might offer more traditional insurance and fee-for-service options). Also assume Palmedico is a provider of average efficiency, and the partial loyalty of its subscribers can be characterized by means of a downward-sloping demand curve (D in **Figure 9-8**, graph A). Associated with this demand curve is an *MR* curve. Palmedico's cost curve will depend on the characteristics of its product: the extent of coverage, the credentials of its staff, its operating hours, the number of satellite clinics it operates, and so on. Initially, assume that Palmedico is a profit-maximizing organization. Given these conditions, it will set its price at the quantity where $MR = MC$. Hence, the price will be around \$750 per subscriber and the enrollment will be 5000.

At this price, Palmedico is earning excess profits, and because it is a representative firm in the industry, presumably others are earning excess profits as well. Because entry is relatively inexpensive, other potential entrants will be attracted by the prospect of high profits. To gain enrollees, these new entrants may reduce price, and may also offer potential enrollees a higher quality product (longer clinic hours or more clinic sites, for example). Palmedico's demand curve will shift to the left unless it responds with an increase in quality and a decrease in price, which in this illustration the assumption is made that it does. As a consequence, Palmedico's costs increase (because of the higher quality). The same forces will affect all firms in the market.

As long as there are any excess profits to be made, this process will continue, and the quality of each firm's product will continue to rise. For each firm, demand will first shift outward in response to its higher quality and then inward in response to the quality and price

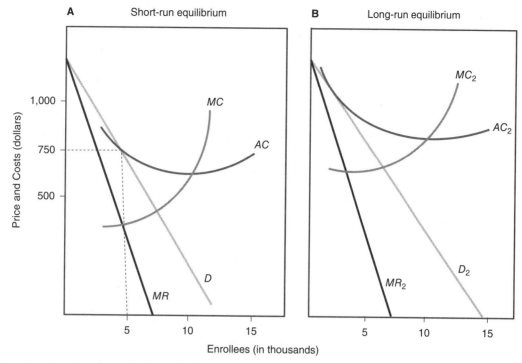

Figure 9-8 Equilibrium in monopolistic competition. In the short run (Graph **A**), the provider's equilibrium price and quantity are set where *MC* = *MR* (at about $750 and 5,000 enrollees). In the long-run (Graph **B**), competitive responses, including increases in quality, lead to an equilibrium where no excess profits are made (price equals average costs).

© Jones & Bartlett Learning.

changes instituted by its competitors. Profit margins (the excess of price over average cost) will continually be lowered as a result of the competition. For any firm, it cannot be predicted whether price will ultimately increase or decrease (i.e., the net result of the competitive process cannot be predicted), because demand has shifted in both directions and costs have changed as well.

For the same reason, the direction of enrollment cannot be predicted. However, the final equilibrium will appear as in Figure 9-8, graph B, where AC_2 just touches the firm's demand curve D_2. The equilibrium quantity is at the point where *MC* = *MR* (i.e., it is the most profitable position Palmedico can have); in this case, Palmedico is just breaking even. Included in the breakeven point, however, is a normal profit accruing to the firm. All that can be said for certain about this equilibrium is that AC_2 represents a higher quality level; it cannot be said for certain whether price and enrollment are higher or lower. For this reason, the monopolistic competition model has been criticized as being incomplete: It fails to make predictions about the direction of some key variables—price and quantity.

Competition between tax-exempt firms would have a similar outcome. If the behavioral assumption was that the firm wants to maximize enrollees,

for example, quality and price competition would still prevail, and the final result would be that each provider breaks even. Models similar to the monopolistic competition model in this section have been used to explain resource-allocation decisions in markets containing numerous HMOs (Christianson & McClure, 1979; Goldberg & Greenberg, 1980) and numerous retail drugstores (Cady, 1976). The importance of nonprice factors (including quality) in these markets has been stressed. Similar models have also been used to explain the diffusion of (high-quality) technological developments in the hospital industry, such as the use of radioisotopes and intensive care units (Baler et al., 2000; Harrison, 2007; Lee & Waldman, 1985; Rapoport, 1978).

9.5.3 Monopolistic Competition and Preferred Provider Organizations

The monopolistic competition model has been used to analyze how preferred provider organizations (PPOs) affect hospital price and quality behavior (Dranove, Satterthwaite, & Sindelar, 1986). The basic model is applied to interhospital competition, and the impact of PPOs on each individual hospital's demand curve is predicted.

A PPO is a subscription-based organization that has been formed to contract with providers in order to obtain discounted prices. The PPO shops around among providers (hospitals and physicians) for lower prices and then contracts with the providers who offer better terms on behalf of insurers and/or employers. The medical providers accept the fee schedule established by the PPO and the guidelines established by the PPO for the provision of care. (The PPO might also institute utilization review.) The discounts are passed on in the form of lower copayments for insureds who choose the preferred providers. In effect, consumers are given incentives to choose providers on the basis of price. This increases the elasticity of demand facing any individual hospital because consumers lose some of their loyalty to "their" hospital.

The enrollees in the PPO have considerable flexibility when seeking care. Unlike a restrictive HMO, individuals enrolled in the PPO can decide to use an in-network or out-of-network provider each time they access the healthcare system. Typically, the fees (prices) paid for services are less when an in-network provider is selected. The providers join a PPO in hopes of gaining access to a larger population base.

Using the monopolistic competition model to analyze this phenomenon, the beginning assumption is that there are many differentiated firms, each facing a downward-sloping demand curve (D_1 in **Figure 9-9**). Assume that each firm has the same demand conditions, and that each firm's demand curve is elastic (although the market curve can be inelastic). The implications of this will be seen in the following paragraphs. Also, each firm has the cost conditions shown in Figure 9-9: marginal cost is constant up to a point, then it starts to increase. The corresponding ATC curve is U-shaped. Initially, assume that short-run equilibrium is at point A, with a price P_0 and quantity Q_0. This is based on the firm's cost conditions, demand conditions, and profit-maximizing objectives.

The change in demand conditions is the crux of this model. The introduction of a PPO will have the effect of increasing the elasticity of each individual hospital's demand (to D_2). That is, the effect of the PPO is to make each hospital more vulnerable to price changes instituted by other hospitals. With its demand elasticity increased, each hospital, assuming it acts as if all else is held constant, will lower its price to increase revenues and profits (this would be a profit-maximizing response of a firm facing an elastic demand curve). However, if all hospitals do the same, each hospital's demand curve will shift down (to D_3), and the new

equilibrium will be at a point such as B (in which each hospital shares in the larger market demand, which has expanded because of the lower price charged by all hospitals). Initially, price will fall, but hospitals in such a market may respond further. If B (on a curve such as D_3) is above the ATC curve, then the hospitals will still be making a profit after the price cut, and no further change will result. On the other hand, if the collective price cuts drive the new demand curve down to D_4 (so that the equilibrium point is at B), the hospitals will all be suffering a loss, and they will have to cut costs (by reducing services, downsizing, etc.) or some will have to leave the market. Cost cutting will shift the cost curves downward, while abandonment of the market by a few hospitals will result in a greater market share for the remaining ones. The final result will be the same: The PPO will have had an impact on hospital services ("quality") and market share.

Note that if the hospitals are operating on the constant portion of their marginal cost curves and no hospitals exit (each hospital's demand thereby remaining the same), then "downsizing" (a reduction in services and thus "quality") will be the outcome.

9.5.4 Increased Concentration

When concentration increases and providers are fewer in number, the probability of price collusion increases. Price collusion involves an explicit agreement or implicit understanding among competitors in a market to limit price competition. If there are only a few suppliers in a market and each understands that the ultimate outcome of price competition is lower prices and profits for all, the likelihood of suppliers refraining from price competition increases.

Explicit agreements to restrict price competition are illegal, but cautious pricing behavior directed at avoiding conflicts in pricing policies among competitors is not. Such cautious behavior is more likely to be found when a market contains a small number of competitors because, as the number of competitors increases, "cheating" is more likely. With fewer suppliers, the cost of detecting cheating is lower. Also, the impact of one supplier's price cuts is less dispersed; that is, each supplier's demand curve is shifted inward more when there are only a few suppliers.

9.5.5 Oligopolistic Markets

In an oligopoly market, a few firms tend to dominate the industry, and new entrants have difficulty establishing a place in the market. In an oligopolistic market, there is a high concentration ratio for the firms

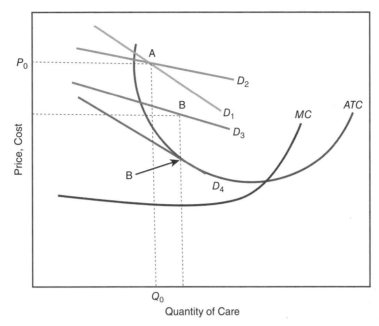

Figure 9-9 Effect of a PPO on a typical hospital's behavior. The initial demand curve facing the hospital (prior to the introduction of the PPO) is D_1, and the cost conditions of the hospital are represented by ATC and MC. The introduction of the PPO will initially increase the elasticity of the hospital's demand curve (to D_2). In response, the hospital will lower its price. All other hospitals are facing the same situation and will do the same. As they do so, each hospital's demand curve will shift inward. The result of these cuts is uncertain, but the demand curve could end up at D_3 (in which case each would operate at a loss). In the latter case, some hospitals would have to cut costs or shut down operations entirely.

© Jones & Bartlett Learning.

in that particular market. While there are a few large firms that dominate the industry, there are usually a large number of small producers, called "competitive fringes," also producing goods and services in the market. The aggregate quantity of output from these small firms typically accounts for less than 25% of the output in the industry, however.

Markets with a small number of suppliers, each of which supplies a significant portion of the industry's output, and a significant degree of producer interdependence are called *oligopolistic*. Although vigorous price competition is not usually a characteristic of an oligopolistic market, quality competition is. In providing higher quality to attract and retain patients, the costs of oligopolistic competitors increase and profits are reduced.

Oligopolistic competition might occur when there are a few HMOs and traditional insurers in a market competing for the business of a large number of enrollees. In this case, rising quality would be expected, but not much price competition (Hay & Leahy, 1984). However, for an oligopolistic market to persist, entry by new competitors must be difficult, and the start-up costs for an HMO may be low enough to make entry easy and attractive. The eventual result might be price

competition. Also, buying power may discourage providers from engaging in oligopolistic behavior. In many markets, businesses play a considerable role in selecting which insurers (including HMOs) will insure their employees. If the buyer's side of the market is dominated by a few large businesses, price competition may become important, despite the low number of providers.

9.5.6 Nonprice Competition

Price competition is sometimes not relevant, especially in the healthcare industry. When patients are fully or substantially insured for a service and have a free choice among suppliers, they will choose suppliers based strictly on nonprice or quality considerations. Quality competition then becomes the major if not only form of competition, and if the supply side of the market is competitive, costs will increase in response to quality improvements until the suppliers reach the break-even point or the limits placed by third-party payers are reached.

Analyses of this type of competitive process have been done for hospital markets (Farley, 1985; Joskow, 1980) and dialysis markets (Held & Pauly, 1983). Studies across hospital markets have shown that, in market areas with greater degrees of competition (measured by the number of hospitals), hospitals are more likely to offer specialized heart surgery (Robinson, Garnick, & McPhee, 1987) and specialized clinical services (Luft, Robinson, Garnick, Maerki, & McPhee, 1986). Although these studies focused strictly on quality measures of output, there is some evidence that quality competition among hospitals is more prevalent than price competition (Noether, 1988).

Evidence (Cooper, Craig, Gaynor, & Van Reenen, 2018) has shown that the mergers and acquisitions of hospitals in the United States has resulted in higher insurance premiums and that the price of healthcare services is much higher in regions with only one or two hospitals. For example, it was found that prices for hospital services like a knee replacement or MRI are, on average, 15% higher in markets, with only one hospital than in regions with at least four hospitals.

Exercises

1. Given the following demand and cost conditions for a monopolistic medical practice, predict the profit-maximizing price and quantity of services utilized. The cost conditions are as follows: fixed costs are $100 and marginal costs are $70 per visit.

Price ($)	Quantity of Visits Demanded
200	0
180	1
160	2
140	3
120	4
100	5
80	6

2. The state Medicaid agency has set a rate of $110 per visit for all Medicaid enrollees who visit a physician. Each physician also has private paying patients. The demand curve for each physician is characterized by the data in the following table, and physicians can be regarded as individual monopolists. Each physician also has a cost schedule that can be characterized by the data in the table.

Price to Private Consumer ($)	Quantity of Visits Demanded	Quantity of Visits Supplied	Total Costs of Production ($)
160	0	0	100
140	1	1	140
120	2	2	220
100	3	3	340
80	4	4	500
60	5	5	700
40	6	6	940
20	7	7	1260

a. If each physician is a profit-maximizing provider, how many visits will he/she provide to public and private patients?
b. What will the number of visits provided be if the Medicaid Agency lowers its rate to $60 per visit but the demand remains the same?

3. A physician practice serves two groups of patients. One group, with limited insurance, has demand represented by Demand Schedule A; the other, with comprehensive insurance, has demand represented by Demand Schedule B in the following table. The cost to produce a visit is $150. The practice wishes to price discriminate in order to maximize revenue. What price should it charge each patient group?

Demand Schedule A		Demand Schedule B	
Price ($)	Number of Visits	Price ($)	Number of Visits
200	1	200	6
180	2	180	7
160	3	160	8
140	4	140	9
120	5	120	10

4. The following table shows hospitals operating in two cities and their annual number of patient days in thousands:

City 1		City 2	
Hospital	Patient Days (000)	Hospital	Patient Days (000)
A	30	H	120
B	170	I	120
C	220	J	108
D	90	K	96
E	140	L	78
F	50	M	78

60	3	160	3
80	4	140	4
100	5	120	5
120	6	100	6
		80	7
		60	8

Compare the concentration of the markets in the two cities using the Herfindahl-Hirschman Index (*HHI*).

5. The data in the following table are the supply schedule faced by a monopsonist and its demand schedule for nurses. Determine how many nurses will be employed and what price will be paid by the monopsonist.

Supply Price ($)	Units Supplied	Demand Price ($)	Units Demanded (Nurse)
20	1	200	1
40	2	180	2

6. What characteristics of market structure make quality competition more likely than price competition? Which type of competition is more desirable from the viewpoint of the consumer? Discuss.

7. Explain why the market for physician services might exhibit some of the behavior of a monopoly market despite an apparently competitive structure.

Bibliography

Baker, L. C., Bundorf, M. K., Royalty, A. B., & Levin, Z. (2014). Physician practice competition and prides paid for private insurance for office visits. *JAMA, 312*(16), 1653–1662.

Baler, C. M., Messmer, P. L, Gyurko, C. C., Domagala, S. E., Conly, F. M., Eads, T. S., … Layne, M. K. (2000). Hospital ownership, performance, and outcomes: Assessing the state-of-the-science. *Journal of Nursing Administration, 30*(5), 227–240.

Barnett, A. H., Beard, T. R., & Kaserman, D. L. (1993). Inefficient pricing can kill: The case of dialysis industry regulation. *Southern Economic Journal, 60*, 393–404.

Beaulieu, N. D. (2004). An economic analysis of health plan conversions: Are they in the public interest? *Frontiers in Health Policy Research, 7*, 129–177.

Blair, R. D., Jackson, J. R., & Vogel, R. J. (1975). Economies of scale in the administration of health insurance. *Review of Economic Statistics, 57*, 185–189.

Cady, J. F. (1976). *Restricted advertising and competition.* Washington, DC: American Enterprise Institute.

Carroll, J. (2011). FTC antitrust rules offer hope of limiting ACO market power. *Managed Care, 20*(5), 5–7.

Cerullo, M., Lee, C., & Offodile II, A. C. (2018). Effect of regional hospital market competition on use patterns of free flap breast reconstruction. *Plastic Reconstructive Surgery, 142*, 1438–1446.

Christianson, J. B., & McClure, W. (1979). Competition in the delivery of medical care. *New England Journal of Medicine, 301*, 812–818.

Clark, R., & Thurston, N. K. (2000). The future of orthopaedics in the United States: An analysis of the effects of managed care in the face of an excess supply of orthopaedic surgeons. *Arthroscopy, 16*(2), 116–120.

Cooper, R., & Kramer, T. R. (2010). Revenue-based cost assignment: A potent but hidden threat to the survival of the multispecialty medical practice. *Academic Medicine, 85*(3), 538–547.

Cooper, Z., Craig, S. V., Gaynor, M., & Van Reenen, J. (2018, May). *The price ain't right? Hospital prices and health spending on the privately insured* (Working Paper 28185). Cambridge, MA: National Bureau of Economic Research.

Cromwell, J., & Mitchell, J. (1984). An economic model of large Medicaid practices. *Health Services Research, 19*, 197–218.

Danzon, P. M. (1982). Hospital "profits." *Journal of Health Economics, 1*, 29–52.

Dobson, A., Davanzo, J., & Sen, N. (2006). The cost-shift payment "hydralic": Foundation, history, and implications. *Health Affairs, 25*(1), 22–33.

Dowless, R. M. (2007). The health care cost-shifting debate: Could both sides be right? *Journal of Health Care Finance, 34*(1), 64–71.

Dranove, D., Satterthwaite, M., & Sindelar, J. (1986). The effect of injecting price competition into the hospital market: The case of preferred provider organizations. *Inquiry, 23*, 419–431.

Einav, L., & Finkelstein, A. (2011). Selection in insurance markets: Theory and empirics in pictures. *Journal of Economic Perspectives, 25*(1), 115–138.

Eisenstadt, D., & Kennedy, T. E. (1981). Control and behavior of nonprofit firms: The case of Blue Shield. *Southern Economic Journal, 48,* 26–36.

Enders, R. J. (1995). Special report on antitrust. Antitrust implications of physician practice affiliations and acquisitions: A question of market power, Part I. *Health Care Law Newsletter, 10*(6), 9–12.

Farley, D. E. (1985). *Competition among hospitals: Market structure and its relation to utilization, costs and financial position.* Hospital Studies Program, Research Note 7. DHHS Publication No. PHS 85–3353. Washington, DC: U.S. Department of Health and Human Services, National Center for Health Services Research and Health Care Technology Assessment.

Feldman, R., & Greenberg, W. (1981a). Blue Cross market share, economies of scale and cost containment efforts. *Health Services Research, 16,* 175–183.

Feldman, R., & Greenberg, W. (1981b). The relation between Blue Cross market share and the Blue Cross "discount" on hospital charges. *Journal of Risk and Insurance, 48,* 235–246.

Filler, B. C. (2007). Coding basics for orthopaedic surgeons. *Clinical Orthopaedics & Related Research, 457,* 105–113.

Foreman, S. E., Wilson, J. A., & Scheffler, R. M. (1996). Monopoly, monopsony and contestability in health insurance: A study of Blue Cross plans. *Economic Inquiry, 34,* 662–677.

Frakt, A. B. (2011). How much do hospitals cost shift? A review of the evidence. *Milbank Quarterly, 89,* 90–130.

Gattuso, C. F. (1997). Negotiating managed care and capitated contracts to minimize risks. *Annals of Thoracic Surgery, 64*(Suppl. 6), S73–S75; discussion S80–S82.

Gaynor, M., & Town, R. J. (2011). Competition in health care markets. In T. McGuire, M. V. Pauly, & P. P. Barros (Eds.), *Handbook of health economics* (2nd ed., pp. 499–638). Amsterdam, The Netherlands: Elsevier Science.

Goldberg, L. G., & Greenberg, W. (1980). The competitive response of Blue Cross to the health maintenance organization. *Economic Inquiry, 18,* 55–68.

Goldberg, L. G., & Greenberg, W. (1985). The dominant firm in health insurance. *Social Science and Medicine, 20,* 719–724.

Goodman, J. C., Villarreal, P., & Jones, B. (2011). The social cost of adverse medical events and what we can do about it. *Health Affairs, 30*(4), 590–595.

Grabowski, D. C. (2002). The economic implications of case-mix Medicaid reimbursement for nursing home care. *Inquiry, 39*(3), 258–278.

Greenberg, D., Peiser, J. G., Peterburg, Y., & Pliskin, J. S. (2001). Reimbursement policies, incentives and disincentives to perform laparoscopic surgery in Israel. *Health Policy, 56*(1), 49–63.

Gulley, O. D., & Santerre, R. E. (2007). Market structure elements: The case of California nursing homes. *Journal of Health Care Finance, 33*(4), 1–16.

Hadley, J. (1979). Physician participation in Medicaid: Evidence from California. *Health Services Research, 14,* 266–280.

Hadley, J., & Lee, R. (1978/1979). Toward a physician payment policy: Evidence from the economic stabilization program. *Policy Sciences, 10,* 105–120.

Harrison, T. D. (2007). Consolidations and closures: An empirical analysis of exits from the hospital industry. *Health Economics, 16*(5), 457–474.

Havighurst, C. C. (1978). Professional restraints on innovation in health care financing. *Duke Law Journal, 1978*(2), 303–388.

Hay, J. W., & Leahy, M. J. (1984). Competition among health plans: Some preliminary evidence. *Southern Economic Journal, 50,* 831–846.

Held, P. J., & Pauly, M. V. (1983). Competition and efficiency in the end stage renal disease program. *Journal of Health Economics, 2,* 95–118.

Karazivan, P., Dumez, P. V., Flora, L., Pomey, M-P., Del Grande, C., Ghadiri, D. P., … Lebel, P. (2015). The patient-as-partner approach in health care: A conceptual framework for a necessary transition. *Academic Medicine, 90*(4), 437–441.

Kessell, R. (1958). Price discrimination in medicine. *Journal of Law and Economics, 1,* 20–53.

Kushman, J. E. (1977). Physician participation in Medicaid. *Western Journal of Agricultural Economics, 2,* 22–33.

Lee, R. H., & Waldman, D. M. (1985). The diffusion of innovations in hospitals. *Journal of Health Economics, 12,* 371–380.

Luft, H. S., Robinson, J. C., Garnick, D. W., Maerki, S. C., & McPhee, S. J. (1986). The role of specialized clinical services in competition among hospitals. *Inquiry, 23,* 83–94.

Newhouse, J. P. (1970). A model of physician pricing. *Southern Economic Journal, 37,* 147–183.

Noether, M. (1988). Competition among hospitals. *Journal of Health Economics, 7,* 259–284.

Paringer, L. (1980, Summer). Medicare assignment rates of physicians: Their responses to changes in reimbursement policy. *Health Care Financing Review, 1,* 75–89.

Pauly, M. V. (1998). Managed care, market power and monopsony. *Health Services Research, 33,* 1439–1460.

Rapoport, J. (1978). Diffusion of technological innovations among non-profit firms. *Journal of Economics and Business, 30,* 108–118.

Rayack, E. (1970). *Professional power and American medicine.* Cleveland, OH: World.

Rice, T. (1984, Summer). Determinants of physician assignment rates by type of service. *Health Care Financing Review, 5,* 33–42.

Robinson, J. C., Garnick, D. W., & McPhee, S. J. (1987). Market and regulatory influences on the availability of coronary angioplasty and bypass surgery in U.S. hospitals. *New England Journal of Medicine, 317,* 85–90.

Sloan, F. A., & Becker, E. (1984). Cross subsidies and payment for hospital care. *Journal of Health Politics, Policy, and Law, 8,* 660–685.

Sloan, F. A., & Ginsburg, P. B. (1984). Hospital cost shifting. *New England Journal of Medicine, 310,* 893–898.

Sloan, F. A., & Steinwald, B. (1978). Physician participation in health insurance plans. *Journal of Human Resources, 13,* 237–263.

Staten, M., Dunkelberg, W., & Umbeck, J. (1987). Market share and the illusion of power: Can Blue Cross force hospitals to discount? *Journal of Health Economics, 6,* 43–58.

Town, R., Feldman, R., & Kralewski, J. (2011). Market power and contract form: Evidence from physician group practices. *International Journal of Health Care Finance & Economics, 11*(2), 115–132.

Trunkey, D. D. (2011). The impact of health care reform on surgery. *Advances in Surgery, 45,* 177–185.

Van Den Bos, J., Rustagi, K., Gray T., Halford, M., Ziemkiewicz, E., & Shreve, J. (2011). The $17.1 billion problem: The annual cost of measurable medical errors. *Health Affairs, 30*(4), 596–603.

Wilder, R. P., & Jacobs, P. (1986). Antitrust considerations for hospital mergers: Market definition and market concentration. *Advances in Health Economics, 7,* 245–262.

Zimmerman, C. (2011). A review of the evidence on hospital cost-shifting. *Findings Brief, Health Care Financing Organization, 14*(3), 1–3.

CHAPTER 10

Health Insurance

OBJECTIVES

1. Explain the basic model of insurance and define the basic terminology.
2. Explain the utility-maximizing model of an individual's demand for health insurance.
3. Explain factors that will influence the demand for insurance.
4. Explain the concept of moral hazard and its influence on the demand for medical care and health insurance.
5. Calculate the elasticity of demand for health insurance and explain its importance.
6. Explain the concept of adverse selection and its implications.
7. Describe the supply function of insurers.
8. Explain what tools insurers have at their disposal to avoid information asymmetry.

10.1 Introduction

Health insurance has a significant influence on markets for medical care. In this chapter, the focus is on the market for health insurance itself. The first step in Section 10.2 is to examine a brief history of health insurance in the United States. The next step, in Section 10.3, is to explain the theory and conditions necessary for an efficiently functioning insurance market. The analytical basis for the discussion of the health insurance market is a theory of decision making in the presence of risk. In Section 10.4, a model of demand for health insurance is presented, focusing on both an individual's demand and then the market demand, including the issue of moral hazard. In Section 10.5, the supply behavior of insurance providers is discussed. In Section 10.6, the existence and implications of adverse selection are discussed. Section 10.7 discusses how the market for health insurance violates the conditions of a true insurance model and the implications of those violations. While much of the chapter applies the basic supply–demand framework in a new context, it also introduces some concepts that are somewhat unique

to health insurance markets, specifically moral hazard and adverse selection.

10.2 Brief History of Health Insurance in the United States

An understanding of the history of health insurance in the United States is critical to understanding the major changes that are currently occurring, driven by government healthcare reforms. Health insurance, similar to any other insurance, is designed to reduce the risk of financial loss from the occurrence of an event. Health insurance, public or private, is intended to reduce the financial risk associated with the occurrence of a health-related event. The first known health insurance in the United States occurred in 1798, when the United States Marine Hospital Service implemented a program that deducted monies from the pay of seamen to cover the medical cost resulting from injuries suffered in the line of duty. During the 1870s, railroads, mining, and other industries provided company physician services funded by payroll deductions from the employees. The first national sick benefit program was introduced in 1877 by the Granite Cutters Union.

Health insurance plans continued to expand in the early 1900s, with Montgomery Ward's entry into one of the first group insurance contracts. In the Northwest and other remote areas, physician services and industrial health plans continued to be established. In 1913, the first union medical services program was started by the International Ladies Garment Workers Union (ILGWU). The stock market crash in 1929 contributed to the start of the first prepaid group plans. In one plan, a group of teachers in Dallas contracted with Baylor Hospital for room, board, and medical services in exchange for a monthly fee. In another plan, consumers formed a medical cooperative in Elk City, Oklahoma, to prepay for health care. And the Ross-Loos medical group in Los Angeles formed the largest group practice on a prepaid basis. As the popularity of health insurance increased during the 1930s and 1940s, several large life insurance companies entered the health insurance field.

In 1932, Blue Cross and Blue Shield, tax-exempt organizations, first offered group health plans. Part of the reasons these tax-exempt organizations were so successful is that in return for promises of increased volume and prompt payment, providers were willing to give discounts to the plans. Also, as tax-exempt organizations, they did not have to pay income taxes. During the 1940s and 1950s, employee benefit plans proliferated, especially after the War Labor Board ruled, in 1943, that fringe benefits were exempt from the wage freeze and the 1954 ruling by the Supreme Court upholding the National Labor Relations Board's decision that employee benefits are subject to collective bargaining. Also, in 1954, the Revenue Act confirmed that employer-paid health benefits were not taxable as employee income.

In 1965 Medicare and Medicaid legislation was enacted and implemented in 1966, insuring a large segment of the population that had not had access to previous insurance plans. In 1968, Firestone Tire and Rubber Company began to self-fund health benefits, soon followed by other large employers. The establishment of self-funding by large companies (in which the companies assumed the financial risk for the healthcare costs of their employees) effectively removed these companies from the requirements and restrictions of the health insurance industry.

In 1973, the Health Maintenance Organization Act was passed, requiring most employers to offer federally qualified HMOs as an option if the plans were available in the area. In 1985, the Budget Act was passed that required employers with 20 or more employees to offer continued health insurance coverage to terminated employees and dependents for 18–36 months. In 1966, the Mental Health Parity Act and the Health Insurance Portability and Accountability Act (HIPAA) were passed, helping individuals maintain insurance between jobs and providing quality improvement strategies. In 1997, the Children's Health Insurance Program (CHIP) was enacted to help provide insurance to low-income children (IOM, 1993).

In 2010, the Patient Protection and Affordable Care Act (commonly referred to as ACA) was passed; this piece of legislation has become known as Obamacare after the signer President Obama. This piece of legislation is over 1000 pages long and contains a wide range of health reforms and extended health insurance coverage to many previously uninsured individuals. One piece of this act was Medicaid expansion. Originally, the ACA mandated states to expand Medicaid coverage to low-income adults if the states wanted to receive existing Medicaid dollars. The Supreme Court ruled that states could not be mandated to provide coverage, but could voluntarily participate in Medicaid expansion. By 2019, 36 states and the District of Columbia participated in Medicaid expansion.

The ACA also imposed individual mandates on all legal residents requiring them to purchase health insurance, except for those individuals that the lowest cost option available would cost more than 8% of their income. A tax penalty was imposed on individuals not purchasing insurance. A succession of legal challenges to the ACA has successfully blocked or reversed a number of its features. Currently, efforts are underway to completely repeal the ACA; whether or not the efforts will be successful remains to be seen (Gruber & Somers, 2019). With all the changes in the healthcare delivery system, and the advances in technologies, pharmaceuticals, medical knowledge, and treatment options, it is difficult to keep the population adequately protected for all the financial costs of their healthcare needs.

10.3 Role of Insurance

Insurance is defined as an economic device transferring the financial consequences of risk from an individual to a company and reducing the uncertainty of risk through pooling of the risk across many individuals (National Association of Insurance Commissioners, 2019). Insurance exists because of risk and risk aversion among individuals. Risk involves uncertainty regarding the occurrence of an event or a state of being. A risk-averse individual will prefer events, or states of being, that involve less uncertainty (more certainty). Insurance enables an individual to manage risk or reduce uncertainty by substituting a known (certain) amount of loss, the insurance premium, for a potential but unknown occurrence of a large loss. Insurance transfers the financial risk associated with the possibility of a loss from one individual to a group of individuals through pooling.

To illustrate, if 10 individuals in a group know that one individual in the group will suffer the occurrence of an event that results in a $10,000 loss, but not which individual will suffer the loss, risk-averse individuals will be willing to pay $1000 (plus a small administrative cost) into a pool to be used to compensate the individual that actually incurred the loss. In this illustration, each individual has a 1-in-10 chance of suffering the loss (9-in-10 chances of not incurring the loss), but does not want to take the risk of suffering a $10,000 loss if the event occurs to him or her. Insurance, then, is a method of pooling resources to mitigate the effects associated with the occurrence of a large, uncertain event. An implied condition in the pooling of risks is that the event being insured against is outside the control of the individuals; it is a random event.

In order for the market for insurance to perform efficiently, certain conditions must exist in the market. First, the event or state being insured against must occur often enough to cause concern, but not occur so often that it becomes routine. It must be possible to determine, with relative accuracy and ease, the probability of the event occurring among the members of the group covered by the insurance. Because the collection of premiums and the payment of benefits involve administrative costs, as well as the financial consequences of the event occurring, insurance premiums needed to cover routine events would exceed the utility derived from purchasing insurance, even by risk-averse individuals.

Second, the event being insured against must be identifiable and well defined to minimize transaction costs associated with determining the occurrence of the event. In addition, the event must have well-established boundaries with ownership able to be easily defined and observable; that is, it must also be possible to establish the value of the loss that will be suffered if the event occurs. Third, the occurrence of the event must generate substantial financial loss so as to have an impact on the income or wealth of the individual. Fourth, the occurrence of the event must be outside the control of the insured individuals; that is, the behavior of the insured regarding the

event does not change just because the event is now covered by insurance.

These market conditions become very important as the market for health insurance is examined and analyzed. As the health insurance market is evaluated, adherence to, or violation of, these conditions are critical in determining the efficiency and effectiveness of market performance.

10.4 Demand for Health Insurance

10.4.1 Individual Demand for Insurance

The simple competitive market analysis of demand for medical care is based on the condition that the consumer knows with certainty what his or her state of health will be during the relevant time period. This underlying assumption of certainty is not plausible for many medical problems. In these cases, a consumer cannot be certain whether or not a health-related problem will occur. The consumer does know, however, that he or she *might* become ill or injured during a particular period of time and might have to visit a physician and even be hospitalized.

In this type of situation, a consumer faces the choice of whether or not to prepare financially for medical contingencies. In this illustration, the individual can prepare for a potentially large loss by purchasing insurance. This action entails an increased outlay of resources (the premium) at the outset of the period followed by reduced outlays of resources should an illness or injury occur. The basic theory of the demand for insurance presents a general overview of how certain underlying variables—tastes and preferences, wealth, price, the likelihood of an illness or injury, and the loss resulting from the illness or injury—can influence the decision to purchase insurance. The following points provide an overview of the basic assumptions regarding the underlying variables in the model.

Consumer tastes and preferences. To characterize consumer tastes and preferences with regard to the alternative situations that may result from an illness or injury, assume that when an illness or injury occurs, it leads to medical care expenses that are sufficient to constitute a noticeable loss of the wealth of the individual. To specify what this loss means to the individual, a concept to characterize the individual's well-being at alternative levels of wealth—the concept of *utility*—must be introduced. Recall that utility represents the amount of satisfaction that an individual receives from possessing or consuming a good or service. In this illustration wealth is a resource possessed.

To illustrate utility, assume one hypothetical individual's taste and preference for wealth is presented in the form of an index of utility in **Table 10-1**. This index shows what level of utility is associated with each specific level of wealth possessed by the individual. Thus, a level of wealth of $10,000 is associated with a level of utility of 100; a level of wealth of $9900 is associated with a level of utility of 99.8; and so on. The size of the specific numbers in the utility index is arbitrary. What is important is that higher wealth gives higher utility (i.e., increased wealth makes the individual "better off" or more satisfied). A further assumption is that the function is characterized by diminishing marginal utility. That

is, in this illustration each additional $100 of wealth results in less additional utility to the individual than the previous $100. For example, if the individual has wealth valued at $8500, then an extra $100 of wealth will yield 3.0 extra units of utility; at $8600, an extra $100 of wealth will yield 2.8 extra units; and so on. It is important to note that while marginal utility declines with the accumulation of wealth, total utility continues to increase. That is, more wealth is preferred to less wealth by the individual.

If wealth has diminishing marginal utility for an individual, that individual is said to be *risk-averse*. The basic idea of being risk-averse is that, for a given wealth level, a loss of a given amount is of greater subjective importance (utility) to the person than would be a gain of an equal amount. Utility is the subjective index of the relative importance of wealth. To illustrate, notice that if our hypothetical individual currently has a wealth valued at $8500, his or her total utility is 76.0. However, if the individual uses $100 so that his or her wealth drops to $8400, his or her total utility falls to 72.6, a change in marginal utility of 3.4 points. However, if the individual had a gain in wealth of $100 to $8600, then total utility would increase to 79.0, and the marginal utility gained would be only 3.0 points.

In this illustration, for simplicity, the utility function contains a single input—wealth. In this model, the utility function $U(W)$ is unique to the individual. Thus, it does not imply that additional wealth means less to a rich person than it does to a low-income person. This kind of comparison, called *interpersonal comparison*, would involve specifying different people's utilities on the same scale. As illustrated by the data in Table 10-1 and Figure 10-1, total utility increases as wealth increases; the first derivative of the utility function is positive. Second, the marginal utility of wealth decreases as wealth increases—this means the second derivative of the utility function is negative. **Figure 10-1** is a graph of the utility function in this illustration.

Level of wealth. The second assumption in this illustration is that the individual has an initial level of wealth of $10,000, with total utility of 100.

Medical expenses in the event of illness. The third assumption in this illustration is that if the individual becomes sick, medical expenses of $1000 will be incurred, which defines the potential magnitude of the loss. This expenditure is assumed to restore the loss in health fully.

Likelihood of illness. A fourth assumption concerns the element of uncertainty. The assumption is that probabilities can be assigned to the various possible

Table 10-1 Relationship Between Wealth and Utility

Wealth ($)	Total Utility	Marginal Utility
8,000	57.0	4.2
8,100	61.2	4.0
8,200	65.2	3.8
8,300	69.0	3.6
8,400	72.6	3.4
8,500	76.0	3.2
8,600	79.0	3.0
8,700	81.8	2.8
8,800	84.4	2.6
8,900	86.8	2.4
9,000	89.0	2.2
9,100	91.0	2.0
9,200	92.8	1.8
9,300	94.4	1.6
9,400	95.8	1.4
9,500	97.0	1.2
9,600	98.0	1.0
9,700	98.8	0.8
9,800	99.4	0.6
9,900	99.8	0.4
10,000	100.0	0.2

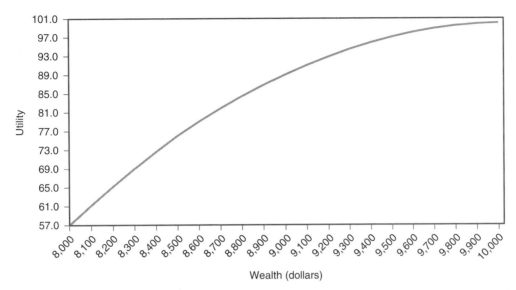

Figure 10-1 Relationship between wealth and utility. The curved line reflects the utility function of wealth for the individual in the illustration presented in the text. It assumes the individual has a guaranteed level of wealth of $8,000, providing a utility level of 57.0 units.

health states the individual may experience. Assuming there is a 0.1 probability of illness (i.e., of 10 people in similar circumstances, one will become ill) and a 0.9 probability the individual will remain well and will not incur any medical costs. These are the only two possibilities in this illustration, so the sum of the probabilities equals 1.

Price of insurance. The individual can shift the risk of loss on to an insurer but will have to pay an insurance premium to do so. In exchange for this premium, the insurer assumes the financial risk (i.e., the insurer will fully pay the $1000, if the person should become ill or injured).

Behavioral assumption. The sixth assumption in this illustration is that the individual wants to maximize the expected value of his or her utility. Thus, the individual will choose that course of action from which the highest level of utility can be expected to be achieved.

The model's conclusions are obtained by determining how, under these assumed conditions, the individual will behave so as to maximize expected utility (i.e., which of the two options, buy insurance or do not buy insurance, will the individual choose). The model predicts that if health insurance is available on the right terms, the risk-averse individual will buy it to reduce financial risk (and hence increase expected utility). To see how this conclusion is derived, it is necessary to examine how much wealth and utility the individual would expect to have with and without purchasing insurance.

The decision problem is summarized with the data in **Table 10-2**. Without insurance, the individual has a 90% chance of having $10,000 in wealth during the period and a 10% chance of having only $9000 in wealth because of having to make the $1000 payout for needed medical care. The expected value of wealth will be 90% of $10,000 plus 10% of 9000, or $9900. This is the sum of the amounts the individual expects to receive under various conditions adjusted for the probabilities that those conditions will arise. Based on the data in Table 10-2, which is derived from the data in Table 10-1, if $10,000 is the level of wealth, the total utility is represented by 100 units. If only $9000 is available because of an illness or injury, the total utility is 89.0 units. But, the individual has only a 90% chance of having 100 units of utility and a 10% chance of having 89.0 units. The expected value of the utility achieved will be 90% of 100 plus 10% of 89, or 98.9 units of utility.

So, without insurance, the expected value of income is $9900, and the expected value of utility is 98.9 units. The utility associated with a *certain* wealth of $9900 is 99.8 units. So a certain wealth of $9900 would be more desirable to the individual than the risky situation (because 99.8 > 98.9). In this illustration a certain wealth of $9900 could be obtained by buying an insurance policy costing $100. The payment of the $100 insurance premium would reduce the initial $10,000 wealth to $9900, but there is then no risk of further financial loss in wealth and utility because, even if illness occurs, the insurance would cover the costs. Thus, the individual in this model would have a demand for insurance at a premium of $100. Note that the premium of $100 here is called the actuarially *fair premium* or *pure premium*. It is the amount an insurer would

Table 10-2 Comparison of "Buy Insurance" and "Do Not Buy" Insurance Options

Price of Insurance ($)	Wealth After Insurance Purchase ($)	Utility After Insurance Purchase	Expected Utility with No Insurance	Decision
100	9990	99.8	98.9	Buy
200	9800	99.4	98.9	Buy
300	9700	98.8	98.9	Marginal
400	9600	98.0	98.9	Do not buy
500	9500	97.0	98.9	Do not buy

© Jones & Bartlett Learning.

have to charge to break even when insuring a large number of people, assuming no administrative costs of operation. The costs associated with the administrative activities involved in managing the insurance process are known as *loading fees*.

In fact, the person in this example would be willing to pay considerably more than $100 for health insurance. Assume that for $200, the individual could buy insurance coverage against the $1000 loss. By buying the insurance, the individual would be certain of having $9800. This is because the individual's wealth would be reduced by the amount of the premium ($200), and if the individual then became ill, the insurer would pay the incurred medical cost. Certainty of having $9800 would yield 99.4 units of utility, which is a higher expected utility than that in the "no insurance" situation. Being a utility maximizer, the individual would buy the insurance on these terms. Indeed, the individual would pay up to almost $300 to avoid the risk of losing wealth due to illness, because at that price slightly below $300, the expected utility with no insurance is approximately equal to the utility of the certain wealth after the purchase of insurance.

Of course, the individual would not buy insurance "at any price." For example, if the premium were $400, the expected utility in the risky no-insurance situation (98.9) is greater than the utility associated with a certain wealth of $9600 (98.0), and the "do not buy insurance" option would be the more attractive one. Insurance demand also depends of course on the size of the possible loss. Assume, in this illustration, that the possible medical expense is not $1000, but rather is $1500, either because the illness is more serious or because the price of medical care is higher. In this situation, the individual faces an expected loss of $1500 if illness occurs, bringing wealth down to $8500. The individual would have an expected

utility of 97.6 units (10% of 76.0 plus 90% of 100) in the "no-insurance" situation. If the individual was certain of having $9600 ($10,000 minus the $400 premium), he or she would be certain of receiving 98.0 units of utility. Therefore, in this case, the individual would be willing to pay something up to $400 for insurance.

The conclusion is that, as the possible loss increases, the amount of money the individual is willing to pay to avert the possible loss increases as well, and the individual will be willing to buy additional insurance coverage if the terms are right. The size of the financial loss in relation to the individual's wealth and the associated utilities is called the *financial vulnerability factor*. A second factor, which is related to the probability of illness, is referred to as the *risk perception factor* (Berki & Ashcraft, 1980). In our example, if the probability of becoming ill increased from 10% to 20%, the expected utility in the "no-insurance" situation would fall to 97.8 (80% of 100 plus 20% of 89.0). This is associated with a wealth level close to $9600, indicating that the individual would be willing to pay up to about $400 to avoid the risk of a $1000 loss.

Figure 10-2 can be used to illustrate how expected utility of an individual will change as the probability of becoming ill or injured changes. Assume first that the individual has a 100% chance of becoming ill so that the probability of becoming ill is equal to 1. In this illustration, the individual's expected utility is equal to the utility gain from a guaranteed income. In this illustration, assume that the guaranteed income is $8400 and is represented by L at 72.6 on the utility curve. Also, assume that the individual has no chance of becoming ill, so that the probability of becoming ill is equal to 0. In this case the individual's income is $10,000 with certainty and utility is represented by H at 100.0 on the utility curve.

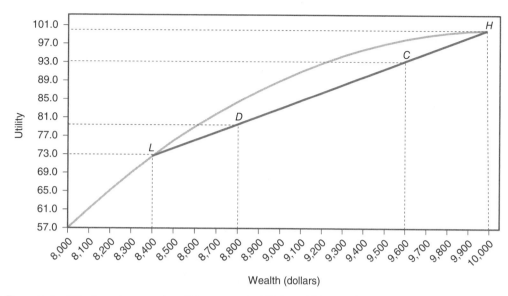

Figure 10-2 Expected utility from income for different probabilities of illness. An individual's expected income and expected utility can be calculated for any probability of illness by moving along the straight-line segment *HL*.

The individual's expected utility then falls on a line between point *L* and point *H*, since *L* and *H* are considered fixed points not impacted by the probability of illness. Now, assume that the individual's probability of becoming ill is between 0 and 100%, at 25% in this illustration. Under these conditions, the individual's expected utility would be located one-fourth of the distance between *H* and *L* at point *C*. Likewise, the individual's expected utility if the probability of becoming ill was 75%, would be three-fourths of the distance between *H* and *L* and reflected at point *D* in Figure 10-2. Notice that expected utility is not derived off the utility curve, but rather from the straight line *H–L*.

The amount an individual is willing to pay for insurance depends on the specific extent of his or her risk aversion. This is represented by the rate at which marginal utility diminishes with increasing wealth. An individual with constant marginal utility would be risk-neutral. For such a person, insurance at the actuarially fair premium would be no more desirable than the "no-insurance" option. The greater the rate of decrease of marginal utility for a person, the more risk-averse the individual is and the more willing the individual is to pay premiums above the actuarially fair premium.

10.4.2 Limitations of the Theory

The theory of insurance demand presented here has the virtue of explicitly organizing some of the variables that are central to the decision of whether or not to purchase insurance. As presented in this illustration,

however, it has important limitations. The following observations may assist in understanding what these limitations are.

First, the reader may find it strange that the utility function, which is supposed to measure satisfaction, does not include medical care. This is, indeed, a shortcoming of the model because well-being can depend on receiving appropriate care, and on taking preventive actions. The model looks only at the financial aspects of the situation, in effect assuming that the care, fully and instantly, restores health to the individual, with no utility implications of either the illness or the process of getting care. Clearly, this is an unrealistic assumption. Including medical care, however, creates a model that is much more complicated and more difficult to apply, and while it is important to understand that the model has been abstracted from reality, this should not detract from the value of the model. The present model has the virtue of focusing on the benefits of risk shifting, which is an economic good distinct from medical care.

Second, insurance has the effect of lowering the direct price of medical care. Under the competitive market model, the expectation would be for the demand for medical care to increase under these circumstances, yet in the basic insurance model, it has been assumed that medical care demand does not change with the lower, post-insurance price to the individual. That is, the model implies that, if an individual becomes ill, he or she will demand the same amount of medical care with or without insurance. This means that the elasticity of demand for medical care is 0, an unlikely scenario for most types of medical care. Again, such an assumption was necessary to simplify the model. If in fact the demand for medical care is affected by the existence of insurance, it violates one of the fundamental principles of the market for insurance.

Third, we have assumed that the individual pays the full amount of the premium. In fact, often a consumer's out-of-pocket premium is substantially less than the total premium received by the insurance company. Many individuals receive their insurance coverage through their place of employment, which pays part, or all, of the premium. This is not to say that the consumer receives "free" insurance. The consumer, through a bargaining unit or via an employer's policy, negotiates for or receives a total compensation package that includes wages (a direct money component) and benefits (e.g., pension rights, paid time off, health insurance, and other fringe benefits). The individual pays taxes on the money portion of compensation, and with after-tax wages, directly pays his or her share of the premiums. Under the Internal Revenue Code, many nonwage benefits received through the employer, including health insurance, are not taxed. Therefore, insurance has a lower price when purchased through employment benefits than if purchased directly by the consumer.

This point is illustrated numerically in **Table 10-3**. In this table, the marginal tax rate of the individual or family is assumed to be 20%, which means that for each $100 in taxable income the employee receives, he or she pays $20 in taxes and takes home $80. Now, assume an individual receives $1250 of additional wage compensation and the individual has no additional deductible expenses. Therefore, the individual will pay $250 (20% of $1250) in taxes and will have $1000 left over to be used to purchase goods or services, including health insurance.

On the other hand, if the $1250 in compensation is in the form of employer-provided health insurance,

then this compensation is not taxed, and $1250 in insurance coverage can be received. A dollar's worth of coverage purchased with after-tax wages is thus worth $(1 - T)$ times the value of the coverage received via employer benefits, in which T is the marginal tax rate. Thus, $(1 - T) \times \$1$ is sometimes called the price of $1 of employer-provided premiums (Taylor & Wilensky, 1983). In terms of this demand model, such tax benefits will lower the cost of health insurance to the individual and thus will increase demand for health insurance.

10.4.3 The Market Demand for Insurance

Insurance availability requires the existence of at least one organization willing to accept the risks associated with an event and pay the costs associated with that event when they arise. To determine under which market conditions this will occur, assume an insurance company is being formed to cover the risks of 1000 people with tastes, incomes, and health experience exactly like those of the representative individual in Section 10.4.1. A more definite meaning can now be given to the "probabilities" assigned to the alternative health states. Assume in this illustration that the insurance company can have 100% certainty that 100 of the 1000 consumers will become ill and require medical care during the covered period. Because pooling a large number of risks yields a considerable degree of certainty regarding an average, it becomes possible to assign a risk to each consumer and evaluate his or her expected loss experience in terms of the group.

The insurance company knows that, in this group of 1000 consumers, 100 will most likely become ill and each of the 100 will require $1000 worth of medical care. Under these conditions, the expected medical expenses total $100,000 for the group. As presented here, the actuarially fair rate (the expected loss per individual participant) is $1000. If each consumer pays a premium of $1000, the expected losses of the group will just be covered. According to the analysis in Section 10.4.1, every individual would be willing to pay a premium equal to the actuarially fair rate to reduce the risk of incurring large losses. Indeed, with diminishing marginal utility, the individuals would be willing to pay a little more.

The insurance company cannot charge just the actuarially fair rate because there are expenses associated with administering an insurance business and some level of profit or surplus must be earned, representing a fair return on investment in the opportunity

Table 10-3 A Comparison of Health Insurance When Purchased by Employer and Employee

	Purchased by Employee ($)	Purchased by Employer ($)
Compensation	1250	1250
Tax	250	0
After-tax money available for purchasing premiums	1000	1250

© Jones & Bartlett Learning.

costs of not investing those resources in the next best option. The insurance company must charge more than the actuarially fair rate to cover these administrative costs and profits. The additional fee charged by the insurance company is called the *loading fee*. The premium each individual pays is thus made up of two components: the fee for benefits received and the loading fee. In this illustration, assume that the insurer has administrative expenses of $7500 in total and desires a profit of $2500; the total loading fee is thus $10,000. The insurance company must charge premiums of $110,000, of which $100,000 will be paid out in benefits. With premiums spread over 1000 consumers, if all pay the same premium rate, the rate will be $110 per individual.

Strictly speaking, the price of insurance is the loading fee, not the premium. In this case, the price of insurance is $10 per insurance consumer. This price can be expressed in several ways, including as a ratio of premiums to benefits ($110/$100 or 1.1), as a cost per policy ($10), or as a ratio of the loading fee to benefits ($10,000/$100,000 or 0.10). The reason the loading fee is the price of insurance is that the product is insurance—the protection from risk—not the provision of medical care. The gains the consumer receives from insurance coverage are the utility gains from the risk reduction. The price of this risk reduction is the loading fee. It is the level of this fee that will determine whether or not the individual will purchase insurance.

The overall market demand will therefore depend on the various factors that influence individual demand and the number of individuals in the market. If all individuals have exactly the same tastes, incomes, sickness profiles, and so on, then they will have the same demand for insurance. In actuality, this is unlikely to be the case. Individuals will differ by illness level, wealth, and degree of risk aversion. Their gains from risk reduction will therefore differ and as the price of *insurance* (the loading fee) increases, some individuals will drop their coverage and market demand will fall off.

10.4.4 Moral Hazard

Once an individual has purchased medical insurance, the direct out-of-pocket price the individual pays for medical care decreases. If the individual has purchased full-coverage insurance, this out-of-pocket price decreases to zero. However, when the direct price of medical care decreases for any reason (including as a result of buying insurance), the quantity demanded will increase given the inverse relationship between price and quantity demanded in the market (i.e., the absolute value of the elasticity of demand is greater than zero). This phenomenon—the existence of an elasticity of demand for medical care in response to insurance coverage—is known in the insurance industry as *moral hazard*. Moral hazard occurs when health insurance coverage causes individuals to take greater risk with their health or to consume more health care than they would if they did not have health insurance. The term suggests that individuals "shirk" their moral responsibilities and consume recklessly or needlessly when they are insured. From the point of view of economics, they are simply behaving in accordance with the principle expressed by the downward-sloping demand curve—as price declines a greater quantity is consumed.

The existence of moral hazard has been used to explain why individuals only partially insure against healthcare risks; that is, why individuals accept copayments, coinsurance, and deductibles rather than purchase full insurance coverage (Feldstein & Friedman, 1977; Friedman, 1974; Kelly & Markowitz, 2009/2010; Pylypchuk, 2010; Steinorth, 2011). Such analyses are more complicated than the basic insurance models presented here, but the essentials involved in the decision-making process can be presented in a fairly simple manner. Assume that an individual has the same utility function as in the model discussed in Section 10.4.1. Other basic assumptions in the model now developed are as follows:

- The probability of being sick is 0.2 and of being well is 0.8. That is, out of each 100 individuals in the group, 20 will get sick.
- If an individual gets sick, the price of each unit of medical care is $500.
- The individual's initial level of wealth is $100,000.

As in the previous model, utility received directly from medical care and health is initially ignored. Now, three options are available to each individual in the group: in Option 1, the individual has no health insurance, but pays the market price ($500) per unit of medical care used; in Option 2, the individual is fully insured and pays a zero price out-of-pocket for medical care consumed; and in Option 3, there is a 20% coinsurance rate and thus a direct price to the individual of $100 per unit of medical care consumed.

Because demand varies with price, the quantity of medical care demanded will vary in the three situations. Assume that in Option 1, in which the direct price is $500, there will be 10 units of medical care demanded. In Option 2, in which the price is 0, there will be 30 units demanded. In Option 3, where the price is $100, there will be 15 units demanded. Now the focus is on the demand for insurance. To simplify the analysis at this time, assume a loading fee of zero (no loading fee), which means that the premium rate will equal the expected loss to the individual. The information for this illustration is summarized in **Table 10-4**.

First, consider Options 1 and 2. Compare the expected utilities, $E(U)$, to determine which provides the highest utility level (and hence which is preferred). If the expected utility in Option 1 is greater than that in Option 2, then the individual will not buy insurance because having no insurance yields a higher expected utility than having full insurance. In fact, under Option 1, the individual faces a 20% chance of becoming sick, paying the full $5000 ($500 per unit times 10 units consumed) in medical costs, and having $95,000 left over. Assume the utility of $95,000 in wealth is 97.0. On the other hand, the individual has an 80% chance of not getting sick, in which case the level of wealth remains at $100,000 and the utility is 100. The $E(U)$ for this situation is 99.4 (80% of 100 plus 20% of 97.0). The $E(U)$ under Option 2 is equal to the utility of the original level of wealth minus the premium (i.e., the utility of $97,000). This amounts to 98.8 units of utility. And because "no insurance" has greater expected utility than full insurance, the individual will demand "no insurance" under these conditions.

Now, bring Option 3 into the picture. First, note that the premium is less than under full insurance, in which 30 units of medical care were demanded. Under Option 3, there will be 15 units demanded, but because of the 20% coinsurance rate, the insurance company pays only $400 per unit, or $6000 in total. The individual, having a 20% probability of becoming sick, will pay a premium of $1200. In addition, if the individual is sick, he or she pays a coinsurance of $100 per unit, or $1500 for the 15 visits. The $E(U)$ for this situation is roughly 99.6 [20% of (100,000 – 1200 – 1500) plus 80% of (100,000 – 1200)]. This is greater than the expected utility of not buying insurance. Now the individual will purchase health insurance.

However, this may not be the preferred option. Other coinsurance rates will have other expected utilities. What is important to note is that the individual will, in some circumstances, prefer insurance with a coinsurance rate to that with full coverage (or no coverage) if the moral hazard is great enough.

A particular shortcoming of this model should be mentioned. Medical care has utility, as does insurance. This fact has been ignored in this model. Indeed, the extra units of medical care consumed in Options 2 and 3 yield extra utility to the individual in their own right. It may well be that the marginal utility of these units would make the full-coverage option preferable to one of lesser coverage. While this may be the case, the point of this discussion is that, if the conditions are right, insurance with a coinsurance may be preferred to all other options.

The typical insurance model views the increase in the demand for medical care by an insured individual as a welfare loss to society. This welfare loss occurs because decisions made by individuals are based on the price paid out of pocket for the service and not on the price the provider receives for the service. As a result, more services are purchased than would be purchased at the full price in the market. Basically, the effect is the same as would occur with an outward shift in the demand curve rather than a movement down the original demand curve with a change in out-of-pocket cost—a larger quantity is now demanded at the original price.

Table 10-4 Example of the Effects of Moral Hazard

	Situation 1 (No Insurance)	Situation 2 (Full Insurance)	Situation 3 (20% Copayment)
Price paid by individual for one unit of care	500	0	100
Units of care demanded	10	30	15
Amount paid by insurance company for care	0	15,000	6,000
Pure premium	–	3,000	1,200
Expected utility	99.4	98.8	99.6

The traditional model views the difference between what the consumer would demand at the original price and the quantity demanded with insurance as a welfare loss to society because the true marginal costs now exceed marginal benefits. The additional medical services consumed by the insured individual are considered to be an inefficient use of society's scarce resources, generating more costs than benefits. If the consumer had to pay full price for these additional services, they would not be consumed.

Figure 10-3 shows an illustration of the social welfare loss to society of moral hazard. In the figure, D_u reflects the original demand without insurance coverage. D_i reflects the new demand with insurance coverage. The distance between P_u and P_i represents the amount of price distortion that occurs because of insurance coverage; that is, it is the decrease in price that would be necessary to entice consumers to purchase the additional units of medical care consumed with insurance. The shaded area in the figure reflects the social welfare loss as a result of moral hazard.

A study by Oakes, Chang, and Segal (2019) examined the overuse of healthcare services in the United States between 2010 and 2015. Overuse was defined as the purchase of care where the potential for harm exceeds the potential for benefit. Such overuse may not only be physically and psychologically harmful to patients, but such wasteful utilization of resources contributes to the high cost of health care in the United States. The authors found that overuse of healthcare services was persistent and varied across regions of the United States. In this study, it was found that rural areas tended to have less systemic overuse of services than their metropolitan counterparts, and that regional systemic overuse of health care remained consistent over time.

Nyman (1999a, 2004) offers a different view, proposing that not all the increase in demand by insured individuals results in welfare loss to society. Nyman (2004) argues that acquiring insurance enables individuals to purchase medical care they could not afford previously, and that much of the increased utilization of services has a substantial impact on the health status of the individual. Because at least some of the increased utilization of services, especially among vulnerable populations, has a positive benefit, it should not be viewed as a welfare loss to society.

Under this model, it is important to separate services into those that have marginal benefits greater than their marginal costs and those that do not. Under Nyman's model, insurance should be viewed as a transfer of income at the time of illness and that the increase in income shifts the demand curve to the right. This shift of the demand curve, rather than a movement down the demand curve because of reduced price, results in much less inefficiency in the market for healthcare services. While Nyman's model does not stipulate that moral hazard is efficient, it does require a separation of the effects of moral hazard into efficient and inefficient categories. In practice, the difficulty arises in determining when marginal costs exceed marginal benefits in health care.

Concern was expressed that the newly covered individuals under the ACA's Medicaid expansion program would increase the demand for health care, possibly overwhelming the system and having

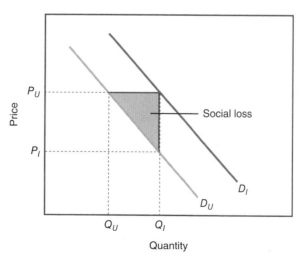

Figure 10-3 Social loss caused by moral hazard. The shaded area reflects the social loss as a result of moral hazard. The distance between P_U and P_i reflects the decrease in price that would be required to persuade the individual to increase to the quantity of medical care demanded with insurance.

a negative spillover effect on access by previously insured individuals. The negative spillover impact that the increased demand could have on the Medicare-covered population was especially concerning to a number of decision makers. However, while Medicaid expansion did increase utilization of healthcare services, a study by Blavin (2019) did not find any adverse effects of it on physician acceptance of new Medicare, Medicaid, or privately insured patients.

Similarly, Admon et al. (2019) examined the impact of Medicaid expansion on hospital utilization and found that Medicaid expansion did not significantly impact hospital utilization based on per capita rates of patient admissions designated as emergent, admitted via the emergency department or clinic, or patients discharged within 1 day, or with length of stay greater than or equal to 7 days. The study also did not find differences in diagnosis at admission, admission severity, comorbidity burden, or mortality associated with Medicaid expansion. The study did find that Medicaid expansion was associated with a shift in payer mix among the nonelderly hospitalized adults, suggesting that Medicaid expansion had reduced uncompensated care without shifting admission practices or acuity among hospitalized adults.

10.4.5 Demand Responsiveness to the Price of Health Insurance

Remember the concept of the elasticity of demand for medical care, which is a measure of how responsive the quantity of medical care is to out-of-pocket price changes. In a similar vein, an elasticity of demand for health insurance showing how buyers will respond to changes in the price of insurance can be estimated. The formula for estimating the price elasticity of the demand for health insurance can be written as follows:

$$E_d = \frac{\left(\text{PREM}_2 - \text{PREM}_1\right)/\left(\text{PREM}_2 + \text{PREM}_1\right)}{\left(P_2 - P_1\right)/\left(P_2 + P_1\right)}$$

in which E_d is the elasticity of demand for insurance coverage, PREM is the dollar amount of premiums demanded (with subscripts 1 and 2 referring to situations 1 and 2), and P is the price of insurance (with subscripts 1 and 2 referring to situations 1 and 2). In the formula the price of insurance is defined as the loading fee, as discussed in the previous section. In the following illustration assume that the loading fee (price of insurance) increases from $800 per policy to $1000 and that, as a result, consumers reduce their demand for insurance, and therefore their premiums

from $10,500 to $9500. Then the elasticity of demand for insurance is calculated as follows:

$$\frac{(\$9500 - \$10500)/(\$9500 + \$10500)}{(\$1000 - \$800)/(\$1000 + \$800)}$$

$$\frac{(-\$1000)/(\$20000)}{(\$200)/(\$1800)} \text{ or } \frac{-0.05}{0.11} \text{ or } -0.45$$

The magnitude of the elasticity of demand for insurance has important implications for policy. The exemption of health insurance benefits from an individual's income tax is equivalent to a reduction in the price of health insurance to the consumer. This exemption has the effect of increasing the demand for health insurance benefits, such as reductions in the coinsurance rates of policies. Lower coinsurance rates increase the quantity of medical care demanded. In the immediate post-World War II era, when the government was trying to encourage the consumption of medical care, this increase in demand was not regarded as a problem. In current times, with the concern over rising medical care costs and concerns with overuse of services, the issue has grown in importance.

Several studies have been undertaken to establish the responsiveness of the demand for insurance to changes in the price of insurance. Taylor and Wilensky (1983) examined how premiums increase as the variable tax rate (1 – marginal tax rate) falls. (This variable was taken to be a proxy for the after-tax price of employer-provided health insurance.) They found the elasticity to be –0.2. In other studies, the value has ranged from –0.2 to –1. There is considerable uncertainty, then, as to the value of this variable. If –0.2 is accepted as the correct figure, then an individual in the 20% marginal tax bracket who received $10,000 in employer-provided premiums has been able to buy $1 in premiums for 80 cents. If the government eliminated this subsidy, the price would rise to $1, and the quantity of insurance demanded (premiums) would fall.

Such a reduction in benefits would mean higher coinsurance and would subsequently translate into less medical care demanded and, with an elastic demand for medical care, into lower medical expenditures. It is important to be aware of the interaction between insurance and medical care markets. What happens in one market influences what happens in the other.

10.4.6 Choice of Health Plan

The purchase of a particular health insurance policy through employment-based insurance requires two decisions, one by the employer and one by the employee. Many employers provide their employees with a selection of health plans and allow them to make their own decisions about the types of coverage and services they will obtain. The plans with more complete coverage will cost more, and for each of these, the insurer will charge a higher premium. Often the employer will pay a fixed contribution toward the premium regardless of the plan chosen, and the employee will pay out of pocket the difference between the premium and the employer's contribution. In such cases, the employee has a choice among alternative types of healthcare coverage. From an economic standpoint, the concern involves discovering what factors influence consumer demand for alternative plans.

Which economic determinants influence the choice of health plan is a topic of considerable importance. If individuals or families with specific characteristics (e.g., people in poor health, young couples with families) prefer one type of plan over another on economic grounds, selection is said to be *biased*, which means that these individuals or families will demand one particular plan systematically. Often the basis for the selection of a plan is economic. In such cases, the selection is a manifestation of demand behavior.

The economic significance of this lies in the fact that, as a result of these selections, different health plans will have different populations with different experiences of healthcare utilization. One plan (e.g., a traditional plan) may appear to be expensive relative to another (e.g., a managed care plan). Some of the difference in price may be due to the enrollment of families with different characteristics in the plan (e.g., older people may tend to enroll in the traditional plan). Any comparison of the cost of the two plans that *did not account for these differences* would be misleading. Thus, these factors and their causes must be considered.

To illustrate the concept of biased selection, the insurance demand model is applied to two alternative situations. In both, there is an employer with 2000 employees. Each employee has one chance in five (i.e., a probability of 0.2) of becoming ill or injured. However, in this illustration the employees can be divided into two groups of 1000 each. Those in the "unhealthy" group will require $2000 in medical care if they become ill or injured; those in the "healthy" group will require only $1000 of medical care. Individuals in both groups have an initial wealth level of $10,000 and the utility function shown in Table 10-1.

The insurance plan in the first situation is a "high-option" plan, in that it covers all expenses in the event of illness. Assume, for simplicity's sake, that the insurance company has no loading fee. The premium is thus equal to the expected loss for the employee.

The total payout will be $400,000 ($2000 × 0.2 × 1000) for the unhealthy employees and $200,000 for the healthy employees ($1000 × 0.2 × 1000). On average, the payout is $300 per employee ([$400,000 + $200,000] / 2000). Assume that all consumers pay according to a *community rating*; that is, each pays the same premium regardless of his or her utilization experience. The full premium therefore is $300. The employer's contribution is assumed to be $200 per employee, and the employee's contribution is $100. It should be remembered that the employer's $200 contribution is employee compensation, and normally there would be tax advantages in receiving compensation in this way. To keep the illustration uncomplicated, these tax benefits will be ignored for now.

With these assumptions specified, the demand for the high-option plan can now be examined. This is done using the utility model of insurance demand that was introduced in previous sections. According to this model, individuals will demand an insurance plan if the expected utility associated with the plan is greater than the expected utility in the absence of the plan. Consider first the unhealthy group. The expected loss for a person in this group, if he or she became sick and had no insurance, would be $2000. The person would be left with $8000 in wealth (yielding a utility of 57.0). However, 80% of the individuals in this group will remain healthy, and each of these individuals will be left with $10,000 and have an associated utility level of 100. The average expected utility for the entire group would be 91.4 (80% of 100 and 20% of 57.0). Similarly, the average expected utility of the healthy group would be 97.8 (80% of the utility of 100 plus 20% of the utility of 80.0), because their costs are only $1000.

To determine the situation of these groups when they have insurance, the premium paid by each group must be known. In this case, under community rating it is $300 per person. This amount is treated as a reduction in employee's wealth, even though some of it may be employer-paid, because more nonwage benefits would mean less wages (and so in the absence of tax considerations, these can be regarded as equivalent). If each employee incurs a premium cost of $300, he or she will be left with wealth of $9700 and have a utility level of 98.8. Because utility with insurance for both groups is greater than utility with no insurance, both groups would demand insurance coverage.

Now, consider a second situation in which there is a low-option plan with the following characteristics. First, there is a limit on the benefits of a maximum of $1000. That is, if anyone becomes ill or injured, the insurance company would cover the first $1000 of expenses, but beyond that, the individual would be responsible. The premium of such a plan would be lower because the insurance company's payout would be limited to only $1000 per episode of illness. In fact, it would be $200 or (0.2 × $1000), since only 20% of the individuals will become ill or injured.

The utility model can again shed light on the choice of plan. First of all, if the individuals joined such a plan, the unhealthy group members would pay the $200 premium plus the excess of illness expenses ($2000) over covered expenses ($1000), or $100 per illness. Their wealth would be $8800 if they were ill and $9800 if they did not become ill, and their expected utility would be 96.4 (20% of 84.4 plus 80% of 99.4).

Utility theory predicts that these individuals would be better off joining the high-option plan (in which the expected utility is 98.8) and so would choose the high-option plan. On the other hand, the healthy group would spend $200 on premiums for the low-option plan and would have no additional out-of-pocket expenses since their costs if they become ill are only $1000. They would retain $9800 whether or not they were ill or injured, and their expected utility would be 99.4. This is greater than under the high-option plan, and so they would choose the low-option plan.

This model thus shows that the characteristics of a group partially dictate the choice of plan. An unhealthy group uses more care and will demand higher coverage. There are a number of reasons why one group might consist of high-cost users: the individuals might be older, have special health problems, be more likely to have children, and so on. For whatever reason, if the group members have higher expected costs, then they will *systematically* select a plan with a higher degree of coverage.

Of course, when biased selection occurs, the rejection of the high-option plan by the healthy group would leave relatively more unhealthy people in that plan, and so the average cost of that plan would increase over time. This is an example of what is called *adverse selection*, and has implications for the functioning of the insurance market, which are discussed next.

There is a very important issue on which the model presented here throws light. As shown earlier, different benefit plans will attract different types of enrollees. In this illustration, a high-option plan will attract individuals who are less healthy and tend to use more care. In a previous section, it was established that individuals with more complete coverage will demand more medical care (because of lower out-of-pocket costs) whatever their health status. If actual data comparing plans are reviewed and it is found that individuals in the higher option plan use more care than in the lower option plan, what can be concluded? In fact, it could be that both the lower out-of-pocket price and the difference in health status contributed to differences in utilization.

This confounding of causal factors in healthcare demand has been a source of conflict in studies comparing utilization among plans. For example, a number of studies have compared utilization between enrollees in HMOs and conventional insurance plans. The general conclusion has been that hospital utilization under HMO coverage is lower than under conventional coverage (Herring & Adams, 2011; Miller & Luft, 1995; Pauly & Herring, 2000). But the issue has been somewhat clouded by the lack of clear evidence that the groups being compared were similar in terms of health status.

10.5 Supply of Health Insurance

10.5.1 Supplier Behavior

The product or output of insurers is the assumption of risks that were initially borne by consumers, including the risk of catastrophic medical costs. An insurer has the choice of accepting or not accepting risks on behalf of consumers, and there are a number of factors that will induce any insurer not to accept certain risks. It is not only consumers who have preferences regarding risk; owners and managers of insurance companies react to risk as well. The insurer is in business to earn profits, which yield utility for its shareholders. Its tastes reflect those of its shareholders. The insurer's wealth (and hence utility) depends on the revenues collected by the insurer and on the insurer's costs, including its payout for covered benefits.

10.5.2 Risk and Size of the Insured Population

The degree of risk of most interest to the insurer is not that faced by any specific individual, but rather the mean (average) risk for the insured population. This is what determines the claims with which the insurer can expect to be faced. However, under normal insurance conditions the insurers are dealing with random events; in any given round of insuring, the actual value of claims the insurer experiences will almost always differ from the mean. Thus, the insurer is concerned with the variability of the insured population's risk; that is, the likelihood that in any given year, it will be very far above or very far below the mean value. Because of such variability, insurers must hold contingency reserves (i.e., funds available for covering claims in years when claims are unusually large).

An important thing to note is that this variability is inversely related to the number of people insured. As additional insured consumers are added, the insurer is less likely to experience a loss for the insured consumer group that is very different from the expected value. In other words, the insurer's risk of large losses is reduced as the size of the insurance pool increases, assuming the loss experiences of individuals are independent. So even if all the consumers face a high degree of risk (i.e., a big spread between financial outcomes), the variability faced by the insurance company can be much smaller because of the effect of large numbers on variation. In statistics, this effect is referred to as the *law of large numbers*.

The actual computation of this effect is beyond the scope of this text. However, the very powerful effect of the number of people insured can be demonstrated using a simple illustration. Assume each person has a risk function as follows: there is a 25% probability of an $8000 loss, a 50% probability of a $7000 loss, and a 25% probability of a $6000 loss. The expected mean loss is thus $7000. In any given year, the actually realized mean of a group's loss will not be exactly $7000, but if the group is large, it will not be very different from the average.

The likelihood of extreme losses for the group as a whole is less than for any individual. For example, for any *one person*, the probability of a loss of $8000 is 0.25. However, for a group of 100 such people with independent loss experiences, it is very unlikely that the *mean* loss would be $8000. Such a result would imply that all 100 people experienced an $8000 loss! Much more likely is the result that some will experience that loss and others will lose $7000 or $6000. The relevant computation shows that for this group of 100 individuals, the mean loss with 25% probability is $7047 or more. If the group size were 1000, a mean loss of $7047 or more would have a probability of only 0.018, and for a group of 10,000, the probability of a mean loss as large as $7047 is virtually zero.

10.5.3 Insurer Costs

The calculation of expected costs involves two components: claims paid out and the insurer's loading fee (administrative expenses and normal profit). The administrative expenses are incurred in the selling of insurance policies and the administration of claims. Economies of scale may play a role in determining administrative costs. If that is the case, larger insurers will have lower per-member administrative costs than smaller insurers. Claims paid out are determined by the price of medical care and the quantity of medical care used by the consumers. To some extent, both of these are outside the control of the insurer.

Prices of medical care are determined in the market for such care, and medical care consumed depends largely on the health status of the insured population. However, an analysis that assumed that both of these are taken as given by the insurer would be seriously flawed for two reasons. First, insurers often have some market power and play a very active role in setting the price of medical care; sophisticated bargaining arrangements exist under ordinary insurance arrangements, as well as under preferred provider organizations, patient-centered medical homes, accountable care organizations, and other managed care arrangements. Second, utilization of care is also subject to a host of forces, including the moral hazard phenomenon and direct insurer–provider relationships under managed care.

10.5.4 Insurer Revenues

The insurer's revenues are the premiums it receives from the plan members. There are two basic ways in which premiums can be set: through experience rating or through community rating. *Experience rating* involves the setting of premiums for individuals or groups according to their risk of loss, based on historical utilization and cost experiences. Healthy, low-risk individuals will be charged lower premiums than unhealthy, high-risk individuals under experience rating. In *community rating*, a single rate is set for the entire insured population based on the average experience of that population. High-risk individuals and low-risk individuals all pay the same rate, regardless of their expected loss.

10.5.5 Predictions About Supply

A simple supply model would show a typical positive relationship between price and quantity supplied. At higher premiums, an insurer would be more willing to take on additional risks. Conclusions can also be drawn about the effect of changes in other variables on the supply schedule of the insurer. Increases in the supply schedule (more risks accepted at a given premium rate) will be related to the following: a less risk-averse utility function on the part of the insurer, a greater initial level of reserves, a reduction in administrative costs, and a drop in the losses that may be experienced by the enrollees. Several additional aspects of supply behavior are worthy of emphasis at this point.

First, if all individuals do not have the same risk function and the insurer can choose between experience rating and community rating, the analysis becomes more complex. Assume there are two groups in the market, one group consists of high-risk individuals and the other consists of low-risk individuals. With experience rating, a premium would be set that reflected each group's loss experience. The insurer would then have to decide for each group whether to supply insurance, a decision that would be based on the premium rate, marginal costs, and so on, for that particular group.

Use of community rating by the insurer would create a different situation. Again, assume there would be two groups (high risk and low risk), each with its own marginal costs. But now there would be a single premium rate, which would fall somewhere between the costs associated with the high-risk group and the costs associated with the low-risk group. An investor-owned insurer would have an incentive to develop criteria to distinguish between high-risk and low-risk individuals and refuse to insure the former (i.e., it would engage in so-called preferred risk selection). In fact, community rating began and evolved as a method in the tax-exempt (not-for-profit) sector, wherein firms follow different objectives than profit maximization. A tax-exempt firm may have as an objective increasing the availability of insurance coverage for higher risk groups. If it did have such an objective, its behavior would differ from the behavior of an investor-owned firm with a profit-maximization objective.

Second, insurers can lower their costs (and increase their profits) in two ways: (1) by reducing the consumers' utilization of insured healthcare services and (2) by lowering the amounts paid to the providers of care. Indemnity insurers have developed a number of utilization-reducing instruments, including such things as preadmission review and rules requiring second opinions for surgery. Indeed, HMOs were developed as a means of controlling the intensity of medical care provided to patients. However, even indemnity insurers have become active in the managed care arena and have resorted to utilization-reducing mechanisms. This is especially true given the incentives offered by the federal government to lower costs and improve quality of care.

Third, whereas previously insurers had played a passive role in the setting of prices, insurers have become increasingly active in contracting with providers and pushing for favorable terms. To illustrate,

in a preferred provider arrangement, insurers have sought to negotiate specified prices and conditions of performance and participation from providers. These organizations have also provided incentives to enrollees, such as lower out-of-pocket costs if the consumers obtain services from the providers on the preferred list. Insurers have also sought to gain a market advantage over providers, so they can either pass the lower prices on to consumers or else can capture the gains as profits for their organization.

10.6 Adverse Selection in Health Insurance Markets

In Section 10.3, the concept of self-selection in insurance coverage was introduced. Insurance plans offering specific types of coverage will attract consumers who will benefit the most from the type of coverage offered. In the presence of information asymmetry, this can create a situation called *adverse selection*, which has the potential to damage an insurance market to such a degree that it ceases to exist. Whereas, in practice, economists have questioned whether this phenomenon is an empirically important one, it has drawn considerable attention in the literature (Buchmueller, 2009; Hirth, Baughman, Chernew, & Shelton, 2006; Jack, 2006; Marquis, Buntin, Escarce, & Kapur, 2007; Marquis & Phelps, 1987; Pauly, 1986).

Adverse selection is based on the ability of consumers to gauge their risk of needing healthcare services more accurately than the insurance company, and to act on the information asymmetry they possess. While insurance companies use general characteristics of the population, such as age, sex, education, and occupation, to calculate the expected healthcare costs of a population, individuals within the population of interest tend to have real information advantages regarding their current and future health status conditions, resulting in a positive risk-coverage correlation. Such adverse selection of insurance coverage can result in a death spiral in the market.

The following illustration can be used to explain this insurance market death spiral. Assume that a large employer offers a choice between two plans to its employees. One plan is a low-cost–low-benefit plan and the other is a high-cost–high-benefit plan. Assume that the employer, because of budget issues, decides to increase the premium of the high-cost–high-benefit plan. The decision of individuals to remain with or leave the plan following this increase in premiums is not random. The individuals that remain with the plan are more likely to be those that anticipate having greater health expenses in the coming enrollment period. The new, smaller high-cost–high-benefit plan now has less healthy and even more expensive enrollees on a per enrolled member. As a result, in the following insurance renewal period, another round of adverse selection would occur, making the plan even more expensive. The final result would be abandonment of the plan by the employer because it becomes too expensive since only the most costly individuals remain in the plan.

The following is an illustration of an adverse selection situation. In this illustration, assume that there are three separate groups of 100 individuals, each with the following demand conditions:

- In group 1, the healthiest group, each individual has a 10% probability of becoming ill and requiring medical care; in group 2, the intermediate group, the probability of becoming ill and requiring medical care is 40%; and in group 3, the least healthy group, the probability is 80%.
- The cost of medical treatment for an individual in any of the groups (i.e., the total amount of the individual's loss in the event of illness) is $1000.
- Individuals have the utility function presented in Table 10-1.

Based on these assumptions, the expected utility of being uninsured for any individual will be the weighted average of the utility of $10,000 (which has a value of 100.0, according to Table 10-1) if the individual stays healthy and the utility associated with $9000 (which has a value of 89.0) if he or she becomes ill and suffers a $1000 medical expense. For group 1 individuals, this is $(0.9 \times 100) + (0.1 \times 89.0)$, or 98.9. The expected utility for group 2 individuals is $(0.6 \times 100) + (0.4 \times 89.0)$ or 95.6, and for group 3 individuals it is $(0.2 \times 100) + (0.8 \times 89.0)$, or 91.2. Each member of group 1 would pay, at most, a premium of approximately $300 (resulting in a utility of 98.9) to be insured. For any premium above this amount, the members would accept the risk and not buy the insurance policy. For any premium lower, they would demand insurance coverage. The indifference premium is approximately $600 for group 2 and approximately $900 for group 3.

Now, turn to the supply side of the insurance market in this illustration. The relevant assumptions for the supplier are as follows:

- The insurance company's administrative costs are $20,000.
- Total insurance company expenses consist of the administrative costs, including a normal profit (loading fee), plus the amount the insurer reimburses for medical care (actuarial costs).

- The insurance company merely wants to break even, so revenues will just equal costs. As for the pricing policy of the insurance company, which is a critical element in the model, there are a number of alternatives available to the company.

One alternative would be to employ an experience-rating methodology, which involves dividing the total pool into subgroups and setting rates according to each subgroup's expected loss. In an experience-rating pricing scheme, groups 1, 2, and 3 in the above illustration would all pay different premiums because they have different levels of expected loss.

The second type of pricing policy is community rating. In a community-rating schema, all individuals pay the same premium. Community rating would probably be the method chosen if the insurer were not able to distinguish among individuals in the three groups. Without the ability to distinguish among the individuals, it would not then be able to charge a different premium based on expected loss.

Assume in this illustration that an information asymmetry does exist. That is, the consumers know which group they belong to, but the insurer does not have accurate health status information. Under this condition, a single community rate would be charged to all individuals in the plan. Now examine how the market might perform over time. Initially, the insurance company, wanting to break even, will charge a premium high enough to cover all the reimbursements for the three groups ($130,000) plus the administrative costs ($20,000). Over the 300 individuals, this rate amounts to $500 per individual. This rate exceeds group 1's indifference premium, and so members of group 1 will choose not to insure, resulting in a reduction of $5000 in premiums collected by the insurance company. Members of groups 2 and 3, on the other hand, will continue to purchase insurance.

With group 1 dropping out of the market, total expenses for groups 2 and 3 are $140,000. Again, the insurance company cannot distinguish between individuals in these two groups and so it must charge a single community premium. This time the premium would be $700 per individual. But this premium will be above the amount members of group 2 are willing to pay since it exceeds their expected utility, and individuals in group 2 will drop out of the market for health insurance, leaving only group 3. The premium will now be raised to $1000 ($80,000 payout plus $20,000 loading fee for the 100 individuals), but this premium now exceeds group 3's indifference premium. The members of group 3 will drop out of the market as well, causing the market to collapse.

This phenomenon is a joint result of adverse selection (those with the highest risks remain in the market) and community rating (chosen as a method because of the information asymmetry).

The popularity of this model might be attributable to its doom-and-gloom prediction of market disappearance, but there is some question as to how well it fits the present market for health insurance. There is some empirical evidence (Buchmueller, 1998; Cutler & Reber, 1998; Monheit, Cantor, Koller & Fox, 2004; Rice & Mays, 1985) to support its applicability, but it has certainly drawn attention to the phenomenon of community rating and its potential role in market failure. And, in fact, in the present model, the market would perform differently if experience rating was used.

To illustrate the application of experience rating, assume that for each group, a premium is set equal to its expected medical costs plus $6667 (which is one-third of the total administrative expenses of $20,000). Then each group would pay a premium that was less than what it would be willing to pay. For example, group 1 individuals would be charged $76.67 in premiums ($1000 + $6667 divided by 100 people). This is below what they would be willing to pay for insurance coverage, and so they would not withdraw from the insurance market. Thus, in this illustration it was the community rating pricing policy that caused the market to fail and disappear.

There have been questions raised as to whether community rating results from informational asymmetry or other factors. Insurance companies have, or can get, considerable amounts of information about potential consumers by looking at age, sex, education, occupation, and medical history and by conducting medical examinations of potential enrollees. In fact, insurance companies use experience rating for pricing policies that they sell to individuals in the market. This being the case, it may not be informational asymmetry that leads to community rating (Feldman, 1987) but other causes. For example, employers may want to be equitable to all employees and so offer a single (community) rate for all—the young, the old, the sick, and so on. Employees, including low-risk employees, may accept this, in part because they are happy with the idea that when they become unhealthy later in life their premiums will be community rated as well.

10.7 Violations of Insurance Conditions

As was discussed at the beginning of this chapter, certain conditions must occur for an insurance market to function effectively. Here, a brief assessment of those conditions in the health insurance market is presented. As discussed, one condition for assessing risk for insurance coverage is that the event being insured against is outside the control of the covered individual—it is a random event. In health care, however, while becoming ill may be considered a random event, outside the immediate control of the individual, how the individual reacts to its occurrence is not an independent factor. If the individual has health insurance, then that individual may be more likely to demand a service that is covered by the policy than a service that is not covered. As a consequence, the existence of insurance coverage may change not only the amount of care utilized but also the type of care used (prescription drugs vs. over-the-counter drugs, inpatient care vs. outpatient care).

A second condition is that the event must occur often enough to raise concern but not often enough to become routine—there needs to be an element of unpredictability to its occurrence. In health care, however, most policies now cover an annual prevention examination, which is routine and totally predictable—the probability of occurring is almost 100%, and so the insurance premium covers not only the medical expense but also a loading fee. This makes the cost of the coverage higher than if the individual had self-insured and saved the money necessary to pay for the known event.

A third condition is that the event being insured against must be identifiable and well defined to minimize transaction costs associated with determining the occurrence of the event. While it may be relatively easy to determine when a certain type of illness or injury occurs after the treatment has occurred, it is often not easy to establish its occurrence earlier. While an X-ray may determine whether or not a bone is broken and therefore establish the boundaries for treatment, such certainty is not known for many other illnesses, especially for early onset of the disease. As a result, establishing a definition of what is included in an episode of illness is difficult, especially for many chronic conditions. The ambiguity in health and health care makes defining a covered event very difficult.

Another condition inherent in the market for insurance is the ability to establish a value for the loss associated with the event being insured. In health care, there is wide variability in approaches to treating an illness or injury, in the prices charged, and in the providers involved in providing the care. Also, because individuals are not standardized, it is very difficult to establish a value for the loss associated with the event.

As this discussion indicates, health insurance is different from insurance purchased for most other events—home, automobile, life, and such. The deviations do not imply that a market for health insurance does not exist, only that the conditions that violate the insurance market requirements must be incorporated into an assessment of the efficiency of the health insurance market and how the violations impact decision making.

Exercises

1. Mrs. Smith's utility function is the same as that shown in Table 10-1. Her initial level of wealth is $10,000. Her annual medical expenses if she becomes ill would be $1200. Her probability of becoming ill (and thus incurring the $1200 medical expenses) is 20% or 0.2. The price of an insurance policy is $300.
   a. If Mrs. Smith were a utility maximizer, should she purchase insurance?
   b. Should she purchase insurance if the price were $600?
   c. Would Mrs. Smith purchase insurance at $600 if her medical expenses, in case she became ill, were $2000?
   d. Is Mrs. Smith risk-averse, risk-neutral, or a risk-taker?
2. Mrs. Rosen has a utility function like that in Table 10-1. There is a 50% probability that she will incur medical expenses of $2000. What is the most Mrs. Rosen would pay for insurance?
3. Health insurance premiums obtained through an employer are not included as taxable income. An individual health insurance policy costs $5000. The personal income tax rate is 30%. An employer provides premiums as a benefit. What is the price to the employee of the insurance?
4. An insurance company has a payout of health benefits of $100,000. Administrative expenses on top of that are $30,000 and profits are $10,000. What is the ratio of premiums to benefits? If there are 100 insureds, what is the premium rate each would pay?

5. Buffalo Systems has 1000 employees, all of whom are insured in the company plan. There are two groups of employees, healthy and unhealthy. Half of the employees are in each category. Persons in both groups have an equal probability of being sick of 20%, an initial wealth level of $10,000, and the utility function shown in Table 10-1. When a healthy person becomes ill, the cost of care is $1000. The cost of care for an unhealthy person is $2000.
   a. If the company plan is community rated, such that each person pays $300, would both groups choose to insure?
   b. Assume that the company introduces a low-cost plan. Those in the plan pay $200. The plan insures up to only $1000. Persons pay any excess out of pocket. Which group would purchase insurance? What would be the total expenditure of each group, including out-of-pocket expenses?
6. How will each of the following affect the supply for insurance:
   a. A larger pool of insured persons
   b. Lower administration costs for insurance companies
   c. Higher premiums (with no change in risk experience)
   d. A greater degree of risk aversion on the part of insurers
7. What is the effect of utilization management on insurance company expenses? Consider both administrative expense and claims expense.
8. What are community rating and experience rating?

Bibliography

Admon, A. J., Valley, T. S., Ayanian, J. Z., Iwashyna, T. J., Cooke, C. R., & Tipirneni, R. (2019). Trends in hospital utilization after Medicaid expansion. *Medical Care, 57*(4), 312–316.

Berki, S. E., & Ashcraft, M. (1980). HMO enrollment: Who joins what and why: A review of the literature. *Milbank Memorial Fund Quarterly, 58,* 588–632.

Blavin, F. (2019). *Impact of the Affordable Care Act's Medicaid expansion on Medicare enrollees access to physician services.* Washington, DC: Urban Institute.

Buchmueller, T. C. (1998). Does a fixed-dollar premium contribution lower spending? *Health Affairs, 17*(6), 228–235.

Buchmueller, T. C. (2009). Consumer-oriented health care reform strategies: A review of the evidence on managed competition and consumer-directed health insurance. *Milbank Quarterly, 87*(4), 820–841.

Cutler, D. M., & Reber, S. J. (1998). Paying for health insurance: The tradeoff between competition and adverse selection. *Quarterly Journal of Economics, 113*(2), 433–466.

Feldman, R. (1987). Health insurance in the United States: Is market failure avoidable? *Journal of Risk and Insurance, 54,* 298–313.

Feldstein, M., & Friedman, B. (1977). Tax subsidies, the rational demand for insurance and the health care crisis. *Journal of Public Economics, 7,* 155–178.

Friedman, B. (1974). Risk aversion and the consumer choice of health insurance option. *Review of Economics and Statistics, 56,* 209–214.

Gruber J., & Somers, B. D. (2019). *The Affordable Care Act's effects on patients, providers, and the economy: What we have learned so far* (NBER Working Paper 25932). Cambridge, MA: National Bureau of Economic Research.

Herring, B., & Adams, E. K. (2011). Using HMOs to serve the Medicaid population: What are the effects on utilization and does the type of HMO matter? *Health Economics, 20*(4), 446–460.

Hirth, R. A., Baughman, R. A., Chernew, M. E., & Shelton, E. C. (2006). Worker preferences, sorting and aggregate patterns of health insurance coverage. *International Journal of Health Care Finance & Economics, 6*(4), 259–277.

Institute of Medicine. (1993). *Employment and health benefits: A connection at risk.* Washington, DC: The National Academies Press.

Jack, W. (2006). Optimal risk adjustment with adverse selection and spatial competition. *Journal of Health Economics, 25*(5), 908–926.

Kelly, I. R., & Markowitz, S. (2009/2010). Incentives in obesity and health insurance. *Inquiry, 46*(4), 418–432.

Marquis, M. S., Buntin, M. B., Escarce, J. J., & Kapur, K. (2007). The role of product design in consumers' choices in the individual insurance market. *Health Services Research, 42*(6, Pt. 1), 2194–2223; discussion 2294–2323.

Marquis, M. S., & Phelps, C. E. (1987). Price elasticity and adverse selection in the demand for supplementary health insurance. *Economic Inquiry, 25,* 299–313.

Miller, R. H., & Luft, H. S. (1995). Estimating health expenditure growth under managed competition. *JAMA, 273,* 656–662.

Monheit, A. C., Cantor, J. C., Koller, M., & Fox, K. S. (2004). Community rating and sustainable individual markets in New Jersey. *Health Affairs, 23*(4), 167–175.

National Association of Insurance Commissioners. (2019, August 24). *Glossary of insurance terms.* Retrieved from https://www.naic.org/consumer_glossary.htm

Nyman, J. A. (1999a). The economics of moral hazard revisited. *Journal of Health Economics, 18*(6), 811–824.

Nyman, J. A. (1999b). The value of health insurance. *Journal of Health Economics, 18,* 141–152.

Nyman, J. A. (2004). Is "moral hazard" inefficient? The policy implications of a new theory. *Health Affairs, 23*(5), 194–199.

Oakes, A. H., Chang, H.-Y., & Segal, J. B. (2019). Systemic overuse of health care in the commercially insured U.S. population, 2010–2015. *BMC Health Services Research, 19,* 280.

Pauly, M. (1986). Taxation, health insurance, and market failure in the medical economy. *Journal of Economic Literature, 26,* 629–675.

Pauly, M. V., & Herring, B. J. (2000). An efficient employer strategy for dealing with adverse selection multiple-plan offerings: An MSA example. *Journal of Health Economics, 19,* 513–528.

Price, J., & Mays, J. (1985). Biased selection in the Federal Employees Health Benefit Program. *Inquiry, 22*(1), 67–77.

Pylypchuk, Y. (2010). Adverse selection and the effect of health insurance on utilization of prescribed medicine among patients with chronic conditions. *Advances in Health Economics & Health Services Research, 22,* 233–272.

Steinorth, P. (2011). Impact of health savings accounts on precautionary savings, demand for health insurance and prevention effort. *Journal of Health Economics, 30*(2), 458–465.

Taylor, A., & Wilensky, G. R. (1983). The effect of tax policies on expenditures for private health insurance. In J. A. Meyer (Ed.), *Market reforms in health care* (pp. 163–184). Washington, DC: American Enterprise Institute for Policy Research.

CHAPTER 11

The Labor Market

OBJECTIVES

1. Define the role of the market for labor and explain how this market is linked to health and health care.
2. Describe a model of the demand for and supply of labor.
3. Explain the factors that affect the determination of wages and total compensation including how health insurance benefits are related to the supply of labor.
4. Explain how a model of the labor market can be used to explain wage and employment figures for healthcare workers.
5. Describe how health status affects workers' compensation.
6. Explain how market power can affect labor market outcomes in the healthcare sector.
7. Introduce budgeting rationale and components.

11.1 Introduction

The market for the workforce in health care is important, especially since the healthcare industry is the largest employer in the United States. Contributing to the growth in employment in health care is the aging of the population—as people age they need more healthcare services, which means a need for increased individuals in health care to provide that care. This employment level in health care results in the healthcare industry accounting for over one-sixth of the Gross Domestic Product (GDP) in the United States.

The labor market is the institution by which workers and employers come together to engage in the production of output. As a result of the interactions of the workers and employers, the amount of labor that is employed and its compensation (wage rate and total income of workers and the expenses of employers) are determined. The number of workers in the healthcare industry and their level of employment depend upon a number of factors. First, they depend upon the number of individuals who choose to enter a health-related profession or career. Second

they depend upon the number of hours the healthcare worker is willing to work and in which geographic area the individual resides or wishes to work. Impacting these decisions are factors such as the wage rate offered, regulatory restrictions, educational opportunities and requirements, and the alternatives available to the individual.

There are a number of health-related issues related to this workforce market. Employers hire and pay workers according to their productivity and, in some instances, a healthy worker will be more productive than an unhealthy one.

Productivity is a key determinant in the employer's demand for labor. A second set of issues is related to labor supply: a worker's health status may influence his or her decision to seek full-time employment, part-time employment, or no employment at all. A third issue is related to total compensation rather than just wages. In the United States, workers receive part of their compensation in the form of fringe benefits, including health insurance that is a nontaxable income to the employee. The demand for health insurance is thus connected with the labor market.

To understand how policies that influence the purchase of health insurance work, it is necessary to understand how labor markets work.

Another set of issues related to the labor market deal with the determination of wages and employment for healthcare workers. Physicians, nurses, technicians, and other professionals and workers perform under the vagaries of the healthcare labor market. Numerous issues have arisen in this market, including shortages of nurses and other health professionals, and rising wages for healthcare workers.

11.2 Demand for Labor

11.2.1 Demand for Labor by the Individual Firm

In this section, an analysis of the demand for a specific resource by an individual provider is developed. The provider could be a healthcare-producing entity, such as a hospital, laboratory, or physician's office, or it could be a nonhealthcare producer. The focus will be on healthcare providers, but the analysis can be applied to any type of institution in which individuals are employed. The dependent variable of interest is the demand for labor input. The labor input can be expressed in time units, such as hours or days. The labor demand curve, or function, is defined as the quantity of labor units that a firm will demand at any given price or wage.

Since health cannot be purchased directly, it is produced using medical care created by health workers, technology, pharmaceuticals, other medical devices and individuals' time as inputs into the production process. In economic terms, this demand for health workers is a derived demand. That is, the firm does not demand labor, or any other input, for its direct value. Rather, any input in the production function is demanded because of the revenue or output it can generate for the firm. In short, the value of an input is derived from the usefulness of the input in achieving some objective of the firm that employs the worker or other input. In traditional economic analysis, this objective is maximizing profits. While healthcare firms may indeed have other objectives than maximizing profits, the profit maximization hypothesis is still a good objective with which to begin the analysis of the demand for labor and other inputs. Even tax-exempt firms must earn a profit (defined as an excess of revenues over expenses) if they are to remain in business over time.

To assist in the analysis of market interactions, an illustration of a commercial laboratory that provides blood tests will be used. The time frame for the initial analysis in this illustration will be a single day. The firm's product (or output) is defined as the number of blood tests produced per day. The firm has a number of inputs into the production process, including the fixed inputs of capital equipment, materials and supplies, and fixed management time, and the variable input of labor time. Indeed, labor units, in the form of lab technician time, are assumed to be the only variable input (although, in reality, reagents and other supplies will also vary with the number of blood tests performed).

11.2.2 Production Function

With inputs and outputs defined above for this illustration, the relationship between inputs and outputs (the production function) is hypothesized. In **Table 11-1**, a numerical example of the relationship for the range of variable inputs from one to seven lab technicians employed per day is presented. In this illustration, with one lab technician, the lab can produce 50 blood tests; with two lab technicians employed, it can produce 110 tests; and so on. As illustrated, this relationship at first exhibits increasing marginal productivity (the additional output produced with the addition of one more technician to the fixed factors of production adds an increasing amount to total output), followed by decreasing marginal productivity (the second technician produces 60 extra tests, but the third technician produces 50 extra tests, the fourth produces 40, and so on).

Marginal productivity is the additional output achieved with the employment of one additional unit of a variable input. Marginal productivity usually initially increases because of the ability to use the fixed resources more efficiently. As more inputs are used by the firm to produce output, marginal productivity will begin to fall as inefficiencies occur from employing less effective units and from difficulties that arise in coordinating activities among the larger workforce, especially in terms of the allocation of workers among the fixed resources (e.g., the capital equipment used to perform the tests).

11.2.3 Revenue Derived from Worker Production

The firm's valuation of technician time rests not on the number of lab tests per se but on the revenue derived from these lab tests. In this illustration, the assumption is that each lab test has a fixed price of $20. Therefore, for each extra lab test produced, the firm brings in $20 in extra revenue. The total revenue

Table 11-1 The Demand for Labor by a Commercial Laboratory

(1) Number of Laboratory Technicians	(2) Number of Laboratory Tests (Total Product)	(3) Additional Tests per Technician (Marginal Product)	(4) Total Revenue from All Units of Production (Price of Product × Number of Units) ($)	(5) Additional Revenue from Addition of One Laboratory Technician (Marginal Value Product) ($)	(6) Laboratory Technician Wage Rate ($)
1	50	50	1000	1000	240
2	110	60	2200	1200	240
3	160	50	3200	1000	240
4	200	40	4000	800	240
5	230	30	4600	600	240
6	250	20	5000	400	240
7	260	10	5200	200	240

© Jones & Bartlett Learning.

from all lab tests at each level of input is shown in the fourth column of Table 11-1 (one technician brings in $1000 in revenues, two bring in $2200, etc.). The fifth column shows the *marginal value product* (MVP) obtained when the firm adds successive technicians. The MVP is defined as the additional revenue obtained from hiring one more unit of input (in this illustration a lab technician). As with marginal productivity, this marginal value product variable at first increases but then decreases. (The first technician has an MVP of $1000, the second has an MVP of $1200, and the MVP of the third is down to $1000). The MVP curve is shown in **Figure 11-1**.

11.2.4 Labor Cost

In this illustration, assume that each lab technician earns $240 per day. As the number of lab technicians hired increases, total labor costs increase. However, because each lab technician is paid the same amount per day, the marginal cost of the input is $240 for each lab technician hired.

11.2.5 Firm's Objectives

The laboratory in this illustration is assumed to have a goal of profit maximization. Profits are defined as total revenue generated minus total costs incurred in the production of the output. The point at which maximum profits are attained occurs when the revenue gained from adding one additional worker is equal to the additional cost of hiring that additional worker.

11.2.6 Predictions of the Model

The predictions of the model in this illustration are as follows. On profitability grounds, the firm would hire the first worker, as the resulting marginal value product ($1000) exceeds the marginal cost ($240). Indeed, the firm would continue to hire workers as long as it was profitable to do so. In this illustration, the firm would hire up to six workers to maximize profits. The laboratory would reduce its profits by hiring the seventh worker. Given the assumptions in the model presented in this illustration, the firm's quantity of labor demanded equals six workers. To the firm the seventh worker would cost $240, but the marginal value product contributed by this seventh lab technician would only be $200.

A demand curve for labor is the graphical representation of the relationship between the quantity of labor inputs a firm wishes to purchase per period of time and the price of that labor, when other things are equal or held constant (ceteris paribus). If the price of a unit of labor input changes, so will the quantity demanded by the producer. In this illustration, a decrease in the wage rate paid to lab technicians by the firm from $240 to $200, will increase the quantity of labor demanded to seven units. On the other hand, an increase in the wage rate will reduce the quantity of labor demanded. The quantity demanded can be traced out by the MVP curve, as this curve shows the additional revenue generated by any given wage rate. Therefore, the MVP curve is the demand curve for the input in a market when the objective is profit maximization.

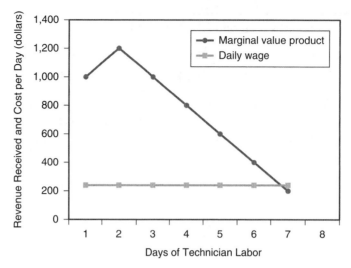

Figure 11-1 Demand curve for labor. The demand curve for labor is based on the additional revenue generated by each additional labor unit (days of technician labor), called the marginal value product (MVP). Firm profitability is determined by comparing the MVP with the marginal price paid for labor.

© Jones & Bartlett Learning.

The demand curve will shift downward and to the right if labor becomes more productive (yielding more output and revenue for the given quantities of labor) or the price per unit of output sold increases. Labor can become more productive if the firm increases its degree of mechanization in its capital equipment. In this illustration, assume the firm purchases more capital equipment, in which case each worker will be able to produce more, since bottlenecks previously experienced on the equipment are reduced. Also, if the price per lab test increases, then each worker will also yield more revenue (although not more output) at the higher price.

To extend the analysis, the effects of benefits as a form of compensation are introduced. Recall that benefits are not included as taxable income to the employee, so each dollar of benefits has more than a dollar of value to the worker. The amount of this added value depends upon the tax bracket in which the individual is located. **Figure 11-2** shows a firm's demand curve for labor at alternative daily wage rates. In this illustration, at a wage rate of $240, the firm will demand 6 labor days. The demand curve for this rate (curve D_n) is based on the assumption that wages are the only form of compensation; that is, the firm does not offer fringe benefits such as health insurance at this time.

Assume, however, the firm agrees to provide $40 worth of fringe benefits per day to its employees. This adds $40 to the total labor compensation for each worker hired by the firm, but it does not add anything to the value of the output (the marginal value product). Therefore, the firm will still be willing to

pay only $240 in total compensation for the 6 labor days—$200 in monetary wages and $40 in fringe benefits. Thus, under the new benefits agreement, the firm would be willing to hire six workers at a wage rate of $200 rather than $240 ($200 in wages plus $40 in benefits is equivalent to $240 in wages with no benefits), and there is a new demand curve for labor. This curve, D_b, is the curve D_n shifted downward to the left by exactly $40 at every quantity of labor. Any further increase in benefits would shift the demand curve further downward and to the left. Furthermore, D_b, like the original demand curve, will shift in response to changes in such factors as the price of output received by the firm and the productivity of labor.

Now, assume that taxes on corporate profits are introduced as a complicating factor into the illustration. Assume that the firm pays a 10% tax on his profits. If an extra worker brings in additional revenues of $400 and costs the firm $240, then the before-tax profits will be $160 for this worker and the after-tax profits will be $144 [$160 × (1 − 0.10)]. If both wages and fringe benefits (insurance premiums) were deductible expenses to the firm, then it would not matter to the firm whether it paid out its compensation to employees in the form of wages or fringe benefits. In this illustration, the imposition of a 10% tax on the firm simply decreases the profits of the firm at each level of output.

Under current tax law, insurance premiums in the fringe benefit package are not taxed as employee income. Thus, this form of compensation is preferred by the employee because insurance purchased with

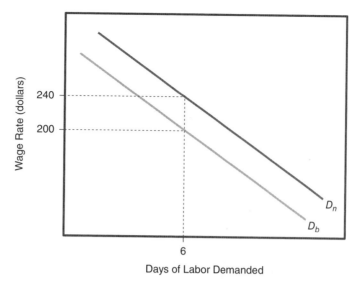

Figure 11-2 The effect of fringe benefits on demand for labor. Curve D_n shows the demand for labor when the firm does not pay fringe benefits. At a wage rate of $240 per day, the firm demands 6 labor days. In this case, the total wage ls the same as total compensation. If fringe benefits for $40 per day are instituted, the demand curve relating the wage rate to the quantity of labor will fall by $40 at every quantity, to D_b. This is because the firm, although still demanding 6 units at an average compensation cost of $240, is now providing each worker only $200 in wages as part of its $240 compensation package.

© Jones & Bartlett Learning.

pre-tax dollars "costs" the employee less than the same amount of insurance coverage purchased individually with after-tax income. Assuming an individual desires health insurance coverage and the individual is in a 20% tax bracket, then taking part of his or her wages in the form of health insurance instead of salary allows additional take-home pay equal to the tax rate of the individual times the value of the insurance premium. In this illustration, the individual would pay 20% of the $240 wage ($48), decreasing his or her take-home pay to $192. If the individual desired insurance, it would then need to be purchased out of the $192. So in this case, the individual would be willing to have wages of $192 and insurance premiums of $48 paid by the employer. This explains, in part, why benefits are so popular as a form of compensation by workers in the United States.

11.2.7 Market Demand for Labor

The market demand for labor or other inputs into the production process can be derived in the same way as other types of market demand. Assume the number of firms demanding labor in a certain market and the demand curve for each firm is known. The quantities demanded for labor at each wage rate can be summed across the individual firms to derive a market demand curve for labor. The assumption is retained that the price of the service or product sold in the market is fixed. The market demand for labor (or other inputs)

is thus a downward-sloping demand curve that shifts with changes in exogenous variables, such as the number of firms demanding labor and the productivity of each worker.

A change in price of labor (the endogenous variable) would simply result in a movement down the demand curve, and not a shift in the demand curve. To illustrate, assume the market demand was for 200 workers at $10 per hour. Then, the minimum wage rate was mandated to increase to $12 per hour. As a result, the workers with marginal value product less than $12 would no longer be demanded in the labor market.

11.3 Labor Supply

11.3.1 Individual Labor Supply

The analysis of the supply of labor focuses on the quantity of labor individuals are willing to supply in order to earn income. The general framework used in this analysis is the consumer demand model. One main assumption of this model is that each consumer has a demand for income (income is needed in order to obtain goods and services) and for leisure time. The individual labor supply model examines how individuals alter their willingness to work in response to changes in labor compensation, such as wages. The end result of the analysis is a supply-of-labor curve graphically relating the quantity of labor supplied to the wage rate.

The unit of observation in this model is the individual consumer (although some analysts have used the household or family as the observation unit because, in many cases, data are collected at the household rather than the individual level), and the dependent variable is the number of hours an individual is willing to work. The assumptions in the analysis are as follows.

Assume a utility-maximizing (satisfaction maximization) individual who has a utility function that encompasses two distinct goods: income (which can be used to purchase desired goods and services) and leisure time (which also provides utility/satisfaction to the consumer). As a greater quantity is obtained of each good, the individual moves to higher levels of utility. It is also assumed that more of either or both of the two goods income and leisure is preferred to less, and so a higher utility level is preferred to a lower level of utility.

In this illustration the quantities of the two goods that will yield the same level of utility (satisfaction) are shown in **Table 11-2**. Assume the individual has 60 hours of time available to allocate between leisure and work. If the individual is willing to spend 60 hours in leisure, then the individual will work zero hours and have no income. This combination of income and leisure will yield the same utility to the individual as 10 hours of work resulting in $400 in income per week and 50 hours of leisure, 18 hours of work at $720 and 42 hours of leisure, and so on. Note that, whereas income increases in equal increments of $40 per hour of work, leisure hours are reduced in successively smaller increments, e.g., 10, 8, 6, etc. This

indicates a diminishing relative valuation placed on income. The individual will give up 10 hours of leisure to get the first $400 in income, but only 8 additional hours of leisure to get the next $320 in income at $40 per hour.

In this illustration, the individual has a total of 60 available hours per week to allocate between work and leisure. If 50 hours are spent on leisure, then 10 hours are available to be spent working. Finally, the individual can work for a wage of $40 per hour for up to 60 hours. Total income earned by the individual equals the product of wages times the hours worked.

The conclusions of the model in this illustration are as follows. The individual will increase the number of work hours from zero as long as the value of lost leisure is less than the wage rate received by the individual. To illustrate, when the individual spends all available time in leisure and has no income, the individual is willing to give up 10 hours of leisure (and work 10 hours) for $400 in wages, a unit value of $40 per hour. However, once the individual has achieved this new allocation of time between work and leisure, then the individual will be willing to give up only an additional 8 hours of leisure for an extra $400 in income. This implies a marginal value of leisure of $50 per hour at the new point since the individual is satisfied with $320 of income instead of another $400. The individual places a lower value on the next $400 increase in income and would be willing to give up only 6 more hours of leisure, implying a marginal value of $67 per hour of leisure. Thus, the individual must be compensated at increasingly higher wage rates to induce him or her to give up more leisure (i.e., to work more).

Assume a wage rate of $60 an hour. The individual is faced with a choice of whether to work and how much to work. In the illustration provided in Table 11-2, the individual will work at least 10 hours because the marginal value of the first 10 hours of work is $40. The individual would also choose to work the next 8 hours because the value of leisure time ($50) is less than the wage rate of $60. Beyond that, the value of lost leisure is greater than the wage rate. Therefore, the individual will choose to work 18 hours. If the wage rate increases, say, to $80, then the individual would be willing to give up 6 more hours of leisure, and work for a total of 24 hours per week because the value of leisure is $67 at that point.

This work–leisure theory illustrates the possible trade-off between potential uses of an individual's time, in which each combination results in the same level of utility (satisfaction) to the individual.

Table 11-2 Income and Leisure Time Combinations at the Same Level of Utility

Hourly Wage Required to Trade Leisure for Work for Income of $400	Leisure Hours per Week (Out of a Total of 60 Available Hours)	Work Hours per Week (Out of a Total of 60 Available Hours)
$0	60	0
$40	50	10
$50	42	18
$67	36	24
$100	32	28
$133	30	30

The positive relationship between wages and work time measures what is called the *substitution effect of income for leisure*. The substitution effect of a wage increase is the increased incentive to work because work time now has a relatively higher reward than leisure time. **Figure 11-3** shows how the quantity of labor changes as the wage rate increases (supply curve S_1). At $8 per hour the individual will work 8 hours. But if the wage increases to $12 per hour the individual will increase work hours to 14 along S_1.

There is also an income effect, which may offset the substitution effect. The income effect of wages reflects the increase in purchasing power associated with more income, enabling the worker to not only purchase more goods and services but also to afford more leisure.

As the wage rate per hour increases, the total income that the individual can receive will increase, and the individual can purchase more goods and services with the increase in income. Therefore, the individual may want to spend more leisure time consuming other goods and services and hence will want to work less. It is possible that this income effect can be strong enough to more than offset the substitution effect, resulting in a backward-bending portion of the labor supply curve, especially at higher wage rates and income levels. However, statistical studies have shown that this is not a common event.

Supply curves for labor can have varying slopes, reflected as steepness. If an individual does not have as strong a willingness to work more as wages increase as the individual did with S_1, then the curve of the second individual will be more steeply sloped (supply curve S_2 in Figure 11-3). An individual more willing to work for small increases will have a curve like supply curve S_1. In Figure 11-3, an increase in wages from $8 to $12 will, depending on the labor supply curve, increase the labor supply to 12 hours (supply curve S_2) or 14 hours (supply curve S_1).

11.3.2 Health Insurance Benefits and Labor Supply

The most common way of financing private health insurance in the United States for individuals under 65 years of age is through the payment of health insurance premiums for individuals in the workplace. Health insurance coverage is a component of total worker compensation, which consists of wages or salaries plus fringe benefits. From the viewpoint of the individual worker, the amount of total compensation is what influences labor supply. However, economists have modeled labor supply decisions using wage rates as the base price rather than total compensation for simplicity. That tradition will be followed in the following illustration.

In **Figure 11-4**, there are two labor supply curves presented, one for the case in which fringe benefits exist and one for the case in which there are no fringe benefits provided. The first analysis is focused on the situation without fringe benefits. Supply curve S_1

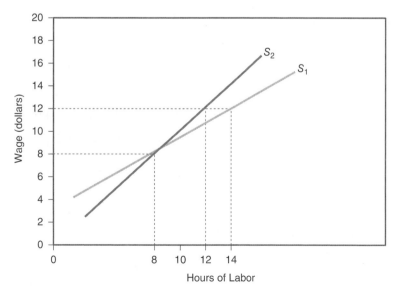

Figure 11-3 Alternative labor supply curves. Supply curve S_1 shows a positive relationship between the wage rate and labor hours. Supply curve S_2 is a curve with a similar direction, but a steeper slope, which means that an increase in the wage rate from $8 to $12 will induce a smaller increase in the number of hours supplied, 12 hours compared to 14 hours.

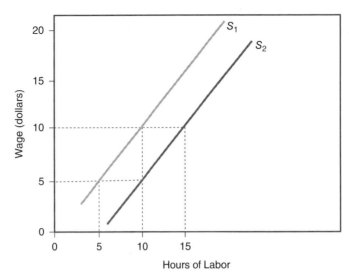

Figure 11-4 Labor supply curves with and without a benefits package. Supply curve S_1 shows the initial relationship between the wage rate and hours of labor supply when there are no fringe benefits. The assumption is made that workers place a $1 value on each $1 of benefits. A $5 benefits package is introduced bringing total compensation to $10. Supply curve of S_2 indicates the new quantity supplied at each wage rate. The reason the curve shifts is: the $5 wage rate now represents $10 in compensation and will induce the same amount of labor as will a $10 wage rate with no benefits. This is true for all wage rates. If, however, $1 in benefits is worth more to the workers than $1 in wages (e.g., benefits aren't taxed), the shift in the curve will be more.

© Jones & Bartlett Learning.

relates the quantity of labor supplied to money wages. At a wage of $5, individuals along supply curve S_1 will supply a total of 10 units of labor; at a wage of $10, the individuals will supply a total of 15 units of labor; and so on.

Now, assume that fringe benefits worth $5 are offered to the individual (an amount independent of hours worked). Assume each worker places a value of $5 on the $5 worth of fringe benefits offered. It is certainly possible of course for a worker to place a value lower than $5 on these benefits, and indeed fringe benefits may be worth very little to some workers who would prefer wages to benefit compensation. Under the current assumption, however, the value of the compensation to the worker is $10 when the wage is $5; when the wage is $10, it is $15; and so on. Put another way, the curve that relates the wage rate to the quantity of labor supplied will shift downward and to the right (supply curve S_2). At a wage of $5 (plus $5 worth of fringe benefits), the supply of labor will be the same as it would be at a wage of $10 without fringe benefits. An additional $5 increase in benefits, wages held constant, will further shift the supply curve downward and to the right. (Of course, if the workers place a lower value on these benefits than their face value, the shift will be less than discussed.)

11.3.3 Market Supply of Labor

The market labor supply is composed of the sum of labor supply curves of all the individuals in the market. As with the demand curve, the labor supply curve of the market comprises the summed quantity for each individual at each wage rate. An increase in the number of individuals in the market will cause the market supply curve to shift downward and to the right. On the other hand, a decrease in the number of individuals in the labor market will cause the market supply curve to shift upward and to the left.

11.4 The Competitive Labor Market

11.4.1 Assumptions

This illustration of labor market analysis will continue to focus on the market for lab technicians. To develop a competitive labor market model, some basic assumptions must be made about market supply and demand factors, and how they interact. The basic demand model is shown graphically in **Figure 11-5**.

The original market demand curve is shown as curve D_1. At a market wage of $20 per day, the firms in

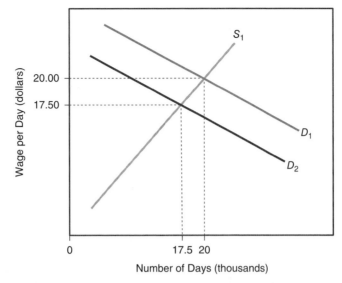

Figure 11-5 Labor market demand and supply. The original demand for labor is shown as curve D_1, and the original supply curve is shown as S_1. The original equilibrium occurs at a wage rate of $20 per day and a quantity of 20,000 labor days. If fringe benefits of $5 a day are introduced, the demand curve shifts down uniformly by $5 (to D_2). The new equilibrium will be at a quantity of 17,500 days and a wage rate of $17.50.

© Jones & Bartlett Learning.

the market demand 20,000 days of lab technician services. At lower wages, the quantity of days demanded from the technicians increases.

The market supply curve is upward sloping, as hypothesized; this curve is shown as S_1 in Figure 11-5. At a market wage of $17.50, a total of 17,500 days of lab technician labor will be supplied in the market. If the wage increases to $20, then 20,000 days will be supplied.

In the competitive model, an equilibrium condition is assumed where quantity supplied and quantity demanded are equal; that is, the quantity supplied is equal to the quantity demanded. As shown in Figure 11-5, the original market equilibrium occurs at 20,000 days demanded and supplied for $20 per day. When wages decreased to $17.50 per day, the new equilibrium quantity is 17,500 days, reflecting the shift in demand when the input costs of labor change.

11.4.2 Predictions
11.4.2.1 Supply, Demand, and Wage Rate

The first prediction of the model in the previous illustration of initial demand and supply conditions (D_1 and S_1) is that there will be a single equilibrium wage set at $20. Bargaining among demanders for and suppliers of labor will result in this single equilibrium price at the equilibrium quantity of 20,000 labor days.

Additionally, the equilibrium quantity and price will change with any changes in the related causal factors.

With regard to shifts in demand, increases in the price of the output produced or the number of firms in the market will result in increased wage rates and increased labor days. Increases in the supply of labor will result in lower wages and higher quantities of labor. This model can assist in analyzing the effect of using health insurance benefits as a form of compensation in the labor market. Assume that the labs pay a $5 health insurance premium per day for each worker. The effect of this is to shift the demand curve uniformly down by $5, to curve D_2 in Figure 11-5. Assume that there is no effect on supply of individuals in the market. The prediction, in this case, is that the wage rate will fall to $17.50 and the quantity of labor employed will be reduced to 17,500 days. In this case, the method of financing total compensation does reduce the quantity of employment.

11.4.2.2 Health and Labor Market Outcomes

Economists have recognized the role of health in labor market outcomes. The topic that has received the most attention has been the impact of health on the supply of labor in the market. The possession of good health by individuals will increase the likelihood that a worker will be employed and that a worker who is employed will work longer hours (e.g., will accept full-time rather than part-time employment) and be more productive when working. In terms of the competitive labor market model, poor health will shift the labor supply curve upward and to the left. At any given wage rate, the quantity of labor supplied will be reduced when health status is decreased. Looking at the workings of the entire market, a reduction (upward and leftward shift) in the supply of labor will reduce the overall amount of employment and result in an increase in the wage rate of the individuals who continue to participate in the labor market. With fewer workers available, firms will compete with each other for the limited number of workers by increasing the wages offered in the market

Much of the evidence of the effect of health status on earnings has come from developing countries (Duraisamy & Sathiyavan, 1998; Jack, 1999). A number of such studies have shown that improved health status, or factors that are associated with health status, such as nutrition and the body mass index, have a positive effect on wages. This finding is as expected, because, in many developing countries, there is a very low general level of health, so improved health status increases the number of workers and their productivity.

However, the same trends have been noted in developed countries as well (Grossmeier, Mangen, Terry, & Haglund-Howieson, 2015; Koopman et al., 2002; van den Berg, Schuring, Avendano, Mackenbach, & Burdorf, 2010). Using a national sample survey of residents in the United States, Kahn (1998) studied the comparative impact of labor market performance of persons with and without diabetes. He found that 64% of males who had diabetes and were between the ages of 50 and 60 were employed; the comparative figure for males without diabetes was 82%. The corresponding statistics for women were 40% and 60%, respectively. Thus, persons with diabetes are 10–20 percentage points less likely to be employed than persons without diabetes. Kahn's statistics indicate that there is a considerable effect of diabetes on labor market behavior, especially with regard to whether persons are employed.

Beck et al. (2011) investigated the relationship between the severity of the symptoms of depression and productivity. They found for every one point increase on the Patient Health Questionnaire 9-item screen (PHQ-9), there was a corresponding 1.65% additional average loss in productivity. In addition, these authors found that a loss in productivity from individuals with symptoms of depression occurred in both full-time and part-time employment, and with self-reported poor or excellent health. This loss in productivity decreases the marginal value of the worker, possibly indicating it would be beneficial for employers to invest in treatment for these individuals.

Alker, Wang, Pbert, Thorsen, and Lemon (2015) found in the study of secondary school staff that three common health conditions (obesity, depressive symptoms, and smoking) were significantly associated with decreased productivity. This decrease in productivity included days of work lost because of health concerns (absenteeism) and decreases in on-the-job productivity because of health concerns (presenteeism).

11.4.2.3 Occupational Risk and Labor Market Outcomes

Injury and mortality rates vary considerably among occupations and industries. In 2010, there were 4547 work-related fatalities in the United States, a rate of 3.5 per 100,000 full-time equivalent (FTE) workers. In 2017, the number of work-related deaths had increased to 5417; the rate was still 3.5 per 100,000 FTE workers. In 2017, the transportation and material-moving group and the construction and extraction occupational group accounted for 47% of worker deaths. On the basis of relative risk, fishers and related fishing workers (99.8 per 100,000 FTE) and logging workers (84.3 per 100,000 FTE) had the highest rates of fatal injuries in 2017. By comparison, workers in education had a fatality rate of 1.0 per 100,000, and workers in healthcare and social assistance had 0.8 per 100,000 FTE workers (U.S. Bureau of Labor Statistics, 2010a, 2018b).

In 2010, the incidence rate of nonfatal occupational injuries and illnesses was 3.5 per 100 full-time workers and by 2017 that had declined to 2.8 per 100 full-time workers. The incidence rate and numbers of nonfatal injuries and illnesses varied by occupation. In 2017, agricultural, forestry, fishing, and hunting had the highest rate at 5.0 per 100 full-time workers, followed by transportation and warehousing at 4.6 per 100 full-time workers, arts, entertainment, and recreation at 4.2 per 100 full-time workers, and health care and social assistance at 4.1 per 100 full-time workers. The two lowest occupations were professional and technical services at 0.8 per 100 full-time workers and finance and insurance at 0.5 per 100 full-time workers. Health care and social assistance had the highest number of workers suffering from an occupational injury and illness at 582,800, but because of the number of workers in that occupation they did not have the highest rate (U.S. Bureau of Labor Statistics, 2010b, 2018a).

If workers correctly perceive differences among risks in different occupations, then according to utility-maximizing principles, individuals will prefer low-risk to high-risk occupations (all other factors held constant). Indeed, starting with a very low-risk occupation (e.g., education with 1.0 deaths per 100,000 FTE workers and health services and social assistance, in which there are 0.8 deaths per 100,000 FTE workers), workers will demand risk premiums in order to induce them to accept occupations with higher risks, such as logging at 84.3 deaths per 100,000 FTE workers (Viscusi, 1978a, b, 1993).

There are widespread differences in wages among occupations. The factors that influence these differences include both demand variables (worker productivity, occupational characteristics, price of the final product) and supply variables (worker age, education, and skill level). The on-the-job risk of mortality is one of many factors that influences the wage rate for any occupation. If adjustments could be made for all factors affecting supply and demand *other than risk*, then the inter-occupational differences in wages would just compensate for differences in risk.

Once measures of that component of inter-occupational wage differentials that reflects differences in occupational risks of mortality have been developed, these measures can be extrapolated to obtain an estimate of the value of a statistical life. To illustrate, assume that there are two occupations with varying risks, but that all other factors are the same. Assume that a 50-year-old male has a life expectancy of 65 years in the absence of a fatal work-related injury. The individual has a choice of two occupations: fishing or healthcare and social assistance. Fishing workers experience 99.8 deaths per 100,000 FTE workers, whereas healthcare and social assistance experience only 0.8 deaths per 100,000 FTE workers. The difference is 99 deaths per 100,000 workers at a rate of 0.00099 per individual. Assume the adjusted wage differential (net of other factors) is $400 annually. A projection can be made of the monetary value for the remainder of the person's lifetime.

Ignoring the discounting factor (i.e., assume the discount rate is 0%), then the wage difference between the two occupations is $6000 (15 years at $400 per year). The value of a statistical life can then be calculated as $6.061 million ($6000 ÷ 0.00099). If more precision is desired, this estimate should be qualified so it can be made more realistic: future years' wages would be discounted, and many characteristics that are difficult to measure would have to be accounted for, such as the pleasantness of the work environment. Having made these adjustments, the estimate would be a better approximation of the valuation of risk that workers actually accept in the marketplace.

Indeed, a considerable number of studies have been conducted to measure the value of life using labor market differentials (Hirth, Chernew, Miller, Fendrick, & Weissert, 2000). These results show a very wide variation in the value of life. For a 40-year-old male, estimates ranged from $923,000 to over $19 million. Such differences are hard to reconcile, and they have created confusion on the part of policy makers. Nevertheless, the importance of the topic for policy-making purposes, including in the healthcare area, ensures that a great deal of additional work needs to be done in this area.

11.5 Market Power in Labor Markets

11.5.1 Buyer's Market Power

In the past, there have been periods of time when widespread nursing shortages were reported by hospitals. A shortage is a situation in which, at the given wage rate offered in the market, the quantity of labor demanded exceeds the quantity supplied. Economists have tried to explain shortages by means of economic models. The model of a hospital's buying power in the market for nurses can be used for this purpose. Assume that there is a single buyer of nursing services, a hospital in a small city. For this single buyer, an economic model is presented to illustrate the prediction of pricing and output decisions.

11.5.1.1 Supplier Costs

With respect to the supply side of the market, assume in this illustration there are a number of nurses available to be hired by the hospital (their supply curve is presented in **Figure 11-6** as supply of nurses). At a wage of $1500 weekly, two nurses will supply their services; if the wage is increased to $2000, three nurses will supply their services; and so on. With respect to the demand side of the market, the successive marginal costs that the single hospital is required to pay additional nurses is also shown in Figure 11-6. The marginal cost reflects the fact that the hospital has to pay all nurses the higher rate, not just the last nurse hired.

11.5.1.2 Revenues

First, assume that hiring additional nurses allows the hospital to treat more patients, but the marginal productivity of these extra nurses declines; and second,

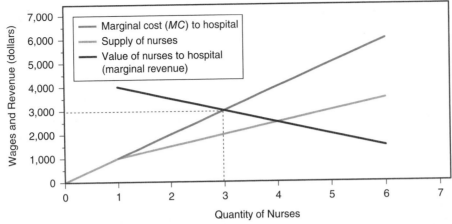

Figure 11-6 Equilibrium wage and number of nurses hired in a monopsony market. The monopsony (single buyer) firm's marginal cost (*MC*) for hiring additional nurses is derived from the schedule of nurses in the market. The value of an additional nurse is based on the amount of output that the hospital can produce with nurses (productivity) and the price of the output (the amount of revenue brought in by hiring an additional nurse). The profit-maximizing hospital will continue to hire nurses up to the point where the marginal cost equals the additional revenue from hiring another nurse.

assume that the price received for each extra patient by the hospital is constant. The hospital's value curve has been derived from the estimated additional revenue that the hospital expects the additional nurses will generate. The marginal revenue (equal to the price of output times the marginal output yielded by an extra nursing unit) is $4000 for the first nurse, $3500 for the second, $3000 for the third, and so on. Note that the total value to the hospital of three nurses is $10,500 ($4000 + $3500 + $3000).

11.5.1.3 Behavioral Assumption

Finally, assume that the hospital wishes to maximize profits. Remember that profit maximization requires production at the point where marginal cost is equal to or less than marginal revenue.

11.5.1.4 Implications of the Model

The implications of this model are that the profit-maximizing hospital will hire additional nurses as long as the marginal cost of doing so is less than or equal to the additional revenue generated by the nurses. But the marginal cost (*MC*) of nurses to the hospital is not the nurses' supply curve. Because the supply of nurses curve is sloped up, each successive nurse wants an additional amount of pay. Assuming that the hospital must pay all nurses the same wage, by hiring the second nurse, it must pay a higher wage to the first nurse as well. As a result, the *MC* curve is more steeply sloped than the supply curve (see Figure 11-6).

To illustrate, the *marginal cost* of the second nurse is $2000, but that of the third nurse is $3000 (the

difference between the total cost of three nurses at $6000 and the total cost of two nurses at $3000). The profit-maximizing hospital will hire three nurses (in Figure 11-6), for then the hospital's added revenue will equal its *marginal cost* for hiring nurses. At such a level of hiring, it will pay a wage of $2000 because that is the wage at which three nurses will supply their services.

In a monopsonistic (single-buyer) market, fewer nurses would be hired than in a competitive market. In a competitive market, competitive forces would drive the wage up to the level at which supply equals demand; more nurses would be hired, and wages would be higher. However, a monopsonistic buyer can prevent more nurses from being hired, thus maintaining its profits. At the same time as it depresses wages, it creates a restriction in supply.

11.5.2 Unions as Monopoly Sellers of Labor

Feldman and Scheffler (1982) stated that in the early 1980s, unions increased nurses' wages by about 8%. A more recent study (Hirsch & Schumacher, 1995) questioned this finding. In 1999, nurses earned $20.86 per hour, compared to $21.53 for librarians and $27.86 for high school teachers (U.S. Bureau of Labor Statistics, 1999), despite the fact that there was a considerable degree of unionism among nurses. In this section, the theoretical argument that unions increase wages is presented.

A union is an organized group of workers that allows individual workers to act as a cohesive unit when bargaining with employers, instead of each individual worker negotiating their own wage rate. In terms of economic analysis, unions allow sellers of labor (in this illustration nurses) to wield monopoly power, raising their wages relative to those of non-union workers. The monopoly model applied to the labor market is used to predict the impact of a union on wage levels.

In **Figure 11-7**, a model of the labor market for nurses is presented, with hospitals as the buyers of nursing labor. Assume that there are several hospitals in the market but only one union supplying nursing labor to the hospitals. The price (wage) is measured along the vertical axis, and the quantity of nurses who are hired monthly by all hospitals in the area is shown along the horizontal axis. The monthly demand for nurses is presented as curve D_L.

The marginal cost curve for nurses is shown as curve *MCL*. As the quantity of nursing time provided increases, the wage that nurses are willing to accept increases as well. Assume that the union's objective is to maximize its "surplus," defined as the total compensation received by the nurse workers. Profits are defined in terms of the entire group of labor suppliers, who are behaving in unison as a labor union.

The union will bargain for a wage at that quantity of labor at which the members' wage income is maximized. The profit-maximizing position is where the demand for nurses equals marginal cost; that is, at the intersection of demand and marginal cost of labor (*MCL*). In Figure 11-7, the profit-maximizing wage is $9000 a month. The union would bargain for that wage and supply 600 nurses to the hospitals. In contrast, the wage in a competitive market would be

$7000 a month, and 800 nurses would be supplied to the hospitals at that price. The prediction of the model then is that unions increase wages for those individuals employed but restricts the number employed.

As stated previously, the question as to whether the union has raised nursing wages is an open one. Other models have been developed that incorporate both hospital and union market power. Under such conditions, the wage would be determined by the relative degree of market power of both bargaining entities, and the same conclusions would not necessarily hold.

11.6 Budgeting

> A budget is a mathematical confirmation of your suspicions.
> ... A. A. Latimer, 1949

11.6.1 Why Budget

A budget is simply a financial plan for a given period of time. A budget is a method of answering the question: "What do I think it will cost me to do what I want to do?" It is used by organizations to define strategic plans of activities to be undertaken in order to achieve an outcome. The budget expresses activities or events in measurable monetary terms.

There are a number of reasons for developing a budget. A budget can outline the process for achieving the goals of the organization by *controlling* activities. The budget is used to set the measures and indicators of performance. These indicators of performance can

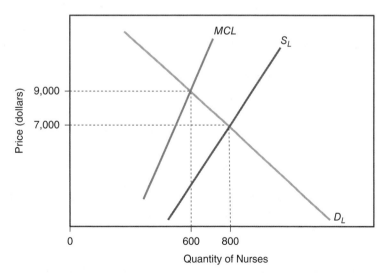

Figure 11-7 Monopoly seller of labor. The marginal labor cost curve (*MCL*) is derived from the seller's supply of labor (S_L). In this illustration, the seller will select the profit maximizing position at 600 nurses at a wage of $9,000, above the market clearing price of $7,000 and 800 nurses.

be used to ensure that the actions being taken are in compliance with the budget that was established; that is, it can be used to determine if the proposed purchase of an item or hiring of additional personnel is an allowable item in the budget. If it is not in the budget, then expenditures on the item can be controlled by denying permission to make the expenditure.

The budget can also be used to *coordinate* activities. This coordination is especially important during the planning phase of the budget. As department heads and managers meet to outline their goals and activities for the coming budget period, attention can be given to how proposed activities overlap across units or are in conflict among departments or units. By identifying potential conflicts or overlap of activities, collaboration to achieve common goals can be undertaken.

Upper levels of management can use the budget to *communicate* important objectives of the organization. In addition, managers can use the budget to communicate important objectives to the staff that will have the day-to-day responsibilities of achieving the objectives. Communicating the objectives and emphasizing the role everyone has in achieving the objectives can help ensure that the goals of the organization are achieved.

Budgets can play an important role in *motivating* personnel in the organization. During the planning stage of budgeting, it is important to solicit input from the individuals that will be critical in and responsible for its implementation. If personnel take ownership of the budget, they will be much more likely to be motivated to ensure the activities needed to meet the budget are performed effectively and efficiently.

Finally, budgets provide a method for *measuring* results. Once the components of the budget are established, it is possible to measure whether or not they are being achieved. Over time, it is possible to use the quantifiable objectives established to measure the progress toward achieving the goals of the organization. In terms of meeting the objectives of the budget, it is possible to use fear as the motivating factor, e.g., your job depends on coming in on or under budget, although most individuals perform better with incentives and support to achieve the goals of the organization. The budget can provide a method for assisting the organization become more efficient and effective by inspiring the staff to focus on outcomes to be achieved.

11.6.2 Key Prerequisites of Budgeting

To be most effective, the budgeting process should focus on outputs to be achieved, not on the inputs to be consumed. The initial step is to decide what the *desired outcome* is that is to be achieved. For example, how many clients can be served in the upcoming budget period? Once the desired outcome has been identified, and quantified, then strategies for achieving the desired outcome can be put in place. These implementation strategies need to be measurable so that it is possible to track progress toward accomplishing the strategies.

11.6.3 Sound Organizational Structure

Within the organization, a *sound structure* is essential. This means that the authority and lines of responsibility need to be clearly defined. Everyone in the organization needs to know who has the responsibility for ensuring that the objectives of the budget are achieved, and that the individual or individuals with the responsibility also has the authority to undertake the activities. Employees of the organization also need to know what their responsibilities are and to whom they report. In turn, the employees need to be granted sufficient authority to perform the tasks they are assigned.

It is important that managers know the scope of the responsibilities and what their authority is within the overall framework of the organization. To be successful, it is essential that the budget is developed in a way that conforms with the existing patterns of authority and responsibility. Assigning responsibility for the achievement of items in the budget without giving authority to implement is a design for disaster.

A second prerequisite is that an appropriate *chart of accounts* exists that conforms to the goals and objectives of the organization. The chart of accounts needs to be designed to accumulate the revenues and expenses according to the unit that has the responsibility for producing the revenue and incurring the expenses. In addition, the revenues of each unit of the organization need to be subclassified by activity source and the expenses of each unit need to be subclassified by the objectives of the expenditure. It is important that historical and budget data conform to the same chart of accounts and that the chart of accounts conforms to the plan of the organization. The chart of accounts is used by accounting to keep track of what the organization has and what it is doing with what it has.

Third, the availability of reliable, nonmonetary *statistical data* is a critical component. These data relate to earlier (historical) volume and scope of service provided by the organization. These previous statistical data on such things as number of clients, number and type of providers, number and type of employees, type and age of equipment, etc., form the basis for establishing future levels of activity in the organization. The statistics compiled about the functioning of the organization need to be accurate and complete, and compiled and classified in a way that is consistent with the chart of accounts.

For the budgeting process to be successful, it is essential to have the support of management. If upper-level management only provides token support, then it will not be possible to obtain the necessary cooperation and interest for successful implementation that is required in lower levels. It is also important to have the support of lower levels of management. To gain acceptance and support, all department managers and supervisors should actively participate in the formulation of the budget, since their future performance, and the future performance of their unit, will be evaluated in terms of compliance with the achievement of the budget.

11.6.4 Effective Performance Measurement

During the budget period, effective *performance measurement* is required on an ongoing periodic basis. As indicated in the previous section, a responsible accounting system is a fundamental component of the process. To be effective, performance standards must be established that provide clear guidance regarding how well the individuals, units, departments, and the organization are doing in meeting the conditions and expectations established in the budget.

In assessing the performance, the ability to do *variance analysis* is vital. Variance analysis is the ability to determine how much difference has occurred between what has actually happened (either over or below budget) compared to the budget established. Not only is it important to know what variance has happened, but also to understand why the difference occurred. Did some unforeseen event happen beyond the control of the responsible unit to cause the variance (e.g., a flood or fire, etc.)? Or was there an inaccuracy in the historical data that caused the budget projections to be inadequate? Or did the unit make expenditures that were outside those contained in the budget?

Developing the budget requires *costs of operations* to be identified and measured: what is the amount and type of resources required in the operation of the organization? In health care, a major resource is *personnel* involved in producing the services of the organization. These personnel are not just the direct patient care individuals, but also those in

maintenance, housekeeping, information technology, public relations, and administration. Data on the salaries and fringe benefits of all personnel are required for the budgeting process.

Data are also needed on the amount and types of *supplies* that are used in the production of services in the organization. As the budget is developed, decisions on the amount of inventory to keep on hand must also be made. In hospitals, it is important to have input from the physicians or medical staff and the nursing staff regarding the types of supplies they prefer in the provision of the services and how individual preferences can be accommodated without too adverse an impact on the efficiency of supply inventory.

Another cost category in the budget process involves the *equipment* and other capital assets needed to provide services. Some of the equipment and capital assets will be specific to the service provided; other equipment and capital assets will be more generic to the physical plant, such as heating and cooling, information technology, backup generators, and dining, laundry, etc. Included in the equipment category are data on depreciation, salvage value, and life expectancy of the equipment. Depreciation is the reduction in the economic value of the equipment and other capital assets of the organization over time. Salvage value is the estimated amount that the equipment and other capital assets of the organization can be sold for at the end of its useful life. Life expectancy is the duration that equipment and other capital assets of the organization is expected to be used.

The expenses (costs) of the *utilities* required to operate the organization must also be included in the budget. The utilities include such items as electricity, water, gas, etc. Total cost data on these items are necessary, as well as an understanding of the method used to allocate these expenses to the various direct cost units. Is the allocation to be done on the amount of square footage the unit occupies, the percentage of the total costs incurred by the unit, or some other method? Whichever method is used, the units impacted need to understand the allocation mechanism in order to develop strategies and monitoring activities that can be used to effect the results.

Finally, *overhead costs* need to be identified and measured. These overhead costs involve activities associated with the administration of the organization. Once the administrative costs have been identified, the costs must be allocated across the revenue-producing units (or else revenue must be allocated to the administrative units). Again, there are a number of methods available for allocating overhead. The important thing is that the units understand the allocative process and have the necessary data provided to them that enable the unit or department managers to understand how the overhead costs will impact the performance of their unit or department. The ability to incorporate the overhead costs is critical to the ability to measure their performance against the budget established.

In addition to the total cost of the various categories of resources, managers need to know the *per unit cost* of each resource. Knowledge about the unit costs of the various resources will enable the decision makers to understand how the use of the resources impacts the budget. If only aggregate cost information is provided, the decision makers have incomplete information for understanding how the costs of their unit or department can be impacted with appropriate substitution among the various resources.

In understanding the budget and the performance of the organization, it is important to know which costs are fixed and which costs are variable. *Fixed costs* are related to those items that do not vary directly with the volume of activity provided by the organization in the short run. These are such items as size of plant capacity, long-term contracts with suppliers, etc. and these items can only be changed by upper management decisions over a longer period of time than is usually included in the budget cycle.

Variable costs are those that, as the name implies, vary directly with the volume of activity performed by the organization. These costs reflect the resources that are directly consumed if, and only if, at least one unit of activity is produced. To illustrate, if the healthcare organization does not provide any services, then there would not need to be any direct healthcare personnel employed. However, as soon as the healthcare organization provides services to the first client, then direct care personnel will need to be employed. And, as the volume of services provided increases, the number of personnel employed would also need to be increased at some point.

Costs can also be classified as either direct costs or indirect costs. *Direct costs* are those that can be traced to a specific service, organizational unit, or individual provider/manager. Direct costs will typically include such items as the supplies directly used in the provision of the service, the labor that directly provides the service, and the portion of the utilities that can be directly measured in the process of providing care. Direct costs are the expenses that can be specifically attributed to a unit or department in the provision of services (the production of output).

Indirect costs are all other costs incurred by the organization that cannot be directly attributed to a specific unit, department, or manager and, therefore, must be allocated to units, departments, or managers by some allocative method. Indirect costs may be either fixed or variable. These indirect costs typically reflect resources that are used by multiple activities and so cannot be directly assigned to a specific activity or objective. Examples of indirect costs include such things as administrative costs, utilities, rent, accounting and legal expenses, overhead, etc. These indirect costs are necessary to operate the business of the organization, but are not necessarily tied to the direct provision of services.

Revenue streams are the sources of income an organization receives from the production and sale of its goods or services. In health care, an organization's revenue can be classified as operating revenue and nonoperating revenue. *Operating revenue* results from the earnings generated by the provision of its core business operations—healthcare services. Operating revenue could be the earnings generated by the provision of healthcare services to the organization's clients or patients. In health care, the revenue can be obtained directly from the individual receiving the service or through an insurance provider on behalf of the patient or client. Operating revenue typically varies with the amount of services produced. Operating revenue can be received from transactions performed, such as a patient visit or a hospital admission. Operating revenue can also be generated by a service performed on a time basis, such as an amount of time a client spends with a mental health professional.

Nonoperating revenue is monies earned from the side activities of the business. Examples of nonoperating revenue may include such items as interest revenue, rent received, dividend revenue, sales in a gift shop, cafeteria sales, etc.

For budgeting purposes, it is important to classify the source of revenue as close as possible to the unit generating the revenue. Since not all units of the organization generate revenue, either these indirect costs must be allocated to revenue-generating units or a mechanism needs to be established that allocates revenue to them. Either way, it is important that detailed data be available on the per-unit revenue generated, since variance from projected revenue needs to be analyzed and reasons identified for the variance.

In the budget process, it is important to keep in mind that balancing the budget is like playing pool. You are behind the eight ball and all you see are empty pockets.

Exercises

1. The Midwest Clinic is a profit-maximizing organization. It has the capacity to hire up to five nurses. Midwest charges a fee of $25 for each clinic visit. It pays nurses $200 a day. The production function for the clinic, in terms of clinic visits, is shown in the accompanying table. What is the quantity of labor demanded by Midwest? What will be the profit-maximizing quantity of labor demanded if the company adds $15 to the wage of each worker to pay for health insurance premiums?

Number of Nursing Hours	Number of Clinic Visits
1	12
2	22
3	30
4	36
5	40

2. What happens to the market supply function of public health nursing labor if
   a. Wages increase in hospitals.
   b. Licensing requirements are made stricter for public health nurses.
   c. Nursing schools close down.
   d. There is a minimum wage imposed on nurses.
   e. The public image of public health nursing is improved.

3. What happens to the demand curve for labor of a clinic if each of the following occurs:
   a. The wage falls.
   b. The clinic purchases equipment that increases worker productivity.
   c. The price of clinic visits increases.
   d. The clinic hires more workers.
   e. The clinic hires better-trained workers who are more productive.
   f. The clinic nurses provide care that is of a higher quality but takes more nursing time.

4. Explain the relationship between the wage rate and the quantity of labor supplied.

5. How does the introduction of health insurance as a benefit influence the supply curve for labor?

6. Assume a competitive model of the market for laboratory technicians in an environment of profit-maximizing laboratories. How will each of the following affect the wage rate for laboratory technicians:
   a. New equipment that increases the productivity of technicians is introduced.
   b. The local university increases the size of the graduating class of technicians.
   c. Technicians take more time in conducting tests in order to be more thorough.
   d. The government issues a generous retirement scheme for technicians over 60.
   e. The government licenses laboratories, restricting their numbers.
   f. Workers bargain for an increase in health insurance benefits; the laboratories provide insurance instead of wages.

7. Using the competitive labor market model, derive a prediction of the impact of poor health on employee wages.

8. The following table provides data on hourly wage rate, quantity of nursing hired, and number of clinic visits produced. Nurses are used by the clinic to provide the clinic visits. Each visit brings in $40 in revenue for the clinic. The provider is assumed to maximize profits. Determine the provider's equilibrium wage and how many nursing hours it will employ. The provider is a monopsonist, which means it is the sole purchaser of labor in the market.

Wage per Hour	Number of Nurses	Number of Clinic Visits
40	1	5
60	2	9
80	3	12
100	4	14
120	5	15
140	6	14

9. What is the purpose of budgeting in an organization?

10. What are the prerequisites for an effective budget?

Bibliography

Alker, H. J., Wang, M. L., Pbert, L., Thorsen, N., & Lemon, S. C. (2015). Impact of school staff health on work productivity in secondary schools in Massachusetts. *Journal of School Health, 85*(6), 398–404.

Beck, A., Crain, A. L., Solberg, L. I., Unutzer, J., Glasgow, R. E., Maciosek, M. V., & Whitebird, R. (2011). Severity of depression and magnitude of productivity loss. *Annals of Family Medicine, 9*(4), 305–311.

Duraisamy, P., & Sathiyavan, D. (1998). Impact of health status on wages and labour supply of men and women. *Indian Journal of Labour Economics, 41*, 67–84.

Feldman, R., & Scheffler, R. (1982). The union impact of hospital wages and fringe benefits. *Industrial and Labor Relations Review, 35*, 196–206.

Grossmeier, J., Mangen, D. J., Terry, P. E., & Haglund-Howieson, L. (2015). Health risk change as a predictor of productivity change. *Journal of Occupational and Environmental Medicine, 57*(4), 347–354.

Hirsch, B. T., & Schumacher, E. J. (1995). Monopsony power and relative wages in the labor market for nurses. *Journal of Health Economics, 14*, 443–476.

Hirth, R. A., Chernew, M. E., Miller, E., Fendrick, A. M., & Weissert, W. G. (2000). Willingness to pay for a quality-adjusted life year. *Medical Decision Making, 20*, 332–342.

Jack, W. (1999). Principles of health economics for developing countries. Washington, DC: World Bank.

Kahn, M. E. (1998). Health and labor market performance: The case of diabetes. *Journal of Labor Economics, 16*, 878–899.

Koopman, C., Pelletier, K. R., Murray, J. F., Sharda, C. E., Berger, M. L., Turpen, R. S., … Bendel, T. (2002). Stanford presenteeism scale: Health status and employee productivity. *Journal of Occupational & Environmental Medicine, 44*(1), 14–20.

U.S. Bureau of Labor Statistics. (1999). *Workplace injuries and illnesses in 1998.* Washington, DC: Bureau of Labor Statistics. Retrieved from https://www.bls.gov/news.release/history/osh_12161999.txt

U.S. Bureau of Labor Statistics. (2010a). Census of fatal occupational injuries (CFOI)—Current and revised data. Retrieved from http://www.bls.gov/iif/oshcfoi1.htm

U.S. Bureau of Labor Statistics. (2010b). Occupational injuries and illnesses by selected characteristics. Retrieved from http://www.bls.gov/news.release/osh2.toc.htm

U.S. Bureau of Labor Statistics. (2018a). *2017 survey of occupational injuries and illnesses chart package.* Washington, DC: U.S. Department of Labor.

U.S. Bureau of Labor Statistics (2018b). National census of fatal occupational injuries in 2017. Retrieved from www.bls.gov

van den Berg, T., Schuring, M., Avendano, M., Mackenbach, J., & Burdorf, A. (2018). The impact of ill health on exit from paid employment in Europe among older workers. *Journal of Occupational and Environmental Medicine, 57*(4), 347–354.

Viscusi, W. K. (1978a). Wealth effects and earnings premiums for job hazards. *Review of Economics and Statistics, 60*, 408–416.

Viscusi, W. K. (1978b). Labor market valuations of life and limb. *Public Policy, 26*, 360–386.

Viscusi, W. K. (1993). The value of risks to life and health. *Journal of Economic Literature, 31*, 1912–1946.

Evaluative Economics

Economic Evaluation of Health Services

OBJECTIVES

1. Identify the main research questions and types of analyses that can be used to address the research question in an economic evaluation.
2. Identify the major types of health outcomes that can be used in economic evaluation analysis.
3. Explain how an economic evaluation analysis can be conducted and provide illustrations using basic information.
4. Explain how to interpret cost-effectiveness ratios and the conclusions that can be drawn from them.
5. Examine how a willingness-to-pay measure can be derived and interpreted.

12.1 Introduction

The practice of assessing changes in outcomes due to an intervention and the resources used to achieve the results is called economic evaluation. Economic evaluation involves the quantification of changes in health resource use and the outcomes achieved due to the use of new or different interventions. The interventions can be a new technology, a different treatment, or a new pharmaceutical product, for example. Policy makers and other decision makers are increasingly turning to these analyses in order to acquire information for making decisions about alternatives in health care. Managers of drug formularies, especially publicly funded ones, resort to economic evaluations in order to determine which drugs to pay for under the insurance plan. Government policy makers use health technology assessments, which are based largely on economic evaluations, to shed light on the economic implications of new interventions.

Economic evaluations are used to inform decisions when there is a concern that a market is not yielding the most efficient or effective allocation of resources. The studies attempt to replace inadequate information or provide missing information on outcomes and their valuations, and on the resources (costs) required for implementation of the interventions. The direct measure of these two factors can provide important insights as to how resources should be allocated among alternatives. Economic evaluations would not be necessary if resources were unlimited and all the interventions could be implemented. However, since resources are limited (scarce), decisions must be made on which alternative use of resources provides the greatest benefits.

In this chapter, the methods that are used in economic evaluation studies are introduced. First, an overview of the subject, indicating the questions that are posed and the tools that have been developed to answer them, is presented. Following this, the guidelines for a sound economic evaluation and the key components of five major types of economic evaluation studies—cost-consequence, cost-minimization, cost-effectiveness (including incremental cost-effectiveness ratios), cost-utility, and cost-benefit studies—are presented.

12.2 The Purposes of Economic Evaluation

There are several distinct reasons to perform economic evaluation studies. *First*, alternative courses of action that are substitute solutions for the same conditions can be compared. For example, two pharmaceutical products available for the treatment of migraine headaches might be compared to determine which product provided the greatest result to determine their relative effectiveness. Or, the use of a pharmaceutical product versus surgery for treating blocked arteries might be compared. Studies have shown that the complications of diabetes can be treated effectively with intensive glucose control, which includes frequent monitoring of glucose levels and frequent clinic visits. The alternative intervention is the more conventional treatment, which includes careful diet and exercise, but less careful monitoring and less frequent insulin doses (Diabetes Complications and Control Group, 1995, 1996). An economic evaluation study would allow a comparison of the benefits of the two treatments.

Second, the question of whether a treatment is worthwhile can be investigated. For example, the question might be asked regarding whether diabetes should be treated at all can be examined. Note that there is an important difference between this second purpose and the first purpose discussed above. In a study of alternatives in the first case, the changes in health that occur as a result of the use of alternative resources would be examined, but the costs associated with the outcomes are not considered. In the second type of study, the question that is asked involves determining the costs of each alternative treatment and the benefits achieved with the costs of each alternative; the goal is to examine which alternative is most cost-effective.

12.3 Steps in Economic Analysis

Regardless of which economic analysis method is employed (cost consequences, cost minimization, cost effectiveness, cost utility, or cost benefit), the same basic steps are employed. The major differences in the five methods are in the magnitude and complexity of the events being evaluated. The *first step* in any analysis is to define the problem to be analyzed clearly and explicitly. The way the problem is defined establishes the boundaries of the viable alternatives—the more broadly the problem is defined, the more alternatives are available for solving the problem. For example, if the problem is defined as alcohol abuse, then the alternatives to address the problem may involve the legal system, the penal system, the educational system, the healthcare system, the mental health system, or the public health system. However, if the problem is defined as the best way to treat the alcohol abuser, then the alternatives are much more limited and involve alternative interventions for rehabilitation.

The *second step* is to explicitly state the degree to which the objectives are to be met. These objectives are quantifiable outcomes associated with the problem being addressed. To illustrate, if the problem identified is the rate of recidivism among alcohol abusers, then the objective of the interventions may be to reduce the recidivism rate from 40% to 20%. The objective in this case is quantifiable and measurable.

The *third step* in any economic analysis is to identify alternatives or options available for achieving the objective or addressing the problem identified. In identifying the alternatives, it is often useful to graph the chronological ordering of the possible sequence of events. The graphing assists in formulating the mathematical model and in identifying the probabilities associated with each decision or outcome in the analysis. In graphing the alternatives, a decision tree can be used in addressing linear-style problems (see **Figure 12-1**), while Markov models are more applicable if the events being analyzed occur repeatedly or over a long period of time (see **Figure 12-2**).

Step four involves identifying the benefits or outcomes to be achieved with the interventions. These benefits can be either direct or indirect. Regardless of the type of benefit, the benefits need to be able to be quantified and measured. To compare benefits across alternatives, the benefits need to be measured in comparable units. While the comparable unit is often monetary, that is not required for any of the approaches; the only thing that is required is that the benefits can be measured and compared with common units (e.g., lives saved, dollars, diseases prevented).

Step five involves identifying and quantifying all expected resources to be expended or consumed. These costs can also be direct and indirect and need to be measured and valued in common units; in other words, don't try to compare apples and oranges. The requirement for common units of measurement enables various alternatives to be compared for decision making.

Step six involves the identification of the perspective from which the analysis is being viewed; the question identified to be answered should determine the perspective to be taken because the benefits and costs

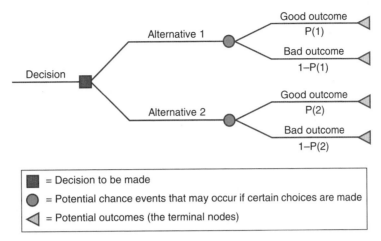

Figure 12-1 Illustration of a decision tree. The decision tree provides a graphical illustration of the decisions that need to be made to achieve the outcome, the alternatives available, and the probabilities associated with each of the outcomes. The sum of the probabilities of the alternatives will equal 1.

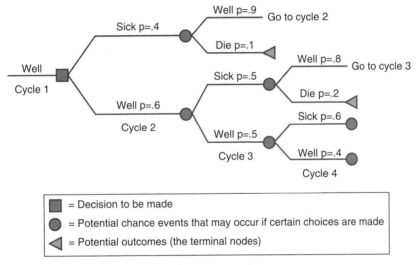

Figure 12-2 Illustration of a Markov model. If events occur repeatedly or over long periods, then a state-transition model, such as a Markov model, may be less cumbersome to use than decision trees.

may be different for each type of entity. Identifying the perspective enables decisions to be made with the best information possible. The perspectives selected could be society, individuals, providers, a payer, any level of government, etc.

In addition to the perspective, it is important to identify the time frame during which the alternatives are being assessed. Unless all costs and benefits occur in the same period of time, then it becomes necessary to perform discounting—*step seven*. Because the value of money or other resources is greater in the present than it is in the future, the preference is to receive the resources (money) as soon as possible, requiring future benefits and costs to be discounted back to the current value. While there is little disagreement regarding the need for discounting, the discount rate to be applied is much more controversial. There is not

a single discount rate appropriate for all situations. In general, the discount rate applied should reflect the best estimate of the risk involved in the situations. If the risks are small, then a low discount rate is appropriate. However, if the risks are great, then a high discount rate should be used.

The *eighth step* involves analyzing the uncertainties associated with the events; this involves performing sensitivity analysis on the key variables to determine the importance of the variables to the results of the analysis. A range of values should be applied to each variable employing the "what if . . ." scenario. If the variation in the value of the key variable is substantial, then the variable will need close scrutiny in the decision-making process, especially closely monitored over time to be sure the decision originally made is still appropriate.

Step nine involves comparing the benefits and costs of the alternatives. The results of this comparison can provide important information regarding the relative impact of the alternatives. This does not imply that the results of the comparison should be the only input into the decision-making process, but rather the analysis can be an important input into the decision-making process. Once the comparative results have been derived, it becomes important to discuss the results with others to check the validity of the assumptions made and to consider the ethical issues surrounding the decision.

The final step, *step nine*, involves monitoring and reevaluating conditions after the decision has been made. This reassessment of the assumptions made and the data used in the original analysis can be used to assist in making any necessary decisions to modify the size or focus of the program implemented, depending on changes that have occurred in the environment or the acquisition of improved data.

An economic evaluation does not provide all the answers, but it does provide explicit consideration of the goals and objectives to be achieved, the perspective taken, the alternatives considered, and the values assigned to costs, benefits, and risks. This explicit consideration should improve the decision-making process.

12.4 Selecting the Right Type of Analysis

Once the purpose of the evaluation to be conducted is clear, the appropriate type of study can be selected. According to Drummond, O'Brien, Stoddart, and Torrance (1997), there are five types of comparative studies in economic evaluation: cost-consequences analysis, cost-minimization analysis, cost-effectiveness analysis, cost-utility analysis, and cost-benefit analysis. A definition of each of these is presented in order to assist in selecting the most appropriate method to achieve the desired purpose.

Cost-consequence analysis (CCA) compares the costs of the program or intervention with its consequences. Unlike the other four types of economic evaluation, CCA does not summarize outcomes into a single result or financial determination. Instead CCA presents outcomes in their natural units and it is up to the decision maker to determine whether the intervention is worth implementing. In CCA, there is a list of the monetary, quantitative, and descriptive consequences presented in which the consequences are not combined with the costs. As a result, CCA does not result in a definite cost-outcome ratio. With this method, the decision maker has to form an opinion concerning the relative importance of costs and outcomes (Bakker, Hidding, van der Linden, & van Doorslaer, 1994).

Cost-minimization analysis (CMA) is used when the alternative interventions have equal effects or outcomes. Cost minimization, therefore, is used to determine the least costly alternative when it has been determined that the results (or outcomes) of either of the alternatives will be the same. To illustrate, if it has been determined that a new pharmaceutical product, A, has the same success in relieving pain and is no more detrimental because of side effects than the traditional pharmaceutical, B, then the goal is to determine the least costly pharmaceutical product.

Cost minimization can also be used when determining if the results of a new medical treatment are worth the cost incurred in its production when treatment for the disease did not previously exist. While the analysis does not provide an absolute answer, it does provide valuable information for decision making. A shortcoming of this method, however, is that there is no consensus as to what the threshold point is when the new treatment is not considered to be worth the additional cost of its production. Historically, medical interventions have been evaluated in terms of improving health or extending life, with very little attention given to costs. What is the maximum cost per additional year of life saved that should be viewed favorably—$50,000? $75,000? Establishing the maximum cost is not designed to place an absolute value on human life. Rather, setting a maximum simply recognizes that resources are limited and that the limited resources have alternative uses that might provide greater value.

Cost-effectiveness analysis (CEA) is used when it is anticipated that the outcomes of the interventions may vary, but that the outcomes of the alternatives can be expressed in some common unit. To illustrate, assume that there are two interventions for controlling hypertension. The two interventions vary in terms of their side effects and other features, but they can be measured in terms of the reduction in diastolic blood pressure achieved. The differences in cost and the differences in outcomes are compared using a ratio of costs to benefits. This cost-effectiveness ratio (CER) is written as:

$$\frac{(c_2 - c_1)}{(b_2 - b_1)}$$

where 1 and 2 refer to the alternative interventions, c is the cost of the interventions, and b is the benefits or outcomes of the interventions. CEA is very useful in assisting in the decision-making process when there are different treatments for a single disease or problem. It is limited in its ability to assist in making choices between interventions for different diseases or problems, since the outcomes may vary and not be conducive to converting the benefits to a common unit. With CEA, for example, it is difficult to compare cases of diabetes and cases of hypertension, especially when there are both morbidity and mortality involved with the two diseases.

Another type or subset of CEA is the incremental cost-effectiveness ratio (ICER). This method of evaluation assesses the difference between cost and effectiveness of two different events or interventions for the same condition. ICER is typically used to compare a new approach to an old approach of treating a disease or problem. As a result, the more general CEA formula is rewritten as:

$$\text{ICER} = \frac{\left(\text{Cost}_{new} - \text{Cost}_{old}\right)}{\left(\text{Effect}_{new} - \text{Effect}_{old}\right)}$$

The ICER ratio is still the difference in cost compared to the difference in outcomes. In health care, this method is useful when a new medical treatment is being considered to replace an existing treatment. In making the comparisons, a number of outcomes are possible.

To illustrate, the new treatment may be less expensive than the old treatment, and it may also be more effective. In this case then, the new treatment is considered to dominate the old treatment and it should be adopted, replacing the old treatment. In another instance, the new treatment may cost less than the old treatment, but it may also be less effective. In this case, neither treatment is dominant, so the decision involves determining if the decrease in health outcomes is worth the savings in cost. In another instance, the new treatment costs more than the old treatment, but it is also more effective. Again, in this case, neither treatment is dominant; the question to be answered is whether the gain in health outcome is worth the increase in costs. In the final instance, the new treatment may be more costly and less effective than the old treatment. In this case, the old treatment is dominant and should not be replaced with the new treatment.

In recent years, efforts have focused on developing a measure of the "utility" of the outcomes achieved in health care. Utility, as discussed earlier in the text, is a measure of the subjective satisfaction that individuals derived from a good or service. Cost-utility analysis (CUA) is a specific type of CEA. In the case of CUA, it refers to the subjective level of well-being expressed by individuals in different states of health. To measure that utility, a number of different scales have been developed, including quality-adjusted life years (QALYs). QALYs combine a subjective measure of quality-of-life with the quantitative measure of years of life to obtain a single universal unit measure of lifetime utility. The focus is on measuring the costs of various interventions in terms of the number of QALYs gained. Another measure that has been developed is the number of disability-adjusted life years (DALYs), which focuses on the number of years of disability avoided in the measure.

In cost-benefit analysis (CBA), the evaluation typically is used to place a monetary value on the benefits of the outcomes. In the analysis, both the resources used and the benefits gained are expressed in monetary terms, since monetary values are a common measure across multiple types of projects. The evaluation in CBA follows the same standard formula as the other types of economic analysis, in that it is comparing costs and benefits ($c_2 - c_1/b_2 - b_1$). Since the results of a CBA are usually stated in monetary terms (although the only requirement is that they be stated in comparable units), then instead of using the ratio of costs to benefits, net benefits may be used.

The net benefit approach compares projects on the basis of the excess of benefits to costs. In this approach, net benefits of each intervention are calculated by subtracting total costs from total benefits and the net benefits are then compared to determine the greatest value of net benefit. In this approach, the project with the greatest net benefit is selected. While the results provide information on the absolute value of net benefits, they ignore the relative magnitude of the projects. To illustrate, a net benefit of $1000 could reflect the difference in total costs of $100 and total benefits of $1100, or it could reflect total costs of $100,000 and total benefits of $101,000.

The cost-benefit ratio approach, on the other hand, compares projects on the basis of the average benefit per unit cost; in this approach, the project with the greatest ratio of benefits to costs is selected. The results of this approach can be impacted by the classification of an event as a cost or a benefit. To illustrate, if a project reduces hospitalization utilization, the reduction in utilization can be viewed as an increase in benefits, thereby increasing the numerator, or as a decrease in costs, thereby decreasing the denominator. Where it is classified will impact the value of the ratio. To illustrate, if the original project had costs of $5000 and benefits of $10,000, then the ratio is 2:1 ($10,000/$5000). Now, assume hospitalization is reduced, decreasing expenditures by $1000. If the reduction is viewed as an increase in benefits, the ratio is now 2.2:1 ($11,000/$5000). However, if the reduction is viewed as a decrease in costs, then the ratio is now 2.5:1 ($10,000/$4000). It is very important, therefore, to state explicitly the assumptions made in the analysis because it will impact the outcomes.

There is an appropriate type of analysis for each study objective. If analysts wish to simply summarize outcomes in their natural units, then a CCA is appropriate. If the goal is to determine which intervention to pursue when the outcomes are the same, the CMA is an appropriate method. If both the costs and benefits can vary but the benefits can be expressed in the same common unit, then cost-effectiveness is the method to be used. If the intervention is a new treatment for an existing problem, then a variation of CEA, then ICER should be used. CUA is used for the comparison when different states of health are the focus and so the comparison is the costs associated with different QALYs. CBA is typically used when it is possible to assign monetary values across multiple types of projects.

12.5 Guidelines for Conducting Economic Evaluations

In the past several years, a number of publications have appeared that provide guidance on what steps to take in conducting an economic evaluation analysis in the healthcare field (Canadian Coordinating Office for Health Technology Assessment, 1997; Cookson, Drummond, & Weatherly, 2009; Drummond et al., 1997; Gold, McCoy, & Siegel, 1996; Higgins & Harris, 2012; Menon, Schubert, & Torrance, 1996; Nixon et al., 2000; Sorenson, Tarricone, Siebert, & Drummond, 2011; Yang et al., 2018; Zhuo et al., 2014). In this section, an outline of the elements of cost-effectiveness and cost-utility analyses in the light of these guideline recommendations is presented. The explanation will be conducted using an illustration of comparing an intensive treatment of diabetes and the conventional treatment for diabetes. First, an example is briefly presented, then the

use of the guidelines to conduct economic evaluation analyses is presented.

The illustration is based on several pivotal clinical trials for diabetes control (Diabetes Complications and Control Trial Research Group, 1995, 1996) in which newly diagnosed diabetes patients were randomized to one of two interventions. In the first intervention, called conventional care, the individual tests his or her glucose level daily, takes one or two insulin injections daily, and visits a clinic every 3 months. In the second intervention, intensive or tight control, the individual tests his or her glucose four times daily, visits a health team often, follows a special diet, exercises regularly, and takes insulin at least four times daily.

Information on deaths and alternative outcomes for the patients in each group are shown in **Table 12-1**. Alternative outcomes are presented in terms of quality of life, willingness to pay, and quality-adjusted life years (QALYs). The annual cost per person is $10,000 for individuals with tight (intensive) glucose control and $3000 for individuals with conventional control.

The details of costs are shown in **Table 12-2**. These include physician visits, inpatient hospitalization, self-care (including the cost of insulin), and adverse events not treated on an inpatient basis. Most of the difference in cost between the two interventions is due to the self-care category. Using this illustration, the various economic evaluation studies that could be conducted are outlined. While the data provided in this illustration are dated, the relative costs and outcomes are still useful for illustrating the application of economic evaluations. A study by Yang et al. (2018) estimated that the total cost of diagnosed diabetes was $327 billion in 2017, including $237 billion in direct costs and $90 billion in reduced productivity. The updated material does not provide data on alternative treatments so the data in the illustration could not be updated; however the illustration is designed to provide an overview of the application of the method, and not to provide information on a current event.

12.5.1 Perspective

Perspective means the viewpoint taken by the investigator. Broadly, there are two types of perspective, private and societal. The private viewpoint is that of any single or group of providers, patients, or payers. If the individuals of interest are patients, the intent is to understand how the intervention impacts these people. If the payer's viewpoint is taken, the concern is with how much of the payer's own resources are used. The societal perspective is the perspective of all

Table 12-1 Outcome Measures for Alternative Interventions in Diabetes Control

	Year 1	Year 2	Year 3
Conventional Care			
Survivors	995	990	984
Deaths	5	5	6
Life years	997.5	992.5	987.0
Quality of life per person	0.8	0.8	0.7
Quality-adjusted life years	798.0	794.0	690.9
Willingness to pay for an additional QALY	$80,000	$80,000	$80,000
Annual cost per person	$3,000	$3,000	$3,000
Annual cost for 1,000 persons	$3,000,000	$3,000,000	$3,000,000
Tight Insulin Control			
Survivors	997	994	990
Deaths	3	3	4
Life years	998.5	995.5	992.0
Quality of life per person	0.9	0.9	0.9
Quality-adjusted life years	898.65	895.50	892.80
Willingness to pay for an additional QALY	$80,000	$80,000	$80,000
Annual cost per person	$10,000	$10,000	$10,000
Annual cost for 1,000 persons	$10,000,000	$10,000,000	$10,000,000

© Jones & Bartlett Learning.

Table 12-2 Annual Cost per Person of Alternative Interventions for Diabetes Control

Category	Calculation Details	Cost per Person ($)
Conventional Care		
Inpatient hospital care	0.10 probability of hospitalization × $5,000 per hospitalization that occurs	500
Outpatient visits	1 annual examination × $500 plus 3 visits × $100 each	800
Self-care expenses	Monitoring supplies, insulin, and supplies for administering insulin per year	1,400
Cost of adverse effects	1 visit to an emergency room per year × $300	300
Total costs		3,000
Intensive Tight Insulin Control		
Inpatient hospital care	0.02 probability of hospitalization × $5,000 per hospitalization that occurs	100
Outpatient visits	1 annual examination × $500 plus 11 visits × $100 each	1,600
Self-care expenses	Monitoring supplies, insulin, and supplies for administering insulin per year	8,270
Cost of adverse effects	0.1 probability of having 1 visit to an emergency room per year × $300 per visit that occurs	30
Total costs		10,000

© Jones & Bartlett Learning.

persons in the population. The societal perspective is an "all resources" perspective, in that it focuses on all resources used by all persons who are involved in the care—providers, patients, and caregivers. In our diabetes illustration, the assumption is an "all health-care resources" perspective, except that it excludes the nonhealthcare indirect resource losses (e.g., lost work time, which in 2017 was estimated to be $90 billion for individuals with diabetes) incurred by unpaid caregivers and patients. Most guidelines recommend taking the broadest societal perspective possible; however, the choice of perspective is a value judgment, and there are uses for studies that take either the private or societal perspective.

12.5.2 Time Horizons

The time horizon is the period over which costs and outcomes are measured. Most guidelines recommend that the analyses incorporate a long enough timeline to take into account all resources and outcome effects, including downstream events. Sometimes, downstream events are hard to identify. To illustrate, if an infant is treated in a neonatal intensive care unit because of prematurity, the individual might experience adverse effects years after the treatment. These events are rarely captured in a study's database, and so the investigators must develop a hypothetical model to estimate the implications of such events. In this illustration, a time horizon of 3 years is assumed.

12.5.3 Outcomes

Outcome measures in this illustration as well as other economic evaluations in healthcare fall into two major categories, as shown in **Table 12-3**. These will be termed *clinical* and *holistic*. Clinical outcome measures are usually used in clinical trials because they provide objective evidence of the illness being evaluated.

Clinical outcome measures do not provide information on patients' perceptions of their own medical conditions. For example, a medical condition may have very little objective medical evidence, such as dyspepsia, but may still be of major importance to the individual because the condition produces discomfort.

As patient and consumer empowerment has increased, there has been a growing interest in developing outcome measures that reflect patients' perceptions of their medical conditions. These measures are termed *holistic measures*, in large part because the concept of a holistic measure is broad, as is the set of the phenomena the concept is designed to characterize and measure. As seen in Table 12-3, measures

Table 12-3 Measures Used in Economic Studies
Clinical Measures (Examples)
Hypertension: Blood pressure measurement
Diabetes: Hemoglobin A1c control
Diabetes: Low-density lipoprotein (LDL) management and control
Diabetes: Diabetic retinopathy examination
Tobacco use assessment
Adult weight screening and follow-up
Influenza immunization for patients 50 years old or older
Childhood immunization status
Holistic Measures
Measures based on mortality
Survival time
Time of survival (life years)
Health-related quality of life measures
Disease-specific indicators
General health indicators
Preference-based measures

© Jones & Bartlett Learning.

based on mortality are included in the holistic category. In fact, they would fit into either category, clinical or holistic. In any case, mortality-related measures are very commonly used because the data are easy to obtain and because mortality is of such importance. Mortality measures include the occurrence of death, as well as the survival time (called *life years*) of the individual.

The indicator of time until death (survival time or life years) illustrates the role that the time dimension plays in outcome analysis. Individuals experience different health states through time, and so the benefits and hardships experienced as a result of these health states should include a time dimension. The time-inclusive counterpart of mortality is the number of years of survival. In this illustration, out of 1000 persons with diabetes who undertook the tight insulin control intensive intervention, there were 997 survivors (three deaths) at the end of the first year, 994 (another three deaths) at the end of the second, and 990 (another four deaths) at the end of the third year (see Table 12-1).

One key outcome to consider would be total deaths within 3 years, which is 10 for the tight insulin control intensive intervention and 16 over the 3-year period for the conventional care intervention population. If the time dimension is added and the number of life years is used as the outcome measure, then, in the first year, there are 998.5 life years in the tight insulin control arm (since specific data are not available, it is assumed that the three individuals who died each lived for 6 months of the year). The total life years for the tight control intensive intervention, therefore, equals 2986 over the 3-year period, and the total life years for the conventional care arm equals 2977.

Life tables have been developed that show, for each age cohort of the population, the probability that a person of that age will not survive until his or her next birthday. From this, it is possible to calculate the probability of surviving any particular year of age, and the remaining life expectancy of people at different ages can also be calculated. To illustrate, in 2017, life expectancy at birth for the U.S. population was 78.6 years. For females the life expectancy in 2017 was 81.1 years and for males it was 76.1 years. At age 65, females in the United States had a life expectancy of another 20.6 years in 2017, while for males the life expectancy in 2017 was only another 18.0 years (Arias & Xu, 2019).

Health-related quality-of-life years may differ from the life expectancy years during any time period because the quality of life that individuals experience can vary considerably. In order to capture the variation in quality of life, a large number of health-related quality-of-life indices have been developed. Some of the indices are specific to a particular disease, some are indices oriented toward health status in general, and some are based on the stated preferences of the consumers. A disease-specific index contains items that are relevant to the particular disease, whether it be asthma, diabetes, or cancer. General health status indices contain items that are relevant to all or at least many conditions experienced by the population.

Both types of indices will contain a number of questions about specific aspects of the health status of the population. To illustrate, a person might be asked to describe or rank on a scale his or her mobility level. The questionnaire might provide five or six levels of mobility (such as none, ability to sit up in bed, ability to stand, etc.), and the individual indicates the level that most closely describes his or her condition. The responses determine the index score for that item, although in some quality-of-life indices there are scores reported for the separate components

not just the aggregate. Guidelines on economic evaluations recommend the inclusion of health-related quality-of-life indices whenever possible.

Health-related quality-of-life indices are usually confined to a patient's health status at a given point in time. Extrapolations from that point can be made to cover intervals between responses. However, if patients die during the measurement interval, then the indices generally do not incorporate this factor into the assessment. In economic evaluations, death (mortality) should be taken into account as a separate indicator. At the same time, mortality measures do not take the quality of life experienced by individuals into account. Additionally, none of the measures that have been discussed so far take into account the consumer's own valuations or preferences for each health state possible.

In order to address these concerns, several different research groups have developed preference-based, or utility, measures of health outcome (see **Table 12-4**). These preference-based measures are each based on a set of health dimensions. In the 15-D (15 dimensions of health) measure (Sintonen, 1981b), each of the 15 health dimensions has five categories, and there is a description for each category. For example, the five descriptions for the Vitality dimension are as follows:

1. I feel healthy and energetic.
2. I feel slightly weary, tired, or feeble.
3. I feel moderately weary, tired, or feeble.
4. I feel weary, tired, or feeble, almost exhausted.
5. I feel extremely weary, tired, or feeble, totally exhausted.

A score for each category was elicited from a sample of interviewees, each of whom placed his or her own valuation on the category.

A second level of weights, sometimes called *importance weights*, was assigned by a sample group to each of the 15 dimensions (see Table 12-4). The importance weights sum to a total value of 1.00 in this index. As a result, the highest possible score on the 15-D measure is 1.00, which is achieved if a respondent scores at the highest level in each of the 15 categories.

Some investigators, both in the 15-D and other preference systems, have assigned a value of 0 to death. This is a very convenient assumption because it allows investigators to score on a single scale those interventions that have both mortality and changes in quality of life as outcomes. Within the context of such systems, the magnitude of QALYs can be calculated, resulting in a very convenient outcome measure. In the diabetes illustration from earlier, in each of the 3 years reported, a QALY value of 0.9 has been

Table 12-4 Health Dimensions in the 15-D Health-Related Quality of Life Index

Dimension	Importance Weight
Breathing	0.075
Mental functioning	0.044
Speech	0.065
Vision	0.075
Mobility	0.046
Usual activities	0.057
Vitality	0.074
Hearing	0.104
Eating	0.040
Eliminating	0.033
Sleeping	0.090
Distress	0.079
Discomfort/symptoms	0.072
Sexual activity	0.084
Depression	0.062
Total	1.000

Based on Sintonen, H. (2001). The 15D instrument of health-related quality of life: Properties and applications. *Annals of Medicine, 33*, 328–335.

assigned to the individuals in the tight insulin intensive control group. Each surviving individual would, therefore, experience a total of 2.7 QALYs over the 3-year period.

In the diabetes illustration, a number of deaths occur each year. In this illustration the QALY valuation for a deceased persons is zero (remember that deaths were assumed to occur at the midpoint in the year). The assignment of a value of zero to death, while convenient, is certainly controversial. When investigators develop weights for alternative health conditions, members of a representative group are usually ask to provide their own values for each of the conditions. If patients who have experienced a specific health state are asked for their evaluations, then a value that is based on an understanding of the condition can be provided. However, most weights have been developed from surveys of the general population, many of whom have not experienced the health states they are asked to value.

In these latter instances, the valuations obtained are projections or estimates of what the respondents believe they might experience in a given state of health. The assignment of a value of zero to death is clearly an instance of projection. Individuals who have been surveyed have not personally experienced the condition, and so its valuation has little factual basis. Indeed, in all quality-of-life valuation surveys, the investigators did not ask respondents about what they thought they might experience in death. The investigators made their own extrapolations of the valuation of death.

An additional issue in preference-based indicators is whose valuations are to be included in the measure of outcome. Investigators have alternatively focused on the values of providers (physicians and nurses), the general population, and specific patient groups. In addition, a number of economists have used introspection (inserting valuations of what they personally think is reasonable), along with performing sensitivity analyses. At present, there is no agreement as to whose values should be incorporated into the weights. The patients are the only ones who have actually experienced many of the conditions, but the impact of decisions made often falls on payers of insurance premiums (employees or employers) or taxpayers.

12.5.4 Efficacy and Effectiveness

When there are two or more interventions available, each of which will achieve a stated purpose, there needs to be a method available to determine the *differences* in outcomes among the interventions. One method is to use experimental techniques, such as randomized controlled trials. Properly set up, these techniques create carefully specified protocols for selected groups of patients, who are randomized to alternative interventions so that the selection of one intervention or another is beyond the control of the investigators. The investigators can then be relatively sure that the two (or more) groups contain comparable patients.

In a randomized controlled trial or other clinical setting, the differences in outcomes achieved between interventions yield a measure called *efficacy*. This term refers only to differences that were obtained between interventions under experimental or controlled clinical conditions. Efficacy measures achieved under these controlled conditions do not always translate the same into everyday practice. Randomized controlled trials usually follow very tight protocols and monitor patients closely. If the trial is not conducted in hospital (and most are not), the trial staff must devote considerable resources to monitoring patient adherence to protocols. In many instances, the treatments for medical conditions have unpleasant side effects, and clinical staff try to ensure that the trial protocols are maintained by the patients (e.g., that they take the medications at the prescribed intervals). No such monitoring is possible for practitioners in everyday circumstances. As a result, efficacy measures obtained from clinical trials or clinical settings are not always good indicators of how an intervention will work in actual practice.

The concept of *effectiveness* is related to differences in outcomes between interventions under non-experimental, or every day, conditions. Effectiveness must be determined from data collected from routine operations. Billing data, collected by insurers, provide information that can be used in many instances to determine effectiveness. However, administrative or billing data usually do not contain information about the quality of life experienced by the patient and often do not contain sufficient clinical information to allow researchers to determine if indeed the patients within each comparison group are truly comparable (which they would be in a clinical trial). Thus, unlike in randomized or clinical setting trials, investigators using statistical studies are less certain that the populations they are comparing are similar. Despite these problems in determining effectiveness, it is this measure of difference, not that of efficacy, that is sought in most cost-effectiveness models. This is because the cost-effectiveness model is used to inform policy or management decisions, both of which are carried out under actual day-to-day conditions.

In the diabetes illustration presented, it is assumed that the measures of outcomes are similar to those that would be obtained in actual practice conditions. Effectiveness, then, is measured by the difference in outcomes observed between interventions. There are several different effectiveness measures in this diabetes illustration. One outcome is the number of lives saved during a given time frame. By the end of year 3, there were 990 survivors in the tight insulin intensive control arm and 984 in the conventional care arm. The difference, six lives, is an effectiveness measure. If all life years in each intervention are summed, then the effectiveness in terms of life years is 9 (2986 − 2977). In terms of QALYs, the effectiveness measure is 404.05 years (2686.95 − 2282.9). It should be noted that in this illustration a QALY occurring in any year is counted as having the same value as a QALYs occurring in any of the other years. Some analysts propose that a discount factor be applied to the benefits that occur in future years. The issue of discounting will be discussed later.

12.5.5 Costs

Economic costs are equivalent to the combined value of all *resources* used in an intervention. Economic costs should be distinguished from transfer payments, which are unrelated to current resources produced, since transfer payments simply move resources from one source to another without goods or services being exchanged for it. Transfer payments include taxes, unemployment insurance payments, social security payments, and so on. From the point of view of the payer, such payments would appear as costs; from the viewpoint of recipients, they would appear as revenues. However, they are not payments for resource use and production and so are not indicators of how the economy's resources are being used.

In most economic evaluations, economic costs are subdivided into direct costs and costs associated with lost productivity (also called indirect costs). Direct costs are equivalent to the combined value of the resources (goods and services) for which payment is received. These costs can be paid for by insurers, governments, or consumers (out of pocket). To be considered a direct cost, the good or service must have involved a resource, and a good or service must have been purchased. Indirect, or lost productivity, costs are the costs of those services that involved resources but were not purchased. If a patient travels to a clinic or sits idly in a waiting room, the individual may be losing valuable productive time and income. In effect, the patient's time, which is a resource, is not being purchased; rather, in this instance they represent payment that has been foregone. The value of time lost cannot be directly observed, but it is real, and an economic value needs to be imputed and assigned to the resource.

Economic evaluation studies often involve different perspectives. To illustrate, an insurer may be interested mainly in what it pays out for goods and services used in the provision of healthcare services. A patient may be interested only in what he or she pays out of pocket for the healthcare service and in the amount of time lost from work. The patient may also be interested in sickness-related transfer payments, as these will reduce the individual's out-of-pocket costs associated with the consumption of healthcare services.

The broadest perspective taken in economic evaluations, called the societal perspective, is from the viewpoint of all societal resources. All resources are included in the societal perspective, including transfer payments. In any other perspective, the costs incurred by individuals in these groups will be the focus of attention. Economic evaluation guidelines generally propose that the broadest viewpoint possibly be taken. However, economic evaluation studies are often initiated by special interest groups, such as governments, pharmaceutical companies, and providers. These groups are usually only secondarily concerned with the societal perspective, however commendable it may be.

The costs that are identified should be the marginal costs of the interventions. These costs are equivalent to the combined value of all additional resources used to deliver the intervention. In the diabetes illustration, the hypothetical marginal cost of two interventions is presented (see Table 12-2). Each cost estimate was separated into four components: inpatient hospitalization from complications of diabetes, routine outpatient visits, self-care, and adverse events that typically led to emergency room treatment.

Hospital costs are the expected costs of hospitalization, and are based on the probability of individuals in the cohort being hospitalized and the resulting cost of a hospitalization. Outpatient costs consist of the physician fees for routine visits. Adverse event costs are the probability of having emergency room visits and the associated costs that might result from complications that do not lead to hospitalization or that precede hospitalization. The costs of self-care include the costs of monitoring glucose levels, insulin, and medical supplies. Many of these costs will be out-of-pocket costs incurred by the patient. The value of lost productivity is excluded in this analysis; therefore, it falls somewhat short of taking a full societal viewpoint.

As seen in Table 12-2, intensive insulin therapy costs $10,000 per person per year, whereas conventional therapy costs $3000 per person per year. The annual difference between the two interventions ($7000) is primarily due to the costs of self-care, which total $8270 for the intensive treatment and $1400 for conventional care, or a difference of $6870 per person per year.

12.5.6 Discounting Future Costs and Benefits

In general, individuals place a higher value on present utilities than on future ones. That is, an individual would prefer to have 1 dollar today than 1 dollar a year from now. The discount rate is used as an expression of the preferences of individuals for present benefits over future benefits. All future period costs should therefore be discounted to make them equivalent to costs in the present time. Continuing with the diabetes illustration, assume a 5% discount rate and assume that all costs occur at the end of each year. Given this assumption (which is typical), the first-year

costs of $3000 are not discounted in the analysis. The discounted costs of the second year for conventional care are $2857 ($3000/1.05). For the third year, these costs are $2722 ($3000/ [1.05]^2). The present value for all 3 years is the sum of these values, or $8578. The discounted costs for all 3 years of the intensive treatment group is $28,594, and the difference in the present value of costs between the two interventions (i.e., $c_2 - c_1$) is $19,991.

There is a controversy over the question of whether to also discount nonmonetary benefits. Investigators who wrote on the issue in the 1970s (Weinstein & Stason, 1977) stated that benefits and costs should be placed on the same plane and both should be discounted. More recently, some investigators (Parsonage & Neuberger, 1992) have claimed that if a discount was applied to the benefits received from such services as health promotion activities, where many of the benefits are not experienced until years after the intervention, the present value would be reduced substantially. For example, the present value of $1000 received in 20 years at a discount rate of 5% is only $376.89. Yet, a gap of 20 years between health promotion activities and health benefits is not unusual. In light of these findings, a debate has occurred over whether to discount health benefits because doing so places many health promotion activities on very shaky ground. The investigators contend that a social time preference discount rate may be less than a private one. In recognition of this, guidelines now recommend conducting a sensitivity analysis that includes a zero (no discount) rate for benefits to determine just how susceptible the results of the calculations are to the use of a discount rate.

12.5.7 Cost-Effectiveness Ratios

In this diabetes illustration, a series of cost-effectiveness ratios can be calculated. Three such ratios are calculated and presented in **Table 12-5**: cost per life saved, cost per life year saved, and cost per quality-adjusted life year saved. Table 12-5 summarizes the costs and outcomes for two groups of 1000 individuals with diabetes. The net discounted costs for 1000 individuals in the intensive treatment group are $28,594,104 and for individuals in the conventional care group net discounted costs are $8,578,231. The net difference in discounted costs ($c_2 - c_1$) is therefore $20,015,873. The difference in the number of deaths equals six, and therefore the cost per life saved is $3,335,979. Similarly, the difference in the number of life years saved is nine, and therefore the cost per life year saved is $2,223,986. The difference in the number of QALYs

Table 12-5 Summary of Data for Alternative Cost–Effectiveness Ratios

Program	Net Discounted Costs for 1000 Persons ($)	Number of Deaths	Cost per Life Saved ($)	Number of Life Years	Cost per Life Year Saved ($)	Number of Quality-Adjusted Life Years (QALYs)	Cost per QALY Saved ($)
Intensive care	28,594,104	10		2,986		2,686.95	
Conventional care	8,578,231	16		2,977		2,282.90	
Difference	20,015,873	6	3,335,979	9	2,223,986	404.05	49,538

saved is 404.05, and therefore the cost per QALY saved is $49,538.

The interpretation of these ratios is as follows. With regard to the QALY outcomes, an additional $49,538 in costs will yield an additional quality-adjusted life year. The ratio by itself does not tell us whether it would be worth it to spend the extra resources, and thus it does not provide all the information that is needed to choose one type of intervention over the other. It merely says what, in physical terms, will be obtained for the money.

12.5.8 Sensitivity Analysis

Most evaluations, even those that are based on randomized clinical trials, will be developed using assumed values for some variables. In this analysis, QALY information may have been obtained from different sources than the information for lives saved. To illustrate, the QALY data may have been extrapolated from another study rather than collected during the current study. If the valuation of QALYs for the two populations was uncertain, then performing a sensitivity analysis to see the effect of making different assumptions could provide valuable information. If the results changed substantially between the two calculations, especially if the new assumptions resulted in different conclusions being reached, then less confidence would be placed on the current analysis (Briggs, Sculpher, & Buxton, 1994).

In the diabetes illustration, assume that the QALY value for the intensive treatment group was 0.85 rather than 0.90 for each of the 3 years. Then the outcome would be 2538.10 QALYs for the 3-year period, not 2686.95. The value of $q_2 - q_1$ would be 255.20 QALYs rather than 404.05, and the cost-effectiveness ratio, if all else remained the same, would be $78,432 per QALY saved. This is considerably more than the original ratio; however, whether it would change the recommendation depends on whether

the cost-effectiveness ratio exceeded some assumed threshold that had been determined. The standard would need to be set to determine what an acceptable cost-effectiveness ratio would be. The following section discusses setting standards.

12.5.9 Interpreting the Results

The cost-effectiveness ratio takes on additional meaning for interpretation if it can be compared to a standard. The development of a standard will require some value judgments to be made about what is an acceptable improvement in cost per QALY. Investigators Laupacis, Feeny, Detsky, and Tugwell (1992) developed a conceptual tool to help interpret such findings. In **Figure 12-3**, the cost-effectiveness results are presented in graphic form, reflecting an illustration of the results of an ICER evaluation. The two axes represent increases (or decreases) in QALYs and increases (or decreases) in cost. The original coordinates are the levels of the discounted cost and the QALY outcome for the conventional care intervention, represented by c_1 and q_1. Let c_1 be $8,578,231 for the 1000 individuals in the conventional care intervention and q_1 be 2282.90 QALYs, reflecting the value for conventional diabetes care in this illustration.

Based on the coordinates in Figure 12-3, there are four quadrants, labeled A, B, C, and D. The origin is c_1 and q_1. Relative to these points, c_2 (the costs of the intensive care intervention group in the diabetes illustration) will be the same as, greater than, or less than c_1; and q_2 will be the same as, greater than, or less than q_1. At any point located in quadrant A, then the intensive treatment intervention would cost less and would produce more QALYs than the conventional intervention. On both cost and outcome results in these circumstances, the intensive care intervention is preferred to the conventional care intervention; it is considered to be *dominant*. On policy grounds, the dominant intensive intervention should therefore

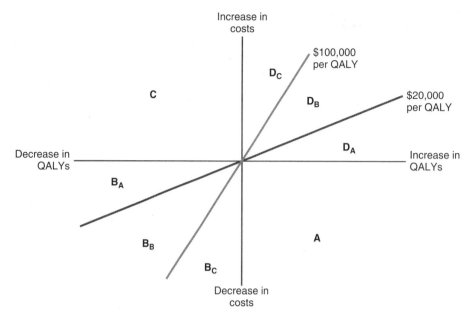

Figure 12-3 Alternative combinations of cost and QALY changes. The position of each point represents a cost-effectiveness ratio. The position of the points will provide a standard that can be interpreted as dominant (quadrants A and C), strong evidence (quadrants D_A and B_A) moderate evidence (quadrants B_B and D_B) and weak evidence (quadrants D_C and B_C).

be adopted. The same type of reasoning holds for any rate that falls into quadrant C; only in this case, the conventional intervention is dominant over the intensive care intervention.

If, relative to c_1 and q_1, the points c_2 and q_2 fall into quadrant D, then the intensive care intervention costs more *but* yields more QALYs than the conventional care intervention. To derive a policy conclusion under these conditions, a value judgment must be used to set a standard for an acceptable cost per QALY. One group of researchers (Laupacis et al., 1992) proposed the following set of value judgments:

- If intervention 2, relative to intervention 1, results in a cost-effectiveness ratio that is less than $20,000 per year, then there is *strong* evidence supporting the adoption of intervention 2.
- If intervention 2, relative to intervention 1, results in a cost-effectiveness ratio that is between $20,000 and $100,000 per year, then there is *moderate* evidence supporting the adoption of intervention 2.
- If intervention 2, relative to intervention 1, results in a cost-effectiveness ratio that is greater than $100,000 per year, then there is *weak* evidence supporting the adoption of intervention 2.

The numbers used in these guidelines were based on 1990 data. In 2018, the average income of individuals in the lowest 50% of wage earners was about $30,000 and the average income of individuals in the highest 5% of wage earners was about $135,000.

As a result, some adjustments might need to be made in the values separating the three groups.

These guidelines are presented graphically in Figure 12-3. The line indicating a cost-effectiveness ratio of $20,000 per QALY separates area D_A from the rest of the quadrant D. The line indicating a cost-effectiveness ratio of $100,000 per QALY separates D_C from the remainder of quadrant D. Thus, quadrant D is now divided into three areas related to the values stated. If the cost-effectiveness ratio falls into the area of D_A (cost-effectiveness ratio below $20,000 per QALY), then this provides strong evidence supporting its adoption. If it falls into area D_B (i.e., it is between $20,000 and $100,000), then there is moderate evidence. And if it falls into area D_C (i.e., it exceeds $100,000), then weak evidence for adoption is provided. Similar reasoning holds for ratios that fall into quadrant B in Figure 12-3.

Analyses such as these make more explicit the value judgments that are related to policy analyses. In this illustration, the standards selected by the researchers were somewhat loosely based on average annual salaries. A low-income person earns about $20,000, and so if the cost per QALY is below that, then the authors conclude that adoption would be warranted.

However, these values are by no means universally accepted. Other investigators have chosen the standard of $50,000 to delineate whether an intervention should be recommended (Hirth, Chernew, Miller, Fendrick, & Weissert, 2000). While the standard of $50,000 still remains in use today, if that value was increased for inflation it would be approximately $90,000 in 2019 (BLS, 2019). A number of investigators have recommended the development and use of community surveys on what the general public is willing to pay for a QALY (Olsen & Donaldson, 1998).

12.6 Cost-Benefit Analysis

CEA and CUA provide information about the differences in outcomes in relation to differences in costs. As already stated, these evaluation methods do not provide information on whether the differences in outcomes are worth the differences in cost. To determine whether they are, either an individual's personal opinion (or someone else's) must be injected into the valuations of the outcomes or else there is a need to determine a monetary valuation of the outcomes.

12.6.1 Valuation of Outcomes

Among the outcomes for health care are improved health, an ability to work or engage in leisure activities, and desired characteristics of the services themselves, such as convenience. In various economic evaluations investigators have attempted to place valuations on all of these characteristics.

12.6.2 Human Capital

One method of outcome valuation, called the *human capital approach*, focuses on lost work and lost leisure time resulting from mortality or morbidity. According to this approach, individuals' lost time from work (or leisure) is valued at the opportunity cost of time. This opportunity cost can be either the value of lost wages or income or the amount an individual must pay someone else to perform the replacement work. To illustrate, an individual is ill or injured and loses 5 days from work; a value can be placed on this time by estimating the per diem wage (e.g., $100 per day) and multiplying this wage by the length of time the individual is unable to work. An alternative way of measuring human capital losses would be through measuring the replacement costs for lost time. To illustrate, if a clinician was ill for 5 days and would not be available to provide office visits, then the loss could be estimated by determining the cost of hiring another clinician to provide the office visits.

The human capital method, once very popular, has fallen out of favor with economists for several reasons. *First*, studies in the Netherlands have questioned whether this method commonly overestimates

productivity losses (Koopmanschap, Rutten, van Ineveld, & van Roijen, 1995). According to their friction-cost analyses, companies may replace individuals who are off the job with others; these replacement workers may have been previously unemployed or underemployed. The value of lost production would then be less than stated by the human capital method. Of course, the ease or difficulty of finding replacement workers would depend on overall economic conditions, such as the prevailing unemployment rate.

Second, if an individual is ill or injured and loses work time and perhaps income because of absenteeism, there are other fringe benefits that may be lost as well. Also, individuals may still work when not feeling well, but the presenteeism effort is at a lower capacity. Or, if an individual cannot work, they may simultaneously lose other benefits that are typically associated with good health. The lost wage from absenteeism therefore is difficult to determine if it is an understatement of the value of the losses to the individuals. Consequently, investigators have sought other means of measuring the value of lost work time.

Third, the theory of human capital incorporates a value system that places emphasis on those who are employed. Retirees and unemployed persons are valued at a very low rate, if at all, under the human capital theory. Yet a large percent of health resources are used to treat those who are not working, including persons who are retired. The human capital approach therefore does not serve as a good method of evaluating lost benefits from interventions that lead to improved health but may not increase work time. Nevertheless, the human capital approach is still widely used, especially in cost-of-illness studies. Proponents of national economic policies espouse the goal of increasing total productivity and per-worker productivity. Improved health can often lead to the achievement of these goals. This may be why the human capital approach has not completely faded away.

12.6.3 Risk Preference

A second method for evaluating lost benefits in an economic evaluation is the "risk preference" approach, which is based on actual market data rather than inferred values, and so it reflects personal preferences. The widest use of this method has been in the applications evaluating the labor market. The economic assumption in the risk preference approach states that individuals will demand a risk premium (higher wages) in order to accept employment in more risky occupations. If the health risks (morbidity and mortality) in various occupations, as well as the wages paid in these occupations, can be quantified, then, after an adjustment has been made for other variables that might also affect wages (e.g., experience, training, and gender), the wage differential observed should be related to the risk differential. Stated differently, the adjusted wage differential measures the extra amount of money that workers demand in return for working in an occupation with a higher risk of injury or death.

This risk preference measure incorporates an estimate of the probability of poor health or death in various occupations and the differential in salaries among the occupations. Somewhat indirectly, a value per QALY can be inferred from the information in the risk preference value. To illustrate, if there is a 10% difference in risk of mortality between two occupations, and the annual pay differential is $5000, then a value of $50,000 for the loss of a life ($5000/0.10) can be inferred. In this way, some of the benefits from an increased probability of improved health can be estimated, namely, those associated with longevity. Many other health-related benefits cannot be dealt with through the use of this concept however.

12.6.4 Contingent Valuation

A third method of measuring benefits is termed *contingent valuation*. In contingent valuation, individuals are asked how much they would hypothetically be willing to pay if the benefits that result from specific interventions could be achieved. To illustrate, assume an individual who undergoes kidney dialysis daily could, with no adverse effects, receive a benefit of having dialysis only twice a week. The individual could be asked to value (in monetary terms) such an occurrence. The stated value could be construed as the individual's willingness to pay for the improved kidney treatments.

In a contingent valuation study, the responses depend on what the respondents are asked and how the question is worded. Much study has gone into this subject. Briefly, the following are some guidelines for achieving a valid valuation of a person's perception:

- The effects of the intervention should be clearly stated and understood by the respondent.
- The questionnaire should stress that there are other goods and services competing for the respondent's money.
- The respondent should be told that there would be a reduction in spending on other things.
- Generally, the respondent should be told that the additional spending for the intervention would be in the form of higher taxes or product prices.

- The interview should include follow-up questions in order to determine the reasons for the respondent's valuations.

12.6.5 Techniques of Valuation

These described valuation techniques have been used by investigators in a number of different contexts. One group of investigators surveyed studies in which respondents expressed a willingness to pay in return for specific reductions in risk that would result in expected increases in QALYs. Using the estimates of these studies, the authors calculated a value of life (Hirth et al., 2000). They estimated the age of persons in each study, the expected life years remaining, the QALYs per life year, and thus the number of QALYs. With this information, the investigators estimated a cost per QALY for each study reviewed. The values arrived at differed widely and results appeared to depend on the research approach taken. According to the human capital approach, the value of cost per QALY was $24,777. Using revealed preference studies, the authors estimated a value of $93,000. And using the contingent valuation approach, they estimated a value of $161,000. Given the large variation among methods, the authors concluded that the goal of determining a cost per QALY was still very elusive.

In theory, the value of a QALY is the most important variable, as it provides a key to answering a central question in economic evaluation. However, the cost per QALY in practice seems to depend on the context of the analysis and on the method used to obtain information. The values arrived at using the method that is closest to revealed preferences—risk preference—cannot be easily linked to specific health states. As well, there are considerable differences in the results of the various studies.

The contingent valuation method suffers from the difficulty of applying it to specific interventions and the difficulty of achieving comparability. This method also elicits responses from individuals based on hypothetical situations; faced with actual situations, individuals may value services differently. It appears that the contingent valuation method is better suited to answering hypothetical questions about health-related programs than questions about the values placed on specific interventions. To be specific, respondents require detailed knowledge about the interventions being evaluated, and their information needs could be too extensive for the interviewing process. A substantial amount of detail about the results of specific interventions can be obtained from health-related quality-of-life indicators, including preference-based indicators. Willingness-to-pay measures cannot provide such detail. In sum, the best instrument to use depends on the purpose of the investigation.

12.6.6 Cost-Benefit Ratio

CBA attempts to answers the question: Are the benefits worth the costs? When examining a specific intervention, this question implies that there is an alternative intervention available, even if the alternative is to "not perform the intervention"—do nothing. The main point to understand is that there are alternative uses of the resources involved, since resources are scarce/limited. In a cost-benefit analysis, the alternative to the proposed intervention should be explicitly considered.

Ignoring discounting at this time, the cost-benefit equation is expressed as

$$NB = b - c \text{ or } Ratio = b / c$$

in which NB refers to net benefits, b refers to the benefits resulting from the intervention, and c refers to the additional costs associated with the intervention. To illustrate, assume that an investor-owned hospital is trying to decide which of two programs to implement, given its limited budget. These programs address two different health issues and probably impact different individuals in the community. One program is a community-wide immunization program and the other program is a community-wide cancer screening program. The planners in the hospital have estimated that the immunization program will cost $40,000 and the screening program will cost $60,000. The planners have also estimated that the immunization program will generate $60,000 in revenue and the screening program will generate $80,000 in revenue.

Given these estimates, the net benefit of the immunization program is $20,000 ($60,000–$40,000) and the net benefit of the screening program is also $20,000 ($80,000–$60,000). Looking only at the net benefit results, neither program is dominant since both programs result in the same net benefit. However, when ratios are calculated, the results are different. The cost-benefit ratio of the immunization program is 1.5:1 ($60,000/$40,000) and the cost-benefit ratio of the screening program is 1.3:1. Since the hospital does not have sufficient resources to undertake both programs at this time, based on the cost-benefit ratios the hospital will implement the immunization program.

Exercises

1. A health economist was asked to compare the outcomes and costs of two diabetes therapies that affected both the severity of the disease and the survival rate. What evaluation concept should be used?

2. A health economist was asked to compare the outcomes and costs for two prophylactic medicines that reduced deaths during surgical operations. The interventions did not influence quality of life. What evaluation concept should be used?

3. Patients who were hospitalized for asthma were placed on a new drug. The drug resulted in an extra day of hospitalization (the length of stay went from 6 to 7 days), the extra day would cost $1600. There were no other differences in the treatment. The drug cost $600 for the dose. Also, administration of the drug and monitoring of the patient after administration took an hour of nursing time (wage = $40 per hour) and $20 in supplies were used in the administration of the drug. The mortality rate was 20 deaths per 100 with the drug and 24 deaths per 100 without it. What is the cost-effectiveness ratio for using the drug?

4. In a population of 1000 persons at the beginning of the year, 40 die during the year. How many life years were there during the year?

5. In 1 year, 30 persons per 1000 die of asthma. A new drug reduces that number to 20 per 1000. How is outcome defined, and what is the "effectiveness" of the drug?

6. An individual with asthma will live for 6 months without taking the medication prescribed. The quality of life of that individual is valued at 0.8. If the asthma medicine is taken as prescribed, the value of the individual's quality of life will increase to 0.9 and the length of survival will increase to 7 months. What is the effectiveness of the medicine?

Bibliography

Arias, E., & Xu, J. (2019). United States life tables, 2017. *National Vital Statistics Report, 66*(4). Hyattsville, MD: National Center for Health Statistics.

Bakker, C., Hidding, A., van der Linden, S., & van Doorslaer, E. (1994). Cost effectiveness of group physical therapy compared to individualized therapy for ankylosing spondylitis. *Journal of Rheumatology, 21*, 264–268.

Briggs, A., Sculpher, M., & Buxton, M. (1994). Uncertainty in the economic evaluation of health care technologies: The role of sensitivity analysis. *Health Economics, 3*, 95–104.

Canadian Coordinating Office for Health Technology Assessment. (1997). *Guidelines for economic evaluation of pharmaceuticals: Canada.* Ottawa: Canadian Coordinating Office for Health Technology Assessment.

Centers for Disease Control and Prevention. (2018). *National diabetes statistics report, 2017.* Atlanta, GA: US Department of Health and Human Services.

Cookson, R., Drummond, M., & Weatherly, H. (2009). Explicit incorporation of equity considerations into economic evaluation of public health interventions. *Health Economics, Policy, & Law, 4*(Pt. 2), 231–245.

Diabetes Control and Complications Trial Research Group (DCCT). (1995). Resource utilization and costs of care in the Diabetes Control and Complications Trial. *Diabetes Care, 18*, 1468–1478.

Diabetes Control and Complications Trial Research Group (DCCT). (1996). Lifetime benefits and costs of intensive therapy as practiced in the Diabetes Control and Complications Trial. *JAMA, 276*, 1409–1415.

Drummond, M. F., O'Brien, B. J., Stoddart, G. L., & Torrance, G. W. (1997). *Methods for the economic evaluation of health care programmes* (2nd ed.). Oxford, England: Oxford University Press.

Gold, M. R., McCoy, K. I., & Siegel, J. E. (1996). *Cost-effectiveness in health and medicine.* New York, NY: Oxford University Press.

Higgins, A. M., & Harris, A. H. (2012). Health economic methods for cost-minimization, cost effectiveness, cost utility, and cost benefit evaluations. *Critical Care Clinics, 28*(1), 11–24.

Hirth, R. A., Chernew, M. E., Miller, E., Fendrick, A. M., & Weissert, W. G. (2000). Willingness to pay for a quality-adjusted life year: In search of a standard. *Medical Decision Making, 20*, 332–342.

Koopmanschap, M. A., Rutten, F. F., van Ineveld, B. M., & van Roijen, L. (1995). The friction cost method for measuring indirect cost of disease. *Journal of Health Economics, 14*, 171–189.

Laupacis, A., Feeny, D., Detsky, A. S., & Tugwell, P. X. (1992). How attractive does a new technology have to be to warrant adoption and utilization? Tentative guidelines for using clinical and economic evaluations. *Canadian Medical Association Journal, 146*, 473–481.

Menon, D., Schubert, F., & Torrance, G. W. (1996). Canada's new guidelines for the economic evaluation of pharmaceuticals. *Medical Care, 34*, DS77–DS86.

Nixon, J., Stoykova, B., Glanville, J., Christie, J., Drummond, M., & Kleijnen, J. (2000). The U.K. NHS economic evaluation database. Economic issues in evaluations of health technology. *International Journal of Technology Assessment in Health Care, 16*(3), 731–742.

Olsen, J. A., & Donaldson, C. (1998). Helicopters, hearts, and hips: Using willingness to pay to set priorities for public sector programmes. *Social Science and Medicine, 46*, 1–12.

Parsonage, M., & Neuberger, H. (1992). Discounting and health benefits. *Health Economics, 1*, 71–79.

Sintonen, H. (1981a). An approach to measuring and valuing health states. *Social Science and Medicine, 15C*, 55–65.

Sintonen, H. (1981b). *The 15-D measure of health related quality of life.* West Heidelberg, Australia: National Centre for Health Program Evaluation.

Sorenson, C., Tarricone, R., Siebert, M., & Drummond, M. (2011). Applying health economics for policy decision making: Do devices differ from drugs? *Europace, 13*(Suppl 2), ii54–ii58.

Thompson, M. S. (1986). Willingness to pay and accept risks to cure chronic disease. *American Journal of Public Health, 76*, 392–397.

U.S. Bureau of Labor Statistics. (2019, October). Table 1. Consumer Price Index for All Urban Consumers (CPI-U): U.S. city average, by expenditure category. Retrieved from https://www.bls.gov/news.release/cpi.t01.htm

Weinstein, M. C., & Stason, W. B. (1977). Foundations of cost-effectiveness analysis for health and medical practices. *New England Journal of Medicine, 296*, 716–721.

Yang, W., Dall, T. M., Beronjic, K., Lin, J., Semilla, A. P., Chakrabartij, R., & Hogan, P. F. (2018). Economic costs of diabetes in the United States in 2017. *Diabetes Care, 41*(5), 917–928.

Zhuo, X., Zhang, P., Barker, L., Albright, A., Thompson, T. J., & Gregg, E. (2014). The lifetime costs of diabetes and its implications for diabetes prevention. *Diabetes Care, 37*, 2557–2564.

CHAPTER 13

Value Judgments and Economic Evaluation

OBJECTIVES

1. Describe what a value judgment is and how it can be used in evaluative economics.
2. Discuss how to identify an efficient level of output in any market.
3. Compare alternative delivery arrangements in terms of their efficiency.
4. Describe how a market for health insurance can be efficient when there is less than complete insurance coverage.
5. Describe the extra-welfarist approach to identifying optimal economic arrangements.
6. Define the concept of equity and identify several alternative measures of equity and their application.

13.1 Introduction

The focus of this chapter is on evaluating alternative possible allocations of resources devoted to health care and the implications of these allocations. In economic evaluation, positive statements are only concerned with what is, what was, or what will be. Expanding the evaluation from what is, was, or will be to include value judgments (normative judgments) involving what should be leads to asking such questions as whether totally free care can be judged "better" than the provision of health care in a competitive market, or whether and in what sense a regulated system may be preferable to an unregulated one. It should be pointed out that many of these normative questions involve public policy issues. Indeed, normative evaluative analysis forms the cornerstone of policy analysis because the ultimate goal of public, as well as private, policy is to bring about improvements in the use of resources.

Before undertaking normative evaluative analysis, the ground rules for conducting a normative evaluation need to be established. Establishing the ground rules for normative evaluative analysis is the purpose of this chapter. In Section 13.2, the importance of having a recognizable and unvarying standard for gauging alternative allocations is discussed. The values that individuals place on specific services can be used as the basis of a social or normative evaluation. One method frequently used by economists for building a social evaluation is discussed in Section 13.3. The standard that results from this method is referred to as an *efficiency criterion*. The efficiency standard derived takes individuals' starting situations as given and therefore bypasses the questions relating to equity and need as determined by clinical or personal criteria. The application of the efficiency criteria to evaluate the performance of the health insurance market is discussed in Section 13.4, and policy goals resulting from this efficiency analysis are presented in Section 13.5. The relevance of the efficiency criteria as the sole benchmark of resource allocation has been questioned by many observers. An alternative approach to address some of the concerns expressed about the efficiency criterion method, called *extra-welfarism*, is presented in Section 13.6. Finally, alternative measures of equity are considered in Section 13.7.

13.2 Values and Standards in Economic Evaluation

An important component in the establishment of value for evaluation is the determination of what is meant by value in terms of a socially optimal outcome. In considering the issue of socially optimal outcomes, the issue of externalities is important. Recall that an externality (either positive or negative) occurs when a third party is affected by the two parties (buyer and seller) directly involved in a transaction or exchange but does not have a direct way of impacting the outcome of the transaction. The presence of externalities plays an important role in determining a socially optimal outcome for society.

In a socially optimal outcome, there can be two types of decisions impacting the outcome. One of these is the private decisions made by individuals in the market about the goods and services they want to consume at the alternative prices. These decisions and the private market reflect only the private costs and benefits gained from the exchanges in the market.

The second type of decision involves incorporating the cost and benefit ramifications of private decisions on the welfare of others. These decisions involve issues of social welfare, and are very important in the healthcare system. In many instances, decisions made by an individual regarding the use of healthcare services may have substantial impacts on the welfare of other individuals.

Some of these transactions may provide benefits to other individuals in the market, such as when a sufficient number of individuals receive immunizations for a contagious disease to provide herd immunity. Within conditions of herd immunity not every individual needs to be vaccinated, only a sufficient number needs to be immunized to prevent the spread of the disease.

Some of these transactions, on the other hand, may cause costs to be incurred by others outside the transactions. For example, coworkers may experience the additional costs of being less productive on the job when an individual takes time off to receive health treatment. In private markets, neither of these external effects factor into market decisions.

If these external effects are present in the market, then the private market will not reach a socially optimal level of transactions and outside intervention will be necessary to achieve maximum social welfare. When the gains to society from the intervention in the private market are greater than the additional costs of the intervention, then a social surplus exists. Alternatively, when losses to society associated with market inefficiency occur, then a social loss exists. The role of a normative evaluation is to assist in ensuring these welfare costs and benefits are incorporated into the decision-making process.

To illustrate social welfare, assume there is a situation in which A has a curable disease but is receiving no health care, and B is healthy but is spending $20,000 on surgical services for a facial lift. Would this be an acceptable allocation of health resources? Many individuals would say it is unfair or unacceptable, but scarcely anybody would take the trouble to set forth the basic standard being used to judge the situation. Assume instead that it was necessary heart surgery that B was receiving instead of the face-lift. Would this change the evaluation of the acceptability of the situation? Would a different standard be used to gauge its fairness in the latter circumstances?

In this illustration, the resources are being allocated differently in the two situations. However, unless there has been a standard established that does not itself vary from situation to situation, it is really not possible to compare the two situations. That is, without an independent scale of fairness or acceptability, there would not be a measure capable of assessing alternative allocations of resources. In this section, a classification of available systems of standards is presented, focusing on the bases on which standards may be formed.

For the purposes of economic evaluation, there are two ways of deriving a system of values and then developing a ranking of alternative uses of resources. In the first method, called *delegatory* or *top-down*, a value system is imposed on the members of society. To illustrate, it might be imposed by a higher entity, such as a deity; by an interpreter of the ultimate word; by an elected body; or by a dictator, who settles on some value system based on personal values. Alternatively, someone can assume the mantle of spokesperson for society, proclaiming "society wants a decent standard of health for all," or some such alleged "truth." Despite the nod toward democracy, any would-be ethical authority who chooses to speak for society without a mandate based on the views of individuals within the society is really imposing personal views on society.

The second method for deriving a system of values is called *participatory* or *bottom-up* decision making. In this method, the views of the members of the community or society play a role. One assumption underlying this method is that *everyone's* values must be taken into account in ranking alternative ways of using resources. Another assumption is that each individual is the best judge of personal welfare.

Attention now turns to the value systems themselves, which can vary tremendously, ranging from very specific values to very vague values. The value system can take the form of specific laws handed down from the top decision maker, or they can be formulated in terms of such general concepts as *fairness*, *liberty*, and *equality*.

The field of analysis in health services contains many examples of writers proposing value systems based on their own view of what seems desirable. For instance, some writers have expressed the view that individuals have a "right" to health or health care. One commentator used the principle of *agape* (emphasizes love for our fellow humans and following the golden rule of doing to others as you would have others do to you) to derive this right (Outka, 1974), whereas another appealed to a strong sense of fairness and equity in the population that this right exists (Mechanic, 1976). This issue of a right to health care was discussed widely in the 2016 and 2020 presidential campaigns.

Even assuming a single value system could be identified, the problem of translating the chosen value system into a gauge or ranking scheme to assess alternative ways of using resources would still need to be established. This translation step can itself be controversial. Because any value system will always be somewhat vague and controversial, different ranking schemes with very different implications can be derived from it.

The next problem encountered would then be the problem of which ranking scheme to choose. To illustrate, the goal of "equality" can be interpreted in many ways—as equality of *health status* or equality of *healthcare utilization*, or equality of *expenditures on health care*. If it is decided that it entails equal use of health care for equal health status, then individuals who have poor health would receive more care than individuals who are basically healthy. This may seem plausible, but how is the decision reached on how much more care people with poor health should get? Also, if the health care given to those in poor health is not effective, should they still receive it? If the individual in better health has a much greater chance of surviving than the individual in poor health, should the individual with poor health receive the intervention?

The last step, after having decided on a ranking scheme, is to apply it to actual or proposed states of resource use (e.g., distributions of health care or levels of health) to determine their desirability from a policy standpoint. It should be stressed here that value systems imposed earlier on society are not necessarily bad or inappropriate. The source of such a system may be a highly respected and beloved authority, and the system may contain laudatory ideals and translate into ranking schemes that seem reasonable and compassionate. Nevertheless, a top-down imposed scheme is not built up from the values of the members of the society and therefore lacks some degree of representativeness of the values of society.

In Sections 13.3 and 13.4, a participatory system of evaluation is developed. This system, well known in economic circles as the *Paretean system* (named after the famous 19th-century sociologist Vilfredo Pareto), allows arrival at an optimum position through examining changes that could be made in resource allocations when started from an initial position. This optimum position holds only with reference to the initial starting point (i.e., the initial endowments each member of society possesses). The starting point is not judged as appropriate or inappropriate, which may or may not be fair, a consideration discussed in Section 13.5.

13.3 Efficient Output Levels

13.3.1 Individual Valuations of Goods and Services or Activities

If individuals' own valuations are accepted as the best indicators of their own welfare, then it must be determined, at least in principle, what these valuations might be. Because this analysis is concerned with specific goods and services (those involved in health care), the task is simplified somewhat. The need in this case is only to determine individuals' valuations with respect to those healthcare goods and services being considered.

Economists have developed a hypothesis regarding an individual's valuation of units of a specific good or service. The hypothesis, which is based on demand analysis, is that the more of any good or service the individual has, the less successive units of the good or service will be worth to him or her (compared with other goods and services)—diminishing marginal value. The analysis can then be conducted using money as the basic unit of value. To do this, it must be assumed that money itself is a constant value. That is, it is assumed in this hypothesis that if an individual gives up $2, that $2 will always represent the same amount of loss to the individual, however much income the individual has. This assumption will hold, at least partially, if the outlay for the good or service in question is a reasonably small portion of the individual's total budget.

If an individual has an income of $50,000, spending $20 or $30 on a good or service is unlikely to cause the valuation of each dollar to change for the individual. However, as the amount that must be given up to obtain a good or service becomes very large relative to income (e.g., $20,000 or $30,000), the utility of, or the subjective valuation placed on, the marginal dollar will change. The assumption being made in this section is that the subjective value of the marginal dollar to the individual does not change. It should be noted that this is a different assumption than often made regarding health insurance demand.

Given the assumption that money income has a constant value for individuals for all relevant ranges of expenditures, the individual valuations of successive units of a good or service in terms of money can be specified. It must be stressed in this situation that these valuations are the individuals' own evaluations of specific units of the good or service, and that these valuations qualify on participatory grounds for inclusion into the overall participatory social evaluation.

13.3.2 Values in a Selfish Market

To simplify the analysis, it is assumed initially in this illustration that there are two individuals in the market, individual A and individual B. Each individual in this illustration has a specific schedule of valuations for his or her own consumption of health care. These valuations of the individuals are referred to as *marginal valuations* (MVs). A marginal valuation is defined as the extra amount of money an individual would be willing to pay for an additional unit of a good or service. Thus, a marginal valuation (MV) is a measure of how much an extra unit of the healthcare good or service is worth to the individual in monetary terms.

In the initial analysis, both A and B derive satisfaction, or value, from their own consumption of healthcare services. The only satisfaction that anyone in society gets from the consumption of health care by A and B is the satisfaction received directly by A and B. In this illustration, assume individual A places a marginal value of $160 on the first unit of health care consumed, $140 on his second unit, and so on, as seen in columns 1 and 2 in **Table 13-1**. Note that the marginal values placed by each individual on successive units of health care consumed diminish; all other factors, such as health status, income, and wealth, are held constant in this illustration (i.e., the initial values of these other variables are held constant). For purposes of social evaluation, then, this is a measure of the social worth of A's consumption of health care (because A is the only individual who values this care).

The assumed relation between marginal value and quantity consumed can be presented graphically as well. In **Figure 13-1**, the curve MV_a represents A's marginal valuation of successive units of health care.

Table 13-1 Values and Costs of Medical Care

(1)	(2)	(3)	(4)	(5)	(6)	(7)
Quantity Consumed by A (Q_a)	A's Marginal Valuation (MV_a) ($)	Quantity Consumed by B (Q_b)	B's Marginal Valuation (MV_b) ($)	Quantity Consumed by A + B (Q_{a+b})	Marginal Social Value of Consumption (MSV) ($)	Marginal Cost of Output at Consumption Level $Q_a + Q_b$ (MC) ($)
1	160	0	0	1	160	70
2	140	0	0	2	140	70
3	120	0	0	3	120	70
4	100	1	90	5	190	70
5	80	2	70	7	150	70
6	60	3	50	9	110	70
7	40	4	30	11	70	70
8	20	5	10	13	30	70
9	0	6	0	15	0	70

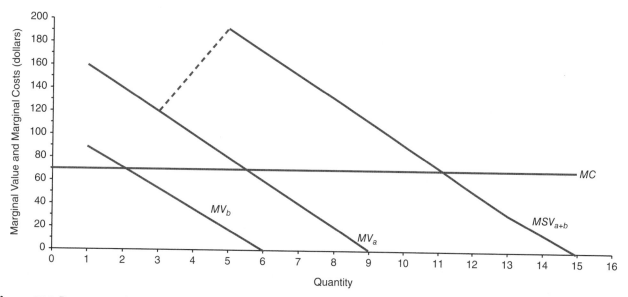

Figure 13-1 Representation of efficient output level when only private valuation is considered. Individuals A and B have private marginal valuations for healthcare (*MV*₍ₐ₎ and *MV*₍ᵦ₎, respectively). Using these, the marginal social value (MSV) curve is calculated, which relates aggregate quantity to the sum of the individuals' valuation. *MC* is the marginal cost of healthcare. The efficient level of output is that quantity at which *MSV* equals the *MC*, or before 11 units (in this illustration it would occur at 9 units since 11 units *MC* exceeds *MSV*).

© Jones & Bartlett Learning.

It is assumed, for ease of graphical presentation, that the units of healthcare can be made very small, so that the *MV* curve becomes smooth. A's valuation of own consumption is referred to as the *private* (or *internal*) valuation of A's consumption. On the assumption that no one else cares about A's consumption, the private valuation of A is the same as the social valuation of healthcare services consumed (the total value placed on A's consumption by all of society).

Similarly, the private valuations of B are presented in Table 13-1, and graphically as *MV*₍ᵦ₎ in Figure 13-1. For whatever reason (B is poorer, healthier, or less well educated), B places a lower value on each unit of health care than does A.

Indeed, B's first unit has an *MV* of $90, her second unit has an *MV* of $70, and so on. These valuations may seem low to A and others, but because B is the ultimate judge of her own welfare, these valuations cannot be questioned; these valuations are simply part of the data.

According to the assumption stated earlier, A and B are the only members of society who participate in the healthcare market in this illustration. The marginal social valuations of healthcare coincide with the marginal private valuations of these two individuals. Column 5 of Table 13-1 lists the aggregated quantities that correspond to each level of *MV* for A and B. To illustrate, at an aggregate quantity of five units of health care (four units used by A and one unit by B), the social marginal value will be $190, the sum of A's and B's marginal valuation. If seven units of health care were consumed (five by A and two by B), each

individual's *MV* would be $150. In this illustration it has now been hypothesized how much each additional unit of health care is worth to each participant in the market.

Furthermore, an aggregate-level relationship has been derived between the quantity of health care and the marginal value to each individual, if the individual was consuming at the level of consumption indicated by the *MV* curve (Figure 13-1). This aggregate curve, called the *MSV* (marginal social value) curve, shows the value to each member of the market if all individuals are consuming at the levels indicated by the curve. Because B does not have an *MV* above $120, for values above $120, the *MSV* curve coincides with A's *MV* curve. Once B enters the market, then the *MSV* curve becomes the sum of A's and B's *MV* curves and so may exceed the *MV* of A, as shown in Figure 13-1.

An implicit assumption of this analysis is that consumer valuations are expressed in terms of health care. But health care may not be valued for its own sake (except perhaps by a hypochondriac); it is usually *health* that is valued, not health care. In fact, each consumer's *MV* is actually made up of two components: a *MV* for health (termed *H*) and the marginal productivity of an additional unit of health care (*M*) in producing health ($\Delta H / \Delta M$), where Δ refers to change. Thus, the valuation of health care is a derivative, stemming from changes in the two components.

Next, the cost of producing health care must be determined. The initial assumption in this illustration is that each level of output is being produced at the minimum or most efficient cost. This assumption is sometimes referred to as the *technical efficiency* assumption. It implies that, given production conditions and input prices, the lowest cost combination of inputs is used at any output level. In column 7 of Table 13-1 and in Figure 13-1, the minimum marginal cost at which providers can produce health care is shown. In this illustration, it is assumed that this minimum marginal cost remains constant at $70 per unit as output increases. In this illustration, therefore, the MC is the additional cost per unit of health care; each additional unit costs $70 to produce, and is reflected as a horizontal line at $70 in Figure 13-1.

One interpretation of MC is that it is the amount of money that must be paid to the inputs in the production process to hire them away from the next-highest valued use. If health care was not produced, something else of value to consumers could be. It can be assumed then that the MC is the amount that would have to be paid to the resources to induce them not to produce that something else. This approach enables being able to put a value on unpaid resources that otherwise would appear to be "valueless" or "free." Thus, the MC is marginally above (and approximates) the value that someone else would have placed on these resources in an alternative use. Viewing the MC in this way means that it is essentially the opportunity cost of the resources used (the value that users of other goods and services would have placed on them).

13.3.3 The Socially Optimum Quantity of Health Care

The next step in this analysis involves the definition and identification of desirable or optimum resource allocations. Because the method of evaluation being used in this illustration is participatory, allocation of resources that would be considered better than other alternatives by all members of the community or society need to be identified. As will be seen presently, it is possible using a participatory method to rank some allocations as superior to others, although every conceivable situation cannot be compared. The criterion here is this: the resources must be used in a way that maximizes social value. That is, if the resources are distributed in such a way that consumers are willing to pay the most for them, then output will be at the "right," or economically efficient, level.

Using the valuations of A and B and the MC of health care in the previous illustration, the market will be at a socially optimal (or economically efficient) level of output if the MVs of A and B equal the MC (i.e., $MV_a + MV_b = MC$). If output is at a level at which

the MVs are greater than MC, say, at an aggregate quantity of 5 in Table 13-1, then an expansion of output to 7 (an increase of 1 for A and 1 for B) would have an MC per unit of output of $70 but would yield $80 extra in value to A and $70 in extra value for B. Similarly, if the MC is greater than the MSV, this indicates that resources are worth more elsewhere, and so output should decrease. In Figure 13-1, the optimal level of health care is 11 units (seven units for A and four units for B) with a social marginal value of $70. Given the assumptions stated earlier, this is how much health care should be produced. As previously stated, the optimal amount occurs where marginal cost just equals marginal benefit. This measure of efficiency—the distribution of output based on utility—is called *allocative efficiency*.

In reality, in a healthcare market, too much or too little (as well as just enough) health care could be produced. Too much could be produced if the government had a policy of financing health care and making it available for no out-of-pocket cost to consumers. In the previous illustration, at a zero price, demand will be at 15 units (when the MVs are zero); the MC of additional units will be well above this if the government is willing to ensure that all that is demanded is provided. The financing of the program could be through the collection of taxes. However, by meeting all demands for health care, the government is clearly providing too much, based on the social marginal value of consumption.

On the other hand, the market may not provide a sufficient amount of health care. If health care was in the hands of a monopolist, the monopolist would set a price well above a point at which MV = MC. If the price was $120, then three units in total would be demanded (all by A). Here, the market would be producing too little care.

In addition, the optimum level of resource use could result in little or even no use of health care by some individuals. The height of the MV curve, which is in effect a demand curve, will depend on the health status of the population, the wealth held, the income earned, and so on. Low-income individuals (e.g., B) may have low MVs for health care. Indeed, if the MC was higher than in the illustration given, a socially optimal quantity of output would be perfectly consistent with no consumption of health care by B. (This is true even though B may have poor health.)

It might be argued that this is unfair or unjust, and indeed, depending on the definition of fairness, it might well be. It should be recognized however that the root cause of the inequitable distribution of health care is the inequitable distribution of wealth or income. A higher income for B would mean higher demand and higher *MV* curves for health care. Of course, as far as the notion of economic efficiency is concerned, initial wealth and income levels for each individual are assumed to be given. A redistribution of income or wealth among individuals might seem fair to many observers, but it would not be evaluated within the bounds of the present notion of economic efficiency. According to Pareto, an outcome is economically efficient when it is not possible to improve the utility of one individual without making another individual worse off in society.

13.3.4 Optimal Output with Altruism

To preserve the present conditions of economic efficiency and to extend the model to cover some distributional issues, the model has been expanded to allow for the concern some individuals have regarding the low healthcare consumption levels of others. Here, the previous illustration is extended to allow for A's external demand for B's consumption of health care. From A's viewpoint, it may well be that B has a level of consumption of health care that is too low. If this is the case, some representation must be found of the value to A of B's healthcare consumption.

It is likely, of course, that A's concern for B's healthcare consumption is not unlimited. A is concerned, but only up to a point, for A has other private and public concerns as well. In fact, as seen in Section 13.4.3, A's valuation of B's health care consumption can be treated as any other good or service; the more B consumes, the less the marginal value to A of an additional unit consumed by B. In **Table 13-2**, A's *MV* for B's consumption is $60 for the first unit, $40 for the second unit, and $20 for the third unit. In this illustration B's consumption of the fourth unit contributes nothing to A's marginal value. In **Figure 13-2**, this external *MV* curve is shown as the short dotted line MV_{ab}.

It may seem strange that A's altruistic concern for B's welfare can be translated into mercenary terms and be given a monetary measure. The ability to do this rests on the assumption that goods and services are scarce, and A must make some choices at the margin. Even if A decided to give all his or her money away and use none of it for his or her family or own personal use, there would still be hard decisions to make. Should the money be donated to the Cancer Society or Heart Association? Should the money go toward the preservation of Newfoundland seals or bald eagles?

Depending on their tastes, even the most altruistic of people must make choices regarding scarcity, and the analysis here is merely a formalization of this fact. Of course, most people will engage in private consumption as well as altruistic consumption; their values can be presented by marginal valuation curves

Table 13-2 Private and Social Values of Consumption of Health Care by A and B

(1) Quantity Consumed by B (Q_b)	(2) Marginal Value to B of Own Consumption (MV_b) ($)	(3) Marginal Value to A of B's Consumption (MV_{ab}) ($)	(4) Marginal Social Value of B's Consumption ($MV_b + MV_{ab}$) ($)	(5) Quantity Consumed by A (Q_a)	(6) Marginal Value to A of Own Consumption (MV_a) ($)	(7) Total Quantity Consumed by A + B (Q_{ab})	(8) Total Marginal Social Value ($TMSV_{ab}$) ($)
0	0	0	0	1	160	1	160
0	0	0	0	2	140	2	140
0	0	0	0	3	120	3	120
1	90	60	150	4	100	5	250
2	70	40	110	5	80	7	190
3	50	20	70	6	60	9	130
4	30	0	30	7	40	11	70
5	10	0	10	8	20	13	30
6	0	0	0	9	0	15	0

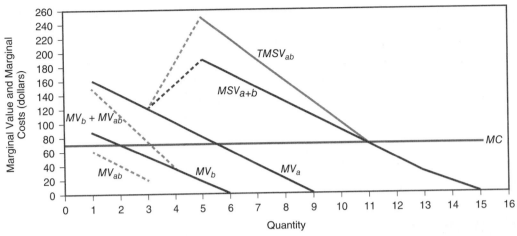

Figure 13-2 Representation of efficient output level when private and social valuations are considered. Individuals A and B have private marginal valuations for healthcare (MV_a and MV_b, respectively). Using these, the marginal social value (MSV) curve is calculated, which relates aggregate quantity to the sum of the individuals' valuation. MC is the marginal cost of healthcare. The efficient level of output is that quantity at which MSV equals the MC, or before 11 units (in this illustration it would occur at 9 units since 11 units MC exceeds MSV).

for both types of activities. The benefits to be obtained from others' consumption will be termed *external benefits*, and the values that people place on these benefits will be termed *external values*.

It is now possible to arrive at a measure of the value that society places on B's healthcare consumption. This value can be called a *social value*, and it is comprised of all individuals' private and external values for the specific good or service being consumed. Thus, the marginal social value for B's consumption of health care can be obtained by summing the values both individuals A and B place on each successive unit of health care that B might consume.

In Table 13-2, society has a marginal valuation of $150 for the first unit of B's health care (equal to the sum of $MV_b + MV_{ab}$), $110 for the second, and so on. These valuations are shown in Figure 13-2 as the dotted line labeled $MV_b + MV_{ab}$, which is the vertical sum of MV_b and MV_{ab}. *Vertical sum* means that each unit of B's consumption has a value to society (individuals A and B) greater than the value placed on it by B alone. Because of this "public" dimension, all values placed on each unit of B's consumption are summed. Because each member's valuation of the good or service is measured along the vertical, or cost, axis, the summation of all members' valuations of this good or service is therefore a vertical sum.

The marginal valuation curve facing the market for health care for A and B is $TMSV_{ab}$, which shows the quantity for all individuals at alternative MSVs for each individual. This curve is much like the MSV curve in Figure 13-1, except it incorporates A's valuation of B's consumption along with the private MVs of both individuals.

The socially optimum level of output is similarly interpreted; the output is optimal at the quantity in which the MSV_{a+b} for all individuals equals the MC. In Figure 13-2, the optimum level of output is 11 units of health care, where the marginal cost of $70 is the same as the total marginal social value of $70. To expand services by one more unit to A and B to a total of 13 units would result in a marginal social value of only $30, less than the MC of $70. Also, the marginal valuation of one more unit of health care to A is only $20 and the marginal value for B is only $10, both less than the marginal cost of $70. This optimum quantity incorporates each individual's private valuations, as well as any external valuations for the poor, the needy, the sick, and so on. The optimum quantity that incorporates the external concerns of A is greater than the optimum quantity if only selfish concerns exist (see Figure 13-1). However, these outcomes are the results of the data, and it may well be that B's optimal consumption is still at a low level.

The results of the extended analysis are consistent with some kind of transfer of funds from A to B for the purposes of increasing B's consumption of health care. However, the analysis does not say what kind of transfer should take place. It may be voluntary (e.g., charitable donations given by A directly to B or to some providing agency) or tax-based (e.g., taxes levied on A might be used to reimburse providers for services provided to B). Although, if taxation is used to raise funds, this analysis implies that it is voluntarily accepted by A. In either case, the optimal solution allows for some transfer, but it should be stressed that a transfer can be too much or too little.

The government can over- or underprovide, based on A's criteria. All that this analysis shows is that *some* transfer is consistent with economic efficiency.

13.3.5 Alternative Delivery Arrangements

Now that an ideal or efficient output level has been identified in this illustration, alternative delivery arrangements can be examined to see how these arrangements compare with the ideal. That is, it becomes possible to determine whether expected output under the alternatives is too little, just enough, or too much.

13.3.5.1 "Free" and Unlimited Care

First, assume that B is given all the health care for free that can be consumed. As column 3 of Table 13-1 indicates, B would choose to consume six units of output, even though the marginal valuation is zero. The social optimum level of consumption is 11 units for A and B, and the MC at this quantity is $70. Optimally, B should consume two units (i.e., when $MSV_b = MC$). For every unit B consumes beyond two, the value of B's consumption is less than the cost to society (everyone). Because someone must bear the burden of this care consumed, and because MC exceeds MSV for all units beyond two, there is a net social loss for these units. B gains handsomely (i.e., B's private benefits exceed B's private costs), but overall, this type of arrangement may lead to a great deal of health care being consumed with very little value attached to it.

13.3.5.2 Competitive Market, No Philanthropy

Another arrangement is now considered, that of a competitive market with no philanthropy or government programs. Equilibrium in a competitive market will occur when marginal private cost equals price. In the example here, A will consume the right amount of health care, but B will not. B's consumption will be less than the socially efficient amount because all society would have been willing to pay more for the first four units of B's consumption than the marginal cost.

The competitive market does not provide a mechanism to express A's external demand for B's care. A freely operating competitive market with no philanthropy will yield less than the optimal level of output when externalities would have justified a larger output. As for a monopolistic market, the output of such a market will be even less than the output of a competitive market, which means it will be even further below the optimal amount (Orzechowski, 2018; Schulman & Milstein, 2019).

13.3.5.3 Competitive Market with Philanthropy

It has been contended that even with philanthropy, a competitive market will not produce the optimal amount of output. To understand why, consider a situation in which there are many donors of health care, each of whom places a value on the consumption of health care by less fortunate individuals. In this case, some social arrangement must be found for ensuring that the values of these donors will be expressed in the market. If each of these potential donors offers to give what the output is worth to him or her, the social value will equal the sum of the private values.

However, if each donor feels that the others will also give, he or she might give less, hoping to get a "free ride," that is, gain the benefit of the others' donations while giving less. It is in the interests of each private donor to initially offer less than the value he or she places on the output in the hope that someone else will donate to cover the costs. If everyone behaves in this way, the total amount given in philanthropy will be less than the socially optimal amount. Analysts who accept the efficiency criterion frequently justify compulsory government programs on the basis that they make everyone pay what the programs are worth. Of course, it is difficult to decide how much a program would be worth to each taxpayer because the individual still has an incentive to understate the value of the program to himself or herself.

Even accepting this justification for government programs, it must still be discovered whether there exists an arrangement that will lead to the correct amount of health care being utilized. As can be seen in Table 13-2 and Figure 13-2, if B was offered subsidized health care, the efficient amount of health care would be utilized. In this case, a charge of $30 per unit of health care to B would lead to B's consumption of the optimal quantity—4 units. The rest of society must now pick up the remainder of the tab. Because the total cost to all members of society of health care consumed by B is $70, and because B will pay $30 of this, some arrangements must be made to collect the remaining $40 from the rest of society. This can be done in the form of taxes. Various arrangements are discussed in the next paragraphs.

It can be concluded from this analysis that some form of cost-sharing arrangement among members of society can lead to the provision of an optimal or efficient amount of the product. However, other arrangements can also be efficient. One is to have less fortunate individuals pay nothing and to impose some form of rationing other than price on these individuals. In practice, this type of arrangement requires that the rationing system used must produce the efficient outcome, and such systems are difficult to design and operate. This analysis can also be extended to a case in which the less fortunate individuals have different levels of income. If their demands differ because of these income levels, a system of variable subsidies tailored to income levels could be designed to have each member consume the right level of output (Pauly, 1972).

What is critical in translating the preceding analysis into a policy prescription is a clear conception of what the external demands might be in actuality. Assuming that external demands for the health care of some groups do exist and are significant, it is essential that it be exactly determined for what services these external demands are. If they are for good health, for example, then the external demanders (the A's in our analysis) may demand preventive care for consumption by the potential recipients of aid (the B's); however, the demands may be much more specific than that.

The demanders might show concern only for individuals who have catastrophic illnesses requiring large financial outlays. In this case, the external demanders will not want to pay for the health care of less fortunate individuals who have sore throats, ingrown toenails, or acne. Very little is known about the nature of healthcare externalities (external demands). From an efficiency point of view however, it is necessary to know what the external demanders are concerned about before designing a delivery system that will incorporate these externalities.

Assuming that the nature of the external demands has been identified, then the preceding analysis can be used to answer the questions as long as the goal of efficiency is kept in mind. Once the demands have been pinpointed, the types of health care that might improve the situation, and the potential recipients, can be identified. The consumer's portion of cost-sharing should be designed to ensure that there is no overuse, which is defined as any quantity beyond which marginal social benefits are less than marginal social costs. The reimbursement mechanism chosen should lead to the least cost output.

13.4 Optimal Health Insurance

The provision of health insurance requires resources and incurs costs. In the same way that there is an optimal quantity of health care, there is an optimal degree of insurance coverage. It is assumed in the following discussion that all individuals are the same in all respects except one—the amount they must pay to obtain insurance.

In this illustration, assume that there are 900 individuals (the number is not important, it is just for an illustrative purpose) who are members of a large group, and 100 individuals who are members of a small group. All individuals have an initial level of wealth of $4000. There is a probability of 10% (0.10) that each individual will become ill (i.e., 10% of each group will become ill). For those individuals who do become ill, the health costs are $800 per patient. The utility function for each member (all have the same tastes and preferences) is shown in **Table 13-3**.

This utility function can be interpreted as a measure of "consumer welfare." With regard to the supply side of the market, it is assumed that there is one insurer that provides insurance at cost to individuals. The loading cost to the insurer of a large group policy is $60, whereas the cost for a small group policy is $120. The objective is to maximize the overall utility of all members without detracting from that of any single member. This is the Paretean criterion.

The framework used focuses on consumer welfare (utility). In general, it is assumed that consumer welfare is maximized by shifting the risk onto the insurer whenever the expected utility with insurance is greater than the utility in the absence of insurance. The post-insurance utility is the net of the economic cost of accepting the risk. Therefore, utility (welfare) is maximized whenever the risk is appropriately shifted.

In this analysis, there are two groups of individuals. Each individual faces an expected loss of $80 (i.e., 10% of $800), and each can obtain insurance at a cost that includes the expected loss ($80) plus the appropriate loading cost. For members of the large group, the full premium, including the loading charge, is $140. For members of the smaller group, the premium is $200. For members of the large group, there is a utility, or welfare, gain by shifting the risk: at a cost of $140, the utility will be 94.4 units, which is less than the expected utility of not insuring, which is 98.0 units [(0.1 × $3200) plus (0.9 × $4000) = $3920]. There is a social loss from shifting the risk.

The same is also true for the members of the smaller group. Because the cost of insurance for them is $200, they would be better off to remain uninsured, with a utility of 98.0 compared to a utility of 89.0 if they purchased insurance. This would be true even if the cost of insurance for the smaller group was subsidized (i.e., if someone else paid part or all of the premiums). This is because the criterion of social efficiency rather than

Table 13-3 Relationship Between Wealth and Utility

Wealth ($)	Total Utility	Marginal Utility
3,600	57.0	—
3,620	61.2	4.2
3,640	65.2	4.0
3,660	69.0	3.8
3,680	72.6	3.6
3,700	76.0	3.4
3,720	79.0	3.0
3,740	81.8	2.8
3,760	84.4	2.6
3,780	86.8	2.4
3,800	89.0	2.2
3,820	91.0	2.0
3,840	92.8	1.8
3,860	94.4	1.6
3,880	95.8	1.4
3,900	97.0	1.2
3,920	98.0	1.0
3,940	98.8	0.8
3,960	99.4	0.6
3,980	99.8	0.4
4,000	100.0	0.2

© Jones & Bartlett Learning.

individual efficiency is being used. When it is recognized that there is a *social* cost of insuring, then it must also be recognized that there is an *optimal* degree of insurance coverage. This optimal degree may be zero if the arrangements for providing insurance are too costly.

It must also be acknowledged that consumers may vary in many respects, including the following: risk of illness, income or wealth level, degree of risk aversion, and circumstances affecting the cost of illness. As each varies, the utility gain from shifting the risk of incurring healthcare expenses will also change. To illustrate, individuals with a high risk of illness will gain more in terms of utility from shifting their risk than individuals with a low risk of illness. Thus, a situation in which individuals who are less healthy have greater insurance coverage could be an optimal

situation. That is, variations in insurance coverage among individuals can be economically efficient.

There is a confounding factor in this analysis: moral hazard. There can be a net welfare gain resulting from the shifting of risk. Once the risk is shifted, the out-of-pocket price of health care to the consumer declines. If there is any elasticity of demand for health care, then moral hazard will come into play and the quantity demanded of health care will increase. If the out-of-pocket price of health care is low enough, the individual might consume care up to the point at which $MC > MSV$. There is a net welfare loss in the healthcare market that occurs when the individual is ill and consumes too much health care. There are, then, two welfare effects of insurance: the welfare gain from shifting the risk and the welfare loss from consuming beyond the optimal point when the individual is ill. True optimality requires that both effects be considered simultaneously (Gianfrancesco, 1978). Usually, investigators focus on the insurance market (Gianfrancesco, 1983; Pauly, 1990) or the healthcare market (Pauly, 1972) in isolation from one another.

13.5 Extra-Welfarism

The framework used until now has included a number of value judgments and principles. A key principle in the previous analysis is that each individual is the best judge of personal welfare. Welfare, in this framework, depends exclusively on the utility of goods and services as valued by the individuals. If there is any "public" component of goods and services, it is introduced through external demand, which is the value some people place on other people's consumption. Beyond this, there is no justification for publicly provided health care that can be derived from the Paretean welfare framework.

The Paretean framework has come under criticism in recent years on the grounds that it does not include everything that people value in life (Culyer, 1990; Rice, 1992). There are other sources of personal well-being besides goods and services. Many of these other sources of well-being are embodied in the characteristics of individuals rather than the characteristics of the goods and services that individuals consume. Individuals value mobility, absence from pain, and absence from distress, and these characteristics are valued for other people as well. While it is true that there are goods and services (including health care) that are linked to these more altruistic sources of well-being, there is no automatic link between them. Consequently, a social evaluation based on goods and services consumed, and nothing else, appears to be too narrow or confining.

"Health" is often viewed as a composite of characteristics of individuals, such as mobility, absence of distress, and so forth. A number of economists have asserted that health is important, and not only because it is desired for ourselves. Individuals regard health as one of several goods and services that "society" recognizes should be made available to everyone (Culyer, 1991; Duckett, 2018; Malbon, Carey, & Meltzer, 2019; Saloner, 2018), regardless of willingness to pay. This position has often appeared in the healthcare literature (Blewett, Planalp, & Alarcon, 2018; Fein, 1972; Outka, 1974; White, 2018). If health really is a socially recognized good, then health *services* cannot be evaluated strictly in terms of their market value. In particular, the distribution of health services must be evaluated on a social basis (Gordon, 2019).

The researchers who hold the position that health care is a socially recognized good or service largely avoid the question of who will be the judge of welfare, a question directly addressed in the Paretean framework. These researchers merely assert that some decision maker, chosen (or elected) by society, should be responsible for conducting the evaluation. Thus, in this extra-welfarist viewpoint, it is no longer clear who the judge of welfare is. Indeed, extra-welfarism is consistent with the use of any social judge other than the consumers; the approach merely posits that there are some goods and services whose social value is determined outside of the consumers themselves. The role of economists is to act as advisors for the distributive organization and uncover the implications of incorporating efficiency and other objectives into the economic analysis. It should be pointed out that the direct evaluations by individuals of their healthcare services can be included in the extra-welfarist economic calculus, as can other (non-direct) evaluations of their health care.

The extra-welfarist position is concerned with how health is distributed among all members of society. Whoever the judge of well-being becomes (the government, a community league, etc.), value judgments must still be made in order to decide how to distribute healthcare goods and services and health. One way to operationalize the extra-welfarist approach (i.e., turn it into an evaluative tool) is to provisionally accept the principle that health care should be distributed according to "need."

If need is defined as the ability to benefit from health services (Culyer, 1995; Fulmer, Mate, & Berman, 2018; Gordon, 2019; King, 2017), then the "decision maker" is faced with the question of how to allocate health services so as to enhance or preserve different individuals' health status. Even if this approach evades the issue (or at least leaves the issue open) of who is to decide on the distribution, it helps make explicit the wide array of distributions that are possible (using the principle of need and other principles as well).

Figure 13-3 is a graph that illustrates the health status of two individuals, A and B, measured along the two axes (Wagstaff, 1991). This curve reflects the utility possibility frontier. The shape of the curve represents the reallocation of resources between the two individuals A and B. To illustrate, if all healthcare resources were allocated to B then B's health status could reach H_{bmax} and A's healthcare status would be at zero. Alternatively, if A received all the healthcare resources, then A's health status could reach H_{amax} and B's health status would be at zero. The outward bend of the curve H reflects the diminishing marginal utility as resources are transferred between the two individuals.

The following (nonvalue-laden) assumptions are made in this illustration: individual A has a self-assessed health status of h_1 and individual B has a self-assessed health status of h_2. The health status of both can be improved, but there is a limit to the resources available to provide health care. Curve H shows the maximum amount of health that can be produced with the finite resources available for health care (assumed to be fixed for society as a whole).

More health can be produced for A, but only at the expense of resources and a decrease in the health of B. With available resources, A's health can be increased up to h_x (with no change in B's health) and B's health can be increased up to h_y (with no change in A's health). The exact shape of the H curve will depend on how effective the additional resources are in improving each individual's health. If very little extra can be done to improve B's health, then the curve will be steeply sloped. The curve in this illustration shows that more can be done for both A and B with the resources available.

Mentioned previously was the principle that health resources should be distributed according to need. There are a number of different ways to express "need."

- *Equal health status.* One value judgment is to allocate resources so that everyone ends up with an equal level of health. If this principle is used, then more resources must be provided to A to ensure

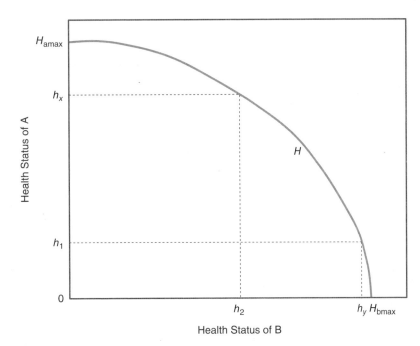

Figure 13-3 Potential health status of two individuals. The health status of A and the health status of B are currently h_1 and h_2, respectively. By expending more resources, their health status can move up to h_x and h_y, respectively. However, since the available resources are finite (limited), the limit of improvement for both individuals combined is shown by curve H.

© Jones & Bartlett Learning.

that, in the end, both A and B are equally healthy. Equal health implies that each person is on a 45° line from the origin.

- *Maximizing total health regardless of its distribution.* In order to implement this criterion, the trade-off in health status between the two individuals must be known. If the health transformation curve, H, favors person A, then resources will be more productive in improving A's health status rather than B's. An optimal point will occur on the H curve above the 45° line when A is favored. The characteristic of the optimal point will be where the additional health per dollar of expenditure will be the same for the two individuals.

- *Equalizing additional health per dollar.* This criterion is most like the Paretean optimum. According to this criterion, the initial starting point (h_1, h_2) is accepted and allocation of additional resources occurs so that the total health gain is as large as possible. The optimum point will at a position northeast (up and to the right) of the initial position on the transformation curve, H.

The usefulness of the extra-welfarist approach is that it allows going further in exploring resource allocation than the Paretean or welfarist position. If society places special importance on such characteristics as health, then alternative distributions of healthcare resources require very careful evaluation.

13.6 Concepts of Equity

Distributional equity is important in analyzing both access to and consumption of health care (e.g., differences in utilization of healthcare goods and services among groups of individuals) and its financing (e.g., differences in payments), and so it is essential to have measures of equity. The focus here is on three types of distributional equity: intergenerational equity, vertical equity, and horizontal equity (Long & Smeeding, 1984).

Intergenerational equity, in a financial context, concerns the distribution of payments among different generations of the population. To illustrate, if the population of the United States is divided into retirees (who are generally 65 or older and eligible for Medicare benefits), those of working age (say, those 18–64), and others, then the classification scheme could be regarded as dividing the population along generational lines. Because the Medicare hospital insurance program is financed largely through the flow of payroll taxes into the Hospital Insurance Trust Fund, these taxes will be borne largely by individuals in the working-age group. In other words, the working-age generation is largely financing the care of the generation of retirees.

The equity implications of this kind of tax are very different than those of the tax used to expand the Medicare program's benefits in 1988. This latter was a 15% tax on the taxable income of the retirees, and it proved to be so unpopular that the program expansion was quickly repealed by Congress. This last type of tax involves a minimal intergenerational transfer of funds. Taxing the income of retirees basically meant this group was financing (at least partially) their own utilization of healthcare services.

Current employment-based private health insurance provides another example of intergenerational transfer. All employees pay a similar health insurance premium, which is based on the average utilization pattern for all workers. According to insurance principles, if workers were rated separately by age group, younger workers would have a lower premium than older workers because their utilization is typically less. The financing method of charging everyone in the plan the same rate (community rating) is, in effect, intergenerationally inequitable.

The second type of equity, vertical equity, concerns the economic burden experienced by different income groups. For example, imagine there are three income groups: those who make under $40,000, those who make from $40,000 to $100,000, and those who make over $100,000. A tax is progressive if members of a higher-income group pay a larger portion of their income in tax than those with a lower-income; it is neutral if the portion is the same for all groups; and it is regressive if members of a lower income group pay a higher portion of their income in tax than those with a higher income.

An illustration of vertical inequity would be a flat tax charged to all individuals regardless of their income level. The original fixed premium for Medicare enrollees was such a tax. Lower-income groups paid the same rate as higher-income groups, and this premium therefore amounted to a higher portion of their income. Recent changes that modified the Medicare premiums to require individuals making above a certain income to pay a surcharge on their premiums has reduced the regressiveness of the Medicare premium somewhat.

Horizontal equity concerns the degree to which equals are taxed equally. An illustration of a horizontally inequitable tax is a tax on specific goods and services such as alcohol, tobacco products, and hospital care. Consumption, or sales, taxes on the former two products fall on groups who use these products more heavily than on nonusers. Such taxes have been a popular means of financing health insurance programs for certain groups of low-income populations. Even though these taxes are horizontally inequitable, it has been argued that because these lower-income individuals are likely to be less

healthy and use the healthcare system more, they should pay higher taxes. That is, if not just taxes but rather the net of healthcare services minus taxes paid are considered, then horizontal *inequity* is not present.

Another type of tax that has been recommended as a way to pay for health care for low-income individuals is a tax on hospital admissions. Such a tax will also be inequitable, although to a large extent it will be less visible because it will be passed on to the third parties who reimburse the providers. (Of course, the insurers in turn will pass the tax on by charging higher health insurance premiums to individuals.)

13.7 Goals of Health Policy

There are a number of different ways that the goals of health policy can be articulated. At one level, a set of environmental conditions can be articulated that will allow for a smoother operating policy. To illustrate, many individuals believe that if consumers are given a range of health plans from which to select, and the freedom to choose among those plans, then social goals will be advanced. At a lower, operational level, there are goals that deal with operating performance, such as efficiency, equity, and public financial constraints.

Finally, social goals can be articulated in terms of the health outcomes of a group of individuals. In order for the policy goal to be operational, policies will still have to specify how each person's health status is to be included (e.g., whether everyone is counted the same). In addition, the policy makers should take into account the economic aspects of the policy goals. There are insufficient resources to allow everyone to maximize their health status, therefore goals have to be set that allow one to rank social measures of health status resulting from different policies.

One option might be to combine policy goals from the different categories mentioned. To illustrate, a policy maker might deem equity of resource use to be important. However, once individuals have equal resources available to them (e.g., through spending vouchers), the policy maker might value freedom of choice to allow individuals to select those types of care that they feel would best suit them. As another example, a policy maker might value a population's health status highly but also want to ensure technical efficiency is achieved. The policy maker would select policies that would promote both objectives. Each of the goals is discussed briefly in the following section.

13.7.1 Environmental Conditions

A competitive market is an institution in which free choice is exercised by the participants who are in pursuit of their own well-being. A social goal that falls under this category is allowing individuals the freedom to seek enrollment in the health plan of their choice. A component could also include a condition that any qualified individual or group who wants to provide health services to the enrollees may do so. Generally, healthcare market opportunities are not extended to everyone who desires to be a provider, through requirements of licensing and certification. These requirements are a reflection of other policy goals, such as the protection of quality and individuals, that are included.

13.7.2 Efficiency

In order to achieve economic efficiency, (1) demand must be at an appropriate level, neither too restrictive (e.g., because of monopolistic prices) nor too low (such that there will be an excessive demand); and (2) providers must produce an adequate supply of services, (3) at an appropriate quality level, and (4) at a low cost of production. Without these conditions being met, the market will not achieve economic efficiency.

13.7.2.1 Demand Barriers

Demand barriers are impediments to receiving health care. Within the context of the market model, price is the prime impediment limiting access to health care. As a result of the price barrier, additional care demanded can be encouraged by lowering the direct price of healthcare services through the purchase of insurance, through public programs, or through charity. To the degree that additional healthcare utilization is thought to be desirable, the extent of financial demand barriers can be measured by the availability of insurance or the direct price faced by individuals.

However, money price is not the only factor related to demand barriers. Waiting costs and travel costs can also obstruct access to health care. If healthcare consumption is to be encouraged, these nonmonetary costs must be addressed, either through subsidies, relocating facilities to lower travel time and expenses, or expanding facilities and increasing operating hours to decrease waiting time. However, it should be remembered that, from an efficiency standpoint, demand can be too great as well as insufficient.

13.7.2.2 Adequacy of Supply

Adequacy of supply refers to the availability of sufficient resources to provide health care at the efficient level (given the desired level of quality). Adequacy of supply depends on the incentive (payment) system developed, the level of payment, and the adequacy of funds. Adequacy of supply also depends on the entry restrictions faced by individuals desiring to become providers

13.7.2.3 Technical Efficiency

Technical efficiency is a measure of the cost of producing a given level and quality of output. Technical efficiency is usually expressed in terms of monetary costs, but care must be taken when comparing costs among facilities to be sure that all other factors (e.g., quality, input prices, and case mix) have been taken into consideration.

13.7.2.4 Quality of Care

On the assumption that quality is not free, it costs more to achieve a higher quality of care. Therefore, like any other characteristic of output, quality can come in too great or too little a quantity. Quality of care is an often-cited policy goal in health care. Regulation and licensing of professionals are often enacted in the name of the protection of quality of care.

13.7.3 Equity

Equity is a very broad concept. Two aspects of equity are considered here: equity of utilization and equity of finance.

13.7.3.1 Equity of Utilization

A service can be provided efficiently, and yet some individuals who could benefit from more of the service simply cannot afford to pay for it. Society or policy makers can set utilization goals above those provided in a market situation. In this case, the direct price or other barriers to care must be reduced or removed. Thus, some efficiency may be lost in order to attain a higher degree of equity.

13.7.3.2 Equity of Finance

Equity of finance can refer to direct out-of-pocket prices as well as taxation and premiums, factors that may not directly affect utilization. Healthcare premiums may be deemed too low, in which case some individuals would be viewed as not paying a fair portion of the cost of health care. Equity of finance would call for an increase in these premiums.

13.7.3.3 Public Financial Constraints

Strictly speaking, the government budget does not fall within the scope of this model. Of course, a transfer of funds from A to B is consistent with a tax on A by a government body and subsequent expenditures on health care for B. But the model says nothing about the size of the tax, the expenditure, or the contribution of excess expenditures over taxes to the budget deficit. In recent years, however, the budget deficit and public spending have come under a great deal of scrutiny, and cutbacks in government programs have been widespread. Typically, the rationale for cutting a program's expenditures is not lack of worthiness of the program but the program's contribution to the overall budget deficit.

To the extent that cutbacks in government programs can be achieved merely through increases in technical efficiency, true savings are provided to society, and there are gains in social efficiency. However, cutbacks may also result in reduced supply and availability of healthcare goods and services. This is not necessarily undesirable if output was greater than the socially optimum level originally. However, if the initial output was at the socially optimum level or below it, cutbacks will lead to reductions in social efficiency because the value of the output that is lost is greater than the savings resulting from the cutbacks.

13.7.3.4 Health Status of the Population

In recent years, many investigators have focused on population-based measures of health status as a goal of policy. Many of the other goals can be viewed as leading to better health, and so these investigators focus on direct measures of health as a policy objective. Of course, the costs of achieving various levels of health status must be considered as well. Thus, the system is confronted with the constrained objective of maximizing population health subject to resource constraints. Additionally, focusing on this goal does not do away with equity considerations. Once there is more than one individual whose health is measured, the problem of how to sum the health status of all the individuals is encountered. These problems have been discussed in this chapter, and they need to be addressed in any policy consideration.

Exercises

1. In a world of completely selfish individuals, if each person's marginal value for own health care could be measured, what conditions must be met in order for the healthcare market to be at an optimal level of output?
2. What is meant by the socially optimal level of health care?
3. In a society with two persons, if one is altruistic and values the other's use of health care, how will this influence the socially optimal quantity of health care that is produced.
4. What is a consumption externality for health care?
5. Will a freely competitive market without philanthropy yield a socially optimal output when there are consumption externalities?
6. If individuals are fully insured for all healthcare services, will this necessarily result in a socially optimal amount of insurance coverage?
7. List and discuss five goals of health policy.
8. Given the following marginal valuation (MV) information, what is the optimal allocation of care according to the Paretean criteria, when the marginal cost of care is constant at $400.

A's Quantity of Care Consumed	A's Marginal Value (MV) (\$)	B's Quantity of Care Consumed	B's Marginal Value (MV) (\$)	Marginal Cost (\$)
1	350	1	300	400
2	300	2	240	400
3	255	3	184	400

4	215	4	132	400
5	180	5	84	400
6	150	6	40	400
7	125	7	0	400
8	105	8	0	400
9	95	9	0	400

Bibliography

Blewett, L. A., Planalp, C., & Alarcon, G. (2018). Affordable care act impact in Kentucky: Increasing access, reducing disparities. *American Journal of Public Health, 108*(7), 929.

Culyer, A. J. (1990). Commodities, characteristics of commodities, characteristics of people, utilities, and the quality of life. In S. Baldwin, C. Godfrey, & C. Propper (Eds.), *Quality of life: Perspectives and problems* (pp. 9–27). London, England: Routledge.

Culyer, A. J. (1991). *Health, health expenditures and equity*. Working Papers 083chedp, Centre for Health Economics, University of York.

Culyer, A. J. (1995). *Equality of what in health policy? Conflicts between the contenders* (Discussion Paper No. 142). York, England: University of York, Center for Health Economics.

Duckett, S. (2018). Expanding the breadth of Medicare: Learning from Australia. *Health Economics, Policy & Law, 13*(3–4), 344–368.

Fein, R. (1972). On achieving access and equity in health care. *The Milbank Quarterly, 50*(4, Pt. 2), 157–190.

Fulmer, T., Mate, K. S., & Berman, A. (2018). The age-friendly health system imperative. *Journal of the American Geriatrics Society, 66*(1), 24.

Gianfrancesco, F. D. (1978). Insurance and medical care expenditure: An analysis of the optimal relationship. *Eastern Economics Journal, 4*, 225–234.

Gianfrancesco, F. D. (1983). A proposal for improving the efficiency of medical insurance. *Journal of Health Economics, 2*, 175–184.

Gordon, D. D. (2019). Medicare for all should not be one size fits all. *Managed Care, 28*(5), 44–46.

King, M. W. (2017). Health care efficiencies: Consolidation and alternative models vs. health care and antitrust regulations–Irreconcilable differences? *American Journal of Law and Medicine, 43*(4), 426–467.

Long, S. H., & Smeeding, T. M. (1984). Alternative Medicare financing sources. *Milbank Quarterly, 62*, 325–348.

Malbon, E., Carey, G., & Meltzer, A. (2019). Personalisation schemes in social care: Are they growing social and health inequalities? *BMC Public Health, 19*(1), 805.

Mechanic, D. (1976). Rationing health care. *Hastings Center Report, 9*(1), 34–37.

Orzechowski, P. E. (2018). The case for a private healthcare insurance monopoly. *Applied Health Economics & Health Policy, 16*(4), 433–443.

Outka, G. (1974). Social justice and equal access to health care. *Journal of Religious Ethics, 2*, 11–32.

Pauly, M. V. (1972). *Medical care at public expense*. New York, NY: Praeger.

Pauly, M. V. (1990). The rational nonpurchase of long-term-care insurance. *Journal of Political Economy, 98*, 153–168.

Rice, T. (1992). An alternative framework for evaluating welfare losses in the health care market. *Journal of Health Economics, 11*, 85–92.

Saloner, B. (2018). Medicaid expansion, chronic disease, and the next chapter of health reform. *Journal of General Internal Medicine, 33*(3), 243–244.

Schulman, K. A., & Milstein, A. (2019). The implications of "Medicare for All" for US hospitals. *JAMA, 321*(17), 1661–1662.

Wagstaff, A. (1991). QALYs and the equity-efficiency trade-off. *Journal of Health Economics, 10*, 21–41.

White, J. (2018). Drawing lessons from Canada's experience with single-payer health insurance. *JAMA Internal Medicine, 178*(9), 1255–1257.

CHAPTER 14

Financing Health Care

OBJECTIVES

1. Identify alternative sources of healthcare funding in the United States.
2. Describe the effects of financing health care through insurance premiums, tax subsidies, and mandated benefits.
3. Compare the effects of financing by insurance premiums, payroll taxes, sales taxes, and income taxes.
4. Discuss the administrative cost of public and private financing mechanisms.
5. Describe the effects of alternative ways of reimbursing providers for services provided.

14.1 Introduction

This chapter examines, conceptually and empirically, the growth in healthcare expenditures and the sources of financing of those expenditures. As spending on healthcare goods and services continues to increase, concerns are increasingly expressed about the increase. It is important to distinguish between absolute expenditures and the relative amount of expenditures on health care. Preliminary estimates indicate that in 2018, the United States spent $3.65 trillion on health care, an increase of 4.4% over 2017. This amount of spending translates into $11,212 per capita, and 17.8% of the gross domestic product (GDP).

The concern should not be focused on the absolute size of spending in the healthcare sector ($3.65 trillion), but rather on the increasing share of total output that the healthcare sector is consuming (17.8% of GDP). As a larger share of total output goes to the healthcare sector, there are fewer resources available for the production of other goods and services in the economy. As a healthcare sector's percent of GDP increases, questions are increasingly being asked about the relative value of the goods and services produced and whether the population might be better off if the resources were reallocated to other sectors. While the United States spends more per capita and a higher

percent of its GDP on healthcare goods and services than any other country, the health status of its population is far from the best. As a result, attention is focused on alternative ways of financing healthcare services in order to try to reduce the rate of increase in spending.

The growth in healthcare spending has implications for the financing of those expenditures and its sustainability. There are three major methods of financing healthcare services—out-of-pocket payments by the consumers, insurance premiums, and taxation—and within each category there are a number of different financing techniques. Out-of-pocket payments by consumers include amounts the insured population pays for deductibles, copayments, coinsurance, and payments for services not covered, and the uninsured are responsible for all services utilized, even though some of the costs of those services become uncompensated care by the providers. Insurance premiums can be paid directly by the consumer, employer, governments, or a combination. Also, taxes can be levied on income or on specific products or services to finance health care. Further, the different financing methods can interact: insurance premiums can be excluded from taxation (as is the case in the United States) or can be taxed; they can be part of a compensation package of employees, or purchased individually with after-tax dollars.

Each method of financing healthcare services will impact differently on groups of the population with different characteristics, such as income level or family size. Determining how the burden of each financing method will fall is not a simple or straightforward matter. To illustrate, the burden of insurance premiums that are paid out of pocket by consumers falls on the consumers directly, but income taxes can influence this burden. When insurance is obtained through the workplace (as is often the case in the United States), the burden of payment is far from clear. Furthermore, different kinds of taxes will have different impacts on different groups within the population, especially due to variations in income levels.

Economic analysis can be a very useful tool for assessing the effects of these various finance methods. The first part of this chapter examines how explanatory economics can be used to analyze the burden of the various financing methods. How these various financing methods can be assessed in terms of specific criteria or policy objectives is also discussed.

Different financing methods can also have substantially different costs. In the case of private insurance, the insurance company will incur the costs of marketing, rating alternative consumer groups, paying providers, and monitoring and enforcing utilization. In the case of government financing, there are the costs of collecting taxes and administering public programs. A debate continues to occur in the United States over whether healthcare coverage for the population should be financed primarily through private markets (with appropriate subsidies when necessary) or through public financing. This chapter illustrates how economic analysis can be used to compare these options.

14.2 Insurance Terminology

A brief discussion of basic insurance concepts and terminology is presented before analyzing the financing of health care. An understanding of these insurance concepts is important since these various concepts also have implications for the variety of methods for financing health care and the burden of healthcare costs.

When utilizing healthcare services, consumers may pay various amounts toward the medical bill associated with those services. Many insurance packages require the consumer to pay a *deductible* before insurance pays anything. This deductible is a flat, or fixed, amount that must be paid by the consumer before the insurance company begins to pay all or part of the remaining amount. To illustrate, an insurance package may require the beneficiary to pay the first $1000 of medical expenses each year before the insurance pays anything.

The use of deductibles has an impact on the administrative costs of the insurance company. Since a deductible eliminates the processing of claims for small amounts, the transaction costs associated with paying small claims are avoided. The higher the deductible the consumer must pay, the fewer the claims that will need to be processed by the insurance company. However, the use of deductibles, especially high deductibles, may be a deterrent to accessing needed medical care for some beneficiaries. In addition, the use of deductibles creates a greater burden on lower-income individuals than on higher-income individuals since the deductible represents a larger percentage of total income for the lower-income beneficiary. Also, if the only feature of the plan is the deductible, then the out-of-pocket cost to the beneficiary drops to zero once the deductible is met. This raises the possibility of overuse of healthcare services once the deductible is met since the consumer faces a zero price in the demand for health care.

Another common feature of insurance is the use of a *copayment*, which requires the beneficiary to pay a fixed amount each time a service is used. To illustrate, an insurance package may require the beneficiary to pay $20 each time a visit is made to a primary care physician, $50 each time a visit is made to a specialist, $75 each time a visit is made to an urgent care clinic, and $150 for each visit to an emergency room. A copayment places similar burdens on lower-income individuals as deductibles since they represent a larger portion of the individual's income. A copayment would not have the same impact on administrative costs as deductibles to the insurer because copayments do not necessarily reduce the number of claims filed.

Coinsurance requires the beneficiary to pay a specified percentage of the price of the medical service, and the insurance company pays the balance. To illustrate, an insurance package may require the individual to pay 20% of the price after any deductible and the insurance company will pay 80%; the copayment amount is not included in the price of the service considered by the insurance company. Assuming that the price of the medical encounter was $1000, if the beneficiary had a $500 deductible and 20% coinsurance rate, then the beneficiary would have to pay $600 ($1000 − $500 + [$500 × 0.2] = $600) and the insurance company would pay $400 ($1000 − $500 − [$500 × 0.8]) = $400. Since the deductible is subtracted from the price of the service first, the insurance company does not pay the full stated percent of the price of the service.

A coinsurance feature lowers the price of the covered medical care by the percentage the insurance company pays; in this case, it lowers the price to the consumer by 80% after the deductible. A coinsurance feature reduces the price of the service, but still provides an incentive to be a cost-conscious consumer, because the consumer pays a percentage of whatever the price is. The actual impact will depend on the price elasticity of demand of the consumer—the more price elastic, the greater the impact on demand.

Many insurance plans included a "stop-loss" feature, which sets an upper limit on the amount the consumer will have to pay. This reduces the risk of a serious medical condition resulting in a catastrophic loss to the individual. To illustrate, an insurance package may contain the provision that once out-of-pocket expenditures of the individual reach a specified amount (e.g., $10,000), then the insurance company will pay all remaining medical expenses associated with covered services. The stop-loss feature is typically an annual condition.

While stop-loss features apply to beneficiaries, insurance companies seek protection by setting maximums and limits. To illustrate, the insurance package may specify a *maximum* annual amount it will cover, such as $250,000 of medical care or 60 days of hospital care. The policy may also contain lifetime *limits* that the insurance company will pay for medical expenses incurred by an individual, such as a limit of $5 million for covered services by the individual. These maximums and limits are not reached by most individuals. However, the presence of the feature can raise the fear that medical bankruptcy is a possibility, even for individuals with good health insurance coverage.

The two basic methods of establishing insurance premiums are *community rating* and *experience rating*. Under the community rating method, all enrollees in the plan are charged the same premium. Even community rating is usually separated into two rates—one covers individuals (single coverage) and the other provides family coverage. Under community rating, high users of healthcare services in the insurance plan are subsidized by low users of healthcare services. If the low users determine that the premiums are too high for the benefits they receive, these individuals may simply drop coverage and become uninsured. Also, the redistribution of resources from low users of healthcare services to high users may actually result in the transfer of income from low-income individuals to high-income

individuals because income level is not considered in establishing the premium. This transfer of income from low-income to high-income individuals is in conflict with most income redistribution policies.

Experience rating relies upon the characteristics of groups of individuals or upon the prior experiences of those groups in establishing the premium to be charged. As a result, different groups within the plan are charged different rates depending upon their expected use of healthcare services. Under this method, individuals possessing characteristics associated with low risk are charged a lower premium for the same package of covered services than other groups with characteristics associated with higher use. Under the experience rating method, the *medical loss ratio*, benefits paid out divided by the premium for each of the groups, is close to 1.0. The loading fee charged for plans using the experience rating may be higher than plans using the community rating because of the administrative costs of determining into which group an individual will be classified. A loading fee is the amount above the pure premium (amount of medical claims paid) that the insurance company charges to cover such things as marketing expenses, administration, claims processing, reserves, and profits.

14.3 Financing Means and Burdens in the United States

Currently, in the United States, a variety of financing mechanisms are used in health care. These mechanisms and the amounts raised through each are shown in **Table 14-1**. As can be seen, a total of $3.492 trillion was spent on health care in 2017. Of this amount, $365.55 billion (about 10.47%) was financed by out-of-pocket payments by consumers. In comparison, in 1965, consumers financed about 43.5% of expenditures out of pocket.

A total of $1.139 trillion (33.9%) was financed through private health insurance in 2017, compared to 23.8% in 1965. A reason for using 1965 as a comparative base is because that was the last full year before the two major government health insurance programs (Medicare and Medicaid) were implemented. Medicare coverage began in January 1966, covering most individuals age 65 and older. Medicaid coverage began in July 1966, covering certain low-income individuals. Medicaid provided coverage to pregnant women, young children, and certain individuals with disabilities with low income. Medicaid did not cover single individuals regardless of income level.

Table 14-1 Sources of Funds for National Health Expenditures, 1965 and 2017

Source of Funds	1965 (in millions of $)	1965 (%)	2017 (in millions of $)	2017 (%)
Private Funds				
Out-of-pocket	18,262	43.50	365,455	10.47
Private health insurance	10,000	23.80	1,183,910	33.90
Other private	694	1.70	–	0.00
Total private funds	*28,956*	69.00	*1,549,365*	44.37
Public Funds				
Medicare		0.00	705,859	20.21
Medicaid				
Federal	–	0.00	361,245	10.34
State and Local	–	0.00	220,619	6.32
CHIP				
Federal	–	0.00	16,594	0.48
State and Local	–	0.00	1,600	0.05
Department of Defense	831	2.00	42,257	1.21
Veterans Affairs	1,120	2.70	72,134	2.07
Other Third-Party Payers				
Worksite Health Care	–		6,914	0.20
Other Private Revenue	–		142,024	4.07
Indian Health Services	–	0.00	3,971	0.11
Workers Compensation	870	2.10	47,396	1.36
General Assistance	122	0.30	5,898	0.17
Maternal/Child Health				
Federal	80	0.20	569	0.02
State and Local	164	0.40	3,203	0.09
Vocational Rehabilitation				
Federal	27	0.10	421	0.01
State and Local	15	0.00	125	0.00
SAMHSA	–	0.00	4,204	0.12
Other Federal Programs	831	2.00	12,023	0.34
Other State and Local	3,389	8.10	33,849	0.97
School Health	168	0.40	5,254	0.15
Public Health Activity				
Federal	214	0.50	13,309	0.38
State and Local	407	1.00	75,625	2.17
Research	1,521	3.60	50,710	1.45
Structures and Programs	3,244	7.70	116,911	3.35
Total Public Funds	*13,001*	31.00	*1,942,714*	55.63
TOTAL HEALTH	*41,957*	100.00	*3,492,077*	100.00

Centers for Medicare & Medicaid Services. National health expenditures by type of service and source of funds, calendar years, 1960–2017. Retrieved from https://www.cms.gov/Research-Statistics -Data-and-Systems/Statistics-Trends-and-Reports/NationalHealthExpendData/index.html?redirect=/NationalHealthExpendData/02_NationalHealthAccountsHistorical.asp#TopOfPage

The percentage of the under-65 population covered by private health insurance declined between 2003 (at 68.9%) and 2010 (at 61.7%) but had increased again to 65.7% in 2017. The majority of the population with private health insurance receive coverage through employment-based insurance (58.2% of the under-65 population, or 88.6% of the privately insured population), with 11.4% of the privately insured purchasing individual policies (Cohen, 2018; DeNavas-Wait, Proctor, & Smith, 2011).

As illustrated in **Table 14-2**, for individuals with employer-based coverage, employers financed 82.8% of the $6896 of premiums for single coverage employees in 2018 and 71.7% of the $19,616 for family coverage. Between 1999 and 2018, both the premiums for insurance coverage and the percentage of

premiums paid by the employee increased. As a result, the employee's cost for single coverage increased from $318 in 1999 to $1186 in 2018, and the employee's cost for family coverage increased from $1543 to $5547 during that period (Claxton, Rae, Long, Damico, & Whitmore, 2018).

As shown by the data presented in Table 14-2 with regard to health insurance provided through the workplace, the majority of the premiums are paid for by employers, with a smaller amount being paid for directly by employees. However, this does not mean that the employers bear the burden of the majority of the health insurance expenses. For one thing, premiums paid for by employers are workplace benefits that are not subject to income tax. Therefore, there is a sizable public subsidy given to employees who

Table 14-2 Average Annual Premiums and Average Annual Worker Premium Contributions Paid by Covered Worker for Single and Family Coverage, 1999–2018

Year	Single Coverage ($)	Single Paid by Worker ($)	Paid by Single Worker (%)	Family Coverage ($)	Family Paid by Worker ($)	Paid by Family Worker (%)
1999	2,196	318	14.5	5,791	1,543	26.6
2000	2,471	334	13.5	6,438	1,619	25.1
2001	2,689	355	13.2	7,061	1,787	25.3
2002	3,083	466	15.1	8,003	2,137	26.7
2003	3,383	508	15.0	9,068	2,412	26.6
2004	3,695	558	15.1	9,950	2,661	26.7
2005	4,024	610	15.2	10,880	2,713	24.9
2006	4,242	627	14.8	11,480	2,973	25.9
2007	4,479	694	15.5	12,106	3,281	27.1
2008	4,704	721	15.3	12,680	3,354	26.5
2009	4,824	779	16.1	13,375	3,515	26.3
2010	5,049	899	17.8	13,770	3,997	29.0
2011	5,429	921	17.0	15,073	4,129	27.4
2012	5,615	951	16.9	15,735	4,316	27.4
2013	5,884	999	17.0	18,351	4,585	25.0
2014	6,025	1081	17.9	16,834	4,823	28.7
2015	6,251	1071	17.1	17,545	4,995	28.5
2016	6,435	1129	17.5	18,142	5,277	29.1
2017	6,690	1213	18.1	18,764	5,714	30.5
2018	6,896	1186	17.2	19,616	5,547	28.3

2018 Employer Health Benefits Survey. Retrieved from https://www.kff.org/report-section/2018-employer-health-benefits-survey-summary-of-findings/

obtain their insurance in this way; their taxes will be lower than if their premiums were taxed at the same rate as their wages. In addition, there is considerable evidence that when all the wage effects are taken into account, the employees do indeed bear a major share of these premium costs through lower direct wages, even if it does not appear that way initially.

The third form of finance that is used is public finance, or programs funded through taxation. In 2017, over $1.94 trillion (55.3%) of total financing for health care involved public programs compared to 31.0% in 1965. Most of this 2017 amount (66.3%) went to pay for the federal Medicare program, which covers individuals 65 and over, those totally and permanently disabled, and those with certain diseases, and the joint federal-state Medicaid program, which is primarily for certain categories of lower-income groups. These two programs are largely, but not entirely, financed by taxation.

With regard to taxation, the major federal tax that pays for the hospital portion (Part A) of Medicare is a payroll tax of 2.9% of all wages, paid equally (1.45%) by employers and employees; self-employed individuals pay the full amount of 2.9%. As of January 2013, individuals filing jointly pay an additional 0.9% on income greater than $250,000 and single individuals pay the additional 0.9% on incomes over $200,000. The employers' tax rate did not increase from 1.45%. In addition, there is a Medicare "premium" paid by enrolled beneficiaries for medical care (physician services) and health maintenance organization (Part B) coverage, which was $135.50 per month in 2019. This $135.50 is a base rate that applies to single

individuals with an income of $85,000 or less and to beneficiaries filing jointly with income of $170,000 or less. **Table 14-3** provides information on the premiums for individuals with incomes above these levels.

Most of the remainder of the federal portion of healthcare expenditures was raised through general taxation, the largest portion from direct income taxation. Of the $1.94 trillion spent by governments on health care, $335.0 billion was raised through state government taxation. Most state taxation is in the form of direct income and indirect sales taxes.

Table 14-1 provides an indication of the sources of the money spent on health care, but Table 14-1 cannot be used directly to assess the "burden" of healthcare financing (defined as the reduction in real income due to payments and taxes). The complexity of the situation and the prominent role played by each of the financing methods calls for a much more detailed analysis. Each financing method imposes different burdens on different groups of the population. The pattern of these burdens will be discussed after examining the burdens from a positive economic perspective.

14.4 Economic Analysis of Alternative Payment Sources

This section presents economic analyses of alternative payment methods. The focus of the analyses is the economic impact of the payment methods on the resource owners (primarily employees and owners of

Table 14-3 Total Medicare Part B Monthly Premiums, 2019

Beneficiaries Who File Individual Tax Returns with Income	Beneficiaries Who File Joint Tax Returns with Income	Income-Related Monthly Adjusted Amount ($)	Total Monthly Premium Amount ($)
Less than or equal to $85,000	Less than or equal to $170,000	0.00	135.50
Greater than $85,000 and less than or equal to $107,000	Greater than $170,000 and less than or equal to $214,000	54.10	189.60
Greater than $107,000 and less than or equal to $133,500	Greater than $214,000 and less than or equal to $267,000	135.40	270.90
Greater than $133,500 and less than or equal to $160,000	Greater than $267,000 and less than or equal to $320,000	216.70	352.20
Greater than $160,000 and less than $500,000	Greater than $320,000 and less than $750,000	297.90	433.40
Greater than or equal to $500,000	Greater than or equal to $750,000	325.00	460.50

CMS.gov. 2019 Medicare Parts A and B premiums and deductibles. *Fact Sheet.* Retrieved October 12, 2018, from https://www.cms.gov/newsroom/fact-sheets/2019-medicare-parts-b-premiums-and-deductibles.

companies). Insurance premiums (in particular, the impact of employer-paid premiums, taxation, and mandated benefits) and taxation (the impact of payroll and sales taxes) are examined.

A primary question relates to the economic impact of a tax, that is, who actually ends up bearing the economic burden. The group that bears the burden of the tax may not be the same group from which the tax was originally collected. To illustrate, a government tax on cigarettes may be collected from tobacco retailers (sellers). However, to the extent that prices of tobacco products are higher because of the tax, the economic burden is on the users of the tobacco, who pay the higher price.

14.4.1 Private Health Insurance

14.4.1.1 Insurance Premiums

Private health insurance can be obtained through the workplace or by direct individual purchase. Health insurance obtained in the workplace can be paid for directly by the employees (through payroll deductions from after-tax dollars), by the employers, or by a combination of employees and employers. There is no controversy over the burden of premiums paid by employees or by individuals; the purchasers bear the cost of their insurance purchases.

The economic burden of employer-paid premiums is more complicated. The cost of insurance benefit packages is viewed by employers as an expense, much like wages are. An employer has a demand curve for labor and will regard the costs of various forms of compensation as monetarily equivalent. To illustrate, if the marginal employee is worth (has a marginal value of) $100 to the employer, then the employer will be willing to pay up to $100 in compensation to the individual, whether the payment is in the form of wages or fringe benefits or a combination (Kreuger & Reinhardt, 1994). If benefits are increased, then the employer will reduce monetary wages. Thus, the economic burden of all health insurance benefits will fall on the employee, either directly (out of pocket) or indirectly (through a lower wage).

14.4.1.2 Taxation and Insurance Premiums

Preferential tax treatment is provided for health insurance that is obtained through the workplace. Both the employer and the employee benefit from payments and contributions made in this system. When the employer pays all or part of the insurance premium for the employees, the employer's payments are excluded from income and payroll taxes the employer pays. In most cases, the amount that the employees pay for their share of the premium is also excluded from income and payroll taxes. In addition, contributions that employers make to certain accounts for employees, such as flexible spending arrangements (FSAs), health reimbursement arrangements (HRAs), and health savings accounts (HSAs), to pay for employee healthcare costs are excluded from income and payroll taxes as well. On average, individuals that receive higher incomes and more expensive health insurance plans receive larger subsidies. It is estimated that the subsidy cost the federal government about $300 billion in foregone revenue in 2018 (CBO, 2018).

Health insurance benefits paid by the employer are exempt from personal income and the payroll taxes of the employee. This reduces the cost to the employee of employer-paid health insurance and increases the quantity demanded for health insurance. However, it cannot be assumed that once a subsidy is put into place, that the quantity demanded and supplied in the insurance market will remain the same. To see why, consider the analysis of a tax subsidy provided in the following illustration.

In **Figure 14-1**, the initial demand curve for health insurance (with no tax subsidies) is D_1. According to this curve, when the premium rate is $1000, a total of 75 individuals will be willing to shift their risks to health insurers. According to the supply curve for insurance (represented by S in Figure 14-1), insurers will be willing to supply 75 insurance policies to individuals at the rate of $1000, and the market is in equilibrium at a quantity of 75 and a price of $1000.

Assume that a 50% subsidy is introduced in the market. The effect of the subsidy is to lower the out-of-pocket price for insurance at every premium rate to potential demanders. Thus, at a premium rate of $1000, the out-of-pocket price to the consumer is now $500, and at this price an additional 25 individuals will be willing to shift their risks to the insurer and purchase an insurance policy, and so the quantity demanded will now be 100 policies. The market demand curve will shift out to D_2.

When demand shifts out to D_2, there is excess quantity demanded from the 25 additional individuals seeking insurance in the subsidized market. In this illustration, interactions will occur in the market forcing changes in the price until a new equilibrium is reached at which insurers are willing to supply 92 policies at a price of $1350 and 92 individuals are willing to pay their 50% of the new subsidized price. Generally, a higher supplier price will be required to induce the insurers to accept more risks.

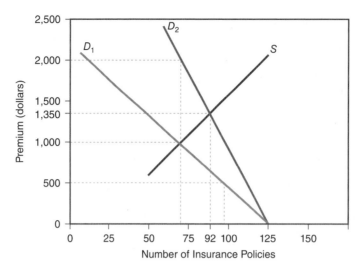

Figure 14-1 Effects of a subsidy on quantity of health insurance. D_1 represents the demand curve for insurance without a subsidy; S represents the supply curve of insurance, and D_2 represents the demand curve with a $500 subsidy for purchasing insurance.

A more detailed explanation of the changes that occur in the illustration is provided here. Initially, assume that there is no tax subsidy for the purchase of insurance. Then 75 risks will be shifted (or individuals insured) at a premium rate of $1000. This is the equilibrium price and quantity as shown in Figure 14-1. Using this position as a base point, a subsidy on premiums of 50% is introduced, reflecting that, the individuals are in a 50% income tax bracket and are allowed to deduct insurance premiums before calculating income taxes (for simplicity, the influence of the payroll taxes is ignored).

A preliminary analysis of the effects of the subsidy indicates that the premium price would remain the same ($1000), but half would be paid ($500) out of pocket by the consumer and the other half would fall on taxpayers (because the individual would get a subsidy of $500 lower taxable income so taxes would be decreased that could have been used to fund a public program). An economic analysis would result in a conclusion that the new quantity on which the subsidy will be based is not the old quantity demanded at a premium of $1000 nor the new quantity demanded at the $500 out-of-pocket cost.

As shown in Figure 14-1, the subsidy raises the quantity demanded at each price, and so more individuals will seek to shift risks at the subsidized premium rate of $1000. However, suppliers (insurers) will require higher premiums in order to accept more risks (issue more policies). The premium rate will rise, and fewer risks (policies issued) will be shifted than were originally indicated by demand conditions alone. In the illustration, the final premium rate will be $1350, and at this price, risks of 92 individuals will be shifted through insurance policies.

The cost of the new premium will be borne half by the consumer and half by the taxpayers under the 50% subsidy assumption. However, the amount of subsidy will be based on the new price of $1350. And the quantity of risks shifted will be the new equilibrium quantity. The final equilibrium (and the burden of the subsidy) will depend on the elasticities of demand and supply. In the extreme, if the supply curve were vertical, indicating no change in risks shifted, then the analysis would indicate that the premium would rise by the full amount of the subsidy. In this extreme case, the taxpayers would pay a subsidy of $1000 based on a new premium of $2000, with the risk of 75 individuals still being shifted. Alternatively, if the supply curve is horizontal, indicating an unlimited supply of risks accepted (policies issued) at a price of $1000, the consumer would get a full $500 subsidy paid for by the taxpayers; in this case, 100 risks would be shifted.

The analysis in this illustration does not take into account subsequent effects of the increased insurance coverage on the healthcare market. Nevertheless, even this simple analysis indicates that the demand-and-supply analysis should be considered when determining the full effects of a tax subsidy on health insurance premiums.

14.4.1.3 Mandated Benefits

Mandated insurance benefits are government-required coverage benefits that individuals must privately purchase or employers must provide. Mandated benefits can have a considerable impact on labor markets depending on how they are viewed by consumers, and this impact will, in turn, affect the incidence of benefits. The Affordable Care Act of 2003 mandated health insurance coverage for individuals in the United States, and those individuals that did not purchase health insurance would be assessed a penalty. Certain individuals were excluded from the penalty if their income was below the threshold for filing a federal income tax return ($10,400 for an individual or $20,800 for a family in 2017), or if an individual or family had to pay more than 8.16% of income for health insurance in 2017 after taking into account any employer contributions or tax credits. Individuals were eligible for a hardship exemption if an application for Medicaid was filed but it was determined to be ineligible due to the state's decision not to expand the program. As of 2019, the penalty would no longer be assessed although coverage is still mandated.

An illustration of an economic analysis of mandated benefits using a labor market analysis is presented in **Figure 14-2**. In the initial situation, there are no mandated benefits and the employer does not provide insurance benefits. In this situation, the demand for labor is shown as D_1, and the supply of labor is shown as $S_{v\,=\,0}$; equilibrium wages are at $80, and equilibrium employment is at 300 workers.

Assume in the illustration that an initial wage of $60 was paid per worker and then mandated insurance benefits that cost $20 per worker are introduced. In terms of total compensation, the employer's demand curve for labor will remain the same because the employer will still value each worker's productivity the same. However, when expressed in terms of the wage rate, the demand curve will shift down by $20, because $20 is added to the wages for each worker to calculate total compensation paid by the employer.

To adjust for the mandated benefits in terms of wages, the new demand curve for labor is shifted down by $20 for each quantity and becomes D_2.

An initial reaction might be to assume that the employees will bear the entire burden of the mandated benefits and be forced to take a $20 reduction in wages. In this situation employment would remain at the same level. This would be the case only if the workers fully value the benefits equally to wages (see curve $S_{v\,=\,b}$). As shown, the new wage price in this situation would be $60, with total compensation valued at $80.

If the workers do not value the benefits at all, there will be a reduction in wages (but not by the full $20 of the benefit). In this illustration, it is assumed wages will decrease to $70 (or some amount, depending on the elasticity of labor supply). There will also be a reduction in employment because of the lower wage. The burden of the mandate will then fall, to some degree, on the workers who lose employment. If benefits are only partially valued (reflected in supply curve $S_{v\,<\,b}$), the net result will be somewhere between these two situations.

In an extreme case, such as a vertical supply curve, there will be no employment effect, but a full wage effect. In fact, an earlier analysis of mandated benefits showed that this result is approximated in reality (Kreuger & Reinhardt, 1994), and so the workers bear the full burden of the mandate. In sum then, mandated benefits may have similar effects to those that might be concluded without a more formal economic analysis. However, this result is the case only if the supply curve of labor is, in reality, close to vertical (zero elasticity) in the relevant ranges.

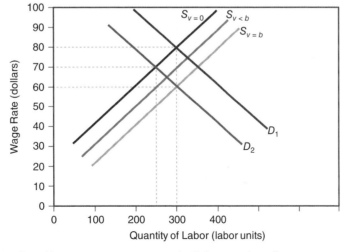

Figure 14-2 The effect of mandated insurance coverage on the labor market. D_1 represents the demand curve for labor without benefits. D_2 represents the demand curve for labor with $20 of benefits. Supply curve $S_{v=0}$ represents the supply of labor that places no value on benefits. Supply curve $S_{v=b}$ represents the supply of labor that values benefits and wages equally. Supply curve $S_{v<b}$ represents the supply of labor that places less than $20 of value on the benefits.

14.4.2 Taxation

Much health care (55.63%) is publicly funded, and much of the funding comes through taxation. Regardless of how taxes are configured, they can be regarded as reductions in income or wealth without any direct corresponding benefits. While it is true that benefits may come as a result of the use of the funds received from taxation, these benefits are not directly linked to payment of the taxes. It is not realistic to attempt to link the benefits resulting from the spending of taxes to the costs of the taxes themselves.

In terms of taxation, the taxing mechanisms can be either direct or indirect. Direct taxes are those that are specifically levied on the income of individuals and businesses. These direct taxes cannot therefore be shifted (i.e., the burden of the tax cannot be made to fall on someone other than the taxpayer). Indirect taxes that are placed on goods and services can be shifted (in essence, avoided) to some degree. Economic analysis is useful in determining the economic impact and burden of taxation. In the next section, the burden of two types of taxes commonly used to finance health care—payroll taxes and sales taxes—are analyzed.

14.4.2.1 Payroll Taxes

A payroll tax is levied on wages. Medicare, for example, uses a payroll (social security) tax of 1.45% of total payroll (the rate is payable by both the employer and employee for a total of 2.9%) to finance the hospital (part A) portion of Medicare. Self-employed individuals are responsible for paying the full 2.9%. The burden of an employee-paid payroll tax is quite clear: it is paid by the worker. However, because it lowers take-home wages, some workers may decide not to supply labor at the lower wage. Employment in the economy will therefore be decreased. The burden of the payroll tax on employees is thus equally shared among workers. The economic effects resulting from the imposition of a payroll tax that is paid by employers is less clear and deserves closer attention.

In **Figure 14-3**, the analysis of the effect of a payroll tax on labor and wages is introduced. In the illustration assume there is a competitive labor market with a given supply of labor (S) and a given demand for labor (D_1). The output measure is labor hours, and, in this market, equilibrium occurs with a wage rate of $40 per unit and a quantity of 300 labor hours. In this illustration a very steep supply curve for labor has been drawn. This steep curve indicates that workers will not change their work habits very much when wages increase or decrease. If the supply curve has been drawn as a vertical line, it would indicate that the workers would not change their employment habits at all. In an economy when many workers do not have the flexibility of reducing hours worked in small increments (e.g., they must either work full-time or only a set number of hours as part time) a vertical supply curve may be more applicable.

In this illustration, assume an employer-paid payroll tax of 100% of wages is introduced. If the employers are in a competitive industry, the price of their output cannot be increased. As a result, their demand-for-labor curve cannot be increased through offering higher prices. Therefore, the employers would have to either absorb the tax or lower wages paid to workers. An initial inclination might be to say that wages would stay at $40, the payroll taxes of $40 would be paid by the employer, and employment numbers would remain the same. This is a very unlikely outcome given the forces behind the employment of labor.

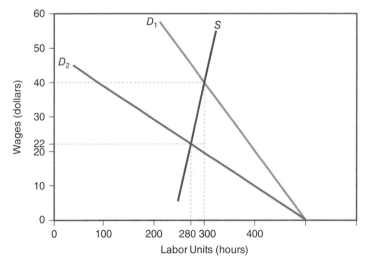

Figure 14-3 Effects of imposing an employer-paid payroll tax. S represents the initial supply of Labor. D_1 represents demand without the payroll tax. D_2 represents demand with a payroll tax. The original equilibrium is 300 hours at $40. The new equilibrium is 280 hours at $22.

Figure 14-3 presents an economic analysis of what would be more likely to happen. The effect of an employer-based payroll tax is to shift down the demand-for-labor curve, which is based on the marginal revenue of the product that labor produces. In this illustration, at a wage of $20, each employer must pay a tax of $20 (which is 100% of the wage). Each worker now costs twice as much as previously to the firm. Therefore, where the employers formerly demanded 300 labor hours when the wage was $40, they will now demand 300 hours of labor at a wage of $20. This last condition occurs because the tax in this illustration is expressed as a percentage of wages. In this situation, the new demand-for-labor curve (in terms of wages) is a fixed percentage lower than the original one. Under this condition of a percentage of wages, the higher the wage, the greater the discrepancy between the original and new demand curves.

With the employers' demand-for-labor curve (in terms of wages) shifting downward and to the left, employees will receive lower wages. In this illustration the new equilibrium volume of labor and the corresponding wage rate are just under 300 hours and just over $22. This means that the quantity of labor will have changed very little, but the wage rate will have fallen by almost the full amount of the tax. The workers have not substituted away from working (working fewer hours) and therefore have borne almost the entire burden of the tax through a reduction in their wage rate. In this case, the supply-of-labor curve is almost vertical, and workers would rather accept lower wages than lose employment.

Other situations in the market for labor are possible with the introduction of a payroll tax. To illustrate, if workers were very sensitive to the wage rates they receive, and the resulting supply-of-labor curve was close to horizontal, the labor supply would decrease when wages declined. In this instance, the workers would avoid the tax entirely by refusing to work at lower wages. At the new wage, the tax would have been shifted to the employers, who also would hire fewer workers because of the increased cost of production.

The effect of the payroll tax then will be to reduce employment and wages. How much of the payroll tax will be borne by the workers (through a decrease in wages) will depend on how much the workers are willing and able to adjust their wages and their work—information that is summarized by the supply-of-labor curve.

14.4.2.2 Sales Taxes

A very similar analysis applies to the use of sales taxes as a mechanism to generate revenue. A sales tax is levied on a good or service sold in the market.

Most states use sales taxes as a major source of revenue. Sales taxes can be general (the taxes placed on all items bought and sold in the market), a modified general sales tax (the taxes placed on most items except, for example, food sold in grocery stores, pharmaceutical products, and children's clothes), or a very specific sales tax (the taxes placed on such items as gasoline, alcohol, tobacco products, etc.). In the case of tobacco and alcohol, these sales taxes may affect consumer behavior with regard to drinking and smoking and thus have an impact on health status (and healthcare demand). This was certainly the rationale provided for a large tobacco tax that the state of Maine imposed in order to pay for more publicly funded healthcare benefits in the 1980s.

In order to analyze the effects of sales taxes, a sales tax on prescription drugs will be used as an illustration. The initial situation, without the imposition of a sales tax, is shown in **Figure 14-4**. The demand for the prescription drugs is shown by the demand curve (D). This represents the demand by consumers for the prescription drugs. There is also a curve for the supply of prescription drugs without the sales tax (represented by S_1). In a competitive market, equilibrium will occur in this illustration at a price of $40 and a quantity of 200 prescriptions filled (at the intersection of D and S_1).

In the illustration assume a sales tax of $20 on each prescription is imposed, to be paid by the pharmacists filling the prescriptions. The initial conclusion might be to assume the pharmacists will simply raise the price of each prescription to $60 and collect the tax on each of the 200 prescriptions filled. Such a result, however, would occur only if the demand curve for prescriptions was vertical and consumers would demand their prescriptions filled regardless of price. Such a situation is not a realistic scenario in the case of prescription drugs or most other goods and services. There is an elasticity of demand for prescription drugs, as indicated by the downward-sloping demand curve.

The sales tax on prescription drugs will cause the prices charged by the pharmacists to increase (if they pay the tax). At first the pharmacists might charge $60 for each prescription filled (although they would receive a net income of $40, as before since they must pay the $20 sales tax). But there is a limit to what consumers will pay for their prescription drugs. In this illustration, some consumers will refuse (or be unable) to fill their prescriptions, thus avoiding the sales tax entirely. In this illustration a new equilibrium will be reached at $50 per prescription filled, and only 150 prescriptions will be filled. The pharmacists will receive a net revenue of only $30 for each prescription and will supply fewer (150 at the net-after-tax price of $30).

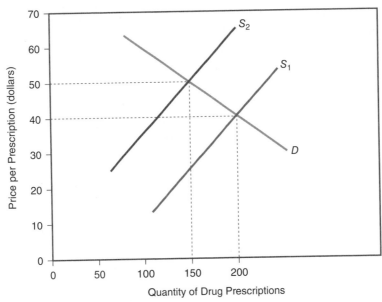

Figure 14-4 The effects of a sales tax. *D* represents the demand curve for prescriptions. *S₁* represents the original supply curve without a sales tax. *S₂* represents the new supply curve with supplier paying the tax. The original equilibrium is at price of $40 and quantity of 200 prescriptions. The new equilibrium is at price of $50 and quantity at 150 prescriptions; the tax is split between pharmacist and consumer.

In this illustration the market will have shifted part of the tax onto the pharmacists, who now pay one-half of it by receiving a lower price. The consumers end up paying $10 of the prescription tax by reducing the quantity they demand. The burden of the sales tax will thus be shared. It should be emphasized that other possible outcomes can occur, depending on the slopes of the supply and demand curves. However, it is not likely that all of the sales tax will be borne by the consumers.

As discussed earlier, sales taxes on a variety of products related to health are very common. Many states impose a tax on health insurance premiums. Such a tax will have an effect on the number of individuals who shift their risks (purchase a health insurance policy) to an insurer, and it can be analyzed using the basic sales tax model.

14.5 The Implications of Alternative Types of Healthcare Financing

In this section, attention turns to the implications of alternative types of healthcare financing. The term *implications* does not have a precise meaning in this context. The term is used to denote the pattern of distribution of burdens of various financing methods (Due, 1957). The focus in this analysis will be on one key characteristic of individuals—their level of income—and four different types of financing:

insurance premiums, income taxes, sales taxes, and payroll taxes. Although highly simplified, the analysis in this section is intended to provide a basic understanding of the major issues involved in using taxes to finance health care.

In evaluating the implications of taxes, the focus is on how regressive the tax is. A tax is considered to be *regressive* if it has a larger relative impact on the income of lower-income individuals than it has on the incomes of higher-income individuals. A tax is considered to be *progressive* if it has a larger relative impact on the incomes of higher-income individuals than on lower-income individuals. A tax is considered to be *neutral* if it has the same relative impact on all income cohorts. The impact of a tax on income is viewed as a relative burden on the various income cohorts.

Assume in this illustration that there are four income groups, and each group includes 100 families (see **Table 14-4**). Each family in the lowest income group has earnings of $20,000; in the next-lowest group, income of $40,000; in the third group, income of $60,000; and in the highest income group, an income of $80,000.

Assume each family, regardless of income group, incurs healthcare expenditures of $5000. There are no differences in healthcare utilization by income level. However, all expenditures are financed by insurance, and the out-of-pocket cost to each family is zero. Total healthcare expenses for all groups is $2 million ($5000 × 400 families = $2,000,000).

Table 14-4 Income and Expenditures for Four Income Groups

Income Group	Earnings per Family ($)	Number of Families	Total Income ($)	Total Consumption Expenditures ($)	Healthcare Expenditures per Family ($)	Total Healthcare Expenditures ($)
A	20,000	100	2,000,000	2,000,000	5,000	500,000
B	40,000	100	4,000,000	3,600,000	5,000	500,000
C	60,000	100	6,000,000	4,800,000	5,000	500,000
D	80,000	100	8,000,000	5,600,000	5,000	500,000
Total		400	20,000,000	16,000,000		2,000,000

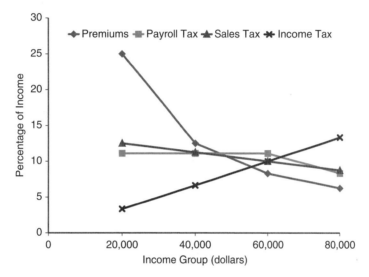

Figure 14-5 Implications of different financing mechanisms. Premiums are the most regressive source of financing. Income tax is the most progressive source of financing. Sales tax and payroll tax fall in between. In this illustration payroll tax and sales tax are still somewhat regressive.

© Jones & Bartlett Learning.

Each family's total consumption of goods and services, including food, utilities, etc., but not health care, is provided in column 5 of Table 14-4. The lowest income group spends all it earns on goods and services, the next group spends 90%, the third group spends 80%, and the highest income group spends 70%. The members of a group save what they do not spend. If they have to pay for health care, they will reduce other expenditures but will not reduce their savings. If they do pay for health care itself it will be paid for through the purchase of insurance.

The financing problem to be resolved is how to pay for the $2 million in healthcare expenses incurred by the population. There are four options available to finance the expenses: insurance premiums, a sales tax, a payroll tax, and an income tax. The task is to determine the impact of each type of financing on the different income groups. The conclusions reached in this illustration are summarized in **Figure 14-5**.

Premiums. Each family in this illustration bears the same risk of incurring $5000 of health expenses, and so it might seem reasonable to simply charge every family the same premium rate (use a community rating). There are 400 families, and $2 million in healthcare funds must be raised (assume no loading fee is collected for simplicity). Therefore, each family will pay a premium of $5000 for insurance coverage.

The burden of this financing method on each family is calculated as the premium paid divided by the family income. This would result in a burden of 25% ($5000 / $20,000) for the lowest income families, 12.5% for the families earning $40,000, a total of 8.3% for the families earning $60,000, and 6.25% for the highest income families. The impact of community rate premiums is such that the burden decreases steadily as income increases.

Payroll Taxes. In the case of a payroll tax, a fixed percentage of wages is charged, but there is usually a cap above which income is not taxed. In this illustration, assume that this cap is $60,000. This means that all wages up to and including $60,000 are taxed. The members of the highest income group (those earning $80,000) will pay taxes on only the first $60,000 of their wages. Total taxable wages are therefore $18 million for all families since $20,000 of each of the 100 families in the highest income group is not taxed. In order to raise the required $2 million, a tax rate of 11.1% ($2 million / $18 million) must be levied on all wages up to $60,000.

The burden of the tax will be the same for the three groups whose members have incomes at or below $60,000; the amounts paid by each of these three groups vary, but the rate is the same at 11.1%. However, the highest income group pays only $6660 in payroll taxes per family, for an effective tax rate of 8.325%. As shown in Figure 14-5, the burden of the payroll tax is the same for the three lowest groups but decreases for the highest income group.

Sales Taxes. Sales taxes can be imposed on any of a variety of consumption expenditures. Assume in this illustration that sales taxes are imposed on all consumption expenditures. Sales taxes are also not imposed on savings, which, as mentioned earlier, vary by income cohort: no savings for families with incomes of $20,000, 10% savings for families with incomes of $40,000, 20% savings for families with incomes of $60,000, and 30% savings for families with incomes of $80,000 Total consumption expenditures for other goods and services for all families therefore equal $16 million. In order to raise the required $2 million in funds, the overall sales tax rate must be 12.5% ($2 million / 16 million). The lowest income group pays $250,000 on its $2 million in expenditures; the next group pays $450,000 on its $3.6 million in expenditures; the next group pays $600,000 on its $4.8 million in expenditures; and the highest income group pays $700,000 on its $5.6 million in expenditures.

Income Taxation. The burden of the income tax will depend on the actual tax rates, and these are subject to policy decisions by Congress. Assume in this illustration that the tax rates are such that the highest income class pays roughly four times the rate of the lowest group. This is very roughly the ratio in the United States today. Specifically, assume in this illustration that given an average overall rate, the lowest group will pay 40% of this rate (i.e., 0.4), the second group will pay 80% of the rate, the third-highest group will pay 120% of the rate, and the highest group will pay 160% of the rate. Let x stand for the overall tax rate. The overall rate can be determined by solving for x in this equation:

$$0.4(\$2 \text{ million})x + 0.8(\$4 \text{ million})$$
$$x + 1.2(\$6 \text{ million})x + 1.6(\$8 \text{ million})x =$$
$$0.8x + 3.2x + 7.2x = 12.8x =$$
$$24x = \$2 \text{ million}$$
$$X = (\$2 \text{ million} / 24) = 8.33\%$$

The $2 million is the amount to be collected by the income tax. If the equation is solved for x, the average overall rate is found to be 8.33%. Based on the ratios determined by "policy," the four groups pay 3.33% (8.33 × 0.4), 6.64%, 9.99%, and 13.33% of income in income taxes, respectively.

The overall impact of the funding methods can be compared. Premiums are the most "regressive" and income taxes are the most "progressive." The other two methods fall in between (under the assumptions in this illustration, the last two methods are mildly regressive).

Omitted from the analysis in this illustration are out-of-pocket expenditures. The use of this type of financing will result in lower overall usage (because of the downward-sloping demand curve for health care). Thus, if families had to pay out of pocket for health care, total expenditures would likely fall below $2 million. The overall burden would depend on the response of each income group.

The assessment of financing options will depend on the policy goals. Much of the focus in evaluating types of financing is on considerations of equity. However, efficiency issues need to be addressed as well.

14.6 The Administrative Cost of Alternative Types of Healthcare Financing

There has been a lively debate in recent years about administrative costs associated with the healthcare financing system in the United States. Much of the debate has been focused on the costs associated with the marketing of health insurance and hospital services; the monitoring of utilization and the regulating of payment by insurers; the billing of third parties by providers; and the collecting of deductibles, coinsurance, and copayments from patients by providers. Because of the complexity of the U.S. system of healthcare finance, more resources are devoted to these functions than in other healthcare systems, such as those of Canada and the United Kingdom. A study conducted using 1987 data estimated that between $96 billion and $120 billion were spent on administration in the United States, out of a total spent of $488 billion for all healthcare-related services (Woolhandler & Himmelstein, 1991). This study primarily added up the money costs of these functions.

Pozen and Cutler (2010) found that the largest difference in spending between the United States and Canada was in administrative costs, with 44% more administrative staff in the United States than in Canada. When all administrative costs were included, they found administrative costs accounted for 39% of the difference between the United States and Canada. Other authors (Blanchfield, Heffernan, Osgood, Sheehan, & Meyer, 2010; Davis et al., 2007; Luxembourg Income Study, 2011) have also found that the United States has many more administrative staff than do other countries. Cutler and Ly (2011) provide an excellent overview of comparative administrative findings.

A paper by Pearson (2018) re-verified that not only does the United States spend more on direct patient care than other countries, but that the United States also spends more on healthcare administration. While it is difficult to identify exactly how much the United States spends on healthcare administration, the consensus is that it is substantial and continuing to grow.

One of the largest subcategories of health administration spending relates to billing and insurance-related (BIR) costs. The Center for American Progress estimated that United States payers and providers will spend $496 billion on billing and insurance-related administrative costs in 2019.

A 2014 study by Himmelstein et al. compared hospital administrative costs in eight nations and found that the costs in the United States exceeded all other countries. They found administrative costs in the United States accounted for 25.3% of the total hospital expenditures. The Netherlands had the next highest expense at 19.8% and England spent 15.5% on hospital administration.

Tseng, Kaplan, Richman, Shah, and Schulman (2018) found that administrative costs associated with physician billing and insurance-related activities in an academic health system accounted for $20 of a primary care visit and $215 for an inpatient surgical procedure. These physician-related administrative costs represented 3%–25% of all professional revenue in 2016–2017. Jiwani, Himmelstein, Woolhandler, and Kahn (2014) investigated BIR costs in the United States and found that these costs were between $330 and $597 billion in 2012. They concluded that the multi-payer system in the United States represented 80% of the difference in cost between the United States and a simplified financing system.

In examining the administrative costs in health care, it is important to keep in mind that sound administration is critical to a well-functioning organization or healthcare system. The United States has a very complex structure for its administration and so careful evaluation needs to be performed to determine the benefits that are associated with the costs. As efforts are undertaken to attempt to control rising costs in health care, the functioning of the administration of the system also needs to be considered. The multi-payer system in the United States adds to the complexity of its administration and providers often have to deal with insurance coverage, eligibility, and billing requirements that vary across payers, requiring additional administrative effort.

14.7 Payment Mechanisms

The healthcare industry has been facing a number of changes in payment systems recently, and indications are that even more changes are looming in the future. A difficulty emerging in the implementation of different payment mechanisms is that there is a disconnect between the external payment systems being implemented and the internal methods that have been used to distribute resources within the organizations. Historically, the healthcare system has been a production-based system, receiving compensation for services produced. The incentive in any production-based system is simply to produce more units, as long as the cost of production is less than the market price received for the unit.

Complicating the production decisions in the healthcare system is the existence of health insurance programs that isolate production decisions from the cost of services utilized and the ability of insurance companies to simply pass the increased costs on to employers and governments, the purchasers of the majority of insurance plans. As healthcare costs began to impinge significantly on the other sectors of the economy, efforts emerged to change the payment incentives in the healthcare industry, especially as the increasing costs did not result in a concomitant improvement in the health status of the population. As attention has focused on controlling the rate of increase in healthcare expenditures, such alternative payment methods as pay for performance, shared savings, bundled payments, and global capitation have been introduced.

14.7.1 Pay for Performance

Pay for performance was introduced to provide incentives to providers to improve the quality of care delivered. This occurred as evidence mounted regarding the underuse, overuse, and misuse of treatments within the healthcare system. The Committee on Redesigning Health Insurance Performance Measures, Payment, and Performance Improvement Programs (2007) defined pay for performance (P4P) as "the systematic and deliberate use of payment incentives that recognize and reward high levels of quality and quality improvement" (p. 5). Pay for performance is designed to offer incentives to encourage the healthcare system to move from its current volume-based structure toward different organizational and individual behaviors. The goal of P4P is to result in better quality and improved outcomes for patients in the population.

In most markets, incentives induce producers and/or consumers to behave or respond in predictable ways. These incentives focus on the identification of desired attributes and provide rewards or penalties in order to stimulate additional production of those attributes. The goal of the P4P model in health care is to motivate constructive change in the system by explicitly linking incentives to the quality and performance of the providers within the healthcare system. The difficulty in implementing P4P is in developing a framework that incorporates the complexity of the clinical situations to be included, the diversity of the environments in which care is provided, and the resources necessary to comply with the requirements of the system.

A critical and difficult issue in any P4P system is the selection of the priority quality dimensions and the establishment of the measures to be used to assess performance and quality. This is especially difficult in health care because focusing on one domain of quality may lead to reductions in other domains of quality. Another aspect to be considered in designing a P4P mechanism for health care is determining whether the focus should be on improvement in quality or on achieving a recognized threshold of desired quality, or both. The P4P system must also be capable of incorporating new measures as the healthcare system evolves; innovations and discoveries in health care should be encouraged. In addition, the incentive created should have a sufficient impact upon the revenues of the provider to influence their decisions, but not be so onerous as to compel providers to leave the system.

Pay-for-performance is a primary tool that has been used to achieve healthcare reform. In the development and implementation of P4P, a number of diverse types with heterogeneous incentives have been implemented, making evaluation of its effects somewhat difficult. In an evaluation by Van Herck et al. (2010) the effect domains assessed were: clinical-effectiveness, access and equity, coordination and continuity, patient-centeredness, and cost-effectiveness. In their review of 128 evaluation studies, the authors concluded that the effects achieved by P4P varied by the design choices and the characteristics of the context in which it was introduced. In their review of these studies, the authors found that process indicators generally yielded higher improvement rates than outcome measures, with intermediate outcome measures yielding rates in between process and outcome measures. The incentives that provided a financial reward appeared to generate more positive effects than did competitive incentives that resulted in winners and losers.

Figueroa, Tsugawa, Zheng, Orav, and Kjha (2016) examined the association between the value-based purchasing pay for performance incentive program introduced by Medicare and the 30-day mortality rate in U.S. hospitals for acute myocardial infarction, heart failure, and pneumonia. They did not find any subgroup of hospitals that implemented the program had better outcomes, including the poor-performing hospitals at baseline. These authors did not find any evidence that the value-based P4P program led to lower mortality rates.

Under the Medicare value-based program hospitals were rewarded or penalized based on their performance on a number of domains of care, including clinical processes and clinical outcomes of the three conditions evaluated as well as patient experiences and cost efficiency. Under this system, which is designed to be budget neutral, Medicare withholds a percentage of inpatient payments to prospectively paid hospitals and then redistributes the money back to hospitals based on their performance. In 2015, 1360 hospitals received penalties and 1700 hospitals received bonus payments.

Another program that has been introduced by Medicare is the hospital readmissions reduction program. This program implemented a financial penalty to reduce payment to hospitals with excessive 30-day inpatient readmissions for pneumonia, acute myocardial infarction, and heart failure. Lu, Huang, and Johnson (2016) found a significant reduction in excessive readmissions for these three conditions between 2013 and 2015, especially in small hospitals, public hospitals, and hospitals located in rural areas.

Medicare has undergone a number of changes in how it pays hospitals, especially since the Affordable Care Act introduced three programs that link

Medicare payment to hospital performance in the areas of quality, efficiency, outcomes, and patient experiences. Earlier the 2003 Medicare Prescription Drug Improvement and Modernization Act initiated the hospital inpatient quality reporting program under which hospitals were required to report on a specified set of quality measures. If a hospital does not report the indicators, they receive a payment reduction. Aggregate hospital performance on required quality measures has improved since the requirement began. In 2012, Medicare began implementing the ACA-mandated Hospital Value-Based Purchasing Program and the Hospital Readmission Reduction Program. In 2015, the Hospital-Acquired Conditions Reduction Program began. With the introduction of these programs, by 2017 hospitals were at risk for losing as much as 6% of base operating payment, or 5% of total operating payments under these three programs. Under the Hospital Acquired Conditions Reduction Program, a 1% reduction in the total inpatient prospective payment system (IPPS) payments is levied against hospitals with scores (based on hospital infection rates and patient safety measures) in the worst-performing quartile of hospitals.

Kahn et al. (2015) evaluated the impact these three programs, taken together, had on hospital performance and payments during FY 2015. The authors concluded that these Medicare pay-for-performance programs have had a significant effect on hospital payments, particularly when the combined effects of the three programs are considered. The performance of hospitals where the various performance matrices are improving is consistent with the incentives created by the programs. The authors point out that appending quality programs to a payment system that is intended to cover the cost of an efficient provider of best care may create onerous outcomes for the providers. Including additional penalties on that payment system, especially with almost two-thirds of hospitals already experiencing negative Medicare patient margins, may be problematic. A more rational approach to aligning payment policy with quality outcomes needs to be considered at this time.

Shih, Nicholas, Thumma, Birkmeyer, and Dimick (2014) examined the incentive design of the second phase of the Medicare P4P program, the Premier Hospital Quality Incentive Demonstration Project, to determine if surgical mortality or complication rates in participating hospitals were reduced. This program, initiated in 2003, was designed to reward high-performing hospitals. Its incentive structure was redesigned in 2006 to also reward hospitals for achieving significant improvement. The authors found that there were lower risk-adjusted mortality rates for both cardiac and orthopedic patients after the incentives were restructured in 2006. However, mortality for CABG or joint replacement did not demonstrate significant improvements. Similarly, significant improvements in serious complications for CABG or joint replacement were not achieved. Also, the worst quintile hospitals targeted in the incentive structure changes did not show a change in mortality or serious complication rates. The authors concluded that significant redesign of the incentives in the program would need to be made in order for the P4P strategy to be successful.

14.7.2 Bundled Payments

The generic term bundled payments is known by a variety of names, such as case rate, global payment, package pricing, episode-based payment, comprehensive care payment, and evidence-based case rate. Regardless of the term used, it is a payment method based on the costs expected to be incurred in the provision of a clinically defined episode of care, adjusted for the severity and complexity of a patient's condition. Bundled payments are viewed as a blend of fee-for-service and capitation payments, discouraging the provision of unnecessary care and encouraging the coordination of care across providers, but not penalizing providers who care for sicker patients in their practice. The goal of bundled payment is to reduce fragmentation of care, thereby improving quality and reducing costs. The use of bundled payments should encourage providers within the system to reorganize how care is delivered so that it is coordinated and responsive to the needs of patients.

Under a bundled payment system, the services that are required by patients during a single illness or a course of treatment for a chronic disease are defined across providers and settings—the services are bundled into a single package of services. Once the required services are defined, a target price is established for the bundle. This target price reflects the total amount that will be paid for the episode of care, and all providers involved in the provision of services are covered under that price. This comprehensive price provides an incentive for the coordination of care in order to keep the costs of producing the services below the price established. Within the provider network, decisions have to be made on how to allocate the global revenue among the participating providers rendering services to the patient.

A number of barriers are encountered in the development of a bundled payment system. A major problem encountered is deciding just when an episode of care begins and ends. For an acute illness of limited duration, this is manageable. For chronic conditions lasting for extended periods of time, this is difficult to determine because, by definition, a chronic condition is a disease or illness that is persistent and long-lasting. Currently, an episode is typically defined for a specified period of time, such as 30–90 days after discharge from an acute care facility or after the first visit to a provider for the condition. The bundled payment is applied only to that particular illness or disease, which differs from capitation, which covers all illnesses experienced by an enrolled member for a specified period of time.

Because the target payment to be made is fixed, providers have an incentive to coordinate care and minimize the provision of any marginal or unnecessary care. A concern raised is that the incentive may encourage providers to underutilize services, negatively impacting the patient's outcome. Careful monitoring is needed to ensure that quality is not negatively impacted and that patients receive necessary care.

In January 2018, the Centers for Medicare and Medicaid (CMS) announced that 1547 providers and suppliers (823 acute care hospitals, 715 physician groups, and 9 "others") had signed agreements to participate in the Bundled Payments for Care Improvement (BPCI)-Advanced model, which builds upon the earlier Bundled Payment for Care Initiative. Under this BPCI-Advanced program, participating hospitals and physician group practices will receive bundled payments for certain episodes of care as an alternative to the traditional fee-for-service payments. Under this BPCI-Advanced program, participants can earn additional payment if all expenditures for a beneficiary's episode of care are less than a spending target. The spending target also incorporates measures of quality. Alternatively, if expenditures exceed the target price, then the participants must repay money to Medicare.

The BPCI-Advanced program expands the original BPCI program to include payments for additional clinical episodes, including outpatient episodes. The participants are provided the target price in advance, so they can plan more effectively how to manage episodes of care. BPCI-Advanced qualifies as an advanced alternative payment model, which means participating clinicians assume the risk for the cost of patient health care and for meeting quality thresholds, potentially qualifying them for other incentive programs and exempting them from the merit-based incentive payment system (MIPS). The stated goal of the program is to accelerate value-based transformation of the healthcare system by offering a range of new payment models so that providers can choose the approach that will work best for them. At this time, the program has not been implemented a sufficient amount of time to enable evaluation.

14.7.3 Value-Based Purchasing

Value-based purchasing (VBP) programs are also sometimes known as shared-savings programs, the goals of which are similar to those of the bundled payment programs: to improve care coordination and redesign the processes of care to produce high-quality and efficient care delivery. Incentives are created within these programs to provide care that has higher value to the patient and to the system; these programs move away from paying providers based only on the volume of services provided to patients. Under these programs, if the provider is able to achieve savings and meet the quality performance standards, then the amount of the savings is shared between the providers and the payer. These programs focus on better care for individuals, better health for the population, and reducing the rate of growth in healthcare expenditures.

Similar to bundled payment systems, value-based purchasing (VBP) programs also require the establishment of clinical measures, measures of effective resource utilization, and incentives within the payment structure to link the two measures to the price paid for services. The focus on these systems is to foster joint clinical and financial accountability within the healthcare system. As with any of the performance-based payment systems, it is critical to have communication among the various providers in order to coordinate care. This communication requires electronic health records with interoperability (the ability to link to each other) capability.

VBP programs are demand-side strategies that impact the utilization of healthcare services by rewarding excellence in healthcare delivery by enhancing revenue through differential payment and by increasing market share by consumer selection. A key component of VBP is the development of standardized performance measures, including involving consumers in changing their lifestyle and self-managing their chronic diseases. The Institute of Medicine (2001) has established the STEEEP—Safe, Timely, Efficient, Effective, Equitable, and Patient-centered—typology of the dimensions of healthcare performance, which need to be incorporated into the system. To be effective, it is necessary to access and aggregate data on these dimensions from different sources and from different providers. As indicated, a key component of this model is patient-centeredness, which involves engaging the consumer in the process.

A number of pieces of legislation, such as the Patient Protection and Affordable Care Act and the Medicare Access and CHIP Reauthorization Act (MACRA) have reinforced the role of value-based purchasing payment in Medicare. In addition, many private insurers are following the lead of Medicare and adopting value-based payment mechanisms. Chee, Ryan, Wasfy, and Borden (2016) conducted a review, summarizing the current state of value-based payment programs and analyzed the strengths, weaknesses, and opportunities for the future. According to these authors, the opportunities to enhance the performance of the value-based payment programs include improving the quality measurement science, strengthening the size and design of incentives, reducing health disparities, choosing appropriate comparison targets, and determining the optimal role of value-based payment relative to alternative payment models. They also indicated that value-based payments serve as an opportunity for providers to build the infrastructure needed for value-oriented care.

14.8 Consumer Engagement

As efforts continue to improve quality and control the costs of health care, attention is focused on ways of influencing consumers to be more informed decision makers. For consumers to become more engaged in the decision-making process, it is necessary for them to have a better understanding of the availability of alternatives and options, and of the quality of care offered, in order to demand and choose appropriate services. As outlined in Aligning Forces for Quality (AF4Q), sponsored by the Robert Wood Johnson Foundation, to be successful in transforming health care, a community-wide consumer-engagement strategy must help consumers to

- Understand their risks or actual conditions, and take actions to manage them.
- Understand and make informed treatment choices.
- Understand the difference between good care and bad care, and demand good care.
- Advocate for public reporting by hospitals and doctors on nationally recognized indicators of quality care.
- Choose providers based on information about their ability to deliver effective care (http://www.rwjf.org/qualityequality/af4q/focusareas/consumer.jsp).

Basically, Aligning Forces for Quality invites the individuals who get care, give care, and pay for care to work together toward common, fundamental objectives that lead to better care. AF4Q showed that progress can be made locally when all stakeholders participate in the process. Effective consumer engagement builds and supports the capacity of consumers to manage their health and health conditions. This also involves the ability to understand, demand, and choose high-quality health care.

For consumers to be informed decision makers in the healthcare system, literacy, and especially health literacy, is critical. A patient's literacy skills are critical in interactions in the healthcare field, impacting the ability of the patient to navigate the services needed and the healthcare delivery system. Literacy skills are also important in enabling the patients to be advocates for their needs within the system, and the role of consumer self-advocacy is increasingly important. The complexity of the healthcare system and the incentives being created in many of the reform activities increasingly requires patients to take a proactive role in the utilization of healthcare services and in the self-management of medical conditions.

As increased emphasis is placed on consumer engagement and access to online information and health information technologies is becoming more widespread, care must be taken that the medically underserved and disadvantaged populations are not further disenfranchised from the system. Health disparities currently exist, and increased reliance on health information technologies for seeking and managing personal health conditions and for communicating between patients and providers may widen the disparity gap rather than solve it. The deployment of health information and health information technology is intended to impact the demand for healthcare services, but care must be taken that this doesn't negatively impact various subgroups of the population.

Patient engagement is also a critical component of the patient-centered medical home model, which involves the provision of quality care that is coordinated, comprehensive, and cost-effective. The patient-centered medical home requires a strong patient–provider relationship through the use of a team approach to care that increases access to care and the continuity of the care provided. In addition to improving quality of care in order to improve health outcomes, the patient-centered medical home is expected to reduce demand for health services through the reduction of duplication of tests, procedures, emergency department visits, hospitalizations, and provider visits as care becomes coordinated across providers.

As the population becomes older and experiences escalating chronic conditions, it is critical that the healthcare delivery system becomes more effective in the management of chronic conditions. New streams of data are necessary to enable better self-management, improve shared decision making, and provide more virtual care. The importance of patient-generated health information, remote monitoring, non-visit-based care, and other innovative care approaches that foster more frequent contact with patients and better management of chronic conditions must become part of the adapting healthcare system (Sands & Wald, 2014).

A study by McFarland, Ornstein, and Holcombe (2015) examined the variation in patient satisfaction as determined by the Hospital Consumer Assessment of Healthcare Providers and Systems (HCAHPS) to determine the factors that predict patient satisfaction scores. The hospital value-based performance program provides incentives for quality performance-based health care and it links payments directly to patient satisfaction scores obtained from the HCAHPS surveys. The authors found that demographic and structural factors can predict patient satisfaction scores. More specifically, they found that hospital size (number of beds) and primary language (non-English-speaking) were the strongest predictors of unfavorable HCAHPS scores. Alternatively, education and white ethnicity were the strongest predictors of favorable HCAHPS scores. Without adjusting for such factors outside the control of hospitals, the value-based purchasing program may unfairly penalize some hospitals and unfairly reward others.

To assist in the improvement of consumer engagement, a new patient engagement measure, the Altarum Consumer Engagement (ACE) instrument, was developed and validated. This instrument was developed to increase the way patient engagement is measured and understood (Duke, Lynch, Smith, & Winstanley, 2015). If consumer engagement is to truly form a foundation for improving the healthcare delivery system and outcomes obtained in the delivery of care, then a mechanism for measuring consumer engagement is essential. Without the ability to measure consumer engagement, the ability to effectively incorporate it into the necessary changes in the healthcare delivery system is limited. To enable consumers to have a significant role in their care through such entities as patient-centered medical homes, coordinated care for chronic disease, and shared decision making, there needs to be a mechanism available for measuring and valuing that engagement. The goal is to lead to safer, more effective, and less expensive health care.

This discussion has served to highlight the fact that a healthcare financing system requires resources and that different systems have different costs. The Canadian system, for example, has lower administrative costs than does the U.S. system. However, the amount of administrative costs is not the only factor that needs to be taken into account when choosing a national healthcare "system." Morra et al. (2011) found that physicians in the United States spend almost four times as much time interacting with payers as do physicians in Canada.

Marketing functions serve to inform potential customers about the characteristics of various health plans. Consumers can better select among health plans if they have more information. Regulation and payment functions serve to help ensure that the care provided is of a high quality and results in good outcomes. Although these functions are not always completely effective, nevertheless, when evaluating a financing system, the benefits of the various financing practices must be examined in addition to the costs.

Exercises

1. What proportion of total health expenses were made by out-of-pocket, government, and health insurance sources of finance in 2017?

2. An employee is worth $100 a week to her employer. The worker demands $20 in health insurance benefits, to be paid by the employer. What would the employer be willing to pay in terms of wages?

3. What is the effect on the market for health insurance of a government tax subsidy on health insurance premiums?

4. What will be the effect of mandated health insurance benefits on the market for labor if the workers do not place any value on these benefits? If they fully value the benefits?

5. What is a payroll tax? How will the imposition of a payroll tax affect the wage rate and the quantity of labor employed?

6. How will the imposition of a sales tax on a commodity affect the price and quantity sold of that commodity? Will the consumer usually bear the entire burden of the tax?

7. How does each of the following methods of financing the healthcare system impact on persons according to their income group?
   a. Income tax
   b. Sales tax
   c. Payroll tax
   d. Insurance premiums

8. Discuss the rationale for the introduction of pay-for-performance mechanisms in health care.
9. What are bundled payments and how are they being used in health care?
10. Why is consumer engagement so important in today's healthcare system?

Bibliography

Blanchfield, B. B., Heffernan, J. L., Osgood, B., Sheehan, R. R., & Meyer, G. S. (2010). Savings billions of dollars—And physicians' time—By streamlining billing practices. *Health Affairs, 29*(6), 1248–1254.

Centers for Medicare & Medicaid Services. (October 12, 2018). 2019 Medicare Part B premiums and deductibles. *Newsroom Fact Sheet.* Retrieved from www.cms.gov/newsroom/fact-sheet /2019-Medicare-Part-B-Premiums-and-Deductibles

Centers for Medicare & Medicaid Services. *National health expenditures by type of service and source of funds, calendar years, 1960–2017.* Retrieved from https://www.cms.gov/Research -Statistics-Data-and-Systems/Statistics-Trends-and-Reports /NationalHealthExpendData/index.html?redirect=/National HealthExpendData/02_NationalHealthAccountsHistorical.asp #TopOfPage

Chee, T. T., Ryan, A. M., Wasfy, J. H., & Borden, W. B. (2016). Current state of value-based purchasing programs. *Circulation, 133*, 2197–2205.

Claxton, G., Rae, M., Long, M., Damico, A., & Whitmore, H. (2018). *Employer Health Benefits 2018 Annual Survey.* San Francisco, CA: Henry J. Kaiser Family Foundation.

Cohen, R. A. (2018). *Long-term trends in health insurance: Estimates from the national health interview survey, United States, 1960–2017.* National Center for Health Statistics. Available from http://www .cdc.gov/nchs/health_policy/coverage_and_access.htm

Committee on Redesigning Health Insurance Performance Measures, Payment, and Performance Improvement Programs. (2007). *Rewarding provider performance: Aligning incentives in Medicare.* Washington, DC: The National Academies Press.

Congressional Budget Office. (2018). Reduce tax subsidies for employment-based health insurance. *Options for Reducing the Budget.* Washington, DC: Author.

Cutler, D., Wilder, E., & Bosch, P. (2012). Reducing administrative costs and improving the health care system. *New England Journal of Medicine, 367*, 1875–1878.

Cutler, D. M., & Ly, D. P. (2011). The (paper) work of medicine: Understanding international medical costs. *Journal of Economic Perspectives, 25*(2), 3–25.

Davis, K., Schoen, C., Schoenbaum, S. C., Doty, M. M., Holmgren, A. L., Kriss, J. L., & Shea, K. K. (2007). Mirror, mirror on the wall: An international update on the comparative performance of American health care. *The Commonwealth Fund.* Retrieved from http://www.commonwealthfund.org/Publications/Fund -Reports/2007/May/Mirror--Mirror-on-the-Wall--An -International-Update-on-the-Comparative-Performance-of -American-Healt.aspx

DeNavas-Wait, C., Proctor, B. D., & Smith, J. C., U.S. Census Bureau. (2011). *Income, poverty, and health insurance coverage in the United States: 2010.* Washington, DC: U.S. Government Printing Office. Retrieved from http://www.census.gov/prod /2011pubs/p60-239.pdf

Due, J. F. (1957). *Sales taxation.* London, England: Routledge and Kegan Paul.

Duke, C. C., Lynch, W. D., Smith, B., & Winstanley, J. (2015). Validity of a new patient engagement measure: The Altarum consumer engagement (ACE) measure. *Patient, 8*, 559–568.

Figueroa, J. F., Tsugawa, Y., Zheng, J., Orav, E. J., & Jha, J. K. (2016). Association between the value-based purchasing pay-for-performance program and patient mortality in US hospitals: Observational study. *British Medical Journal, 353*, i2214. Retrieved from http://dx.doi.org/10.1136/bmj.i2214

Himmelstein, D. U., Jun, M., Busse, R., Chevreul, K., Geissler, A., Jeurissen, P., … Woolhandler, S. (2014). A comparison of hospital administrative costs in 8 nations. US costs exceed all others by far. *Health Affairs, 33*(9), 1586–1594.

Institute of Medicine. (2001). *Crossing the Quality Chasm: A New Health System for the 21st Century.* Washington, DC: National Academies Press.

Jiwani, A., Himmelstein, D., Woolhandler, S., & Kahn, J. G. (2014). Billing and insurance-related administrative costs in United States health care: Synthesis of micro-costing evidence. *BMC Health Services Research, 14*, 556–565.

Kahn, C. N., Ault, T., Potetz, L., Walke, T., Chambers, J. H., & Burch, S. (2015). Assessing Medicare's hospital pay-for-performance and whether they are achieving their goals. *Health Affairs, 34*(8), doi:10.1377/hlthaff.2015.0158

Kreuger, A., & Reinhardt, U. E. (1994). Economics of employer versus individual mandates. *Health Affairs, 13*, 34–54.

Lu, N., Huang, K. C., & Johnson, J. A. (2016). Reducing excess readmissions: Promising effect of hospital readmissions reduction program in US hospitals. *International Journal for Quality in Health Care, 28*(1), 53–58.

Luxembourg Income Study (LIS). (2011). *Database.* Retrieved from http://www.lisproject.org/techdoc.htm

McFarland, D. C., Ornstein, K. A., & Holcombe, R. F. (2015). Demographic factors and hospital size predict patient satisfaction variance—Implications for hospital value-based purchasing. *Journal of Hospital Medicine, 10*(8), 503–509.

Morra, D., Nicholson, S., Levinson, W., Gans, D. N., Hammons, T., & Casalino, L. P. (2011). US physician practices versus Canadians: Spending nearly four times as much money interacting with payers. *Health Affairs, 30*(8), 1443–1450.

Papanicolas, I., Woskie, L. R., & Jha, A. K. (2018). Health care spending in the US and other high-income countries. *JAMA, 319*(10), 1024–1039.

Pearson, E. (2018). How much is too much? What does the US actually spend on health care administration. *The Incidental Economist.* Retrieved from https://theincidentaleconomist.com

/wordpress/how-much-is-too-much-what-does-the-us
-actually-spend-on-health-care-administration/

Pozen, A., & Cutler, D. M. (2010). Medical spending differences in the United States and Canada: The role of prices, procedures, and administrative expenses. *Inquiry, 47*(2), 124–134.

Robert Woods Johnson Foundation. *Aligning Forces for Quality*. Retrieved from http://rwjf.org/qualityequality/af4q/focusareas /consumer.jsp

Sands, D. Z., & Wald, J. S. (2014). Transforming health care delivery through consumer engagement, health data transparency, and patient-generated health information. *Yearbook of Medical Informatics, 23*(01), 175–176.

Shih, T., Nicholas, L. H., Thumma, J. R., Birkmeyer, J. D., & Dimick, J. B. (2014). Does pay-for-performance improve surgical outcomes? An evaluation of phase 2 of the premier hospital quality incentive demonstration. *Annals of Surgery, 259*(4), 677–681.

Tseng, P., Kaplan, R. S., Richman, B. D., Shah, K. P., & Schulman, K. D. (2018). Administrative costs associated with physician-billing and insurance-related activities of an academic health care system. *JAMA, 319*(7), 691–697.

Van Herck, P., De Smedt, D., Annemans, L., Remmen, R., Rosenthal, M. R., & Sermeus, W. (2010). Systematic review: Effects, design choices, and context of pay-for-performance in health care. *BMC Health Services Research,* 10. Article number 247.

Woolhandler, S., Campbell, T., & Himmelstein, D. U. (2004). Health care administration in the United States and Canada: Micromanagement, macro costs. *International Journal of Health Services, 34*(1), 65–78.

Woolhandler, S., & Himmelstein, D. U. (1991). The deteriorating administrative efficiency of the U.S. healthcare system. *New England Journal of Medicine, 324,* 1253–1258.

CHAPTER 15

Public Health Insurance

OBJECTIVES

1. Identify the key policy goals of public health insurance plans.
2. Describe the Medicare and Medicaid programs in terms of populations covered, services included, financing arrangements, reimbursement strategies, and pro-competition policies.
3. Explain some of the key issues surrounding public health insurance.
4. Identify the key types of policies required for the delivery of a public health insurance program and indicate their effect on the achievement of social goals.

15.1 Introduction

This chapter presents an economic framework that can be used to analyze selected aspects of public health insurance coverage in the United States. Health insurance coverage is a critical element of the healthcare system, and public policies related to health insurance influence the functioning of the healthcare market. In this chapter, a discussion of how the economic framework can be used to analyze policy choices, a discussion of policy goals in relation to the economic framework, and an assessment of policy choices in terms of the social objectives are provided.

In Section 15.2, an overview of public health insurance in the United States is presented. The focus is on the Medicare and Medicaid programs, two of the major national public health insurance plans in the U.S. In Section 15.3, the issue of health insurance coverage is discussed. In Section 15.4, information on recent trends in public health insurance is presented. In Section 15.5, the social goals of Medicare are discussed. In Section 15.6, a sample of solutions proposed in recent years is described and discussion on how each solution contributes to or obstructs the achievement of specific health policy goals is described. Section 15.7 considers alternatives to

Medicaid as approaches to addressing issues of inequity and access to needed healthcare services.

15.2 Public Health Insurance

Public health insurance in the United States for nonmilitary populations involves two key programs aimed at specific target populations. These are the federal Medicare program and the state-federal Medicaid programs. The majority of states also participate in Medicaid expansion. Some states also provide additional public health insurance programs. Often these additional state programs will be tied in some way to Medicaid, but in some circumstances they are not. In this chapter, the focus is on Medicare and Medicaid, including Medicaid expansion.

15.2.1 Medicare

15.2.1.1 Who Is Covered

Medicare is a national health insurance program for a subset of the U.S. population. Medicare was established in 1965 under Title XVIII of the Social Security Act and began coverage of beneficiaries on

January 1, 1966. Originally, Medicare covered individuals 65 years of age or older, regardless of income or medical history, as long as they or their spouse contributed to Social Security for at least 10 years (40 quarters), Railroad Retirement, or federal retirement programs. In 1972, Medicare was expanded to cover individuals under 65 with certain permanent disabilities or who had end-stage renal disease (ESRD), the permanent failure of kidneys requiring dialysis or a transplanted kidney. Medicare was again expanded in 2001 to cover individuals with amyotrophic lateral sclerosis (ALS, or Lou Gehrig's disease).

In 2019, Medicare covered about 64 million people of which 22 million, or almost 34%, were enrolled in Medicare Advantage plans. Of the individuals covered by Medicare, about 85% were 65 and older and 15% were disabled. Medicare covered about 18% of the total population (Annual Report of the Boards of Trustees, 2019; Kaiser Family Foundation, 2019). Between 1966 and 2000, the population covered by Medicare doubled and is projected to double again to about 80 million by 2030.

The population served is also diverse. For example, in 2017, about 55% of the beneficiaries were female, 75% were White, and 12% were under 100% of the national poverty level and another 20% were between 100% and 199% of the federal poverty level. As the characteristics of the population change over time, the diversity of the covered population will become more racially and ethnically diverse. About 25% of beneficiaries reported only fair to poor health in 2017, with disproportionate representation in the nonelderly, Black, Hispanic, and lower-income populations. Also, about 90% of noninstitutionalized Medicare beneficiaries have one or more chronic illnesses, with 68% with two or more chronic conditions, and 17% with six or more chronic conditions (CMS, 2018).

15.2.1.2 What Is Covered?

Medicare consists of four parts: Part A, Hospital Insurance; Part B, Supplemental Medical Insurance; Part C, Medicare Advantage; and Part D, Prescription Drugs. Each of these will be discussed in more detail in the following paragraphs.

Part A, Hospital Insurance (HI), covers inpatient hospital services, limited skilled-nursing facility services for rehabilitation, home health care, and hospice services. Most individuals are automatically eligible for Part A coverage if they are a U.S. citizen or permanent resident, if they or their spouse are eligible for Social Security payments, have made payroll tax contributions for 40 quarters (10 years), and are age 65 or older.

These individuals are eligible regardless of income or asset level or any preexisting medical condition.

Individuals under age 65 qualify for Medicare Part A if they have received Social Security Disability Income (SSDI) payments for at least 24 months; these individuals do not have to have made payroll tax contributions for 40 quarters. In addition, people with end-stage renal disease or Lou Gehrig's disease are eligible for Medicare as soon as they begin receiving SSDI payments. Individuals age 65 and older not eligible (e.g., who have not contributed to payroll tax for 40 quarters) can enroll in Part A by paying a monthly premium.

Individuals who are eligible for Medicare Part A do not pay a premium. Part A beneficiaries on original Medicare (not Medicare Advantage) are responsible for a deductible before Medicare begins to pay; in 2019, the Part A deductible was $1364 for each episode or "spell of illness" for an in-hospital stay during the benefit period. In addition, beneficiaries generally pay a coinsurance amount for extended hospital stays (days 61–90) or skilled-nursing facility stays (days 21–100). In 2019, the cost per day of extended hospital stay was $341.04 for days 61–90 and $682 for each lifetime reserve day after day 90 (up to 60 days over the beneficiary's lifetime). Beyond the lifetime reserve days the beneficiary is responsible for all costs. For extended nursing facility stay beneficiaries paid $175.50 per day for days 21–100, and were responsible for all costs beyond 100 days. If an individual is enrolled in a Medicare Advantage Plan, the rules may differ, but the plan must provide at least the same coverage as original Medicare.

If an individual has Part A (hospital insurance), then the individual is eligible for hospice care. To qualify for hospice care, a physician must certify that the individual is terminally ill with a life expectancy of 6 months or less. And, the individual agrees to accept palliative care instead of curative care, and the individual signs a statement choosing hospice instead of other Medicare-covered benefits to treat the terminal illness and related conditions. Then, the beneficiary pays nothing for hospice care. There may be a copayment of 5 dollars for each prescription drug and other similar products for pain relief and symptom control while at home. The individual may, however, be required to pay 5% of the Medicare-average amount for inpatient respite care. Respite care is short-term inpatient care provided to the beneficiary in order to relieve family members or other caregivers that are caring for the beneficiary at home. It is reimbursed for no more than five consecutive days per respite period. Medicare does not cover room and board for hospice care in the home or other facility (like a nursing home).

Part B, Supplementary Medical Insurance (SMI), Original Medicare assists beneficiaries paying for medically necessary physician services, outpatient services, home health services, preventive services, ambulance services, clinical laboratory services, durable medical equipment (DME), kidney supply and services, outpatient, inpatient, and partial hospitalization for mental health services, and diagnostic tests. In addition, it covers an annual comprehensive wellness visit and personalized prevention plan. Beneficiaries pay nothing for preventive services if the provider accepts assignment. Assignment means that the provider agrees (or is required by law) to accept the Medicare-approved amount as full payment for covered services. Unlike Part A, however, Part B is voluntary and beneficiaries are required to pay a premium for the program (in 2019 the base premium was $135.50 per month, and additional premium amounts were charged for individuals with higher incomes).

About 95% of the rate of increase in the premium is limited to the cost-of-living increase in Social Security benefits. Also, the premium paid is related to income; single individuals with an income greater than $85,000, or couples filing separately with income greater than $85,000, or couples with an income greater than $170,000 in 2019 pay a higher premium, ranging from $189.60 to $460.50 per month. Part B benefits are also subject to annual deductibles ($185 in 2019) and a 20% coinsurance rate, although the preventative services are exempt from the coinsurance and deductible. Over 90% of eligible beneficiaries enroll in Part B.

Part C, Medicare Advantage plans, are alternatives to the Original Medicare plan. Part C allows beneficiaries to enroll in a private plan, such as a health maintenance organization (HMO), preferred provider organization (PPO) or a private fee-for-service plan with specific characteristics, such as an accountable care organization. These Medicare Advantage plans contract with Medicare and must cover all of the medically necessary services that Original Medicare covers, although Original Medicare still covers the cost of hospice care, some new Medicare benefits, and some costs of clinical research studies. In addition, most Medicare Advantage plans offer coverage for items not covered under Original Medicare, such as vision, hearing, dental, and some wellness programs like gym memberships. Many of the plans cover other health-related services that promote health and wellness. Most include Medicare prescription drug (Part D) coverage. In addition to the Part B plan, most plans charge an additional premium.

Part D, Outpatient Prescription Drug Benefit, is a relatively recent addition to Medicare, implemented in 2006. It is an optional benefit offered to all Medicare beneficiaries. If an individual does not enroll in Part D when first eligible, then usually a late enrollment penalty is required for the delayed enrollment, which is applied as long as the individual is enrolled in the prescription drug coverage. Private plans contract with Medicare to provide coverage to voluntarily enrolled beneficiaries. Beneficiaries enrolled in the plan typically pay a monthly premium, and individuals with modest income and assets are eligible for assistance. Beginning in 2011, the health reform law establishes a new Part D premium program similar to the Part B program and gradually phases in coverage of the Part D coverage gap (the donut hole) by 2020. Beneficiaries then pay 100% of drug costs until they have spent $4550 out-of-pocket for prescriptions. Both original Medicare and Medicare Advantage plans offer Part D coverage.

Each Part D drug plan under Medicare is required to provide at least a standard level of coverage set by Medicare. Plans are permitted to vary the list of prescription drugs they cover (their formulary) and how they place drugs in two different "tiers" on their formulary. These formularies cover both generic and brand-name prescription drugs. The formularies are required to include at least two drugs in the most commonly prescribed categories and classes, but can select which specific drugs are covered. Beginning in 2019, drug plans that meet certain requirements can immediately remove brand-name drugs from the formularies and replace them with new generic drugs or change the cost of coverage rules for brand names when adding new generic drugs. **Table 15-1** provides information on the premiums for Part D coverage in 2019. The additional paid above the plan's premium is paid directly to Medicare, and not to a Medicare Advantage plan.

Deductibles charged by plans vary across the plans, but the maximum deductible in 2019 was $415. Some plans do not have a deductible. Many plans also have a copayment per tier (a fixed amount) or a coinsurance rate (percent of the cost of the drug) per prescription.

15.2.1.3 Financing Medicare

The primary sources of Medicare funding are general revenues (43%), payroll tax revenues (36%), and premiums (15%) paid by beneficiaries. In addition, taxation of Social Security benefits (2%), transfers from states (1%), and other sources, such as interest (1%) also help fund Medicare.

Part A, the Hospital Insurance Trust Fund, receives funding through a dedicated tax levied against earnings (88%). This tax (2.9%) is paid

Table 15-1 Filing Status and Yearly Income in 2017*

File an Individual Tax Return	File a Joint Tax Return	File Married but Separate Tax Return	Payment Each Month in 2019 in Addition to Plan Premium ($)
$85,000 or less	$170,000 or less	$85,000 or less	12.40 plus premium
More than $85,000–$107,000	More than $170,000–$214,000	N/A	31.90 plus premium
More than $107,000–$133,500	More than $214,000–$267,000	N/A	51.40 plus premium
More than $133,500–$160,000	More than $267,000–$320,000	N/A	70.90 plus premium
More than $160,000 but less than $500,000	More than $320,000 but less than $750,000	More than $85,000 but less than $415,000	77.40 plus premium
$500,000 or more	$750,000 or more	$415,000 or more	

*IRS tax returns from 2 years previously are used.
Modified from Monthly premium for drug plans, Retrieved from www.Medicare.gov/drug-coverage-part-D/costs-for-Medicare-drug-coverage/monthly-premium-for-drug-plans

equally by employers and employees (1.45% each), with self-employed individuals paying both parts. Beginning in 2013, the health reform law increases the tax for higher-income individuals (greater than $200,000 per individual and greater than $250,000 per couple) to 2.35% from 1.45%. This tax is levied against earnings (salary and wages), not total income. Part A receives about 1% from premiums, 8% from taxation of Social Security benefits, 2% from interest, and 1% from other sources.

Part B, the Supplementary Medical Insurance Trust Fund, is financed in part from general revenues (72%) and in part by premiums (26%) paid by beneficiaries voluntarily enrolled in the program. The goal is to have premiums to cover about 25% of the costs of Part B, and general revenues cover about 75%, interest and other sources cover approximately 1% each. Higher-income individuals pay a larger share toward the premiums.

Part C, the Medicare Advantage program, is not separately funded. It provides benefits under Parts A, B, and D and so receives its funding through these sources.

Part D, the Prescription Drug program, receives funding from general revenues (71%), premiums from beneficiaries (17%), and state payments for dual eligible individuals (12%). The monthly premiums from beneficiaries are established to cover 25.5% of the costs of the standard plan and Medicare funds the other 74.5%. As under Part B, higher-income individuals pay a larger share of the coverage and therefore receive a smaller subsidy from Medicare.

Financing the Medicare program continues to face a number of challenges. These challenges include rising healthcare costs, a population that continues to age, and a declining ratio of workers contributing to the system to beneficiaries enrolled in the program. Efforts to control the costs of Medicare remain a federal priority because it accounted for about 15% of the total federal budget in 2018 and is projected to increase to 18% in 2029 (Cubanski, Neuman, & Freed, 2019; Potetz, Cubanski, & Neuman, 2011).

15.2.1.4 Paying Providers

Except for Medicare Advantage (Part C) arrangements, Medicare pays most providers on a fee-for-service basis, with bundling of services occurring under the hospital prospective payment system with MS-DRGs. Physician fees include an aggregation of elements under the RBRVS system, and home health is paid a bundled, capitated amount. Medicare has implemented a number of programs to improve quality and control costs that will be discussed later.

Medicare benefit payments totaled $731 billion in 2018, up from $462 billion in 2008. During this period spending on Part A benefits decreased from 50% to 41%, while Part B spending increased from 39% to 46%. Spending on Part D increased from 11% to 13%. Medicare financed about 20% of total national healthcare expenditures in 2017, with its share varying by the type of service. For example, Medicare funded about 23% of the total spending on physician services. The most rapidly growing service funded by Medicare is prescription drugs, in which Medicare financed about 30% of national retail drug sales in 2017, compared to only 3% in 2005, the year prior to implementation of Part D. Hospitals received about 25% of their funding from Medicare in 2017 (Cubanski, Neuman, & Freed, 2019).

Payments to Medicare Advantage plans have increased substantially in recent years as more and more beneficiaries have elected to enroll in these plans instead of Original Medicare. In 2018, 34% of Medicare beneficiaries were enrolled in Medicare Advantage plans. Payments to Medicare Advantage plans for Parts A and B benefits increased from $99 billion (21%) in $2008 to $233 billion (32%) in 2018. Total Part D benefit payments increased from $49 billion (11%) in 2008 to $95 billion (13%) in 2018.

Medicare has experienced slower growth in spending in recent years, mainly because of the implementation of the Patient Protection and Affordable Care Act (ACA) and the Budget Control Act (BCA) of 2011. The ACA introduced system reforms to improve efficiency and quality of patient care and reduce costs. These reforms included Accountable Care Organizations (ACOs), medical homes, bundled payments, and value-based purchasing initiatives. The ACA also included reductions in payments to plans and providers. The BCA, through sequestration, reduced payments to providers and plans by 2% beginning in 2013. And while Medicare has seen an increase in enrollment as the "baby boomer" generation begins to age into the Medicare program, these individuals tend to help lower the average age of the Medicare population and are healthier (Cubanski, Neuman, & Freed, 2019).

15.2.1.5 Supplemental Insurance Coverage

Because of the risk of substantial out-of-pocket costs to Medicare beneficiaries through deductibles, coinsurance, and uncovered services, about 90% of Medicare beneficiaries have purchased supplemental insurance coverage (a.k.a. Medigap plans). This supplemental coverage takes several forms, but the goal is to assist the beneficiaries in covering the relatively high cost-sharing expenses of Medicare and also to cover benefits that Medicare does not cover currently. While traditionally the primary source of supplemental coverage was employer-sponsored benefits, large employers offering retiree health benefits have declined substantially due to rising costs and the economic environment. However, the number of beneficiaries enrolled in Medicare Advantage plans has been increasing, and the additional coverage offered by these plans has helped to cushion some of these changes.

Another source of supplemental coverage comes from state Medicaid programs, which provide some assistance to low-income Medicare beneficiaries who also have modest assets. The Medicaid programs often

pay the Parts B and D premiums for these eligible beneficiaries to ensure they have coverage under these voluntary programs. Medicaid may also pay premiums for individuals who don't qualify for subsidized enrollment but are eligible to pay premiums to join the program. More about these "dual-eligible" beneficiaries will be provided in the Medicaid section.

Medicare beneficiaries also have the ability to purchase supplemental private insurance plans, usually called Medigap plans. These Medigap policies help cover the cost-sharing requirements of Medicare and fill in the gaps in the benefits. These policies are designed to cover the deductibles, coinsurance, and copayments associated with Medicare-covered services. While these plans reduce financial burdens to the beneficiaries, they do reduce the typical incentives associated with having beneficiaries retain some financial responsibility, impacting the price consciousness of consumers. In general, these Medigap policies must conform to 1 of 10 standard benefit packages. Each of these packages offers coverage of a different set of benefits from which the beneficiaries can select. The monthly premium charged varies by the benefits covered, the insurer, the age of the beneficiary, and the place of residence. Beginning in 2020, Medigap plans purchased by new Medicare enrollees will not be allowed to cover the Part B deductible.

Some beneficiaries enroll in multiple supplementary plans to provide more complete coverage of medical expenses. Even with all these supplemental policies, many Medicare beneficiaries still experience substantial out-of-pocket expenses. For example, Medicare beneficiaries spent over 14% of their income out-of-pocket for health care in 2013, and that percentage has been increasing with economic conditions and changes in premiums and services covered. In 2013, one-fourth of Original Medicare enrollees spent about 30% of their income on out-of-pocket cost, even with Medigap coverage. As out-of-pocket costs increase, Medicare beneficiaries face additional challenges to maintaining daily necessities. As cost-sharing increases, more Medicare beneficiaries may have to choose between basic necessities and health care, with the results being adversely impacted health.

15.2.2 Medicaid
15.2.2.1 Who Is Covered?

Medicaid is another public insurance program. Medicaid was established in 1965 as part of the "Great Society" program under Title XIX of the Social Security Act; it was implemented as of July 1, 1966. Medicaid was established as an entitlement program to provide financial assistance for healthcare services and long-term care services for certain low-income individuals and families who were receiving cash assistance (welfare recipients). However, since its beginning, it has been expanded to increase eligibility to cover additional individuals living below or near the poverty level. Today, Medicaid covers both working and jobless families and children, pregnant women, individuals with a variety of physical and mental conditions, and elderly individuals. The role of Medicaid has expanded substantially under health reform.

Unlike Medicare, which is a federal program operated under guidelines established by the Social Security Administration and administered through the Centers for Medicare and Medicaid Services (CMS), Medicaid is a state-federal partnership program. The administration of Medicaid is at the state level, according to federal requirements. Medicaid participation by states is voluntary, although all states currently participate in the original Medicaid program, and it is financed jointly by federal and state governments, with the federal government "matching" dollars expended by the states. The federal match rate (Federal Medical Assistance Percentage, or FMAP) to the states varies and is based on average state per capita income relative to the national average. By law, FMAP is at least 50% (meaning that for every dollar the state spends on Medicaid, the federal government will provide another dollar for Medicaid services) and reached as high as 74.94% for the fiscal year 2020. The higher the FMAP, the greater the percentage of total Medicaid costs that are financed by the federal government.

In 2009, the American Recovery and Reinvestment Act temporarily increased the FMAP, and for 2010, the FMAP ranged from 50% to 85%. This increased the federal share of total Medicaid spending in 2010 from 57% to 66%, enabling states to cover additional individuals due to the economic conditions.

Because most private insurance is obtained through place of employment, when individuals lose employment, they also usually lose insurance coverage. The expansion in Medicaid during the period covered by the American Recovery and Reinvestment Act was designed to provide financial assistance to individuals until they became reemployed and began receiving insurance coverage again (Doty, Collins, Robertson, & Garber, 2011).

Under the partnership, Medicaid is administered by the states under broad federal guidelines and oversight by CMS. The broad federal guidelines enable states to exercise considerable variation in the design of their programs. While state participation in Medicaid is voluntary, currently all states participate.

The federal government defines minimum requirements that states must meet, but the states have broad authority to establish eligibility criteria, benefits covered, provider payments, delivery systems, and a number of other conditions for their program. As a result, the percentage of the population covered across states varies widely.

In addition, states may request a waiver from the federal government, enabling them to design and operate their program outside the federal guidelines. A typical reason for requesting a waiver is to adopt a new model of coverage and delivery system for their low-income population. The waiver capability and the inherent flexibility of the Medicaid program have enabled states to adapt and evolve to meet the needs of their populations better. States can adjust more quickly to changing economic conditions or medical conditions (such as the HIV/AIDS pandemic) to coordinate and manage the health of their populations. The flexibility also means that there is substantial diversity in who is covered across the states.

In general terms, not only must an individual qualify based on financial criteria, but the individual must also belong to a group designated as "categorically" eligible for coverage. The federal government mandates that pregnant women and children under 6 with family incomes less than 133% of the federal poverty level (FPL) be covered. In addition, children age 6–18 with family income below 100% of the FPL must be covered, as must parents below states' 1996 welfare eligibility levels. Most elderly populations and individuals with disabilities and on SSI must also be covered. States do, however, have flexibility in determining what counts as income for the program, with most states including assets in the measure. In addition to the minimum mandatory groups, states have the option of expanding coverage to additional groups. These optional groups covered typically extend the upper income levels for covered groups.

Medicaid is an entitlement program. Once a state has established the eligibility criteria for its Medicaid program, then all individuals in the state meeting the criteria have a federal right to Medicaid coverage; the individuals are entitled to coverage, and enrollment cannot be limited by the state, nor can waiting lists be applied. One federal criterion is that individuals must be American citizens or specific categories of lawfully residing immigrants who have resided in the United States for 5 years.

Medicaid is currently core to the financing structure of the U.S. healthcare system and expanded substantially under health reform. Currently, more children are covered under Medicaid than any other source. Also, the majority of adults who are covered under Medicaid are in working families, holding low-paying jobs without access to employer-based health insurance. Many nonelderly individuals with disabilities unable to obtain coverage in the private market or for whom the coverage available does not meet all their needs, rely on Medicaid. Medicaid also covers pregnant women, with about 40% of all births occurring to Medicaid mothers.

Another group of enrollees in Medicaid are the low-income individuals on Medicare, the "dual-eligible" individuals. In 2017, there were 12 million individuals dually enrolled. The dual-eligible populations are poorer than the other Medicare populations and also tend to have poorer health, with higher rates of chronic illness, require more long-term care needs, and have greater social risk factors. In 2017, 41% of the dually enrolled individuals had at least one mental health diagnosis.

About one in six Medicare beneficiaries are also enrolled in Medicaid, which assists enrollees in paying their premiums for Parts B and D, cover the cost-sharing obligations of Medicare, and cover services not covered under Medicare, especially custodial long-term care in nursing facilities. Because of poorer health and services needed, these individuals place greater financial strain on the Medicaid program than the typical Medicaid recipient. Typically, Medicare pays for covered services first, with Medicaid the payer of last resort. Medicaid may also pay for services Medicare does not cover and will pay the premium for those individuals to enroll in Medicare Parts B and D plans.

In 1997, the Children's Health Insurance Program (CHIP) was created under Title XXI of the Social Security Act. CHIP is another insurance program that provides federal matching funds to states to provide health coverage to children in families that have incomes that are too high to allow them to qualify for Medicaid but do not have sufficient income to enable them to purchase private health insurance coverage. CHIP allowed states substantial flexibility in the expansion of insurance coverage of children, but every state now covers children and families to at least 200% of the federal poverty level.

This program can either be included with the state's Medicaid program or established as an independent program or as a combination. The independent design allows states more flexibility and requires states to describe the characteristics of their program in a state health plan. If the state includes CHIP in their Medicaid program, then the same rules apply as to other recipients, although eligibility is extended to higher-income individuals. As eligibility for coverage became more expansive, concerns were raised that the public insurance program would "crowd out" private insurance coverage. The concern was that the lower, subsidized premium of CHIP would cause parents to drop dependent children from their private insurance plan and enroll them in the public program.

The goal of the Affordable Care Act (ACA) was to reduce the number of uninsured individuals in the United States by providing a number of affordable care options through Medicaid and the health insurance marketplace. The ACA authorized states to expand Medicaid eligibility if they wished to enroll individuals under 65 and families with incomes below 138% of the federal poverty level (FPL). It also standardized the rules for determining eligibility and providing benefits through Medicaid, CHIP, and the health insurance marketplace. In June 2012, the Supreme Court ruled that participation by states to expand Medicaid coverage had to be voluntary.

Under Medicaid expansion, the cost-share of the new enrollees covered was financed 100% by the federal government for the years 2014 through 2017, and then gradually declining until it reached 90% federal share in 2022 and beyond. This federal share percent is much more generous than the 50%–75% (averaging 57%) for existing Medicaid expenditures. As of 2019, 14 states were still not participating in Medicaid expansion.

Even with the expanded coverage under Medicaid, there are still groups, or categories, of individuals who are not eligible for Medicaid, regardless of income level. Low income is a necessary condition but not a sufficient condition for coverage. One group of the uninsured is the parents of children who are on Medicaid because the income requirements are more restrictive for adults than for children. Another group is adults without dependent children, who no matter how low their income is, unless they are pregnant or disabled, do not qualify for Medicaid. This latter group was the primary focus of the Medicaid expansion program. Most states do not cover lawfully resident immigrants during their first 5 years in the United States. Federal law prohibits undocumented immigrants from being covered by Medicaid.

15.2.2.2 What Is Covered?

Medicaid covers a broad array of services, both mandatory and optional. The federal government mandates each state offer a specific set of services in order to participate in the program. The federal government also allows states to cover additional optional services under the Medicaid allowable services. These optional services qualify for the same federal match as the mandated services. The specific optional services covered vary across states.

Because of the rather diverse needs of the Medicaid population, not only are the typical benefits covered under private insurance provided, but Medicaid programs also typically cover dental, vision, transportation, translation services, and long-term care services and support. **Table 15-2** provides a list of mandatory services as well as typical optional services covered. States employ a number of strategies to limit utilization of services, such as concurrent and retrospective utilization review, prior authorization, restrictive definitions of medical necessity, and case management, especially for high-risk/high-cost cases.

For children under 21, the mandatory coverage of Early and Periodic Screening, Diagnostic, and Treatment (EPSDT) benefit provides a very comprehensive set of services to correct or ameliorate acute and chronic physical and mental health conditions. The services covered under the EPSDT benefit are broader than most private insurance plans and are especially important for children with disabilities.

Also not widely provided under private health insurance are the long-term services and support provided under Medicaid, although individuals can purchase long-term care policies privately. Medicaid includes services provided in skilled and intermediate-level nursing homes, as well as such community-based services as home health, rehabilitation therapy, medical equipment, adult daycare, and respite care for caregivers, to enable individuals to live as independently as possible. Medicaid is the largest public payer of mental health care, and Medicaid also covers about two-thirds of all nursing home residents and about 40% of individuals with HIV.

15.2.2.3 Financing Medicaid

The federal-state partnership organizational structure of Medicaid results in financing also shared between the two. There is a statutory formula that dictates how the federal government matches the spending of each state. The federal match rate, FMAP, is based on a state's per capita income relative to the national average—the lower a state's per capita income, the higher the rate paid by the federal government. There is not a limit on total Medicaid expenditures, but expenditures are limited by the ability of the state to generate its share of the expenses. This creates a barrier for many states that are required to balance their budgets, because states must first spend the Medicaid monies paying providers and then get reimbursed

retrospectively from the federal government for their share.

The Basic Health Program was part of the ACA and provides states an option to establish health benefit programs for low-income residents who would otherwise be eligible to purchase coverage through the health insurance marketplace. The Basic Health Program is designed to provide affordable coverage and better continuity of care for people whose income fluctuates above and below Medicaid and CHIP levels. States may offer coverage to individuals with incomes between 133% and 200% of the federal poverty level.

For most states, Medicaid is the largest source of federal revenue for the state, while it tends to be the second-largest sector of a state's budget, behind education. Because most states must balance their budgets, generating revenue to support Medicaid can be difficult, especially in economic downturns, when state revenues decline while the enrollment in Medicaid increases. However, because increased Medicaid spending by the state results in an influx of federal dollars, it increases the multiplier effect of those dollars, as businesses and residents generate successive rounds of earnings and purchases. This influx of federal dollars into the state's economy provides an incentive for states to focus on health care and not necessarily reduce coverage of their populations, although states are forced to control costs to balance their budget.

15.2.3 Paying the Providers
15.2.3.1 Fee-For-Service

There are two generic types of healthcare financial coverage for providers under Medicare: fee-for-service and per capita (or capitation) payment, although recently Medicare has implemented a blended strategy combining the two types of payment. In the fee-for-service plan, the Medicare program sets prices for individual patient contacts or encounters. Medicare has developed systems for classifying services of providers for most types of care supplied; these systems now include inpatient hospitalization, outpatient care, home care, and skilled-nursing facility care. Any classification system can divide cases or patients into groups of patients or encounters; the patients within each group are assumed to use a similar amount of resources. Each group is assigned a *relative weight*, and a dollar value is assigned to a weighted unit. Medicare adjusts the monetary prices for a variety of factors, including whether the provider is in an urban or rural area, area wage and cost-of-living levels, and provider characteristics (e.g., teaching versus nonteaching

Table 15-2 Services Covered by Medicaid Programs

Mandatory Services	Commonly Offered Optional Services
Inpatient hospital services	Prescription drugs
Outpatient hospital services	Clinic services
Early and periodic screening, diagnostic, and treatment (EPSDT) services for individuals under 21 years of age	Physical therapy
Nursing facility services	Occupational therapy
Home health services	Speech, hearing, and language disorder services
Physician services	Respiratory care services
Rural health clinic services	Other diagnostic, screening, preventive, and rehabilitative services
Federally qualified health center services	Podiatry services
Laboratory and X-ray services	Optometry services
Family planning services	Dental services
Nurse midwife services	TB-related services
Certified pediatric and family nurse practitioner services	Dentures
Freestanding birth center services (when licenses or otherwise recognized by the state)	Prosthetics
Transportation to medical care	Eyeglasses
Tobacco cessation counseling for pregnant women	Chiropractic services
Tobacco cessation, www.governing.com/news/state/gov-Study-Medicaid-Anti-Smoking-Programs-Lead-to-Significant-Savings.html	Other practitioner services
	Private duty nursing services
	Personal care
	Hospice
	Case management
	Services for individuals age 65 or older in an Institution for Mental Disease (IMD)
	Services in an intermediate care facility for the mentally retarded
	State plan home-and-community based services 1915(i)
	Self-directed personal assistance services 1915(i)
	Community first choice option 1915(k)
	Inpatient psychiatric services for individuals under age 21
	Health homes for enrollees with chronic conditions—Section 1945
	Other services approved by the secretary*

*This includes services furnished in a religious nonmedical healthcare institution, inpatient psychiatric services for individuals under age 21, emergency hospital services by a non-Medicare certified hospital, and critical access hospital (CAH).
Mandatory & Optional Medicaid Benefits. Retrieved from https://www.medicaid.gov/medicaid/benefits/list-of-benefits/index.html

units). The result is a complex array of prices that are being paid for patients with the same diagnosis.

The inpatient hospital stays under Medicare Part A are paid a prospectively set rate and the payments system is referred to as the inpatient prospective payment system (IPPS). Under IPPS, hospitals are paid according to the Medicare Severity Diagnosis Related Group (MS-DRG) system. The original DRG system was implemented in 1983, with 467 DRGs; the system was modified to incorporate the severity of cases within the DRGs in 2007, with over 700 groups established. In 2019 there were over 750 groups established. Each group is assigned a basic weighted rate that is then multiplied by the conversion rate to obtain the amount paid for patients hospitalized in that group. The group reflects the average resources used to treat Medicare patients in that MS-DRG.

This payment rate is divided into two components: labor-related and nonlabor-related, with proportions based on the wage index. In defining the service area of hospitals to be used in the labor-related adjustment, a commuting ratio of workers commuting from home to work is used in defining the hospital's labor market. For 2020, the base rate was $5654.75 per admission. If the wage index was greater than one, then the labor share accounted for 68.3% of the relative weight, or $3862.19 per unit, and the nonlabor share accounted for 31.7%, or $1792.56 per unit. If the wage index was equal to or less than one, then the labor share was 62.0%, or $3505.95 per unit, and the nonlabor share was 38.0%, or $2148.80 per unit. These base rates are multiplied by the relative weight of the MS-DRG to obtain the amount the hospital will receive for a patient hospitalized with that diagnosis.

Under programs established by the ACA, additional adjustments to the labor and nonlabor wage index numbers are made. For hospitals that submitted quality data and were a meaningful user of an electronic health record (EHR) then the amounts they were paid for the labor and nonlabor wage index components were increased by 2.2%. If the hospitals submitted quality data but were not a meaningful user of an EHR, their amounts were increased by 0.35%. If the hospitals did not submit quality data but were a meaningful EHR user, the amounts were increased by 1.85%. For hospitals that did not submit quality data and were not a meaningful user of an EHR, their amounts were decreased by 0.4%.

Hospitals may receive an add-on payment to the base payment if they treat a high percentage of low-income patients, known as the disproportionate share hospital (DSH) adjustment. The ACA modified how hospitals are reimbursed for serving a disproportionate share of low-income patients. Beginning in FY 2014, hospitals receive 25% of the amount they previously would have received under the current statutory formulas for Medicare DSH. The remaining 75% of what would have been paid as Medicare DSH becomes available for uncompensated care payments after the amount is reduced for changes in the percentage of individuals that are uninsured in the hospital's service area.

If a hospital is an approved teaching hospital, then it receives an indirect medical education (IME) adjustment percentage add-on payment. This rate depends upon the ratio of residents-to-beds for operating costs and on the ratio of residents to average daily census for capital costs.

The final adjustment is made for unusually costly patients—the outlier adjustment. This adjustment is designed to protect hospitals from unusually expensive cases. The total payment hospitals receive for a patient in a MS-DRG then, reflects the base payment plus DSH adjustment, plus IME adjustment, plus outlier adjustment (see https://www.cms.gov/AcuteInpatientPPS /01_overview.asp#TopOfPage). Hospitals can also receive additional payments for treating patients with certain new expensive technologies under the capital payment rate. For 2020 the national rate was $462.61.

The IPPS payment to hospitals is also adjusted for the hospitals participating in the value-based purchasing (VBP) program, the hospital readmission reduction program (HRRP), and the hospital-acquired conditions (HAC) reduction program. The hospital's VBP can result in the rate being adjusted upward, downward, or remaining neutral based on the performance on a set of quality measures. The VBP program provides incentive payments to participating hospitals that exceed performance standards and/or improve performance during the period. Beginning in 2017 the reduction to base operating MS-DRG payment amounts decreased by 2.0% for those hospitals not meeting the standards.

The HRRP allows an adjustment to the base payment to hospitals to account for excessive readmissions for the conditions of acute myocardial infarction, heart failure, pneumonia, chronic obstructive pulmonary disease (COPD), total hip/knee arthroplasty, and coronary artery bypass graft surgery (CABG). Hospitals ranking in the lowest performing hospital-acquired conditions (HAC) reduction program quartile will receive payment equal to 99% of what the IPPS would normally pay the hospital.

Medicare has also implemented a prospective payment system for post-acute home care. A classification system was developed that is based on the patient's diagnosis, clinical factors, functional factors, and on therapeutic needs (physical therapy [PT], speech-language pathology therapy [SLP], and occupational therapy [OT]), medical social services, routine and nonroutine medical supplies, and home health services (Liu, Gage, Harvell, Stevenson, & Brennan, 1999; Medicare Learning Network, 2018). As with inpatient care, a weight is assigned to each group in the class, and a price per weighted unit is set. There were 153 case-mix groups in 2018 and the rate is established to cover a 60-day period. The Medicare home care payment system replaced a system by which home care providers billed for individual services. It thus represents a bundling of services, in comparison with the payment system prior to 1999, when the prospective payment system was introduced. The price includes a wage adjustment factor. Outliers are also permitted for additional payment. The ACA places an limit on home health services so that no more than 1% of a home health agency's (HHA's) total payments are paid as outliers.

Unlike hospital and home care reimbursement, the payment for physicians under Medicare remains on an individual service basis. Physicians are paid by fee category, called *Current Procedural Terminology* (CPT). There are over 10,000 CPT codes currently. Each service is assigned a weight; currently, the weighting system is called the *Resource-Based Relative Value System* (RBRVS). The RBRVS contains separate component weights that reflect work performed, practice expenses, liability insurance, and regional cost variations. A dollar value is assigned by Medicare, which converts the resource-based weights to dollar payments. In 2019, this conversion figure was $36.0391. CMS has established 89 physician fee schedule (PFS) localities reflecting geographical cost variation to adjust the payment rates for physicians.

15.2.3.2 Additional ACA Programs

In July 2014, the Medicaid Innovation Accelerator Program (IAP) began. This program is a collaboration between the Center for Medicaid and CHIP Services (CMCS) and the Center for Medicare and Medicaid Innovation (CMMI). Under this program, support is provided to state Medicaid agencies to build capacity in key program functional areas by offering targeted technical support, tool development, and cross-state learning opportunities. The programs in which technical support is being offered include: reducing substance use disorder; improving care for Medicaid beneficiaries with complex care needs and high cost;

promoting community integration through long-term services and supports; and supporting physical and mental health integration. IAP also works with states through its functional areas for Medicaid delivery system reform: data analytics, performance improvement, quality measurement, and value-based payment of financial simulations.

Another feature of the ACA was the creation of the Health Insurance Marketplace, also known as the Health Insurance Exchange program. The health insurance marketplace program is a service that helps people shop for and enroll in affordable health insurance. These are plans offered by private insurance companies with a range of prices and features accessed through the federal government, although some states operate their own program. Individuals who qualify may be eligible for a premium tax credit and other savings that would lower monthly insurance bills and allow extra savings for out-of-pocket costs like deductibles, coinsurance, and copayments. The premiums under the health insurance marketplace program are based on estimated income of the enrollee.

Under the Medicare Shared Savings Program providers that participate in an Accountable Care Organization (ACO) continue to receive traditional Medicare fee-for-service payments under Parts A and B. However, the ACO may be eligible to receive a shared savings payment if it meets specified quality and savings requirements. This program was a one-sided program in that the ACOs could receive bonus payments, but were not at risk for excess costs. Under the new Pathways to Success Program the direction of the shared savings program is redesigned to encourage participating ACOs to transition to a two-sided model. Under this new model, ACOs continue to be able to share in savings, but are now accountable for repaying shared losses.

The objectives of the Pathways to Success Program are to: increase savings for the Trust Fund and mitigate losses, reduce gaming opportunities, promote flexible regulatory requirements, and promote free-market principles. Under this program, CMS introduced additional access to telehealth services provided in a patient's place of residence (home or long-term care facility). Also, the ACO can offer new incentive payments to beneficiaries for taking steps to achieve better health. For the ACOs taking on the risk for spending increases above the cost targets, they are held responsible for paying back to CMS up to at least 2% of the revenue or 1% of their cost targets. In return for accepting the risk, they are eligible for higher levels of shared savings.

15.3 Uncovered Care

Despite the existence of Medicare, Medicaid, the Medicaid expansion program, and the mandated health insurance requirement, many individuals either have no health insurance coverage at all or have large gaps in coverage. According to estimates by the U.S. Bureau of the Census, 16.3% of all individuals (about 49.9 million) had no insurance coverage in 2010 (DeNavas-Walt, Proctor, & Smith, 2011). In 2017, the number of uninsured increased to 28.0 million from the 27.3 million in 2016, still much lower than the 49.9 million in 2010 (Berchick, 2018). Most uninsured individuals (84.6%) were 19–64 years of age. The uninsured were disproportionately located in the south, where participation in Medicaid expansion was low. The uninsured have lower education and are more likely to live in poverty than the insured population. Most uninsured have at least one individual in the family working, which poses a problem because employment is the usual route through which health insurance is obtained.

It should be pointed out that *uninsured* is not the same thing as *unserved*. Many individuals with no insurance still receive medical care: they either pay the full price for this care or receive subsidized or charity care. What is likely, however, is that they receive less care than they would if they had insurance coverage.

In addition to those with no coverage, a substantial number of individuals have gaps in coverage. The Medicare deductibles and copayments can add up to a substantial amount, and individuals who are covered by Medicare but do not have additional private (Medigap) or Medicaid coverage can, if they become ill, incur substantial out-of-pocket costs. This is especially true for individuals who need nursing home care. There is very little in the way of long-term care insurance coverage at present, although private policies are available, and so individuals in nursing homes (especially intermediate-care facilities) will be required to pay for such care themselves, unless they "spend down" to the point at which, if married, both incomes (less medical expenses) and their assets are below the state Medicaid limits.

15.4 Some Trends in Public Health Insurance

In recent years, several public insurance trends have captured interest in the public policy arena. In this section, these trends are reviewed briefly.

15.4.1 Disbursements of the Hospital Insurance Trust Fund

Medicare's HI funding is tied to the growth of the portion of the Social Security tax that is earmarked for the Hospital Insurance Trust Fund. However, there is no automatic link between the growth of trust fund revenues and the growth of fund expenditures, which primarily go to reimburse hospitals (Iglehart, 1999; Wolkstein, 1984). The revenues are based on a percentage of payrolls and so cannot be increased by more than the increase in payrolls, unless the Social Security tax rate is increased or, as happened recently, the base on which the tax is levied is increased (i.e., employment and wages have increased). In the absence of such increases in tax revenues, large deficits in the fund had been experienced, and until very recently, increasingly large deficits had been predicted.

According to the 2018 Annual Report of the Board of Trustees of the Federal Hospital Insurance and Federal Supplementary Medical Insurance Trust Funds, expenditures from the HI Trust Fund exceeded revenues by $1.8 billion. Deficits in the Trust Fund are projected to continue, requiring redemption of Trust Fund assets to pay expenditures. It is estimated that Trust Fund assets will be depleted/exhausted in 2026.

15.4.2 Medicare's SMI Revenues and Expenditures

SMI funds come from two main sources: premiums paid directly by the enrollees (or by Medicaid for those qualifying for Medicaid coverage) for Parts B and D revenue funds and from general revenue funds. Parts B and D are maintained in separate accounts in the SMI. Originally, the premium rate for Part B was set so that premium revenues of the SMI trust fund were one-half of all revenues. From 1973, the growth of premiums was mandated to be no greater than the growth of Social Security cash benefits. As a result, since then, the premium share of total fund revenues in Part B has fallen to about 30%. The nature of financing for both Parts B and D is similar, with premiums and the transfer from general revenues for each part established annually at a level sufficient to cover the following year's estimated expenditures. Accordingly, each account within SMI is automatically financially balanced each year. As in the case of the Hospital Insurance Trust Fund, this growth in expenditures has been a major cause of concern. However, unlike Hospital Insurance Trust Fund outlays, Medical Insurance Trust Fund expenditures can be increased by government appropriations.

According to the Trustee's Report (2019), expenditures for Parts B and D grew at an average annual rate of 6.6% and 3.6%, respectively, over the past 5 years. Part B cost increases are projected to grow at an annual rate of 8.3% and Part D costs are projected to grow at an annual rate of 7.3% over the next 5 years. A "hold harmless" provision does not allow Part B premium increases to cause a beneficiary's net Social Security benefits to decrease, limiting the amount of revenue generated from premiums.

15.5 Goals of Medicare

In order to discover what the policy issues are with Medicare, the social goals of Medicare need to be examined. It was relatively recently that these goals were stated explicitly (Cutler, 2000; U.S. General Accounting Office, 1999). Among these stated goals were affordability, equity, adequacy, feasibility, and acceptance. The definitions of these concepts given here are those of the U.S. Government Accounting Office (GAO), which differ from the standard economic definitions.

Affordability refers to the total costs incurred by the program. When stating this goal, the GAO is referring to the public component of the program and its burden on public spending. *Equity* refers to the burden of payments on specific groups. Individuals can be viewed as paying too much if they don't have sufficient coverage or if their premiums are too high. Individuals can also be paying too little for premiums and copayments; with low direct costs, they would be using too much care (from a strict efficiency viewpoint). *Adequacy* refers to the availability of care. *Feasibility* refers to the ability of Medicare to actually implement changes in policy. *Acceptance* refers to the acceptability of the program to consumers, intermediaries, and providers.

These goals bear some resemblance to the following very general economic goals of health policy: economic efficiency (which has demand, technical efficiency, and adequacy-of-supply aspects), equity in utilization and equity in payment, quality of care, and public expenditure control. The economic goal of public expenditure control translates into the GAO goal of affordability. The economic goal of equity of payment translates into the GAO goal of equity. The economic goals of equity in utilization and adequacy of supply translate into the GAO goal of adequacy. The economic goals of quality of care and technical efficiency are not directly addressed in the GAO goals, although quality assurance activities are a very important component of Medicare activities (Medicare Payment Advisory Commission, 2000, 2019). The GAO goals of feasibility and acceptance are not directly addressed in the general economic goals.

In order to assess Medicare policies, Medicare performance must be evaluated in light of the policy goals. The major issues facing Medicare include rising expenditures, hospital trust-fund deficits, and large out-of-pocket payments for some groups of beneficiaries. These phenomena are related to the goals of affordability, equity of payment, and adequacy of supply. Most importantly, the goals may well conflict with each other (otherwise there would not be an economic problem). In the late 1990s, the Health Care Financing Administration (the agency that administered Medicare at that time) and the Congress instituted a series of reforms designed to address the goal achievement balance under Medicare. The policy initiatives were Medicare Part C and the Balanced Budget Act of 1997. In the following section, an overview of the policies that are available to Medicare is provided.

15.6 Policy Alternatives for Medicare

15.6.1 Economic Analysis and Alternative Solutions

Six basic types of policies can be identified that can be used to help achieve policy goals. The first set of policies deals with the setting of the broad outline of the program. For example, Medicare can change who is entitled to benefits or what benefits individuals receive. The second set of policies deals with health insurance premiums. Medicare can change Part B premiums, and it can change the out-of-pocket price of supplementary private insurance premiums. As well, Medicare can arrange for supplementary coverage in other programs, such as Medicaid.

The third set deals with the direct price of care. Medicare can change the deductibles and copayments paid by enrollees and, in the process, impact the demand for care (subject, of course, to the purchase of supplementary insurance). The fourth set deals with provider reimbursement. Medicare can change the basis of reimbursement. For example, home health care was formerly funded on the basis of individual services. Most recently, Medicare developed a home healthcare classification system that bundled individual services within diagnostic and needs-based groups. In addition to changing the definition of what output they will cover, Medicare can change the rate of payment.

Fifth, Medicare can introduce competitive practices into its reimbursement mechanism. It can fund care on the basis of vouchers, encouraging individuals to shop around for their care. And sixth, Medicare can regulate the behavior of providers (i.e., make them provide care based on specific norms set by the program).

15.6.2 The Scope of the Program

Currently, Medicare's main line of business is to provide insurance coverage for persons 65 years of age and older. In 1997, Congress set up the Medicare Payment Advisory Commission to make recommendations about policies that could affect the future of Medicare. One of the policies recommended by the two committee chairs was to increase the age of Medicare beneficiaries to 67 to have it in line with the age requirement for Social Security benefits. This proposal did not achieve policy status, but it is an obvious way of changing the number of beneficiaries in the system. One proposal intended to extend the Medicaid mandate to Medicare was to provide prescription drug insurance coverage (Davis, Poisal, Chulis, Zarabozo, & Cooper, 1999; Soumerai & Ross-Degnan, 1999). Prescription drug coverage was implemented in 2006 with a wide variety of features, including additional premiums, copayments and deductibles, prescription limits, and so forth. Its inclusion added a new dimension to the program, and administrative costs increased considerably.

15.6.3 Insurance Premiums

Individuals and groups have proposed policies that would both increase and decrease health insurance premiums. Concern over the growth in first-dollar coverage has led some observers to propose a premium tax on Medigap policies. The introduction of such a tax would raise the price of Medigap coverage and reduce the amount of coverage purchased. The reduction in such coverage would lead to a reduction in the use of medical services in the short run.

There is a premium only for Parts B and D Medicare. The premiums under Part C are set by the insurance plans in which the beneficiaries are enrolled. About one-quarter of Part B revenues come from this premium and the rest from general government revenues. The Balanced Budget Act of 1997, which overhauled Medicare's finances, did not substantially increase the premium; however, the premium is based on Social Security payments, and as such payments increase, so will the Part B premium.

In 2000, the premium was $45.50 per month; by 2012, it increased to $99.90 (or $115.40 for those not under the Social Security cap). In 2019, the base premium was $135.50, with individuals having higher incomes paying between $54.10 and $325.00 more per month. An increase in the premium influences the goal of equity in payment.

15.6.4 Copayments, Coinsurance, and Deductibles

Copayments, coinsurance, and deductibles serve to regulate demand for covered healthcare services and to reduce government expenditures. Coinsurance is fixed as a percentage of medical charges, and it increases as charges rise. Copayments and deductibles are based on usage and are not always predictable. Individuals seek predictability by purchasing Medigap insurance coverage, which pays for the copayments and deductibles. The deductible in 2019 was $1364 for Part A and $185 for Part B. There was also 20% coinsurance for Part B. These payments have increased annually, but they have not been a major part of Medicare's cost-cutting plans. Higher copayments, deductibles, and coinsurance reduce availability.

15.6.5 Provider Payments

In 1983, Medicare began paying for inpatient hospitalization on a DRG basis, and expanded to MS-DRG in 2007. A price is applied to the MS-DRG weighted units to obtain a given price per weighted unit, which is what the hospitals receive. Every year, this price is increased by a given update factor in order to account for inflation and technological change. The update factor is supposed to cover changes in capital input prices, technology changes, and any real changes in the case-mix factor. The Balanced Budget Act of 1997 made changes to Medicare that were projected to result in $116 billion in savings between 1998 and 2002. Two-thirds of these savings were to come from limits in the update factors for inpatient care (Moon, Gage, & Evans, 1997). For the first year, there was a freeze on payment rates (Levit et al., 2000).

The Medicare Part A payment strategy also included a switch from fee-for-service to prospective payment systems for home health care and outpatient care. Classification systems have been developed for home health care (Goldberg, Delargy, Schmitz, Moore, & Wrobel, 1999) and outpatient care (Health Care Financing Administration, 2000). Such systems are expected to increase control over spending in these areas by Medicare. They may also reduce availability.

15.6.6 Managed Care and Competition

In the original Medicare scheme for HMO coverage, the fees paid to HMOs were based on total medical care expenditures per beneficiary. Using the adjusted average per capita cost (AAPCC) method of rate setting, fees were set at 95% of the total medical costs for persons in the geographic area (usually the county). Included in the rate was the enrollee's Part B premium. The health plan decided on any benefit package in excess of the standard Medicare A and B coverage (e.g., whether to include drug coverage), additional premiums (if any), and copayments for medical visits. The basic rate was risk-adjusted for age, gender, eligibility for Medicaid supplemental coverage, and whether the enrollee was institutionalized.

In 1998, Congress enacted a new Part C of Title XVIII of the Social Security Act, creating the Medicare + Choice program. The program had two new features. First, it created a blended national-regional rate for the managed care premium. In this rate, Medicare combined a national rate ($398 per month) with the county rates (the old AAPCC rates). There was to be a floor below which no county-specific rate would fall. This resulted in a severing of the link between fee-for-service costs and managed care rates (McClellan, 2000).

Second, Congress instituted a new risk-adjustment variable, called the *Principal Inpatient Diagnostic Cost Group* (PIP-DCG). According to the PIP-DCG, a patient who is hospitalized in the previous year for a specific (serious) condition will fall into a higher risk category, and the HMO will receive a higher rate adjustment for this patient. The intent of these changes was to encourage HMOs to establish programs in areas that are now poorly served and to accept higher risk patients who have been hospitalized for serious conditions. Other features of the Medicare risk system remained. These include the variable benefits package, additional premiums tied to the benefits package, and consumer premiums and copayments.

In 2003, the Medicare Modernization Act renamed Medicare + Choice to Medicare Advantage (MA). The focus of MA became one of expanding access to private plans and providing additional benefits to private plan enrollees rather than cost control. The result is that Medicare pays more per enrollee in these plans than it does per enrollee in the traditional Medicare plan. In 2010, the Health Reform Act caused another shift by beginning to reduce payments to MA plans in an effort to bring their costs back in line with the fee-for-service Medicare system. A bonus system was also introduced into the MA program in which bonuses would be paid according to quality ratings for the plan. In addition, by 2014, the plans would be required to maintain a medical loss ratio of at least 85%, limiting administrative expenses and profits to 15%. By 2018, 21.1 million beneficiaries were enrolled in the MA plans. In electing to enroll in an MA, individuals are making the determination that such a plan is best for them.

Medicare Advantage plans are paid a capitated amount to provide all Parts A and B benefits. A separate amount is paid to cover Part D. The rate paid is established in a bidding process based on estimated costs per enrollee for covered services. All bids that meet the necessary condition are accepted. The bids are compared to a benchmark amount, and the benchmarks become the maximum amount Medicare will pay a plan in a given area. If the bid from a plan is higher than the benchmark, then enrollees pay the difference in the form of a monthly premium. If it is lower, the plan and Medicare split the difference. The plan's share is known as a rebate and must be used to offer supplemental benefits to enrollees. Medicare's payments to plans reflect the enrollees' risk profile. The 2010 health reform law reversed the methodology for paying plans and reduced the benchmarks. The amount of the rebate in the future will depend upon the quality rating of the plan.

In the coming years, there will be many reform proposals seeking to push Medicare toward becoming a competitive system. It is questionable whether such reforms would solve the problems associated with introducing managed care principles into the Medicare program. Medicare enrollees still join HMOs individually and have high and variable costs. The very significant incentive to select healthier cases will remain as long as the risk-adjustment tools do not permit the identification of high-risk individuals.

As well, any attempt to regulate competitive practices will result in an extremely complex set of rules. However, the set of rules may not be any more complex than the set of current fee-for-service rules, in which a multitude of prices and adjustments have been introduced within a complicated regulatory framework. Further, the definition and regulation of the basic product characteristics will prove to be a daunting task. Medical care is a service with many aspects, and the between-patient and between-provider differences are very subtle.

A successful capitation program will better allow Medicare to achieve a greater degree of control over public expenditures. Competition should lead to a greater degree of efficiency in the market. The achievement of the other social goals may be more controversial. The ability of Medicare to ensure uniformly high-quality services is still open to question. And the availability of care may be hampered by the continual attempt by managed care plans to enroll low-cost patients. Nevertheless, any system must be judged by comparing it to other feasible systems. Currently, fee-for-service is the alternative to Medicare Advantage. Fee-for-service may perform better in terms of availability and quality of care, but it is lacking in regard to the goals of efficiency and expenditure control. In the end, the policy maker is faced with a trade-off, and the choice of system will depend on the degree of importance given to each of the social goals.

15.7 Policy Alternatives for Medicaid

Medicaid programs are run by the states under federal requirements and financed by states and the federal government. Individual states have a great deal of discretion in the policies they institute to govern the programs, which indeed exhibit substantial variability. Part of this variability is due to the fact that Medicaid serves several very different populations, including the poor aged, poor families with dependent children, and the blind and disabled.

Medicaid's problems are somewhat different from those of Medicare. To begin with, there are a number of uninsured children in the United States who are eligible for coverage under the Accountable Care Act but who have not been enrolled for one reason or another. In addition, there are many persons 65 years of age and older who have low incomes but no supplementary coverage and who are thus at risk for considerable out-of-pocket expenditures. In 2018, about 15% of the Medicaid population was 65 years old and older and had joint Medicare-Medicaid coverage (Berchick, Barnett, & Upton, 2019).

Until 1990, the growth in total expenditures for Medicaid was moderate. However, beginning in 1990, following the expansion of the program to cover children and women whose incomes were above the poverty level but still low, the growth in expenditures was substantial, although in 1996 and 1997, expenditure growth leveled off. At its inception, the Medicaid program accounted for 2.9% of all national health expenditures. In 2017 state and federal outlays for Medicaid totaled $581.9 billion, accounting for 16.7% of the nation's health expenditures.

15.7.1 Scope of the Program

Until 1987, only low-income women (under age 65 and not blind or disabled) and their children who were receiving Aid to Families with Dependent Children (AFDC) payments were eligible for Medicaid enrollment. The Medicaid program expanded eligibility in 1987 to include low-income women and children who were not on the AFDC program. At their discretion, states could offer coverage to families whose incomes reached 185% of the poverty level. This expansion of coverage led to a rapid increase in Medicaid enrollment and expenditures beginning in 1990 (Cutler & Gruber, 1996a, b). If states enrolled in the Medicaid expansion program, then all individuals with incomes at or below 138% of the federal poverty level are eligible for Medicaid. This increased the number of individuals enrolled in Medicaid in those states, leaving a substantial number of individuals uninsured in the states not enrolling in Medicaid expansion.

Medicaid's scope of coverage is very broad. It usually includes outpatient drugs and dental care. Because the breadth of coverage is wider than that for Medicare, Medicaid also enrolls low-income Medicare enrollees who do not have supplementary coverage.

Although the variety of services was not affected, the state of Oregon instituted a benefit limitation policy in 1994. It created a ranking of the costs and benefits of alternative medical procedures and proposed to pay for only those procedures whose cost–benefit ratios ranked above a certain cut-off point. Near the top of the list were treatments for disorders such as bone cancer and multiple sclerosis, which, it was claimed, yield substantial benefits per dollar of cure. Lower on the list were disorders whose treatments have a lower rate of return, including chronic ulcers and sleep disorders. Thus, the scope of the services was to be limited by type of treatment. This program was quite controversial and has generated a great deal of discussion.

15.7.2 Copayments

Generally, Medicaid does not charge recipients for their services. However, states can institute a copayment for some services. As of 2004, some 41 states had copayments for prescription drugs, usually ranging from $0.50 to $1.00 per prescription. In addition, some states have mandated limits on the quantity of drugs prescribed and the number of refills. After the enrollee reaches these limits, the drugs are no longer covered. There is evidence that these copayments affect the utilization of drugs, and there is only limited evidence that health status is adversely affected (Stuart & Zacker, 1999).

15.7.3 Provider Payments

Medicaid programs are noted for the low levels of fees paid to providers (Gruber, 1997). Low fee levels discourage providers from serving Medicaid enrollees and thus reduce availability. This is a problem often noted when Medicaid is discussed.

15.7.4 Competitive Bidding by Suppliers

Competitive bidding, which has been implemented by the California and Arizona Medicaid programs, has the objective of providing cost-effective care for indigents. If the buyer has a considerable degree of market power, it can extract a lower price from competitive sellers, and if there is any room for cost reductions, either through increasing efficiency or lowering quality, the reductions will be incorporated into the providers' bids. However, the bidding process is a complex one and may not automatically lead to savings.

15.7.5 Managed Care

Many states are looking to managed care programs in order to consolidate their efforts at provision of services to their populations. In 1998, about 53% of the Medicaid population was enrolled in managed care plans, while by 2017, approximately 83% were enrolled in some type of managed care plan. The proportion of persons who were enrolled in managed care varied by group.

Many older individuals receive long-term care coverage through Medicaid (as well as through their Medicare coverage). Long-term care utilization, for those who need it, is less controllable than other types of care (acute care), and long-term care is thus less amenable to managed care-type coverage. Older Medicaid long-term care patients would therefore tend not to be enrolled in a Medicaid managed care plan. Indeed, only 4.9% of Medicaid enrollees who are served by managed care are age 65 or older. The majority of Medicaid-managed care enrollees are children and parents.

Under Medicaid, managed care organizations face the same issues as under Medicare. There is a wide variation in fee-setting practices and in fees among states (Holahan, 1999). In addition, as in the fee-for-service sector, managed care rates in general are quite low (Bruen & Holahan, 1999). As well, risk-adjustment factors have not been well developed, and so biased selection in membership may be a problem. In short, Medicaid has problems enrolling members and maintaining the provision of care for these individuals. Since managed care organizations are paid a capitated fee per enrolled member per month, the movement of individuals on and off the Medicaid roles makes it difficult to keep track of and manage the care of these individuals. This policy has the effect of reducing the availability of care for these populations.

15.8 Pay-For-Performance Initiatives

A number of different pay-for-performance (P4P) models have been proposed and tried in recent years. The Centers for Medicare and Medicaid Services (CMS) have supported a number of demonstration projects to evaluate their effectiveness in improving quality and decreasing costs. The health reform law also calls for a number of additional demonstrations to incorporate value-based purchasing into the payment system.

Basically, P4P links the payment system to the accomplishment of predefined performance measures. These performance measures can contain either positive incentives or disincentives. An example of a positive incentive is to link the amount paid to the provider to the documented achievement of a certain level of preventive services performed (e.g., the percentage of women in the practice over age 50 who have received mammography screenings in the last 2 years). The provider receives higher payment if his/her practice percentage is equal to or greater than the desired, predefined percentage. A disincentive establishes a penalty for the occurrence or nonoccurrence of certain events (Cromwell, Trisolini, Pope, Mitchell, & Greenwald, 2011). For example, Medicare has established a policy that it will no longer pay providers for the increased costs associated with medical errors or hospital-acquired infections. Another area being carefully scrutinized currently is the rate of readmission to hospitals in less than 30 days, especially for the same diagnosis or for diagnoses related to the original admission.

An issue that needs to be carefully considered in the development of incentives and/or disincentives is the potential negative impacts on patients. Will a P4P incentive encourage adverse selection of patients that will assist the provider in reaching the desired goal? How will patients who have serious and complex conditions be treated in a P4P system when the patient interacts with multiple providers in multiple locations. Will a P4P system decrease access to care for the sickest, most vulnerable populations? In the complex, fragmented delivery system, can a P4P model be developed that can accurately and appropriately attribute responsibility for the outcome of care for complex patients?

Pay-for-performance models and demonstration projects have been undertaken and supported by CMS in an effort to transform itself from a passive payer for services delivered to its beneficiaries to an active, value-based purchaser of higher quality, affordable healthcare services. To become a value-based purchaser, CMS is attempting to establish incentives and disincentives designed to change the behavior of providers by linking effective resource utilization and clinical measures to a redesigned payment system, increasing joint clinical and financial accountability in the healthcare system.

When evaluating the transformation of the system to achieve value in the healthcare system, Christianson, Leatherman, and Sutherland (2007) provide a number of issues that require consideration and answers. First, is the goal of the incentive/disincentive to achieve improvement or attainment? If the goal is improvement, then rewarding change may maximize the potential improvements in quality, because the low-performing providers can improve the most. On the other hand, rewarding achievements would tend to focus and reward the providers who were delivering superior care.

The second issue revolves around deciding if the goal is to reward achievement of an absolute value or standard or to achieve a relative rating or percentage of a target. Establishing an absolute value to be achieved can be difficult and expensive to establish the correct benchmark and keep it up to date. It can also be expensive, if most providers surpass the threshold established. A relative rating (such as using quartiles), can be easier to calculate, but may not be very informative if there is very little variation among the providers; if the first quartile and the fourth quartile are clustered close together, then differentiating between them for payment is relatively worthless.

Third, how should risk adjustments or exemptions/exclusions be handled? Risk adjustments are typically undertaken to reflect differences in case mix or severity of patients in a panel or practice. Determining and appropriately measuring the risk and establishing a valid adjustment factor is difficult, or even not applicable to certain metrics (e.g., immunizations).

On the other hand, if exemptions or exclusions for certain patients or providers are allowed based on pre-determined/prespecified conditions or characteristics, then opportunities for gaming the system are increased.

Another issue encountered in applying P4P criteria to individual physicians is the small sample size of eligible patients or procedures. If a practice has very few patients, procedures, or conditions eligible to be scored in the metric, then a single outlier can significantly impact the results, making them uninformative. As a result, these providers can either be excluded from the P4P system, or multiple years of data combined to achieve larger numbers. A problem with using multiple years is that it may camouflage important changes over time.

When patients see multiple providers, it is especially difficult to obtain outcome measures that can be attributed to an individual provider. This ties into the next issue of obtaining physician engagement to improve care processes: if the physician doesn't see the relevancy to their own activities, it is hard to get him/her motivated to participate and change behavior.

P4P may also have unintended consequences. For example, the selection of the measurement criteria may lead to better documentation rather than an actual improvement in the outcome being measured. Physicians could also either move practices or select patients that are more likely to manage their own care, thereby reducing access to services for certain groups of patients. Providers could also focus on the areas that are included in the incentives and let other areas decline because they are not being measured. Coordination of care could also decrease for patients with multiple conditions, and administrative costs could increase, as additional time is needed to comply with the quality metrics, document care provided, or track rewards to individual providers in a group.

As this discussion indicates, implementing a value-based, pay-for-performance system is not without problems. However, careful evaluation of incentives/disincentives created will enable Medicare and other purchasers to become more prudent purchasers, not just payers.

Exercises

1. What populations and what services are covered by Medicare?
2. What are the major sources of funding for Medicare?
3. What populations and what services are covered by Medicaid?
4. What are the major sources of funding for Medicaid?

5. What is Medigap and what purpose does it serve?
6. What are the goals of Medicare?
7. List five policies for Medicare and identify what goal(s) each address.

8. What are the most important problems faced by Medicaid and what policies might be used to help solve them?

Bibliography

2011 Annual Report of the Boards of Trustees of the Federal Hospital Insurance and Federal Supplementary Medical Insurance Trust Funds. Retrieved from https://www.cms.gov/Research-Statistics-Data-and-Systems/Statistics-Trends-and-Reports/ReportsTrustFunds/downloads/tr2011.pdf

2019 Annual Report of the Boards of Trustees of the Federal Hospital Insurance and Federal Supplementary Medical Insurance Trust Funds. Retrieved from https://www.cms.gov/Research-Statistics-Data-and-Systems/Statistics-Trends-and-Reports/ReportsTrustFunds/Downloads/TR2019.pdf

Berchick, E. (2018). *Most uninsured were working age adults*. Washington, DC: U.S. Census Bureau.

Berchick, E., Barnett, J. C., & Upton, R. D. (2019). *Health insurance coverage in the United States: 2018*. Washington, DC: U.S. Government Printing Office.

Bruen, B., & Holahan, J. (1999). *Slow growth in Medicaid spending continues in 1997*. Issue paper. Washington, DC: Kaiser Commission on Medicaid and the Uninsured.

Centers for Medicare and Medicaid Services. (2018). Chronic conditions charts. Retrieved from www.cma.gov/Research-Statistics-Data-and-Systems/Statistics-Trends-and-Reports/Chronic-Conditions/Chartbook_Charts.html

Christianson, J. B., Leatherman, S., & Sutherland, K. (2007). *Paying for quality: Understanding and assessing physician pay-for-performance initiatives*. Princeton, NJ: Robert Wood Johnson Foundation, The Synthesis Project, Issue 13.

Cromwell, J., Trisolini, M. G., Pope, G. C., Mitchell, J. B., & Greenwald, L. M. (2011). *Pay for performance in health care: Methods and approaches*. Research Triangle Park, NC: RTI Press Publications. Retrieved January 26, 2012, from https://www.rti.org/pubs/bk-0002-1103-mitchell.pdf

Cubanski, J., Neuman, T., & Freed, M. (2019, August 20). The facts on Medicare spending and finance. *Issue Brief*. San Francisco: KFF.org.

Cutler, D. M. (2000). Walking the tightrope on Medicare reform. *Journal of Economic Perspectives, 14*, 45–56.

Cutler, D. M., & Gruber, J. (1996a). The effect of Medicaid expansions on public insurance, private insurance, and redistribution. *American Economic Review, 86*, 378–383.

Cutler, D. M., & Gruber, J. (1996b). Does public insurance crowd out private insurance? *Quarterly Journal of Economics, 110*, 391–426.

Data.Medicaid.Gov. (2019). 2017 managed care enrollment summary. Retrieved from https://data.medicaid.gov/Enrollment/2017-Managed-Care-Enrollment-Summary/uw3d-3r25

Davis, M., Poisal, J., Chulis, G., Zarabozo, C., & Cooper, B. (1999). Prescription drug coverage, utilization, and spending among Medicare beneficiaries. *Health Affairs, 18*(1), 231–243.

DeNavas-Walt, C., Proctor, B. D., & Smith, J. C. (2011). *US census bureau, current population reports, P60-239, income, poverty, and health insurance coverage in the United States: 2010*. Washington, DC: US Government Printing Office.

Doty, M. M., Collins, S. R., Robertson, R., & Garber, T. (2011). Realizing health reform's potential: When unemployed means uninsured: The toll of job loss on health coverage, and how the affordable care act will help. *Issue Brief (Commonwealth Fund), 18*, 1–18.

Goldberg, H. B., Delargy, D., Schmitz, R. J., Moore, T., & Wrobel, M. (1999). *Case mix adjustment for a national home health prospective payment system: Second interim report*. Cambridge, MA: Abt Associates.

Gruber, J. (1997). Medicaid and uninsured women and children. *Journal of Economic Perspectives, 11*, 199–208.

Health Care Financing Administration. (2000, April 7). Medicare program prospective payment system for hospital outpatient services. Final rule. *Federal Register, 65*(68), 18433–18820.

Holahan, J. (1999). *Medicaid managed care payment methods and capitation rates*. Washington, DC: Urban Institute.

Iglehart, J. K. (1999). The American health care system–Medicaid. *New England Journal of Medicine, 340*(5), 403–408.

Kaiser Family Foundation. (2019). State health facts. Retrieved from www.kff.org/state-category/Medicare/

Levit, K., Cowan, C., Lazenby, H., Sensenig, A., McDonnell, P., Stiller, J., ... Health Accounts Team. (2000). Health spending in 1998: Signals of change. *Health Affairs, 19*(1), 124–132.

Liu, K., Gage, B., Harvell, J., Stevenson, D., & Brennan, N. (1999). *Medicare's post-acute care benefit*. Washington, DC: Urban Institute.

McClellan, M. (2000). Medicare reform: Fundamental problems, incremental steps. *Journal of Economic Perspectives, 14*, 21–44.

Medicaid.gov. (2019). Mandatory and optional Medicaid benefits. Retrieved from https://www.medicaid.gov/medicaid/benefits/list-of-benefits/index.html

Medicare Learning Network. (2018, March). *Home health prospective payment system*. Washington, DC: U.S. Department of Health and Human Services.

Medicare Payment Advisory Commission. (2000). *Report to Congress*. Washington, DC: Medicare Payment Advisory Commission.

Moon, M., Gage, B., & Evans, A. (1997). *An examination of key Medicare provisions in the balanced budget act of 1997*. Washington, DC: Urban Institute.

Potetz, L., Cubanski, J., & Neuman, T. (2011). *Medicare spending and financing: A primer*. Menlo Park, CA: The Henry J. Kaiser Family Foundation.

Soumerai, S., & Ross-Degnan, D. (1999). Inadequate prescription drug coverage for Medicare enrollees. *New England Journal of Medicine, 340*, 722–728.

Stuart, B., & Zacker, C. (1999). Who bears the burden of Medicaid drug copayment policies? *Health Affairs, 18*(2), 201–212.

U.S. Bureau of the Census. (1999). *Health insurance coverage, 1998*. Washington, DC: U.S. Bureau of the Census.

U.S. General Accounting Office. (1999). *Medicare and budget surpluses* (Publication No. GAO/TAIMD/HEHS-99-113). Washington, DC: Government Accounting Office.

Wolkstein, I. (1984). Medicare's financial status: How did we get here? *Milbank Quarterly, 62*, 183–206.

CHAPTER 16

Regulation and Antitrust Policy in Health Care

OBJECTIVES

1. Define regulation and describe two different views on why governments regulate markets.
2. Describe the variables that regulators focus on when regulating health care.
3. Explain the rationale for antitrust policy and describe market changes that have taken place in health care, and explain how these might affect antitrust enforcement.
4. Describe the key provisions of antitrust legislation in the United States.
5. Explain how antitrust legislation regulates price-fixing and mergers.
6. Explain how quality issues in health care affect antitrust policy.

16.1 Introduction

The healthcare industry is one of the most highly regulated industries in the United States. Not only must the healthcare industry comply with general regulatory requirements, but also a large number of regulations have been implemented specifically for one or more components of the healthcare industry. The regulation of markets takes three general forms. *Direct regulation* refers to intervention in markets by regulatory agencies to control price, quantity, or quality by direct action, such as instituting price controls, establishing professional licensure requirements, or assessing and regulating the quality of services. *Indirect regulation* refers to regulatory activities that affect price, quantity, or quality by enforcing the competitive behavior of firms in the market or by changing the structure of the market. Antitrust policy is the leading example of indirect regulation.

Governments also intervene in markets through *public ownership* and operation of healthcare facilities and services (Santerre & Neun, 1996). Examples of public ownership include public utilities, public hospitals and other facilities, Veterans Administration healthcare system, and the Indian Health Services system. In this chapter, the use of the term *regulation* will generally refer to direct regulation. The chapter will focus mainly on regulation of private sector healthcare providers in the United States. The public ownership of healthcare facilities, which is more common in other nations, will only be addressed briefly in this chapter.

16.1.1 The Concept of Economic Regulation

Economic systems that are based on competitive markets and private enterprise are characteristic of most of the nations of the world, including the United States. In private enterprise systems, scarce resources are allocated and income is distributed primarily on the basis of supply and demand in markets and the resulting price, income, and profitability signals. In these systems, largely unrestricted free markets are the principal determinants of economic outcomes. Almost all of the free-market systems today are a blend of free enterprise, private ownership, and public regulations.

Under conditions of perfect competition and complete information, the economic outcome of these systems meets the social welfare standards of Pareto optimality. In other words, changes in the allocation of resources in the systems could not improve the welfare of some members of society without reducing the welfare of other members of society.

In some instances, including the market for health care, outcomes achieved in these competitive markets may be viewed as suboptimal by society in general. Situations in which a market's price, quantity, or product quality does not meet social welfare norms are said, by economists, to be cases of market failure. A market failure results in an inefficient distribution of goods and services in a free or competitive market. In a market failure, the incentives/disincentives present in the market do not lead to rational, market-clearing outcomes for the market. While each individual makes a rational self-interest decision in terms of individual preferences and outcomes, the decisions made by the individual do not lead to the correct outcomes for the group. In a market failure, the social benefits (total benefits to society) diverge from the private benefits to individuals and the social cost (total cost to society) diverges from the private cost to individuals. There are a number of different types of reasons for a market failure.

One form of market failure occurs when prices in a market are above marginal costs as a result of monopoly power. Monopoly power typically occurs when there are increasing economies of scale in the production process so that it is more efficient to have a single producer of the good or service. This allows the monopolist to set a price higher than a competitive market, leading to a suboptimal level of production and consumption. Monopoly power may be a result of factor immobility in the production process. A good example of factor immobility is when individuals are unable to move to another location without incurring unacceptable personal costs and so the employer is unable to hire sufficient highly trained individuals in the new location.

Another type of market failure occurs when the external effects (externalities) of the production or consumption of a product, such as pollution, are not captured in the product's price, creating a wedge between the price and social costs or social benefits of the product. Because the free market has not captured the consequences of externalities (either positive or negative) the market signals result in a suboptimal production of the good or service. If the externality results in consequences that are beneficial to society, it will have too little of the good or service consumed because the price is higher than it should be since the price does not capture the additional benefits to society. If the externality results in consequences that are harmful to society, there will be too much of the good or service consumed because the price is lower than it should be since the price does not capture the additional cost to society. In both cases, the existence of an externality will cause the market to reach an inefficient level of production and consumption of the good or service because it has allocated resources without considering the externalities.

A third form, especially important for healthcare markets, results from imperfect information. In a market with a low level of information, consumers find it difficult to evaluate the quality of goods and services, and therefore it is difficult to make decisions regarding whether or not to purchase the goods and services at an appropriate level. This lack of information results in consumers and producers unable to make informed decisions in the market. And again, inefficiencies in the allocation of resources result. Market failure may also result from the situation when agents have different objectives than the principles and information asymmetries lead to suboptimal decisions by the principles.

Another form of market failure is the result of the presence of merit goods in the market. A merit good or service is one that is judged to have value that an individual or society should have based on some concept of need rather than on the willingness and ability of individuals to pay for the good or service in the market. The merit good or service would be underproduced and underconsumed in free-market systems because its consumption creates positive externalities and also because individuals make decisions based on short-term utility and do not always take into consideration the long-term benefits of the good or service.

The final form of market failure involves the existence of public goods or services in the market. A public good or service is one that has the characteristics of being nonrivalous and nonexcludable. The nonrivalous characteristic means that the consumption of the good or service by an individual does not reduce the amount available for consumption by another individual. The nonexcludable characteristic means that an individual cannot be excluded from using the good or service. For example, it would be very costly or impossible to exclude one individual from receiving the benefits of national defense. Also, the consumption of national defense by one individual does not reduce the amount of national defense available to another individual in society.

A problem encountered in the provision of a public good in the free market arises from the free-rider phenomenon. A free rider is an individual who receives the benefits of the good or service without paying for it. As a result, the good or service may be underproduced. For goods that the consumption by one individual does not prevent simultaneous consumption by another and when it is very difficult if not impossible to prevent individuals who have not paid for the good or service from having access to it, then the free market lacks adequate features to ensure inefficiencies do not occur in its production and consumption.

Economic regulation consists of governmental interventions intended to affect market outcomes in some manner. There are two different views of why economic regulation exists. According to the first view, economic regulation is generally motivated by the objective of reducing the extent of market failure. According to the second view, it is the result of producers or consumers working through the political process to further their own interests.

16.1.2 Regulation of Health Care

The regulation of health care in the United States and Canada is extensive. Much of this activity is directed toward information and quality issues. Quality-of-care regulation frequently takes the form of control of entry into the market, such as requiring that healthcare professionals be licensed or certified before performing services and that new drugs and medical devices be approved by a regulatory agency before they can be offered for sale in the market. Entry by hospitals into the market is also commonly regulated through policy instruments, such as the certificate of need (CON) programs, which give permission to a healthcare firm to develop the infrastructure to provide care to specific populations. The regulation of price in health care is generally carried out indirectly through antitrust policy and through the effects of government reimbursement rules on the prices of healthcare services.

16.1.3 Regulation as a Means of Correcting Market Failure

Healthcare markets are characterized by imperfect information on the price and quality of many healthcare services. The problem of inadequate information on health care can take a number of forms. Consumers tend to have incomplete information about the quality of healthcare services available from alternative providers. And consumers also have incomplete information about the probability of a successful outcome for procedures that involve risk. For example, consumers may have incomplete information on the relationship between the volume of surgical procedures performed and the success rate of the surgeon. Consumers may also have incomplete information about price because the out-of-pocket price to consumers may be the result of negotiations between providers and third-party payers. Since the out-of-pocket price for many healthcare services and goods represents a very small portion of the total value of resources used in the production process, overutilization of healthcare goods and services may occur.

Information can also be impaired as a result of relationships in which a principal delegates responsibility to an agent. One inherent difficulty with such relationships is that the agent possesses information not available to the principal (the person with ultimate authority), and may have different objectives than the principal. An example of an agency relationship is that between a physician and a patient. In health care, the physician is both a healthcare provider and an agent of the consumer. The physician's incentives in the provider role may not be aligned with the incentives of the consumer. In addition, the patient may possess information not shared with the provider that impacts the decision regarding production or consumption of the healthcare good or service.

This agency relationship between physician and consumer is complicated further by the relationship between the physician and the third-party payer or managed care organization, which also involves agency relationships. This complexity of relationships has led at least one writer to use the phrase "the doctor as double agent" (Blomqvist, 1991). When the physician serves as both a provider of services and a demander of services in the role of the patient's agent, then the independent relationship between demand and supply is broken and market failure can occur.

Consumers may be handicapped by the lack of information about quality of healthcare services and about quality of alternative providers. Thus, incomplete information may prevent socially optimal outcomes in healthcare markets. The agency relationships between a consumer and his or her physician and between the consumer and other providers may also lead to over- or underconsumption of healthcare services relative to the socially optimum amount that would be achievable with complete information.

Therefore, the direct regulation of healthcare providers may be a response of governments to the perception that the consumer lacks adequate information about quality of providers and healthcare services and thus that the workings of competitive, private-enterprise healthcare markets may not produce the best outcomes in terms of social welfare. Another possibility, as mentioned earlier, is that regulation is fostered as a means for providers to further their private interests instead of, or in addition to, protection of the public.

16.1.4 Regulation as a Political Good

In his seminal work on the economic theory of regulation, George Stigler (1971), supplemented by the work by Peltzman (1976) and others, pointed out that regulatory legislation may be pursued in an effort to redistribute wealth. This effect of regulation is important, given that the behavior of legislators is likely to be motivated and influenced by their wish to remain in office. If there is competition among special interest groups in the democratic system, that competition may take the form of exchanges of political support from the group in terms of donations for legislation favorable to the objectives of the interest groups. If the political process works in this manner, well-organized interest groups, with a high per capita stake in the outcomes of legislation, will tend to dominate larger interest groups with a smaller per capita stake.

The economic theory of regulation as a political good suggests that providers may be able to dominate the legislative and regulatory process because they have a concentrated interest in the outcome, while the general population has a diffused interest. This suggestion is a hypothesis and not a conclusion of the economic theory of regulation. What the actual healthcare-related outcomes of real-world legislative and regulatory processes are is an empirical question. Very active lobbying activities are pursued by healthcare provider groups, as well as healthcare consumer groups.

16.2 Regulation of Health Care

Regulation of health care takes a number of different forms of the regulation of price, quantity (or utilization), and quality. Sometimes, the quality objectives are achieved through control of entry, such as the licensure of physicians and other healthcare professionals and facilities. In other instances, quality is regulated by the setting of technical standards, as in the regulation of pharmaceuticals and medical devices. In the following sections, the regulation of hospitals and long-term care facilities, physician services, and pharmaceuticals are discussed separately. Indirect regulation through antitrust policy is also considered in the final sections.

16.2.1 Regulation of Hospitals and Long-Term Care Facilities

Community hospitals are the major providers of acute medical and surgical care. Many hospitals in the United States are tax-exempt not-for-profit institutions, supported by government or by charitable organizations. In the United States, there has been an increase in the importance of investor-owned hospitals in the provision of inpatient medical and surgical services. In addition, there has been a large number of hospital mergers, acquisitions, and partnerships, as well as formal and informal vertical combinations among hospitals, insurance and managed care companies, and physician groups (Gaynor & Haas-Wilson, 1999; Kim & McCue, 2012; Russo, Calo, Harrison, Mahoney, & Zavotsky, 2018; Trepanier, Crenshaw, & Yoder-Wise, 2016).

Direct regulation of hospitals includes supply-side measures such as certificate-of-need requirements for the entry of new hospitals or the expansion of additional services in existing hospitals. Demand-side regulations include price controls imposed through the payment practices of government programs such as Medicare and Medicaid. Price controls may also affect the supply side by motivating greater efficiency and reducing lengths of stay. Regulation of hospital service quality includes licensure, peer review, utilization review, and pay-for-performance systems.

16.2.2 Regulation of Hospital Quality

Hospitals, both tax-exempt and investor-owned, are licensed by a state licensing agency, typically located in the state department of health. The license to operate the hospital requires that a minimum level of facilities, services, and personnel be present; the intent of these requirements is to ensure the quality of services delivered is safe, cost-effective, and compliant with all state and federal laws. In addition to this direct regulation by state governments, hospitals often participate in self-regulation by seeking accreditation from The Joint Commission (TJC), formerly known as the Joint Commission on Accreditation of Healthcare Organizations (JCAHO). By the end of 2018,

The Joint Commission accredited or certified over 22,000 healthcare organizations and programs in the United States, including hospitals, physician offices, office space, surgery centers, behavior health treatment facilities, and home care providers (Joint Commission, 2019). The Healthcare Facilities Accreditation Program (HFAP) grew out of a former hospital approval process of the American Osteopathic Association and encompasses acute care hospitals, critical access hospitals, outpatient clinics, and laboratories.

Hospital quality is also regulated by quality improvement organizations (QIOs), which were originally established as peer-review organizations (PROs) under the Tax Equity and Fiscal Responsibility Act (TEFRA) of 1982, an act that made numerous changes to Medicare. The QIO program is dedicated to improving quality for Medicare beneficiaries and is an integral part of the U.S. Department of Health and Human Services national quality strategy for providing better care and health at lower costs. The mission of the QIO program is to improve the effectiveness, efficiency, economy, and quality of services delivered to Medicare beneficiaries. The Centers for Medicare and Medicaid Services (CMS) identify the core functions of the QIO program as:

- Improving quality of care to beneficiaries;
- Protecting the integrity of the Medicare Trust Fund by ensuring that Medicare pays only for services and goods that are reasonable and necessary, and that are provided in the most appropriate setting; and
- Protecting beneficiaries by expeditiously addressing individual complaints, such as beneficiary complaints, provider-based notice appeals, violations of the Emergency Medical Treatment and Labor Act (EMTALA), and other related responsibilities as articulated in QIO-related laws. (http://cms.gov/Medicare/quality-initiatives-patient-assessment-instruments/qualityimprovementorgs/index.HTML.)

There are two types of QIOs that work under the direction of CMS in support of the QIO program. One is the Beneficiary and Family Centered Care (BFCC) QIOs to help Medicare beneficiaries exercise their right to high-quality health care. These QIOs manage all beneficiary complaints and quality of care reviews to ensure consistency in the review process. Two designated BSCC-QIOs serve all 50 states and three territories.

The other type of QIO is the Quality and Innovation Network (QIN)-QIOs which bring Medicare beneficiaries, providers, and communities together in data-driven initiatives that increase patient safety, make communities healthier, ensure better coordinated post-hospital care, and improve clinical quality. There are 14 QIN-QIOs serving the 50 states and the three territories (http://cms.gov/Medicare/quality-initiatives-patient-assessment-instruments/qualityimprovementorgs/index.HTML).

Throughout the history of PROs and QIOs, efforts have been directed to advance national efforts to motivate providers to improve quality. They have also focused on measuring and improving outcome quality. The transformation of the QIOs into two separate types was intended to enhance quality by separating the case review function from the quality improvement function. The thought was that separating the punitive case review side from the quality improvement side would enhance participation by providers.

16.2.3 Supply-Side Regulation of Hospitals

The quality improvement organizations, in addition to regulating quality, also review utilization of care. Utilization deemed inappropriate would be denied payment by Medicare. Since the advent of the prospective payment system, however, and the restructuring of the program, the QIOs have been more focused on quality of service and quality improvement than on excessive utilization by providers.

Certificate-of-need regulation is a form of supply-side regulation. Its stated purpose is to restrain health facility costs and allow coordinated planning of new services and construction in order to prevent duplication of facilities or excessive capital expenditures. The program was designed to ensure demand was sufficient to allow for new or expanded construction. Certificate-of-need regulation for hospitals played an extensive role during the 1970s and 1980s, but the federal requirement that states have certificate-of-need regulation ended in 1986. Since then, several states have ended certificate-of-need regulation for hospitals. Currently, 35 states and the District of Columbia have retained some type of CON law.

A retrospective study of the consequences of ending certificate-of-need regulation found that such regulation had only a modest containing effect on hospital costs (Conover & Sloan, 1998). A 2009 study by Hellenger found that CON laws reduced the number of hospital beds by about 10% and healthcare expenditures by almost 2%. A 2017 study by Bailey, Hamami, and McCorry did not find a statistically significant difference in the prices of hospitals in states with CON laws compared to those without such laws. A study by Rosko and Mutter (2014) found that cost inefficiency was less in CON states (8.10%) than in non-CON states (12.46%) suggesting that CON may be an effective policy instrument in an era of a new medical arms race.

16.2.4 Demand-Side Regulation of Hospitals

Hospital prices and charges are subject to extensive regulation. Rate regulation at the state level was widely practiced during the 1970s and 1980s but has since largely disappeared. Medicare's prospective payment system (PPS), established in the early 1980s, controls hospital charges nationwide, but for Medicare patients only. In addition to their direct effect on hospital charges, Medicare payment rules may influence the charges paid by other payers, such as health insurance companies and managed care organizations.

Studies of the effectiveness of price regulation of hospitals have generally found that hospitals entered a new competitive era in the early 1980s, as Medicare's PPS, which paid providers prospectively based on diagnosis rather than retrospectively, tended to reduce days of stay and hospital occupancy rates and increase price competition among hospitals (Dranove, Shanley, & White, 1993). The increase in price competition was reinforced by the rapid development of managed care and the greater purchasing power of large payer groups.

The use of hospital price competition has continued to evolve as Medicare has implemented a number of mandatory and voluntary programs to control the rate of increase in healthcare costs and improve the quality of healthcare services. While Medicare continues to use the prospective payment system based on patient diagnosis to pay hospitals for services provided to Medicare beneficiaries, CMS has also introduced a number of incentive systems designed to control costs and improve quality of care. One of the recent systems introduced is the Pathways to Success Program. This program redesigns Medicare's Accountable Care Organizations to advance the goals of accountability, competition, engagement, integrity, and quality.

Under the current Shared Savings Program, the ACOs do not face financial consequences when costs increase, although they share in any savings they achieve in reducing costs. The Pathways to Success Program will have the ACOs accept real risk, as well as give them more flexibility to coordinate and innovate. The Pathways to Success Program provides higher shared savings rates as ACOs transition and accept greater levels of risk. While ACOs have the ability to share in greater savings, they will also now have to accept the possibility of having to pay money back to Medicare if they are unable to reach a target in the costs of care provided to their beneficiaries.

16.2.5 Regulation of Long-Term Care Facilities

Long-term care in the United States is provided in tax-exempt and investor-owned nursing homes. These long-term care facilities are regulated by state and federal agencies. Licensing is by state agencies, usually located in the states' health departments. Nursing homes may also pursue additional self-regulation by seeking accreditation through The Joint Commission.

Nursing homes, like hospitals, are regulated on the supply side by state CON regulation, which restricts construction and capacity increases. Certificate-of-need regulation was most important in the years directly after Medicare and Medicaid began to cover nursing home costs for some patients. It limited the expansion of nursing home providers and hence the financial burden on states, which finance Medicaid jointly with the federal government (Getzen, 1997). A 2016 article by Rahman, Galarraga, Zinn, Grabowski, and Mor found that states with CON laws compared to states without had faster growth in Medicare and Medicaid spending on nursing home care and slower growth in home healthcare expenditures, leading to a domination of the long-term care market by nursing homes in those states.

Whatever price regulation of nursing homes exists is primarily a result of the reimbursement systems used by Medicare and especially Medicaid. Medicaid, which covers mainly low-income individuals requiring institutionalization, generally pays a flat rate per day for Medicaid recipients in nursing homes. Some states have moved to adopt a system in which payment to nursing homes is based on the health status of the patient. Medicare covers skilled nursing services for a very limited period of time after certain hospitalizations for Medicare beneficiaries. Since the changes introduced by the 1997 Balanced Budget Amendments, Medicare uses a prospective payment system in which the daily rate depends on the health status of the patient (Folland, Goodman, & Stano, 2001). This prospective rate creates an incentive to keep the costs of providing for the residents below the rate (Walshe, 2001).

Quality of care in nursing homes has been a concern for many years, and a number of regulations have been introduced in efforts to address the problem. In order to receive Medicare and Medicaid payments for residents, nursing homes are required to meet certain standards and to provide certain services to residents. Failure to comply with these requirements can result in penalties that include fines, imposed staffing training, increased monitoring, temporary outside management, and loss of Medicare and Medicaid certification. Currently, nursing homes are required to conduct comprehensive and accurate assessment of each resident's functional capacity, develop a comprehensive care plan for each resident, and promote quality of life for all residents, among other things. The increased requirements are viewed as necessary since individuals and families needing nursing home care lack sufficient information to judge the quality of care provided in these facilities.

16.2.6 Regulation of Physician Services

Physicians play a central role in the provision of health care. Physicians have total or partial control of hospital admissions, specialist referrals, and drug prescriptions, accounting for a high proportion of healthcare expenditures. Physicians also advise patients on the necessity or potential benefit of medical services. Traditionally, physicians were paid on a fee-for-service basis for the services provided. A fee-for-service system creates incentives based on volume production, not quality production. Currently, 80%–90% of physician fees are paid by third-party payers, who possess some control over price and utilization. Physicians are also subject to regulations intended to ensure high quality of care and control costs.

16.2.7 Regulation of Physician Quality and Utilization

Regulation of physicians typically focuses on three issues: how physicians compete; how physicians are paid for services; and the structure of their practices and joint ventures. The primary direct regulation of physician quality is through state licensure—the granting of licenses to practice medicine to those who meet specific criteria. Because state legislatures appoint state licensing boards with input from the state medical associations, licensing is a form of self-regulation by the profession. When a state issues a license to a physician, it is a document enabling the physician to practice medicine in the state. The license is for the general practice of medicine and does not license the physician in a specific specialty. The specialty declared by the physician is not part of the licensing process. State licensing boards also have responsibility for monitoring and taking such actions as revoking or suspending licenses of physicians if the physicians are found to be incompetent or have performed in ways that are dangerous to patients or have resulted in injury to patients.

Quality Improvement Organizations monitor the utilization patterns and the professional quality of hospitals and physicians. In 1986, Congress enacted the Health Care Quality Improvement Act, which provides legal protections to those participating in peer reviews by granting immunity from testifying in malpractice lawsuits. In addition, the act established the National Practitioner Data Base, which is an information clearinghouse that gathers information on malpractice judgments, disciplinary actions, and license suspensions and revocations. Scheutzow (1999) reviewed the practice of peer-review organizations and concluded that because of the failure to report incidents and other problems, the peer-review process at that time was ineffective. In the early 1990s, the earlier PROs were converted to QIOs, with more emphasis placed on improving quality of care and outcomes. As discussed in an earlier section, increased emphasis is being placed on improving measures of quality and assisting providers to achieve these measures.

16.2.8 Regulation of Physician Pricing

Medicare and Medicaid reimburse physicians on a modified fee-for-service basis. In the early years of Medicare and Medicaid, fees were screened on the basis of usual, customary, and reasonable (UCR) payments. The UCR system included the range of fees charged by other physicians in the same geographic area. In 1992, Medicare began using a new method of physician payment. This method, which utilizes the Resource-Based Relative Value Scale (RBRVS), includes components for physician time and skill, practice expenses, and professional liability insurance (Medicare Payment Advisory Commission, 2000). The reimbursement rules amount to price controls on the services provided to patients covered by Medicare, and in fact they have an effect on the prices charged by managed care plans and private insurance plans that insure large numbers of private patients.

In general, there are four key healthcare laws that are especially relevant to physicians. One of these is the Stark law, which is a federal law that prohibits a provider from referring Medicare and Medicaid patients for designated health services if the provider (or an immediate family member) has a financial relationship with the entity to which the patient is referred.

The provider also cannot establish a plan of care that includes a designated health service for providers with which the referring provider has a financial relationship. The designated health services do not cover all health services but do include many laboratory tests, therapy services, radiology services, imaging services, medical equipment and supplies, home health services and supplies, outpatient prescription drugs, and inpatient and outpatient hospital services.

Another important law is the federal criminal Anti-kickback Statute that prohibits the exchange of anything of value in an effort to induce the referral of Medicare or Medicaid business. The statute is broad and establishes penalties for both the giving and receiving individuals. If convicted, the provider is excluded from participating in Medicare and Medicaid programs. In recognition of the broad range of transactions that may violate the anti-kickback statute, certain types of payments are allowed under safe harbors established by the Department of Health and Human Services.

The False Claims Act covers individuals and groups that defraud government programs. The general violation areas in health care include upcoding for medical procedures and performing or ordering unnecessary procedures. The law includes a Qui Tam provision that allows people who are not affiliated with the government to file actions on behalf of the government, commonly known as whistleblowing.

The Health Insurance Portability and Accountability Act (HIPAA) protects the privacy of individually identifiable health information. It applies to patients who are transferred to or maintained by a healthcare provider, including email, electronic, fax, paper, oral and voicemail records, as well as phone conversations. The rules protect the information itself, not the record in which the information appears. HIPAA also requires entities and business associates to provide notification following a breach of unsecured protected health information. Also, the confidentiality provision of the patient safety rule protects identifiable information from being used to analyze patient safety events and improve patient safety.

16.2.9 Regulation of the Pharmaceutical Industry

The production of pharmaceuticals is regulated at the federal level by the Food and Drug Administration (FDA). The distribution and dispensing of pharmaceuticals are regulated at the state level by the licensing of pharmacists and by requirements that apply to pharmacy operations. At the present time, the prices of pharmaceuticals are not directly controlled, but government agencies, such as Medicaid, and other large purchasers, use their purchasing power to obtain lower prices than those paid by noninsured consumers.

In some instances, lower prices are negotiated through the design of drug formularies, which are lists of drugs eligible for prescription under a managed care plan or other insurer, including Medicare. Drug formularies help lower the cost to insurance companies and patients. Patients and providers often rely on formularies, and information on efficacy, for decisions regarding medically appropriate and cost-conscious prescriptions. These formularies are usually updated at least annually to provide better therapy options and lower costs. In order to have a drug included on the formulary, the pharmaceutical manufacturer must agree to charge a discounted price (Abbott, 1997).

16.2.10 Food and Drug Administration Regulation of Drugs

The FDA, founded in 1906, is one of the oldest federal regulatory agencies in the U.S. The FDA is responsible for protecting the public's health by assuring the safety, efficacy, and security of human and veterinary drugs, biological products, food supply, cosmetics, and products that emit radiation. The FDA also provides science-based information to the public. Prior to 1962, the FDA regulated drugs for safety, although there existed a strong element of self-regulation. The 1962 Drug Amendments strengthened the FDA's regulation of drugs for safety and extended its focus to include effectiveness.

The approval of a new drug requires extensive testing by the manufacturer and submission of drug studies to the FDA, so that the agency can evaluate the drug and reach a judgment as to whether its benefits outweigh its risks. Most new drugs are initially approved as prescription medicines, which means their purchase requires a physician's authorization, or other professional with prescribing authorization. The FDA also regulates generic drugs (which compete with brand-name products at the end of the life of drug patents) and over-the-counter drugs (those available without a prescription) (U.S. Food and Drug Administration, 2000).

The competition from generic drugs was promoted by a 1984 law that greatly reduced the testing required of generics. Prior to 1984, generic producers were often required to perform tests for safety and effectiveness as part of the approval process. After 1984, they were required only to show the generics were bioequivalent to the name brands. This change promoted the entry of generics and led to lower prices within a relatively short period after patent expiration (Grabowski & Vernon, 1992; Kesselheim et al., 2008).

Patents on new drugs provide a monopoly position for a period of time that may extend beyond the 20-year standard for American patents (the possibility of extension is to allow for the considerable time required by the regulatory process). The patent right provides an incentive for manufacturers to develop and test new drugs. This incentive must be balanced against the length of time it takes to develop drugs and the risk of failure. The total time lag from the beginning of research and development of a new drug to bringing it to market may be 10–15 years, and the total development cost may run over a billion dollars, and the inclusion of the cost of failed drug development brings the number to as high as $11 billion (Herper, 2012; Pharmaceutical Research and Manufacturers of America, 2011).

16.2.11 State Regulation of Pharmacists

In addition to their commercial role as sellers of pharmaceutical products, pharmacists perform a professional role in monitoring prescriptions and educating patients. State boards of pharmacy regulate registered pharmacists. In most states, the members of the state board are appointed by the governor, and registered pharmacists generally make up the majority of the members. The state boards regulate pharmacist quality through licensure and through requirements for continuing education. The increasing importance of mail-order pharmacies may restrict the ability of state boards to control the quality of dispensing within state boundaries (Conlan, 1997).

16.2.12 Regulation of Health Insurance and Managed Care

In the United States, regulation of insurance is practiced at the state level. This federalist tradition means that state insurance commissions regulate private health insurance companies, both investor-owned and tax-exempt. The state insurance commissions have oversight control regarding entry and prices for commercial health insurance. Changes in healthcare markets have increased competition in these markets. The growing tendency of large employers to self-insure, assuming the financial risk for their employees, and utilize third-party administrators is a significant trend. As a result of this trend, a larger portion of the market escapes much of the insurance industry regulation. While the trend for self-insuring increased to 40.7% in 2016, there was a decrease to 38.2% in 2018 (Frech, 1993; Rodriquez, 2019).

In fact, more and more, state regulators have turned their attention to regulating the behavior of managed care organizations. During the 1990s and early 2000s, many state legislatures enacted bills intended to influence the practices of these organizations. Among the provisions were some that placed restrictions on physician communication with patients, placed restrictions on lengths of hospital stay, and mandated the creation of external grievance processes for dissatisfied patients. Many of these restrictions had been discontinued by 2019, as new programs and experiences occurred.

A number of Patient's Bill of Rights exist. In 2010, a new Patient's Bill of Rights was created along with the Affordable Care Act, which extends the federal role in the regulation of private health insurance. Earlier bills focused on the right of patients to sue and the ability of managed care organizations to override the professional judgments of physicians (Pear, 2000). Federal regulation of health insurance traditionally has been restricted mostly to Medicare and Medicaid, which are public health insurance programs.

The Employee Retirement Income Security Act of 1974 (ERISA) preempts state law related to benefit plans, including health insurance plans, offered by employers. One effect of ERISA has been to free employer self-insured health plans from most state regulatory restrictions, thereby contributing both to the growth of employer-provided plans and to complaints about the lack of patient rights (Havighurst, 2000). Currently, the Patient's Bill of Rights included alongside the 2010 Accountable Care Act addresses eight key areas: information for patients about quality, choice of providers and plans, access to emergency services, taking part in treatment decisions, respect and nondiscrimination, confidentiality (privacy) of health information, complaints and appeals, and consumer responsibilities. In addition, some states have their own bill of rights.

16.3 Antitrust Policy

16.3.1 Conceptual Framework

The economist's model of perfect competition is generally used as a benchmark in evaluating market outcomes. The perfectly competitive market, with large numbers of buyers and sellers, free entry and exit, and homogeneous products, yields a long-run competitive equilibrium in which all firms in the market are producing at the minimum long-run average cost and in which price is equal to marginal cost. This market equilibrium yields both technical efficiency and economic efficiency. (*Technical efficiency* refers to the tendency of firms in a market to produce goods and services at the minimum long-run average cost, a result of the price competition among firms and of the relatively small scale of each firm in comparison to market demand. *Economic efficiency* refers to the equality of price and marginal cost, which suggests that the allocation of resources could not be improved in a perfectly competitive world by moving resources from their present use to a different one.)

A second benchmark in examining market outcomes is found in the monopoly market model. In this market structure, because there is a single seller with blocked entry, long-run market equilibrium may yield a price greater than marginal cost. If the monopolist is a profit maximizer, productive efficiency is still achieved (in the sense that average cost is at the lowest level possible given the monopolist's choice of output). However, the monopolist may not produce at the lowest average cost possible, independent of the rate of output selected.

Monopoly markets also raise the possibility of shifts in the distribution of income, compared with a perfectly competitive organization of the market. Under restrictive assumptions, a competitive market in long-run equilibrium that is transformed into a monopoly market as a result of cartelization or merger would be changed in the way shown in **Figure 16-1**. Total market output would decline from Q_c to Q_m as a result of monopolization. The corresponding equilibrium price would increase from P_c to P_m. Monopoly profits would appear in the amount shown by area ABDE, while the consumer surplus would decrease from the amount reflected by area FCD under perfect competition to area FAE under monopoly.

The consumer surplus is the difference between the sum of the marginal valuations over all quantities of the service and the prices paid over all quantities. It is a reflection of the welfare gains made by the consumer from purchasing the product. The difference between these two levels of consumer surplus, measured by area ABC, is traditionally called the *deadweight loss due to monopoly*. In sum, the adverse effects of monopoly market structures are related directly to the reduction in market output from Q_c to Q_m. The reduced market output causes redistribution between consumers and producers, as well as allocative effects in the form of deadweight loss.

Many real-world markets, including most healthcare markets, are structured as oligopoly markets. Paucity of sellers and generally large numbers of buyers characterize oligopoly markets. Some healthcare markets are oligopolies on both sides of the market (i.e., both buyers and sellers are few in number). Economic models of markets structured as oligopolies tend not to yield general predictions about market outcome. Depending on whether sellers attempt to engage in price collusion and if not, how they react to one another's price changes, the outcome in oligopoly markets may cover the entire outcome range from monopoly on one extreme to perfect competition on the other.

Antitrust policy economic analysis has traditionally made an attempt to analytically define the boundaries of product markets and geographic markets and to consider whether the structure of markets so defined is close enough to a monopoly structure to suspect that performance in these markets is adversely affected. This approach is reflected, for example, in the merger guidelines that have been developed by the U.S. Department of Justice and the Federal Trade Commission. More recently, antitrust economists have begun to use simulation as a means of predicting the likely outcome of changes in market structure due to horizontal mergers.

It should be noted that, in the previous discussion of competitive and monopoly markets, perfect information on the part of consumers as well as producers is generally assumed. Complete information implies that there is no uncertainty on the part of the consumers regarding product quality. Furthermore, because products are assumed to be homogeneous in a given market, price is the major decision variable for consumers.

Clearly, healthcare markets do not meet this information requirement, partly because of the imperfect ability of consumers to link the acquisition of healthcare services with improvements in health status and to compare the quality of alternative providers. Additionally, because third-party payers are dominant in most healthcare markets, the price of a particular healthcare service may be relatively unimportant to the ultimate consumer of that service. The market structure is further complicated by the role of the physician as the agent of the patient in making decisions about whether a particular service should be purchased.

As a result of these differences between healthcare markets and markets for standard consumer goods, a discussion of antitrust policy in healthcare markets must take into account their particular economic characteristics. The point of view expressed here favors

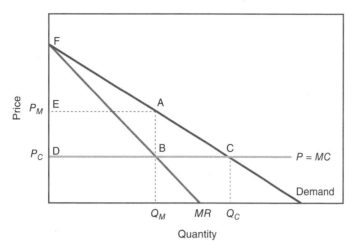

Figure 16-1 Economic analysis of monopolization effects. Under perfect competition, the price is P_C and the quantity is Q_C. Under monopoly, the price is P_M and the quantity is Q_M. Competition yields no monopoly profit and a consumer surplus of FCD. Monopoly yields monopoly profits of EABD, a consumer surplus of FAE, and a deadweight loss of ABC.

public policies that oppose monopoly power and promote competitive market structures. In the case of healthcare markets, however, there are even more caveats concerning this generalization than is true of traditional markets for consumer goods. It is often asserted that, in markets for traditional goods and services, economies of scale and the possibly greater propensity of firms with monopoly power to engage in research and development may justify market concentration. In healthcare markets, in addition to those two factors, high seller concentration may also be justified on the basis of access-to-care or quality-of-care considerations.

16.3.2 The Structure of Healthcare Markets

16.3.2.1 Hospitals

Hospital services in the United States and Canada have historically been provided by private community hospitals, which have traditionally been tax-exempt hospitals sponsored by religious organizations, local governments, and charitable organizations. One major structural trend in the 1980s and 1990s in the United States was the rapid growth of investor-owned hospital corporations.

Another strong trend in the 1980s and 1990s among U.S. hospitals was the increasing rate of mergers. Many of the mergers were related to the rise of investor-owned hospital corporations. Other mergers have occurred among tax-exempt hospitals in response to the rise of investor-owned hospital corporations, or to the increasing market power (on the buyer side) of managed care networks (Schactman & Altman, 1995). The total number of hospital

mergers in 2018 was 90, down from 115 in 2017. Another 27 occurred in the first quarter of 2019, with 22 announced in the second quarter of 2019. But the recent mergers were larger, with the trend in megamergers increasing (Reed, 2019).

The economic analysis of mergers suggests that mergers may be motivated by the pursuit of increased market power, the pursuit of increased efficiency, or both. The effects of changes in Medicare payment policies after the early 1980s provided a ready source of efficiency gains from mergers. The shift to prospective payment for Medicare resulted in shorter inpatient stays and a shift from inpatient to outpatient treatment. The general effect of these shifts was to create overcapacity in many hospitals, increasing the likelihood that efficiency gains could be realized from mergers, especially mergers within the same geographic market. Such horizontal mergers also increase market power in given geographic markets, raising the issue of whether hospital mergers are in the public interest (Gaynor & Haas-Wilson, 1999).

The healthcare industry is facing a tremendous amount of uncertainty and volatility as hospitals and health systems assume an increasing amount of risk under new payment programs, while operating on very thin margins. As systems attempt to find more sustainable platforms, new revenue streams are being explored. In other cases, systems are selling one or more hospitals to other systems. Investor-owned health systems and hospitals accounted for five of seven divestitures in the second quarter of 2019. The view is that health systems are increasingly aware of what is needed to achieve strategic growth, whether that is to divest hospitals outside the system's major market, or acquire hospitals to fill gaps in capabilities or market coverage (LaPointe, 2019).

Value-based purchasing is putting pressure on hospitals and healthcare systems to become more efficient, control costs, and become sustainable. Mergers and acquisitions are the strategy many healthcare systems are pursuing to achieve these outcomes. Megamergers with values in the billions of dollars are undertaken to provide greater scale to reduce costs, offer additional services, and create a larger footprint in the local market.

Healthcare systems are also increasingly acquiring physician practices to extend their reach into the community and to capture more of the care continuum. These types of changes result in transformative change in the healthcare system rather than incremental changes; these transformative changes are much more disruptive. These changes include managing the health of populations, and introducing innovations in health care. Questions are beginning to arise in terms of what these mergers and acquisitions are going to mean for healthcare costs and quality.

Value-based care forces providers to control costs and outcomes for an entire episode of care. ACOs and other alternative payment models also force providers to be responsible for a patient's entire healthcare journey, so providers are seeking ways to prevent costly services and conditions. Through these mergers and acquisitions, healthcare organizations are seeking economies of scale to obtain cost and care efficiencies to succeed under value-based care.

The Federal Trade Commission (FTC) and state officials closely scrutinize proposed mergers and acquisitions to ensure the results do not create a monopoly in a particular market. Attention is also given to the amount of market power that will result from the merger or acquisition, therefore impacting the bargaining power with private payers, increasing the ability to negotiate a higher claims reimbursement rate.

16.3.2.2 Physician Services

Physician services have traditionally been produced by physicians practicing alone or in small-group practices. Before 1980, when cost containment was less prominent in the healthcare sector, physicians played the dominant role in the management of hospitals, as well as in the management of physician group practices. The cost-containment trend in hospitals has led to the increased power of hospital administrators in hospital management.

The development of managed care networks also tended to reduce the discretionary power of physicians in determining the price and quality of service.

One response of physicians to these trends is to form larger practices and other physician networks. Regional and even national physician practice corporations have been established. As in the case of hospitals, the combining of physicians into large networks raises issues of efficiency versus market power. The formation of ACOs will increase the pressure on physicians to work in teams in order to achieve economies of scope and improve efficiency in the delivery of care.

16.3.2.3 Health Insurers and Managed Care Plans

Employers have traditionally provided health insurance in the United States as a tax-exempt fringe benefit. Before about 1980, most Americans were covered by traditional health insurance, which supported fee-for-service transactions with providers. Health insurers competed with one another to obtain insurance contracts with employers, who provided health insurance as a fringe benefit. Until the 1980s, healthcare cost containment had a relatively low priority in the U.S. system.

The early 1980s saw the rise of two important healthcare cost-containment mechanisms. First, Medicare's prospective payment system allowed the program to use its purchasing power to control the pricing and utilization of hospital services and physician services. Second, some states, beginning with California in 1982, began to allow payers to contract selectively with providers. Selective contracting enabled payers to negotiate reduced rates from providers in exchange for volume. Greater coordination of care, utilization review, and other changes caused health maintenance organizations (HMOs) and other forms of managed care to grow rapidly. As of 2010, HMOs enrolled about 77 million Americans, or about 25% of the population (Sanofi-Aventis, 2012). By 2017, HMO enrollment grew to 94.8 million or over 29% of the population (Sanofi-Aventis, 2018).

The structural change in the payers' markets has important implications for healthcare competition. In effect, increased market power on the buyer side has evolved in response to market power on the provider side, or to rapid price inflation in healthcare markets resulting from the absence of economizing by consumers due to the existence of third-party payers. Mergers and consolidation among payers also raise potential issues of market power versus efficiency.

16.3.2.4 Pharmaceuticals

The pharmaceutical industry is an oligopoly that includes a relatively small number of large multinational firms with broad product lines, along with a large number of small companies with limited product lines. A major competitive dimension is research and development competition—the search for new drugs with broad potential usage. The main incentive for new product development is the patent system, which grants the holder of a patent monopoly rights to manufacture and sell the product for about 20 years. Pharmacy retailers and pharmacy benefits-management companies carry out the distribution of pharmaceuticals, with registered pharmacists usually licensed by state departments of health.

16.3.3 Antitrust Policy: History and Institutions

The most prominent piece of antitrust legislation in the United States is the Sherman Act of 1890, which was a legislative response to rapid changes occurring in American industry. In the last two decades of the 19th century, innovations in transportation and communication led to the transformation of local and regional markets into national markets. Business consolidation was a major trend, and near-monopoly conditions arose in some markets. The Sherman Act, building on common law traditions against conspiracy and monopolization, had two major sections:

1. Every contract, combination in the form of trust or otherwise, or conspiracy, in restraint of trade or commerce among the several states, or with foreign nations, is declared to be illegal.
2. Every person who shall monopolize, or attempt to monopolize, or combine or conspire with any other person or persons, to monopolize any part of the trade or commerce among the several states, or with foreign nations, shall be deemed guilty of a felony.

The Clayton Act of 1914, with subsequent amendments, is the other major antitrust legislation in the United States. Two of the more important provisions of the Clayton Act are found in Sections 2 and 7, quoted, in part, as follows:

2a) It shall be unlawful for any person engaged in commerce in the course of such commerce, either directly or indirectly, to discriminate in price between different purchasers of commodities of like grade and quality . . . where the effect of such discrimination may be substantially to lessen competition or tend to create a monopoly.

7) No person engaged in commerce or in activity affecting commerce shall acquire, directly or indirectly, the whole or any part of the stock or other share capital and no person . . . shall acquire the whole or any part of the assets of another person engaged also in commerce . . . where in any line of commerce in any section of the country, the effect of such acquisition may be substantially to lessen competition, or to tend to create a monopoly.

The Federal Trade Commission Act, also passed in 1914, established the Federal Trade Commission (FTC). The FTC shares in the enforcement of the Clayton Act and enforces Section 5A1 of the FTC Act, which holds that "unfair methods of competition in or affecting commerce, and unfair or deceptive acts or practices in or affecting commerce, are declared unlawful."

There are two federal agencies that share the enforcement of antitrust law: the Antitrust Division of the U.S. Department of Justice and the Federal Trade Commission. The Department of Justice has primary responsibility for public enforcement of the Sherman Act; the FTC has primary responsibility for enforcement of the Federal Trade Commission Act and of Section 2 of the Clayton Act. The two agencies combine in enforcing the merger provisions of the Clayton Act. In addition, there are areas of overlap in which the agencies share jurisdiction.

In addition to public enforcement of the antitrust laws, private enforcement is also important. The importance of private enforcement is related directly to Section 4 of the Clayton Act, which provides that those injured as a result of "anything forbidden in the antitrust laws" may bring private suit and recover triple damages, including attorney's fees. The triple damages provision provides a strong incentive for injured parties to bring private suits, including class action suits.

Because of the time and expense of fully developing cases and bringing them to trial, the majority of antitrust cases are settled by consent decrees. In a consent decree settlement, a court-supervised agreement is worked out between the parties. In the case of criminal suits, a settlement sometimes involves the use of a no-contest plea in order that the defendant may avoid pleading guilty. In private civil cases, financial settlements, generally involving amounts less than those initially requested by the plaintiffs, are common.

16.3.4 Price-Fixing and Conspiracy in Restraint of Trade in Healthcare Markets

Section 1 of the Sherman Act concerns conspiracy in restraint of trade. The legal tradition in the enforcement of this section is that evidence of direct communication among competitors is sufficient to find a violation. This principle is referred to as the "per se rule." The U.S. Supreme Court has strongly stated that whether or not the prices established by conspiracy are reasonable is *not* an issue.

Despite the strong *per se* tradition in enforcing price-fixing, legal precedent was relatively slow in extending the range of antitrust law to the professions. A landmark case in this regard is *Goldfarb v. Virginia State Bar* (1975), in which the Supreme Court stated that the professions are not exempt from the Sherman Act's prohibition of price-fixing. The *Goldfarb* case involved fee schedules set for legal fees by a bar association.

That the *per se* rule also applies to price-fixing among physicians was forcefully stated in the U.S. Supreme Court's decision in the case of *Arizona v. Maricopa County Medical Society* (1982). In this case, two physician groups utilized relative value schedules to establish maximum prices for medical services. The Court ruled that this approach to setting maximum physician fees was subject to the *per se* rule against price-fixing.

The *Maricopa* case clearly establishes that the healthcare professions fall under the *per se* rule concerning price-fixing and conspiracy in restraint of trade. This is not to say that physicians and other health professionals may not form professional associations and discuss issues of mutual concern. Trade association activities, including some exchange of pricing information, generally do not constitute a violation. However, the use of a common fee schedule setting either maximum or minimum fees would likely be a violation of the Sherman Act.

16.3.5 Mergers in Healthcare Markets

A merger is a partial or total combination of two separate business firms. Partial mergers include such combinations as joint ventures and intercorporate stock purchases. Complete mergers are more common. A complete merger involves the purchase of assets or stock in one corporation by a separate corporation and typically results in the blending of identities and the creation of a single succeeding firm.

Mergers are generally described as falling into one of three categories. The first type of merger is the horizontal merger, which is the combination of two firms that compete in the same product market and geographic market. A merger of two community hospitals in the same metropolitan area would be an example of a horizontal merger. The second type of merger is

the vertical merger, which involves firms that have a buyer–seller relationship. The acquisition of a physician group practice by a managed-care company, a healthcare system, or a hospital would be an example of a vertical merger. The third type of merger is the conglomerate merger, which unites firms that are neither horizontally nor vertically related. The acquisition of a community hospital by a banking corporation would be an example of a conglomerate merger.

Mergers and joint ventures have become very common in healthcare markets. Investor-owned hospital corporations, such as Tenet Healthcare Corp., have expanded in size and in geographic scope, primarily through merger. Presently, many investor-owned systems have divested many of their hospitals in an effort to reduce their debt load resulting from their earlier acquisition activities. Mergers have also been common in physician group practices, as solo practitioners combine to form local and regional group practices. These larger groups enable economies of scale and negotiation leverage with payers.

The enforcement of Section 7 of the Clayton Act by the Department of Justice and Federal Trade Commission focuses on the seller concentration in the market before and after prospective mergers. The Hart-Scott-Rodino Act of 1976 requires that mergers above a threshold size ($100 million in sales or assets on the part of one premerger firm and $10 million for the other party) must notify the Federal Trade Commission and Department of Justice in advance of the merger. This provision of the law allows the antitrust authorities to intervene before the merger actually occurs rather than wait until asset ownership has changed hands. This provision also allows for modification of the assets to be acquired if seller concentration in certain markets raises objections to parts of the merger.

Hospital markets tended to be local or regional in scope, although recent mergers have led to the establishment of large nationwide systems. In addition, because hospitals differ with respect to the array of services offered, the analysis of hospital mergers must consider both product market definition and geographic market definition. The definitions of geographic market and product market for hospitals are based on the interchangeability or cross-price elasticity of the services offered, as viewed by consumers. Two or more hospitals are in the same geographic market if consumers (or their physician agents) consider the hospitals to be reasonably interchangeable when making decisions regarding where to seek care. Two or more hospitals are in the same product market if consumers consider their offerings of a given service to be reasonably interchangeable (Wilder & Jacobs, 1987).

As noted earlier, the Clayton Act prohibits mergers when "the effect of such acquisition may be substantially to lessen competition, or to tend to create a monopoly." In the case of hospital mergers, a potential anticompetitive effect exists if there is overlap in the product and geographic markets of the hospitals prior to the merger. In general, the question of whether two hospitals are in the same geographic and product markets may be more complicated for hospitals than for nonhealthcare service firms. The geographic market definition is likely to vary depending on the medical procedure in question. Because patients are likely to be willing to travel greater distances for more complicated, more expensive procedures, the geographic market definition for hospitals is not independent of the procedure in question. In general, the geographic market is much wider for complicated procedures than for simple procedures, or for tertiary care than for primary care (Wilder & Jacobs, 1987).

Antitrust aspects of hospital mergers must be considered in the light of merger history. During the period 1950–1980, enforcement agencies treated horizontal mergers very strictly, and modest market concentration levels and modest increases in concentration were often sufficient for horizontal mergers to be successfully challenged. After 1980, horizontal merger enforcement became more lenient, as reflected in the Department of Justice and Federal Trade Commission merger guidelines, the most recent version of which was released in 2018.

In evaluating horizontal mergers, the Justice Department guidelines use the Herfindahl-Hirschman Index (HHI) of market concentration. The HHI is defined as the sum of the squares of the individual market shares of all firms in the market, wherein market shares are expressed in percentages. For example, one hospital in a market would result in an HHI of 10,000 (100^2). Two hospitals of equal size would result in an HHI of 5000 ($50^2 + 50^2$). Ten hospitals of equal size would result in an HHI of 1000. According to the guidelines, in evaluating a proposed merger, the Justice Department and Federal Trade Commission consider both the market concentration and the increase in concentration that would result from the merger. The guidelines establish three categories of horizontal mergers:

1. Post-Merger HHI Below 1500: The agency regards markets in this region to be unconcentrated. Mergers resulting in unconcentrated markets are unlikely to have adverse competitive effects and ordinarily require no further analysis.
2. Post-Merger HHI Between 1500 and 2500: The agency regards markets in this region to be moderately concentrated. Mergers producing an increase in the HHI of less than 100 points in moderately concentrated markets post-merger are unlikely to have adverse competitive consequences and ordinarily require no further analysis. Mergers producing an increase in the HHI of more than 100 points in moderately concentrated markets post-merger potentially raise significant competitive concerns.
3. Post-Merger HHI Above 2500: The agency regards markets in this region to be highly concentrated. Mergers producing an increase in the HHI of less than 100 points, even in highly concentrated markets post-merger, are unlikely to have adverse competitive consequences and ordinarily require no further analysis. Mergers producing an increase in the HHI of more than 100 points in highly concentrated markets post-merger potentially raise significant competitive concerns, depending on the factors set forth in [other sections] of the guidelines. Where the post-merger HHI exceeds 2500, it will be presumed that mergers producing an increase in the HHI of more than 200 points are likely to create or enhance market power or facilitate its exercise (U.S. Department of Justice and Federal Trade Commission, 2018).

Hospital mergers have occurred at a rapid rate since 1980. Blackstone and Fuhr (1992) state that 40–60 hospital mergers per year occurred in the 1980s, but that the Department of Justice and Federal Trade Commission challenged fewer than 10 hospital mergers during this decade. In some cases, mergers were not challenged because the hospitals were not in the same geographic market. Many of the mergers and acquisitions were part of the hospital consolidation involved in the formation and growth of such firms as Columbia/HCA. Even when hospital mergers were truly horizontal, the Justice Department and Federal Trade Commission applied somewhat different standards to these mergers than to other horizontal mergers.

The variation in standards is apparent in the Department of Justice-Federal Trade Commission Antitrust Guidelines for the Business of Health Care, which were released initially in 1993 and updated in August 2010. The purpose of the guidelines is to provide information concerning the types of mergers, joint ventures, and other competition-related actions that might be challenged by the antitrust authorities. In the area of mergers, the guidelines state that the merger of two small hospitals with low occupancy rates, even if they are in the same geographic market, would not be challenged. The guidelines also state that two or more hospitals of any size could engage in joint ventures to buy high-technology equipment, if each hospital by itself could not fully utilize the equipment.

For mergers between larger hospitals, the antitrust agencies state that they will use the "rule of reason" in analyzing mergers. The rule of reason approach considers whether mergers may have a substantial anticompetitive effect and, if so, whether the anticompetitive effect is offset by procompetitive efficiencies (Steiger, 1995).

One reason for the relatively lenient antitrust policy toward hospital mergers is the possibility of efficiency gains. Gaynor and Haas-Wilson (1999) point out that some mergers are rational responses to excess capacity and empty hospital beds resulting from the shift to increased use of outpatient treatment. Mergers may also be driven by changes in payment practices, such as the Medicare Pathway to Success Program and Accountable Care Organizations, that shift more risk to the provider.

The pharmaceutical industry has a relatively high seller concentration in some drug submarkets, but the level of concentration in the broadly defined pharmaceutical preparations industry is relatively low. An example of an FTC merger complaint is that issued by the agency regarding the Hoechst AG and Rhone-Poulenc merger. This complaint argued that Hoechst's acquisition of Rhone-Poulenc would reduce competition in the market for agents used to treat blood-clotting diseases. A consent decree in 2000 allowed the merger subject to the transfer of Rhone-Poulenc's product in this submarket to a separate firm (U.S. Federal Trade Commission, 2000). This case illustrates that the relevant product market in pharmaceutical antitrust cases may be defined quite narrowly.

16.3.6 Antitrust Policy: Monopolization

Section 2 of the Sherman Act makes it illegal to "monopolize, or attempt to monopolize." The use of the verb *monopolize* rather than the noun *monopoly* suggests one of the difficulties in enforcing monopoly laws. Conceptually, a monopoly is a single firm with exclusive possession of a market for a good or service. As a practical matter, however, pure monopoly status is highly unusual. Markets with high seller concentration resulting in partial or near-monopoly market structures are the more common objects of monopoly inquiries. As a result, the enforcement of monopoly laws tends to focus on market definition, market share, and specific acts that suggest monopolistic intent.

A good summary of the enforcement tradition in monopoly cases may be found in the U.S. Supreme Court decision in the *Grinnell* case, in which Justice Douglas stated that the offense of monopoly "has two elements: (1) possession of monopoly power in the relevant market and; (2) willful acquisition or maintenance of that power" (*U.S. v. Grinnell Corporation*, 384US 563 [1966]).

Relatively little of the antitrust enforcement activity in health care has involved monopolization issues directly. Instead, most enforcement activity has taken place under the conspiracy statute (Section 1 of the Sherman Act) or the antimerger statute (Section 7 of the Clayton Act). However, as national hospital corporations and healthcare provider networks grow more important in the United States, the likelihood that monopolization issues will become more important will increase.

The major reason that monopolization issues have been less important than other antitrust issues is that the level of seller concentration in most hospital or physician services markets, while relatively high in some instances, does not approach the level that indicates monopoly on the basis of case law. In the most direct statement on the connection between market share and monopoly status, the *Aluminum Company of America* case, Judge Hand stated that a market share over 90% "is enough to constitute a monopoly; it is doubtful whether 60 or 64 percent would be enough; and certainly 33 percent is not" (*U.S. vs. Aluminum Company of America*, 148F. 2nd 416 [1945]).

Since the *Aluminum Company of America* case in the 1940s, the only very large national corporation whose monopoly status was broken up by antitrust action was AT&T, in a case settled through a consent decree in 1982. A monopolization case against IBM by the Justice Department was dropped at about the same time (in the early 1980s). Because neither of these cases reached the Supreme Court, there is no clear recent judicial statement interpreting monopoly law for today's world.

There are at least three principal market areas within health care in which monopoly issues may come to the fore. First, as national hospital corporations grow and as tax-exempt community hospitals merge and engage in joint ventures, the market structure in some local hospital markets may evolve in such a way that a group of jointly owned hospitals will reach a market share of 60%. Such market evolution could then make monopolization enforcement under Section 2 of the Sherman Act relevant in some hospital markets.

Physician networks may also become subject to monopolization enforcement. Physicians have been rapidly forming networks that operate as unified firms. Such networks may increasingly accumulate market shares in relevant geographic markets in the 60% range or greater. As such market shares arise through continued consolidation, antimonopoly law may become directed toward the larger networks.

HMOs and other managed care organizations may also become the target of monopolization statutes. These organizations tend to increase concentration on the buyer side in markets for hospital and physician services. As the market penetration of managed care organizations increases, the potential for high market shares on the buyer side of healthcare markets also increases. Some observers believe that the rapid growth of physician networks and the increasing number of hospital mergers and joint ventures are partly responses to the increased purchasing power of managed care organizations.

The 1996 Department of Justice and Federal Trade Commission statement on healthcare and antitrust laws addresses the interaction of physician networks and multi-provider networks. In general, the statement indicates that multi-provider networks might violate antitrust laws if the exclusion of some physicians from a dominant network in a local market makes it impossible for them to practice medicine. A similar argument could be directed at a dominant multi-provider network that excludes hospitals in a local market. Efficiency gains may be an offsetting virtue of provider coordination and combination. Antitrust cases considering monopolization issues would also consider efficiency effects.

16.3.7 Quality Competition and Antitrust Policy

Nonprice competition is particularly important in most sectors of the healthcare market. Quality competition among insurers or managed care organizations is related to such attributes as access to specialists, freedom of choice among providers, and treatment capacity. Quality competition among providers is based on such attributes as credentials, location, and treatment outcomes (Sage & Hammer, 1999). Because of incomplete information in healthcare markets, consumers may be poorly informed about the quality of service. This information problem could mean that antitrust policies that encourage price competition may lead to the provision of lower quality service than is socially optimal (Gaynor & Haas-Wilson, 1999).

16.3.8 Antitrust Issues Related to Managed Care

One of the most important trends in the healthcare sector during the 1980s and 1990s was the rise of managed care plans, selective contracting, and integrated health networks. In a nutshell, what happened is that the market power in the hands of the physicians and hospitals (the suppliers of health care) was met by the growth of market power on the buyer side. The growth of managed care appears to have promoted competitive efficiencies in health care and likely reduced the rate of increase in healthcare costs. At the same time, the rise of managed care could eventually result in increased market power on the part of buyers or sellers of health care and ultimately lead to an increase in the prices paid by consumers (Schactman & Altman, 1995).

16.3.9 Federal Antitrust Policy Guidelines

A major landmark in healthcare antitrust policy was the issuing of the *Statements of Enforcement Policy and Analytical Principles Relating to Health Care and Antitrust* by the Department of Justice and Federal Trade Commission in 1993 (revised in 1994 and 1996). The revisions in 2011 specifically addressed ACOs participating in Medicare's Shared Savings Program. These statements reflect the complexity of markets and provider and purchaser institutions in health care. They also indicate that the antitrust authorities are seeking to adapt antitrust policy, which was developed for broad applicability, to the particular economic characteristics of healthcare markets.

The purpose of the statements is to reduce uncertainty concerning antitrust policy and to establish "antitrust safety zones" (market conditions under which business conduct will not be challenged). For example, the merger of two small hospitals with low occupancy rates would fall into one of the safety zones. A physician network might attract antitrust scrutiny by collusive agreement on price or by excluding some physicians, making it impossible for them to practice in the market.

The healthcare system in the United States has been transformed by structural change, including the rise of managed care, selective contracting, provider networks, and numerous large mergers. These changes have the potential to increase productive efficiency and to slow the rate of healthcare price inflation. At the same time, the changes may increase market power in some product or geographic markets and may lead to higher consumer prices. In addition, there is increasing concern regarding the quality of healthcare services, leading to such developments as congressional debates on the legal rights of physicians to form unions and on the patient bill of rights. It is likely that as greater consolidation among providers and purchasers occurs and as quality-competition tradeoffs are discussed widely, regulation and antitrust issues will become even more important. As changes occur in payment models and the organizational structure of the healthcare system, modifications to modernize the antitrust laws as they apply to health care are likely to continue to evolve.

Exercises

1. Why are physicians sometimes described as "double agents?"
2. How can consumers of healthcare services obtain more information about service quality?
3. Explain how the patent right provides a financial incentive for pharmaceutical manufacturers to develop new drugs.
4. Suppose that you overhear a foursome of physicians on the golf course discussing the prices they charge for an office visit. Suppose further that you hear them reach an agreement to all charge a fee of $100 for an office visit. What is such an agreement called in antitrust policy, and what antitrust law may have been violated?
5. Suppose that emergency room services in the city of Hibiscus are provided by three hospitals. Two of the hospitals each have a market share of 40% and the third hospital has a market share of 20%. The two largest hospitals plan to merge.
   a. Compute the pre-merger and post-merger HHI for this market.
   b. Based on the 1992 merger guidelines, would this merger likely be challenged by the antitrust authorities?
6. What is a market failure and its potential consequences in the market?
7. What is a public good and what are the potential market effects of a public good?
8. Describe the Pathways to Success Program and its potential impact on providers.

Bibliography

Abbott, T. (1997). The pharmaceutical industry. In T. E. Getzen (Ed.), *Health economics*. New York, NY: Wiley.

Bailey, J., Hamami, T., & McCorry, D. (2017). Certificate of need laws and health care prices. *Journal of Health Care Finance, 43*(4), 1–7.

Blackstone, E., & Fuhr, J. P. (1992). An antitrust analysis of non-profit hospital mergers. *Review of Industrial Organization, 8,* 473–490.

Blomqvist, A. (1991). The doctor as double agent: Information asymmetry, health insurance, and medical care. *Journal of Health Economics, 10,* 411–432.

Conlan, M. (1997). Board games. *Drug Topics, 17*(November), 58–63.

Conover, C., & Sloan, F. (1998). Does removing certificate-of-need regulation lead to a surge in health care spending? *Journal of Health Politics, Policy and Law, 23,* 455–481.

Dranove, D., Shanley, M., & White, W. D. (1993). Price and concentration in hospital markets: The switch from patient-driven to payer-driven competition. *Journal of Law and Economics, 36,* 179–204.

Folland, S., Goodman. A. C., & Stano, M. (2001). *The economics of health and health care* (3rd ed.). Englewood Cliffs, NJ: Prentice Hall.

Frech, H. E., III. (1993). Health insurance: Designing products to reduce costs. In L. Deutsch (Ed.), *Industry studies*. Englewood Cliffs, NJ: Prentice Hall.

Gaynor, M., & Haas-Wilson, D. (1999). Change, consolidation and competition in health care markets. *Journal of Economic Perspectives, 13,* 141–164.

Getzen, T. E. (1997). *Health economics*. New York, NY: Wiley.

Grabowski, H., & Vernon, J. (1992). Brand loyalty, entry, and price competition in pharmaceuticals after the 1984 Drug Act. *Journal of Law and Economics, 35,* 331–350.

Havighurst, C. (2000). American health care and the law—We need to talk! *Health Affairs, 19*(4), 84–106.

Hellinger, F. J. (2009). The effect of certificate-of-need laws on hospital beds and healthcare expenditures: An empirical analysis. *American Journal of Managed Care, 15*(10), 737–744.

Herper, M. (2012). The truly staggering cost of inventing new drugs. *Forbes*. Retrieved from https://www.forbes.com/sites/matthewherper/2012/02/10/the-truly-staggering-cost-of-inventing-new-drugs/#77c170574a94

Joint Commission. (2012). *Facts about the Joint Commission.* Retrieved from http://www.jointcommission.org/about_us/fact_sheets.aspx

Joint Commission. (2019). *Facts about the Joint Commission.* Retrieved from http://www.jointcommission.org/about_us/fact_sheets.aspx

Kesselheim, A. S., Misono, A. S., Llee, J. L., Stedman, M. R., Brookhart, M. A., Choudhry, N. K., & Shrank, W. H. (2008). Clinical equivalence of generic and brand-name drugs used in cardiovascular disease: A systematic review and meta-analysis. *JAMA, 300*(21), 2514–2526.

Kim, T. H., & McCue, M. J. (2012). The performance of the leveraged buyout of the Hospital Corporation of America, Inc. *Health Care Management Review, 37*(3), 214–222.

Kirchheimer, B. (2000). Move over Columbia, HCA is back. *Modern Healthcare, 19*(June).

LaPointe, J. (2019, July 23). Hospital merger and acquisition activity. *Revcycle Intelligence Practice Management News.*

Medicare Payment Advisory Commission. (2000). Report to Congress: Medicare payment policy. Retrieved from http://www.medpac.gov

Pear, R. (1996). Doctors may get leeway to rival large companies. *New York Times,* 8 April.

Peltzman, S. (1976). Toward a more general theory of regulation. *Journal of Law and Economics, 19,* 211–240.

Pharmaceutical Research and Manufacturers of America. (2011). *Pharmaceutical Industry Profile 2011.* Washington, DC: PhRMA.

Rahman, M., Galarraga, O., Zinn, J. S., Grabowski, D. C., & Mor, V. (2016). The impact of certificate-of-need laws on nursing home and home health care expenditures. *Medical Care Research and Review, 73*(1), 85–105.

Reed, T. (2019, January 15). Hospital mergers and acquisitions in 2018 were fewer but larger. *Fierce Health Care.* Retrieved from https://www.fiercehealthcare.com/hositals

Rodriquez, A. (2019, September 23). Percentage of private-sector employers with at least one self-insured health plan has decreased. *American Journal of Managed Care Newsroom.*

Rosko, M. D., & Mutter, R. L. (2014). The association of hospital cost-inefficiency with certificate-of-need regulation. *Medical Care Research and Review, 71*(3), 280–298.

Russo, C., Calo, O., Harrison, G., Mahoney, K., & Zavotsky, K. E. (2018). Resilience and coping after hospital mergers. *Clinical Nurse Specialist, 32*(2), 97–102. Retrieved from www.cns-journals.com

Sage, W. M., & Hammer, P. J. (1999). Competing on quality of care: The need to develop a competition policy for health care markets. *University of Michigan Journal of Law Reform, 32,* 1069–1118.

Sanofi-Aventis. (2012). *Managed care digest series, HMO-PPO digest, 2011–2012.* Bridgewater, NJ: Sanofi.

Sanofi-Aventis. (2018). *Managed care digest series, payer digest, 2018.* Bridgewater, NJ: Sanofi.

Santerre, R. E., & Neun, S. (1996). *Health economics: Theories, insights and industry studies.* Chicago, IL: Dryden.

Schactman, D., & Altman, S. H. (1995). *Market consolidation, antitrust, and public policy in the health care industry: Agenda for future research.* Princeton, NJ: Robert Wood Johnson Foundation.

Scheutzow, S. O. (1999). State medical peer review: High cost but no benefit—Is it time for a change? *American Journal of Law and Medicine, 25*(1), 7–60.

Steiger, J. D. (1995, November 9). *Health care enforcement issues.* Prepared remarks of Commissioner Janet D. Steiger, Federal Trade Commission, before the Health Trustee Institute, Cleveland, OH.

Stigler, G. (1971). The theory of economic regulation. *Bell Journal of Economics, 2,* 3–21.

Trepanier, S., Crenshaw, J. T., & Yoder-Wise, P. S. (2016). Risk taking: A required competency for merger, acquisitions, and partnerships. *Nursing Administration Quarterly, 49*(4), 307–311.

U. S. Department of Justice and Federal Trade Commission. (1993). *Horizontal merger guidelines,* Washington, DC.

U. S. Department of Justice and Federal Trade Commission. (1994). *Horizontal merger guidelines,* Washington, DC.

U. S. Department of Justice and Federal Trade Commission. (1996). *Statements of antitrust enforcement policy in health care.* Washington, DC.

U. S. Department of Justice and Federal Trade Commission. (2018). *Horizontal merger guidelines,* Washington, DC.

U. S. Federal Trade Commission. (2000). *FTC antitrust actions in pharmaceutical services and products.* Retrieved from http://www.ftc.gov

U.S. Food and Drug Administration. (2000). *About the Center for Drug Evaluation and Research.* Retrieved from http://www.fda.gov/cder

Walshe, K. (2001). Regulating U.S. nursing homes: Are we learning from experience? *Health Affairs, 20*(6), 128–144.

Wilder, R. P., & Jacobs, P. (1987). Antitrust considerations for hospital mergers: Market definition and market concentration. In R. M. Scheffler & L. F. Rossiter (Eds.), *Advances in health economics and health services research.* Stamford, CT: JAI Press.

CHAPTER 17

Reform of the Healthcare Market

OBJECTIVES

1. Review reasons stimulating healthcare reform.
2. Define the concept of healthcare market reform and explain the need for reform in the context of health care and health insurance markets.
3. Define each of the following policies and describe their effects in terms of equity and efficiency: premium subsidies, cooperative pools, community rating, mandates, and limits on selection.
4. Define managed care, its characteristics, and its effects.
5. Define *selection bias* and explain how it might cause a managed care organization to misleadingly appear more efficient than fee-for-service healthcare provision.
6. Compare the effects of managed care with the effects of fee-for-service on resource use and quality of care.
7. Explain the conceptual role of consumer sovereignty in hospital markets and identify several reasons why early attempts to achieve it were controversial.

17.1 Introduction

17.1.1 Issues Facing the Healthcare System

The healthcare industry is a major sector in the economy of the United States, accounting for almost 18% of the gross domestic product (GDP). Because the healthcare industry represents such a substantial portion of economic activities, it both impacts and is impacted by the general economy. As the healthcare industry continues to grow and evolve, a number of transformational changes are occurring in its organizational structure and in the arrangements of healthcare providers, in its financial systems, in new technologies and advances in medical science, and in the introduction and implementation of new and modifications of existing healthcare policies. Consequently, the healthcare industry continues to present a dynamic environment for the application of economic evaluation and analysis.

The passage of the Patient Protection and Affordable Care Act (P.L. 111-148) in 2010 stimulated significant activity in the healthcare system, as each sector of the healthcare industry reacted to and prepared for the implementation of the various features of the act. A major contributor to the passage of the act was the continued rapid rise in healthcare expenditures and the projections regarding the growth in those expenditures. As the data in **Figure 17-1** illustrate, healthcare costs were projected to continue consuming an ever-increasing percentage of the GDP in the United States.

Every sector of the healthcare industry is facing tremendous pressure to cut costs, improve quality, and prepare for fundamental change in how health care is provided, financed, and consumed. An initial reaction in the hospital industry has been to acquire and merge organizations, and to purchase or develop extensive

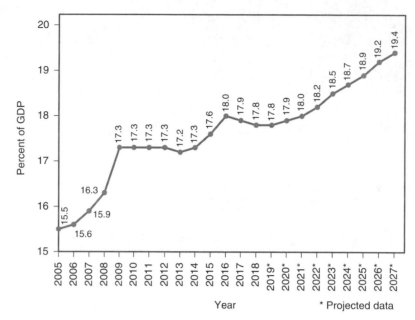

Figure 17-1 Actual and projected healthcare expenditures as percent of GDP. Note the rapid increase in percent of GDP between 2008 and 2009 and the slight decrease between 2012 and 2013.

Modified from CMS.Gov, Historical National Health Expenditures, Table 01 and National Health Expenditures Projections 2018–2027, Table 01.

physician networks as the hospital industry assumes more financial risk. As hospital organizations grow, they have also begun to undertake direct approaches with employers with insurance-like options, eliminating the health insurance plan in the middle.

Vertical collaborative arrangements have also been undertaken to integrate better control over the coordination of care across providers and institutions. In addition, insurance plans have increased direct involvement with providers, and employers are seeking different ways to reduce benefit costs for their employees. Government programs are seeking alternative payment methods and reducing payment schedules to providers. Pressures continue to mount to control costs, increase access, and improve the quality of care delivered in the healthcare system.

A major contributor to the growth of healthcare expenditures has been the rapid development and widespread diffusion of new medical technologies and services; this is expected to continue or even increase in the future. These procedure, equipment, and process innovations enable the diagnosis and treatment of previously untreatable terminal conditions and acute healthcare problems, and change the diagnosis and treatment of existing healthcare problems by identifying secondary conditions and expanding the indications for treatment.

Many of these new innovations require costly new pharmaceuticals, expensive equipment, and a more highly skilled healthcare workforce. These innovations also enable the expansion of the scope of medical interventions into areas outside previous boundaries

of the healthcare system (Carecloud, 2019; Jones, 2018; KFF, 2007). Unlike other industries in which the adoption of new innovations typically reduces the per-unit cost of output, many of these innovations in health care usually increase the costs of the output. Consequently, economics has an important role in assisting in the evaluation of the value-added of existing and new technologies.

In addition to determining the impact of existing and new innovations on the per-unit cost of output, determining the impact of the innovation on the total healthcare expenditures is another crucial role for economics. In examining the impact, it is important to determine if the innovation supplements an existing treatment, or if it is a partial or total substitute for an existing treatment, and then if the use of the innovation results in higher or lower expenditures for each patient treated.

It is also important to examine the number of patients treated by the new innovation. For example, does the new innovation enable the provision of services to a broader population, either because access is increased or because previously unidentified or untreatable individuals now receive services? Does the innovation allow new populations to be diagnosed for existing treatments, or does it extend existing treatments for new conditions in the population? Or does the new innovation reduce utilization by improving screening and diagnosis capacity, allowing more targeted treatments to be provided to the population?

While it is often possible to identify new innovations and determine when they were first introduced into the healthcare system, it is usually very difficult to measure the impact that the technology has on the costs of health care. One reason for this difficulty is that the introduction and adoption of innovations do not occur in a linear fashion or in similar ways in organizations or systems. Oftentimes, multiple innovations are introduced into the healthcare system in a short time span, and the impacts of the different innovations are often interrelated, making measurement of the impact of a single innovation difficult, if not impossible. (See **Table 17-1** for a list of 20 technologies introduced just in 2018.)

In addition, the wide diversity of the innovations and of the structure and organization of the healthcare delivery system makes direct measurement of the impact of a single innovation on the entire system difficult, although assessing the impact of the adoption and implementation on a single organization or practice is more manageable. Economic tools are certainly appropriate and applicable on the micro level, and also make valuable contributions at the macro level.

One of the technologies changing the healthcare industry is health information technology. The introduction of health information technologies to digitize health records was established as a national priority in efforts to assist in the improvement of quality, safety, and efficiency in health care. As electronic health records (EHRs) are adopted, implemented, and used by practices and organizations, they will increase the complexity of changes occurring in the healthcare system. The EHR provides support for clinical decision making and enables the delivery of health care in remote or inaccessible areas. The focus and incentives provided for the adoption and use of EHRs create particular problems for individual and small practices because they often have very limited resources, small staff numbers, and lack the expertise to deploy and integrate these EHRs into their practices. As health

Table 17-1 Top 20 Healthcare Technology Advances in 2018

1	Discovery of the genes that make cancer metastasize
2	A DNA test that predicts the likelihood of drug-based side effects
3	A simulation to aid in successful cardiac surgeries
4	An inexpensive way to diagnose hepatitis B
5	Progress with artificial ovaries
6	Changing brain chemical imbalances in drug addicts
7	More user-friendly and specialized applications
8	Using common bacteria for medical imaging processes
9	Marijuana-based epilepsy drug earns FDA approval
10	The continued widespread adoption of EHRs
11	The possibility of using drugs to treat hearing loss
12	More applications of virtual reality in medicine
13	Increased uses for big data
14	A proactive way to identify instances of spastic cerebral palsy
15	An injection for migraine headaches that reduces frequencies
16	Scientists find brain cells responsible for anxiety levels
17	A pill that may eliminate type 1 diabetes injections
18	An oral treatment that reduces peanut allergy effects
19	A fast-acting influenza pill
20	A simpler way to detect cognitive decline

Data from Carecloud Corp. (2019). Top 20 healthcare technology advances in 2018. *Continuum*. Retrieved from https://www.carecloud.com/continuum/top-20-healthcare-technology-advances/

information exchanges continue to expand and create the need for interoperability of automated data systems, the expectation is that the sharing of information across organizations will reduce the number of laboratory and imaging procedures, emergency department visits, and the number of provider visits, especially referrals to specialists, significantly impacting the processes of healthcare delivery and outcomes.

If EHRs are to be deployed successfully so that providers achieve meaningful use, then a good understanding of the current processes of delivering care is needed. These processes must be mapped so that they can be changed to adapt to the new requirements of the EHR system. To be successful, support for the technical aspects of the EHR is needed, as well as support for change management within the practices or organizations. Much of this support will need to come from outside sources because the necessary human capital is often not available internally, especially in small practices or small organizations.

In addition to the EHR, health information technology is also expected to reduce the current lengthy process of translating scientific findings into general clinical practice. Part of these translations into generalizable results involves performing comparative effectiveness research. The tools of health economics are especially relevant in this environment, as the processes, tools, and resources needed for the successful transformation of the healthcare industry must be employed in the translation.

17.1.2 Healthcare Reform

Healthcare reform is a term that has been applied to insurance and healthcare markets, as well as to the total constellation of health services. In the case of insurance markets, the term refers to specific ways to make the markets perform more like a competitive market, such as by setting rules to prevent insurers from engaging in "biased risk selection," a key factor in market failure, and trying to ensure that insurance is available at a "reasonable" price to those who want it.

In the case of the healthcare market, the main goal of reform has been to increase consumer choice and become more patient-centered (i.e., to make the healthcare markets more sensitive to consumer rather than provider demands). One of the key efforts has been to increase the degree of competition so that the markets perform more like the textbook model of a competitive market, recognizing that certain characteristics of the healthcare system will interfere in accomplishing these efforts.

A competitive market has a number of specific characteristics that impact its performance and efficiency. For one, a competitive market contains a large number of buyers and sellers, with each acting independently. This characteristic means that no one buyer or seller can individually impact the market for the product or service. The interactions of buyers and sellers in the market determine the price and quantity that will result in market equilibrium. In a competitive market a supplier can sell all desired quantity of its product or service at the established market price. All suppliers are providing homogeneous products. Both buyers and sellers possess complete information about the market. Consumer sovereignty prevails in a competitive market, with consumer preferences determining the services offered in the market. While the healthcare market violates many, if not all, of these conditions, incentives and penalties can still be designed to impact the healthcare system, making it react in a more competitive manner.

The goals that market reforms seek to achieve include equity and efficiency. The insurance market reforms have focused largely on equity (i.e., making insurance affordable to those who want it). A possible strategy includes subsidies for high-risk consumers. The early reforms were only secondarily concerned with increasing provider efficiency or consumer choice. More recent insurance market reforms have focused more on increasing provider efficiency in the production of healthcare services. Healthcare market reforms as opposed to health insurance market reforms have tended to be focused more on efficiency—on making the markets more like the competitive ideal.

This chapter examines reforms in healthcare markets and insurance markets and considers the integration of the insurance and healthcare delivery functions into managed care. Section 17.2 reviews insurance market reforms, focusing on alternative mechanisms that have been proposed to make insurance markets more sensitive to consumer wants. Section 17.3 looks at the role of managed care in changing provider and buyer incentives to promote greater efficiency and limit cost increases. Finally, Section 17.4 describes some of the developments in information and consumer orientation that have affected healthcare markets.

17.2 Insurance Market Reform

17.2.1 The Need for Reform

The performance of insurance markets can be judged from the vantage point of efficiency or equity. In looking at economic efficiency performance criteria, the essential question being asked is whether an optimal degree of risk is being shifted by consumers to insurers. This degree is related to the value or benefits of risk shifting to the consumers and the cost of risk shifting to insurers. If individuals are willing to pay for greater amounts of coverage (e.g., coverage for more expensive services), and there are insurers who are willing to provide this coverage at the desired price, but there are some impediments to the shifting of the risks so that it does not take place, then the degree of insurance coverage is not optimal. By the same token, if the value to consumers of shifting additional risks is low (below the cost to insurers of accepting these risks), but consumers purchase insurance anyway because of subsidized out-of-pocket prices or lack of good information, then an excess of coverage will result.

Under these conditions, an efficient degree of coverage may mean no coverage at all for healthcare expenditures, especially for some individuals. If individuals value risk shifting less than they do the cost of insurance, then they will simply not insure. However, these individuals may be very high-risk and/or low-income individuals, or may work for small companies that do not provide benefits, and other society members may think it is inequitable for these individuals to go without insurance coverage. On the grounds of equity, it could be decided that something should be done to remedy the situation. This section will examine the causes of market failure in insurance markets and the remedies that have been proposed. The analysis using a simple economic model to illustrate the essential features of insurance market failure and market reform is presented.

17.2.2 The Basic Model

A basic model of a health insurance market is presented, in which there are seven individuals, each with a given degree of risk of becoming ill. The expected loss for each of these individuals is shown in **Table 17-2**. Individual 1, the least healthy of the lot, has an expected loss of $120; individual 2 has an expected loss of $80; and so on.

The assumptions about the demand for insurance are now introduced in this illustration. Each individual has a certain willingness to pay for health insurance coverage. Individual 1 is willing to pay $120, which would indicate that he or she is risk neutral (i.e., puts no additional value on the size of the loss). Individual 2 is willing to pay $100 for coverage, individual 3 is willing to pay $90, and so on. Note that individual 1 might be a high-risk person with limited means to pay for health insurance.

In addition to the individuals' demands, the personal characteristics or circumstances that will affect the insurance market in a systematic way are specified. One such characteristic is age. In this illustration, two separate age groups are specified—individuals older than 50 and individuals 50 or younger. In general, the expectation is that an individual whose age is above 50 will have greater expected healthcare costs

Table 17-2 The Value and Price of Insurance for Individuals

	Individual						
	1	**2**	**3**	**4**	**5**	**6**	**7**
Willingness to pay for insurance coverage ($)	120.00	100.00	90.00	80.00	70.00	60.00	50.00
Expected loss due to illness ($)	120.00	80.00	70.00	60.00	50.00	40.00	30.00
Age	>50	>50	>50	≤50	≤50	≤50	≤50
Employment group type (N = no group, L = large group, S = small group)	N	L	L	L	L	L	S
Cost of administering insurance in the absence of pool membership ($)	30.00	10.00	10.00	10.00	10.00	10.00	30.00
Model 1 prices (experience rating in the absence of pool membership) ($)	150.00	90.00	80.00	70.00	60.00	50.00	60.00
Model 2 prices (complete information asymmetry, first round) ($)	80.00	80.00	80.00	80.00	80.00	80.00	80.00
Model 3 prices (25% subsidy provided to all individuals, experience rating, and information symmetry) ($)	112.50	67.50	60.00	52.50	45.00	37.50	45.00

because of declining health status due to age. Age is a piece of information that may be used by insurers in setting premium rates.

Also specified in this illustration are the individuals' work circumstances, as these are a prime determinant of the cost of providing health insurance and thus of the loading charge of the insurer. It costs less to provide insurance coverage to individuals in a large group than to individuals who are employed by small companies, who are self-employed, or who are not employed at all. An insurance company will basically incur the same selling cost to a large group in which a large number of insurance policies are sold as it will with a small group in which only a small number of insurance policies are sold. In this example, it is assumed that it costs $10 to supply insurance coverage to individuals in a large group and $30 to individuals in smaller employment groups or to those who must purchase insurance individually.

With regard to the supply side of the market, it is assumed that there is a single supplier of insurance. This supplier knows the risk for each person (a situation referred to as *information symmetry*). The supplier sets a price for each person based strictly on his or her expected loss plus the cost of administration (i.e., the supplier engages in experience rating). Thus, for individual 1, the price will be $150 (the expected loss plus the $30 administrative cost). It is also assumed that the insurer has sufficient capacity to insure all consumers who are willing to shift their risks.

The conclusions of this model regarding the availability of insurance can now be examined. Each individual will purchase insurance as long as the premium rate is less than or equal to what the individual is willing to pay. In this model, individuals 1 and 7 are not willing to pay the premium rates that would be charged by the insurer. Individuals 2–6 will obtain insurance at the given premium rates. For all individuals, the outcome is the result of rational decisions. Further, this outcome is economically efficient, in that the net benefits from insurance coverage are maximized. If any additional insurance coverage was secured, the result (given the assumptions in this illustration) would result in a net social loss.

However, just because the outcome is economically efficient does not mean that it is "fair," "equitable," or even "socially acceptable." All individuals in society (1–7) may agree that this outcome is unacceptable and that some solution must be found to ensure that all individuals have some degree of insurance coverage. The focus now is on a number of these

solutions in subsequent sections of this chapter. However, the focus is first on one of the critical assumptions of this analysis—the assumption of information symmetry. There is considerable literature on what happens when this assumption does not hold. This simple model will be changed to take the assumption of information asymmetry into account.

17.2.3 Information Asymmetry and Adverse Selection

In a state of information asymmetry, one group of individuals (potentially) engaged in a transaction has better information than another group (potentially) engaged in the transaction. Such a situation can lead to market failure, such that a transaction benefiting both parties never actually takes place. To see how market failure might occur, focus on the previous model, except that it is now assumed that information asymmetry exists. In this illustration, the information is about the expected loss of the potential purchasers of health insurance. The assumption made is that the consumers have full information about their risks, but the insurer knows nothing about the health status and risks of individual consumers; it only knows about the risks associated with the entire population.

Given this assumption, the insurer cannot distinguish among the potentially insureds in terms of their health status, and it will therefore have to charge each insured the same premium (a community rating method). In total, expected costs in this illustration are $450, and administrative costs are still the same, $110 for all individuals. Therefore, the insurer must collect $560, or $80 per person, since the insurer has no way of distinguishing among individuals with regard to their risk.

At a price of $80 per person, only individuals 1–4 will purchase insurance, as the price of $80 exceeds the willingness to pay for potential insureds 5–7. If this situation occurs, then the expected loss per person will be determined by the loss experience of the members 1–4 who remain in the market, $390. The market will now insure individuals 1–2 because with the other members dropping out the price will have to increase to $97.50 to cover the $390 of cost of insuring these individuals. Indeed, the entire market can eventually disappear as people successively drop out. It should be noted that, except for individual 1, each individual would be willing to pay for the cost of his or her insurance. However, the insurer has no way of finding out each person's risk, and so it must charge a community or group rate.

17.2.4 Underwriting and Group Rating

The phenomenon of adverse selection occurs in extreme cases of information asymmetry. In fact, insurers or underwriters have numerous ways of distinguishing between high- and low-risk insureds. Insurers know, or can obtain information on, many characteristics associated with the risk of loss, such as age, gender, and employment (Giacomini, Luft, & Robinson, 1995). Insurers can also resort to physical exams and tests to determine if individuals have certain conditions that might lead to costly health care. In addition, insurers have access to the past health records of individuals enrolled with them in the past, and these are often good predictors of future usage. Based on such risk-related information, rates can be set that reflect individual expected costs. Insurers do not have to know exactly how much each person will spend on health care; they must only be able to form separate risk pools and estimate average costs in each pool.

In cases in which there are large groups, insurers need only predict the experience of the entire group. For very large groups, healthcare costs are quite predictable, and therefore information asymmetry does not pose a problem. Indeed, many large employers have realized this and so they self-insure. Of course, this does not solve the problem of those who are not members of large groups.

Nevertheless, these phenomena raise the issue of how relevant adverse selection is. Certainly, if information on projected utilization was not available to insurers, this would be a major problem in the market. But the main problem does not seem to be an absence of information; rather it appears to be what happens when insurers *do* have accurate information about the projected utilization of potential insureds. If the insurer knows about preexisting conditions, then very high rates that consumers cannot afford (i.e., are not willing to pay) can be established. This leads to a situation in which some individuals are selectively excluded from the insurance market. This situation, called "preferred risk selection," will be discussed in subsequent sections.

17.2.5 Subsidies

The absence of insurance coverage can come about in markets with information symmetry or information asymmetry. Attention now focuses on when there is complete information on the part of both groups. In Section 17.2.2, it was concluded (under assumed conditions in the illustration) that two individuals—1 and 7—would not purchase insurance. While this situation was efficient, it was not considered equitable. Consequently, some solution needs to be devised to increase the purchase of insurance by the uninsured individuals.

Assume the market is a mechanism for ensuring that individuals have access to health care when they become ill or injured. Also assume the policy goal of total population insurance coverage is to be achieved. However, because the "unfettered" market excludes some individuals, a solution must be found allowing all individuals to obtain insurance coverage. One such solution, widely used in the United States, is an insurance premium subsidy provided by governments to individuals who purchase health insurance. An example of such a subsidy is the income tax deduction for employer-paid health insurance premiums. Such a deduction reduces the cost of the premium by the individual's personal income tax rate. Some states also provide subsidies directly to smaller employers in order to induce them to purchase health insurance for their employees.

In this illustration, a subsidy of 25% of the premium paid by the individual is introduced so each person pays 25% less than previously. The postsubsidy premium rates for each individual are shown in Table 17-2. Under the initial assumption of experience rating, individual 1 now pays $112.50 (three-quarters of what was paid before), individual 2 pays $67.50, and so on. In this illustration, all individuals will purchase health insurance. The subsidy is successful in achieving full coverage.

However, the postsubsidy situation may not be efficient from a social point of view. If the cost of insuring exceeds the individual's willingness to pay in the absence of the subsidy, the social cost of insurance will exceed the social value. Only now, the cost has been shifted to the taxpayer, and so the true cost of insurance coverage is hidden. A second problem with subsidies is that they may not be successful. Studies of subsidies provided to small employers in New York State indicated that even large subsidies may be insufficient to induce firms to provide the desired increases in health insurance coverage (Thorpe, Hendricks, Garnick, Donelan, & Newhose, 1992). In the New York program, the subsidy was only to last for 2 years, after which time the employers would be required to continue providing insurance and to pay the entire amount to cover their employees. With the greater eventual financial burden, employers were deterred from providing the health insurance coverage.

17.2.6 Cooperative Pools

The provision of insurance is less expensive when it is done in the context of a large group, such as large employers or professional associations. Individual and small-group policies are much more expensive to administer. As a result, the loading charge for individual and small-group policies is greater than it is for large-group policies.

There has been a recent trend toward the formation of cooperatives or insurance-purchasing groups that individuals or smaller employers could join. These are called health insurance purchasing cooperatives (HIPCs). By forming a cooperative, smaller groups can be rated together as a unit and therefore receive the same rate that a larger group with the same risk profile would receive. Purchasing cooperatives have become commonplace, and a number of market reform proposals focus on this trend (Hall, 1994; Reinhardt, 1993).

The Patient Protection and Affordable Care Act (ACA) of 2010 mandated health insurance coverage for most individuals in the United States and it created the health insurance exchanges (or healthcare marketplaces) program in every state to assist individuals fulfill the mandate. A health insurance exchange is a comparison-shopping area for health insurance; it is a platform for purchasing insurance from an insurance company. Under this program, private health insurance companies list their health plans with the exchange, and then individuals can compare plans listed on the exchange. The plans listed on the exchange must be compliant with the ACA requirements in terms of services covered. These exchanges are also the only place people can obtain premium subsidies and cost-sharing subsidies to reduce premiums and out-of-pocket costs for eligible enrollees.

In the exchange, health insurance plans compete for the business of potential enrollees. This direct competition is intended to reduce the cost of health insurance premiums and make it easier for individuals to compare the policies being offered. The exchanges are available to individuals who do not have health insurance through a private insurance plan, Medicare, Medicaid, the Children's Health Insurance Program (CHIP), or another source that provides qualified health insurance coverage.

The Tax Cut and Jobs Act of 2018 repealed the mandated coverage requirement of the ACA as of 2019. As a result of Trump's instruction to the IRS to ignore taxpayers who do not prove they have insurance, healthier individuals have been dropping coverage, leaving insurance companies with a higher proportion of individuals with poorer health. Because of the need to now charge higher premiums to cover these individuals, some plans are withdrawing from the exchanges (Amadeo, 2019a).

In this analysis of the previous illustration, assume that individuals 1 and 7 can join the main group. If they join the group, the administrative cost of providing them with health insurance falls to $10. If the assumption of experience rating by individual risk is retained, then individual 1, at least, would remain uninsured. Individual 1 would still not be willing to pay $130, the necessary premium. However, the cooperative would have increased insurance coverage (by extending coverage to individual 7) through lowering the cost of provision. This would be an efficient solution and would increase equity.

17.2.7 Community Rating and Biased Selection

One feature that has been included in some health insurance reform proposals is a requirement for community rating. To determine the effects of community rating, return to the original model presented (see Section 17.2.2). It is initially assumed that everyone pays the same premium to a single insurer. If the insurer has only to meet its full costs, including its loading fees, and if all individuals are enrolled, then the single community rate would be $80. At this single community rate, individuals 5, 6, and 7 will not purchase the insurance. This may start a spiral that leads to the eventual demise of the entire market.

There is another consideration in community rating. Assume that there are two insurers, A and B, and they are competing for business at the community rate. Another assumption is also changed: assume that the insurers want to maximize their profits. The implications of these changes in the illustration are as follows. In order to maximize profits, each of the two insurers will seek out individuals with a low risk of loss and low administrative expenses. They will avoid providing insurance to other individuals. A number of ways exist enabling the insurers to do this. The insurer can screen applicants and, if provision is not mandatory, refuse to sell insurance to high-risk individuals. Alternatively, they could make it difficult for potentially high-risk individuals to reach them by locating in areas where younger, healthier individuals live (Light, 1992).

The incentive for insurers to select low-risk individuals is powerful, and its relevance needs to be emphasized. A key way for insurers to contain their costs is to make certain that their clients are initially low risk. Numerous health insurance reform proposals have been put forward, and most of them at least try to address this issue. However, under community rating, this issue is especially difficult to address because it relates directly to the profits that the insurers can earn. The ACA has helped in that it forbids the exclusion of individuals based on pre-existing health conditions.

Another issue relating to community rating is that if each individual's premium is fixed, there is no incentive to reduce their risk through health promotion and disease prevention activities. Under experience rating, individuals can be offered incentives (lower premiums) to engage in behaviors that lead to better health (e.g., no smoking). Such incentives do not exist when everyone pays the same premium.

Community rating can now be evaluated on two grounds: equity and efficiency. From one point of view, community rating can appear to be the most equitable rating method since everyone pays the same rate. However, if everyone is not in the same health risk category, then community rating involves the subsidization of the unhealthy by the healthy. Issues of equity may arise if the unhealthy individuals have higher-income than the healthy individuals, then the lower-income healthy individuals will be subsidizing the higher-income individuals. Typically, the goal of many public policies try to achieve greater equity across populations by transferring resources from higher-income individuals to lower-income individuals. If equity is assumed to be based on the premise that equals should pay equally and unequals should pay unequally, then community rating may not be an equitable method. Alternatively, if all individuals are viewed as "equals" (in the sense that, no matter how healthy or unhealthy, they are all human beings), then community rating will appear equitable.

On efficiency grounds, little can be found in favor of community rating. Community rating discourages health promotion activities when the social costs warrant them. Cost savings from such activities are not passed on to the individuals who engage in them. In addition, community rating encourages insurers to seek out the lowest risk individuals, and this can cause individuals who would otherwise buy insurance to be unable to purchase it, which eventually could lead to a demise of the health insurance market. In response to these problems, two additional innovations have been introduced. One is a mandate requiring individuals or employers to obtain insurance. The second is risk rating—the assignment of individuals to groups according to their risks, and the requirement that they pay different premiums based on these risks.

17.2.8 Mandates

A mandate is a legal requirement that some action be taken, such as the purchasing of health insurance coverage. One purpose of a mandate to purchase insurance is to block individuals from leaving the health insurance market. It is maintained that some individuals (primarily low-risk individuals) will not insure until the risk of using services increases. Only then do they insure and "take advantage" of their coverage. When low-risk individuals do not participate in the market, this causes higher group premiums and could even result in the eventual disappearance of the market. Under a mandate, everyone must purchase insurance.

The Patient Protection and Affordable Care Act, more commonly known as the Affordable Care Act (ACA), passed in 2010, contained mandatory coverage provisions (Cogan, 2011). To provide coverage for most Americans meant the population must participate to avoid substantial increases in premiums. The ACA contained a number of provisions designed to transform the health insurance market in the United States, and to expand insurance coverage to about 95% of the population.

Under the ACA, discriminatory practices that exclude individuals from coverage because of pre-existing conditions were eliminated. Also, lifetime and unreasonable annual limits on benefits were eliminated, and policies were prohibited from being rescinded because of health status. In addition, policies were required to develop uniform coverage documents, so comparisons could be easily made. Insurance companies were prohibited from setting rates or denying coverage based on health status, medical condition, claims experience, genetic information, or other health-related factors.

Under the ACA, most individuals would be required to maintain insurance for minimum essential coverage or pay a penalty, with individuals under 18 paying half the established premium. Certain limited exceptions to the mandate were allowed. Employers with more than 200 employees were required to automatically enroll new full-time employees, and any employer with more than 50 employees not offering coverage must pay a penalty for each employee, if at least one full-time employee receives the premium assistance tax credit under the health insurance exchange program. If the employer of more than 50 employees offers a plan deemed unaffordable or that does not meet the standard for minimum essential coverage and has at least one employee receiving the premium tax credit under the health insurance exchange program, then the employer pays a penalty per employee (Hardcastle, Record, Jacobson, & Goston, 2011).

Starting with our original illustration, a community rating is assumed and a mandate that all individuals purchase insurance. The premium rate will be $80, and all individuals are mandated to pay this rate.

Such a premium rate might impose a considerable burden on low-income individuals, and so few proposals stop at a mandate. One way to reduce the burden is to provide a subsidy for individuals who are designated as low income. The combined reforms would ensure that all individuals were insured and could afford insurance because those who could not otherwise afford it would be subsidized.

The Affordable Care Act stipulates that insurance premiums will vary only because of family structure, geography, actuarial value, tobacco use, participation in health promotion programs, and age. To ensure the mandatory insurance coverage is affordable, out-of-pocket costs are limited. Coverage is offered at four levels, with actuarial values defining how much the insurer pays, ranging from 90% to 60%. A low-benefit catastrophic plan is available to individuals under 30. States must establish a Health Insurance Exchange to assist individuals and small employers obtain coverage. The ACA establishes new, refundable, sliding-scale tax credits for Americans with incomes between 100% and 400% of the federal poverty level. In addition, a new tax credit is available for employers with fewer than 25 workers for up to 50% of the total premium cost. The ACA allows the expansion of Medicaid and the Children's Health Insurance Plan (CHIP) eligibility to low-income individuals and families. Not all states participate in Medicaid expansion and the mandate has been effectively removed under the Trump Administration.

One objection to a mandate is that it imposes a welfare loss on some individuals. For example, individuals 5, 6, and 7 are not willing to pay $80 for health insurance coverage. Under a mandate, they would have to pay and suffer an added burden in order for higher risk and/or lower-income individuals to be able to obtain insurance (Hall, 1994). In addition, the mandate does not eliminate the powerful incentive insurance companies have to "cherry pick," or engage in other competitive practices that enable them to select low-risk individuals. Other elements of health insurance reform occur to curb these practices. The most prominent of these options is risk adjustment.

17.2.9 Risk Selection Limitation and Risk Adjustment

Some government policies directly limit insurers' ability to select individual risks. Because past or current health may be a good predictor of future health, a decision to accept a person for coverage, or renew a policy, may involve examination of the applicant's current health or past claim experience. The existence of a chronic health condition, or large past expenses, could be the basis for denying coverage. In such cases, decisions to deny coverage have generated significant media and political attention because they can be seen as refusing coverage to people who need it most. In 1996, federal legislation directly addressed this issue by requiring companies to sell insurance policies to groups willing to purchase them and guaranteeing individuals or groups the right to renew policies. This legislation did not however address the premiums that could be charged for such policies. The ACA further addressed the issue of preexisting conditions, but only addressed premiums indirectly.

Risk adjustment is a technique used to modify payments made to prepaid plans on the basis of characteristics of the entire group. The rationale behind this technique is that certain subgroups are more costly to treat (because they use more services) and that health plans should be appropriately compensated for accepting these subgroups as members. Among the variables that have been used in risk-adjustment formulas are age, gender, self-reported health status, and prior period healthcare use (Frank & Welch, 1985).

A problem with risk adjustment is that identification of a variable related to healthcare utilization could enable the health plan to profit by selecting low-risk individuals. For example, if body weight was associated with utilization, then a health plan could select members, at least partly, on the basis of their body weight. Assuming it was successful, it would benefit from having lower costs. A number of risk factors not included in the risk-adjustment techniques commonly used provides opportunities for health plans to invest in techniques that will identify potentially heavy healthcare users and avoid them. Such actions could reduce the effectiveness of market reforms.

17.3 Managed Care

17.3.1 Introduction

Managed care is a system of healthcare insurance and delivery by which the payer attempts to exert direct influence over the economic behavior of the suppliers.

Managed care focuses on efforts to coordinate, rationalize, and channel utilization to achieve desired outcomes and costs. Growth of managed care has been a central aspect of healthcare reform in the United States. In the 1970s, federal legislation endorsed and encouraged the growth of health maintenance organizations (HMOs).

Rapid growth of HMO membership occurred during the 1980s, along with the development of other types of managed care organizations and the adoption by traditional insurers of some of the techniques of cost control that had been introduced by HMOs. By the 1990s, managed care was a major part of the healthcare delivery system, as well as an important segment of financial markets. A "backlash" developed as state and federal governments became aware of growing concerns about quality of care and the restriction on consumer choice in the managed care context. Part of the awareness by state and federal governments was the result of providers becoming unhappy with the requirements of the managed care organizations and so lobbied legislatures to intervene in their behalf.

Integration of the insurance function with the healthcare delivery function in one organization changes incentives for use of resources. Under traditional insurance and fee-for-service medical practice, the providers have little reason to be concerned with the cost consequences of their treatment decisions, because the payers bear all the risks of the providers' actions. On the other hand, a managed care organization receives prepayment for members' health care. Because the plan's surplus (profit) is the difference between the prepaid amount and the amount spent on health care, it has a clear incentive to provide care as inexpensively as possible. The acceptance of a predefined financial payment for a set of defined benefits for its members places the managed care organization at financial risk. Managed care was initially seen as a possible means of enhancing two types of economic efficiency.

Improvements in *productive efficiency* could result from using different combinations of inputs to produce a given output level (e.g., the substitution of nonphysician providers of care for physicians and the substitution of outpatient treatment for hospitalization). Greater *allocative efficiency* could result from more careful weighing of the marginal health benefits against the marginal costs of particular treatments. Further, competition among HMOs, and between HMOs and traditional insurers, had the potential of reducing healthcare costs through price competition. It was also anticipated that HMOs would shift the emphasis from short-term acute care for illness to prevention and long-term health maintenance. The next section reviews some of the economic issues associated with the development of managed care.

17.3.2 Types of Managed Care Organizations

All managed care organizations (MCOs) employ some form of prepayment and some degree of integration of financial risk bearing with healthcare delivery. All MCOs contract to provide fairly comprehensive health services to members in exchange for an annual premium and often small copayments. However, they differ importantly in their relationships with the healthcare providers and in the arrangements for dispensing care. In terms of ability to control provider decision making, the "tightest" type of plan is the staff-model HMO, in which physicians are employees of the HMO.

A group-model HMO is similar, except that the health plan and the physician group are separate legal entities. Usually, HMO members make up all or a great majority of the physician group's practice, and the plan and the physician group are in fact managed jointly in many respects. Members of a staff-model or group-model HMO receive care at one of the HMO's medical office locations, which typically have a number of primary care providers and often some specialty care providers under one roof.

An independent practice association (IPA) type of HMO provides a contrast in several respects. In an IPA, the physicians practice in their own offices as solo practitioners or small groups. The health plan contracts with the physicians to provide care for HMO members. Members of the HMO typically would account for only a small proportion of any physician's practice. Indeed, the physician might well be a provider for several different HMOs. Compared with a staff- or group-model HMO, an IPA usually offers members a larger number of providers and a larger number of office locations among which to choose.

A preferred provider organization (PPO) is an arrangement whereby the insurer designates a selected list of providers, including physicians and hospitals. If a patient seeks care from a provider on the list, the insurance coverage will be extensive, with a small or zero copayment. However, a patient may choose to seek treatment from providers not on the list. In that case, there will still be some insurance coverage, but the patient will bear a larger share of the cost.

As the industry evolves, there have emerged various mixed models. The term *network model* is often applied to these. For example, an HMO might offer care through its own health centers and also from a list of physicians in the community. Increasingly popular in HMO contracts is a point-of-service (POS) provision. This provision enables the HMO member to seek care from providers other than the HMO providers but at greater cost. Membership in HMOs and PPOs is presented in **Figure 17-2**.

Medicare has recently introduced a number of programs that have incorporated various features of managed care. The Medicare Advantage Plans (Part C) incorporate many of the features of PPOs. While beneficiaries are able to select the providers of their choice and to see specialists without a specific referral, their copayments, coinsurance, and deductibles are lower when in-plan providers are used.

The patient-centered medical home (PCMH) program is a model of primary care that is patient-centered, comprehensive, team-based, integrated and coordinated, accessible, and focused on quality and safety. The patient-centered medical home model is based on the fundamental tenets of primary care: (1) first direct access, comprehensiveness, coordination, and relationships involving standard partnerships; (2) new ways of organizing practices: (3) development of practices' internal capabilities; and (4) related healthcare systems and reimbursement changes. The focus is on increasing the value of health care. It has been shown that systems with a focus on primary care have better quality, lower cost, less inequality in healthcare and health, and better population health when compared with systems based on other approaches to health care (Stang et al., 2010).

Medicare makes upfront quarterly payments to medical homes for their beneficiaries based on expected costs of primary care services. Medicare also pays an average care management fee per beneficiary per month. The program may risk adjust care management fees based on patient health status. If medical homes meet specified requirements, they may share in savings with Medicare. These specified requirements include patient experience, clinical quality, and expenditures. Medical homes may share in losses with Medicare if they exceed specified spending targets. Medicare also pays medical homes flat bonuses per beneficiary per month. These payments are recouped if quality and spending targets are not met. Beginning in 2019, physicians affiliated with medical homes are eligible for automatic 5% bonuses when quality and spending targets are met (KFF, 2018).

In Medicare's bundled payment models, a total budget for all services provided to a beneficiary during a given episode of care is established. If the spending on services during that episode of care is less than the budget, the provider shares in Medicare savings. If the provider's costs exceed the budget, then the provider incurs a loss. In many of the models, the episode of care covered is triggered by hospitalization. The bundled payment includes inpatient hospital stays, postacute care, and physician and other related services up to a predefined number of clinical episodes.

17.3.3 Control of Resource Use

While the overall incentive for a managed care organization is to minimize costs, the specific ways to accomplish this make a large difference in the public and political acceptance of this type of organization. Proponents of managed care point to the elimination of unnecessary or low marginal benefit care, the selection of more cost-effective treatment approaches, the encouragement of

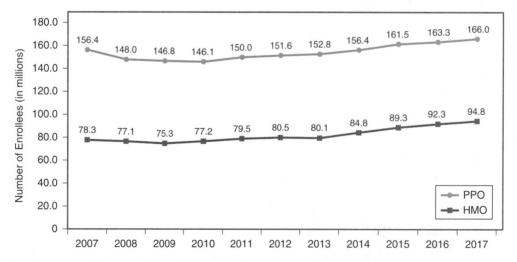

Figure 17-2 Enrollment in HMOs and PPOs, 2007–2017. Note the decline in enrollment in HMOs between 2007 and 2009 and PPOs between 2007 and 2010 with steady increases between 2013 and 2017 in both.

Sanofi-Aventis. (2018). *Managed care digest series, payer digest, 2018.* Bridgewater, NJ: Sanofi-Company.

wellness, and increased access to care through elimination of financial barriers. Critics note the lack of choice of provider and fear that the cost incentives can lead to lower quality care through the elimination or restriction of necessary treatments (Berchtold, Kunzi, & Busato, 2011). A position in this controversy is not presented here, but rather some of the factors used in the managed care environment are described.

Incentives provided to both physicians and patients are relevant. The initial decision to seek care is a patient decision. Specific treatment choices require both physician recommendation and patient consent. Decisions with major resource-use implications, such as hospitalization or surgery, are complex, and the physician is still a major decision maker, although patients are becoming more informed and more involved in the decisions made (Deom, Agoritsas, Bovier, & Perneger, 2010).

The method of physician compensation plays an important role and is best viewed in an agency context. Under fee-for-service compensation, the physician earns more by using more services and seeing more patients. This type of compensation can lead to supplier-induced demand and treatments of low marginal benefit. While some managed care organizations (typically IPAs or PPOs) use fee-for-service payment, alternative forms of compensation are common.

One payment method is to provide a straight salary to providers. Under salary compensation, a physician's income is not affected by treatment choices made. Capitation is another payment method. Under capitation, a physician receives a certain sum per assigned patient, irrespective of what services are provided to the patient. A more extreme form of capitation would pay a primary care physician (PCP) a certain sum per patient and the PCP would then be financially responsible for all care the patient received during the time period, including specialty or hospital care. This provides a very strong incentive to limit the care provided and puts the physician at great financial risk if a patient should need treatment for catastrophic illness. The risk is somewhat mitigated if the capitation payment goes to a physician group rather than individual providers, and capitation of this type is often used to pay the physician group in a group-model HMO. Individual providers in the group could then be compensated by salary, fees for service, or some other method. The patient-centered medical home described earlier focuses on the use of primary care providers to manage the health of a population.

Different combinations of compensation schemes are also in use. For example, physicians in an HMO might be paid fees in return for services but have a certain portion of the fees held back by the HMO until the end of the financial year, at which time an amount would be returned to the physician based on the HMO's surplus; or salary payment could be supplemented by a year-end bonus related to the HMO's financial results. As discussed earlier, Medicare's bundled payment program incorporates a number of these features.

Under a typical traditional insurance plan, copayments, coinsurance, and deductibles, to some extent, deter utilization of services. For some types of services (e.g., preventive services), coverage may not be included at all, and patients would have to pay the full cost. Under the ACA, the reverse is true with certain preventive services provided free of charge. Managed care tends to rely less on financial incentives to limit utilization and more on administrative arrangements, especially for influencing the use of specialized referral services. In contrast to traditional insurance, in which a patient can self-refer to a specialist, many managed care plans will have the primary care provider play a "gatekeeper" role. That is, a referral to a specialist must be authorized by the member's primary care provider in order for the expense to be covered by the managed care plan. The referral may be limited to a small number of visits to the specialist, after which time the patient care responsibility is returned to the primary care provider. Concurrent utilization review for hospitalized patients is another example of a managed care strategy that has the potential to influence utilization more than the relatively laissez-faire role of the traditional insurer, although most traditional insurers have adopted many of the utilization controls introduced by managed care.

As discussed, it is difficult to generalize about the effects of managed care. Some of the early findings on resource savings attributable to managed care have not held up in the later work. It is also apparent that the worst fears of managed care critics about quality effects are not borne out by research findings. Not all of the possible economic effects of managed care can be captured by the type of study that compares individual managed care organizations to traditional insurance plans, however. The presence of managed care in a market may affect the economic behavior of other market participants and change the nature of competition.

17.3.4 Evaluating Managed Care

When attempting to evaluate the efficiency and effectiveness of managed care compared to traditionally insured populations, a number of key features must be considered. One of the first issues is that of selection bias by the managed care organization: are the members of the managed care organization different from the population with traditional insurance in terms of health status. If the managed care population is healthier, then this status needs to be incorporated into the evaluation of the efficiency, effectiveness, and costs of managed care (Kolbasorsky, 2011).

Another issue involves the quality of care provided to the two groups. A concern has been expressed that the financial incentives in managed care might lead to a deterioration in quality in order to maximize profits. A counterargument is that the removal of financial barriers to early treatment and emphasis on wellness could lead to higher quality of care in managed care. In efforts to evaluate quality, it is important to incorporate risk adjustments associated with population into the analysis.

When attempting to evaluate access to care between the managed care population and the traditional insurance population, a difficulty arises in defining an appropriate level of access. Concerns have been expressed that the incentives under traditional insurance encourages overutilization of health care both from the providers' incentives of fee-for-service and the incentives created by low out-of-pocket cost to consumers. There has also been concern expressed about the financial incentives created under managed care to underutilize health care because of barriers in place to limit access to providers—location of providers, hours of operation, etc. These features need to also be incorporated into comparative evaluations in order to obtain valid results.

17.3.5 Managed Care in the Market

The entry of new participants into a market can change the structure of the market and the nature of buyer–seller interactions in it. The specific nature of the change will depend of course on what the market structure and conduct were like before the entry of the new participants. Managed care represents vertical integration of insurance with service delivery and thus has possible effects on two types of market, the market for health insurance and the market for medical care.

In the early years of managed care growth (the 1970s and 1980s), the major issue and subject of research was the effect of managed care market entry on traditional insurers. In a simple theoretical model, entry of new sellers to the insurance market would be expected to shift the supply curve outward and to the right and result in lower prices. If preentry market power was held by the established firms, price competition would be expected to drive prices down. If the entrants had lower costs than established firms, further downward pressure on price would occur, as established firms imitated lower-cost technology and the competition forced prices to reflect the marginal costs of production.

In markets with the possibility of nonprice competition, such as markets able to employ product differentiate, the rivalry among firms may not take the form of price competition, in which case lower costs and prices would not result (McLaughlin, 1988). The new entrant into the market may price its products somewhat below the established firms and not fully exploit its cost advantage to lower prices further. In the case of managed care entry into the market, a more comprehensive benefits package and lower cost-sharing were offered. As a consequence, considerable pressure is placed on established health insurers to adopt organizational and product innovations, such as expanded benefits packages and utilization review techniques to control costs (Frank & Welch, 1985).

In terms of the medical care market, managed care enters as a buyer of services, including hospital and physician services. If the buyer side of these markets was initially competitive (i.e., there were many small buyers), the entry of managed care as a large buyer would introduce monopsony power into the market. Here, theory predicts a downward pressure on price as well as a lower quantity of output. The effects of managed care on hospital costs might occur for two reasons. First, managed care organizations might simply decrease the use of hospital care, substituting outpatient for inpatient care or reducing lengths of stay through administrative techniques, such as utilization review. Second, managed care organizations might engage in selective contracting (i.e., directing patients to less expensive and more efficient hospitals).

One methodology to examine the impact of managed care on hospitals is to examine the relationship between managed care penetration in a market and the rate of hospital cost inflation. As managed care gains market share, what happens to hospital costs? Another type of medical care market in which changes might result from the increased presence of managed care is the market for specialized, expensive, high-technology services. Do the incentives and controls in managed care decrease the demand for such services (Hill & Wolfe, 1997)? Does an increase in managed care enrollment create pressure for hospitals to cooperate more in the acquisition of expensive technologies rather than underutilize the technologies if all hospitals acquire it? One possible effect on market structure results from the pressures of selective contracting by managed care organizations. If managed care organizations search for the low-cost providers and channel business to them, there is a powerful incentive for other providers to seek out and realize economies of scale.

17.4 Information and Consumer Choice

In a well-functioning competitive market, the principle of "consumer sovereignty" prevails (i.e., the products to be produced are determined by consumer preferences, and appropriate incentives are in place for economic efficiency to be achieved). This market result, however, depends on consumers having adequate information about prices and product characteristics to be able to choose appropriately among alternatives (Vranceanu & Ring, 2011). If market-oriented reforms in health care, particularly managed care, are to be effective, potential buyers must be able to assess the characteristics of managed care products. During the period when managed care was experiencing rapid growth, the technology used for developing and disseminating statistical information also advanced greatly. The combination of these changes resulted in a number of initiatives designed to make information about healthcare organizations more available to consumers, with the goal of improving their decision making and at the same time improving market outcomes. This section reviews some of those developments and the issues they raise.

The characteristic of healthcare organization performance that is perhaps most difficult for consumers to understand is quality, so not surprisingly, that characteristic has received the most attention. A number of reporting or rating systems have been introduced that attempt to define quality in a measurable way, develop statistical information about the quality of specific healthcare organizations, and disseminate that information widely to consumers and employers, often in the form of "report cards." Some of these efforts have been by government agencies, while others have taken place in the private sector. Ratings or reports have been developed for such healthcare providers as hospitals or individual physicians, as well as for managed care organizations.

One of the earliest attempts to report widely on hospital performance was the dissemination by the Health Care Financing Administration (HCFA), beginning in 1986, of hospital mortality rates for all hospitals in the United States. These annual reports provided for each hospital the actual mortality rate of Medicare patients, as well as that predicted statistically based on characteristics of the admitted patients. Frequently, the performance of a particular hospital was the subject of local media attention if it appeared to have an unusually low or high mortality rate compared with other hospitals. The reporting program gave rise to a great deal of controversy and was ended in 1992. Several aspects of the controversy are of continuing interest because they apply to other similar programs.

First, critics questioned whether the statistical methodology used was adequate to adjust for severity of illness. Certainly, hospitals with sicker patients would be expected to have more deaths, so a higher mortality rate in such hospitals would not be indicative of a quality difference but rather a case-mix difference. Indeed, it may be that higher quality hospitals attract the sickest and most difficult to treat patients and have higher mortality rates for that reason.

Second, there is a question as to whether it makes sense to consider the hospital's patient population as a whole or whether the analysis should be conducted for individual patient groups. For example, a hospital may be very successful at treating cardiac surgery patients but have less than average success treating cancer patients. An overall assessment would miss these important details.

Third, administrative data may not capture clinical information accurately. There may be data errors that occur in the transition from a patient chart to a hospital information system. Moreover, administrative datasets, developed mostly for financial or operational purposes, may not reflect fully the clinical complexity of a patient's illness and treatment. Finally, of course, there is the question of whether the information provided actually influences the choices of consumers and healthcare providers.

Although much effort has gone into developing systems for analyzing health plan performance, creating statistical reports on performance, and disseminating these reports, the actual effect of these activities is, as yet, unclear. From an economic standpoint, the important question is whether actual market decisions are made using such information. It is important to recall here that the health plan enrollment decision is mainly a two-stage process: first, the employer decides to offer particular plans to its employees as choices, and second, each employee chooses a particular plan from among those in the benefits package.

It is reasonable to think that an employer's decision to include a plan in the benefits package would be influenced by performance data, at least in the case of a large employer with sophisticated benefits administrators who have the time and expertise to evaluate the data. Whether smaller employers and individual consumers have the ability and incentive to use such information is less evident. Furthermore, it is hard to know whether the variables chosen by "experts" as measures of plan performance are really what individual consumers care about.

17.5 Consumer-Focused Health Care

17.5.1 Patient-Centered Medical Homes

The United States continues to explore and experiment with strategies and designs to transform the functioning of the healthcare system to improve outcomes and control costs. There is increasing recognition of the role that consumers can play in improving the healthcare system. Not only is the system recognizing the consumers' role in improving or maintaining their own health, but also the important role consumers play in the health of the population of the community. In recognition of the need to focus on consumers, experimentation with the patient-centered medical home (PCMH) model was undertaken.

The term *medical home* was coined by the Academy of Pediatrics in 1967 and has since evolved into the concept of patient-centered medical home. PCMH is a supply-side market intervention method to enable clinicians to provide care of a higher quality in a more efficient manner. Conceptually, it promotes better relationships between patients and providers, resulting in better access, increased quality, and improved consistency in care. PCMH focuses on and rewards ongoing patient–physician relationships and high-quality coordinated care. PCMHs require healthcare providers to reorganize practices into more effective systems in order to deliver high-quality efficient care.

Patient-centered medical homes are designed to offer care that is consistent with the needs and expectations of patients. The provision of needed care is enabled by technology and delivery systems that coordinate care safely. A key component of PCMHs is a payment system aligned to compensate providers for the infrastructure and time costs necessary for the coordination and delivery of patient-centered care. In addition to the reorganization of care delivered, PCMHs also focus on self-management strategies for the patient (Bertakis & Azari, 2011). These

last strategies are designed to decrease reliance on the healthcare system and increase patient responsibility for their own health outcomes.

The Centers for Medicare and Medicaid Services (CMS) sponsored demonstration projects to create and implement medical homes to provide continuous and coordinated family-centered medical care. The focus on family-centered rather than just patient-centered care recognized the important role families have in improving health outcomes. The focus of the medical home is on coordinated and integrated health care that is managed by primary care physicians. The integrated care is expected to increase preventive care, to enhance patient adherence to a treatment plan, and to avoid unnecessary hospitalizations, office visits, tests, and procedures. PCMHs are also expected to increase the use of less expensive technologies and biologicals when appropriate and reduce the risks to patients that are inherent in a fragmented system that results in inconsistent treatment decisions.

CMS has identified six domains of medical services that must be present in a medical home. These are continuity of care; clinical information systems; delivery system design to promote access and communication; decision support; patient/family engagement; and coordination. Criteria are established for each of these domains, and the performance of the practice is measured against these criteria. Providers receive additional funding per member per month to participate; and for aggregate savings to Medicare, the providers receive a share of the savings.

As PCMHs evolve and expand, the focus on comprehensive care provided by a team of providers increases. The team approach relies heavily on the easy flow of information, reducing redundancy of tests and information, and improving coordinated decision making. As the concept evolves, increased recognition of the role of the patient and family as team members has occurred. The information exchanged among *all* team members is critical to the success of the PCMH.

For PCMHs to achieve their potential, the payment system will need to be restructured to incorporate appropriate incentives and rewards. The current fee-for-service system rewards providers for delivering more curative services and pays little or nothing for preventive care. In general, physicians receive payment for services delivered, even if the services provided omit some or many of the clinical practice guidelines. Fragmentation is rewarded in the current system because multiple providers are paid for multiple tests on the same patient.

Providers are not rewarded for efforts to manage the health of the patient between visits in the current system, only for services delivered during the visit. In addition, in the current system, patients do not have financial incentives to adhere to preventive or disease-management recommendations, and insurers lack mechanisms for directing patients to higher value providers. The payment system developed for PCMHs must incorporate features to address the shortcomings of the current payment system if they are to achieve their goals of increased efficiency, better outcomes, and controlled costs (Butcher, 2011).

Medicare and the private system have recognized that one model is not appropriate for all areas and so a number of different models have evolved incorporating key design features. Included in the redesign has been upfront payments for the costs of infrastructure changes needed to adapt to the new requirements. When appropriate, providers are asked to assume more financial risk in return for potentially greater financial benefits from savings achieved. The medical homes are also recognizing the valuable contributions patients and families can make, and so are including them on committees, boards, and other decision-making teams. As the PCMH evolves, blended payments and other reimbursement strategies are being tested to redistribute resources to the primary care functions that provide the greatest value.

17.5.2 Accountable Care Organizations

Another concept that is being used to improve quality and slow the growth in healthcare costs is Accountable Care Organizations (ACOs). The ACO concept involves considerable flexibility in how ACOs can be organized, which will enable them to develop more quickly and require fewer resources. Also, ACOs are paid on a shared-savings basis, which reflects a percentage of the difference between a benchmark or target established by the Secretary of Health and Human Services and the costs to Medicare for services provided to ACO-assigned beneficiaries. The ACO faces less financial risk than under a fixed-amount capitation system, which pays the same amount per member regardless of the amount of services actually used. Under the ACO model, the standard Medicare payment level for beneficiaries using services is generally guaranteed, although the ACO can suffer a loss if expenditures for beneficiaries are too high.

In general, an ACO is defined as a local organization with a related set of providers (at least primary care physicians, specialists, and hospitals) that can be held accountable for costs and quality of care delivered to a defined population. The defined population can be either a subset of Medicare beneficiaries or subscribers in health insurance plans. The organization must be able to provide services and manage patients across a continuum of care, have sufficient financial resources to assume risk, and have sufficient volume to support comprehensive, valid, and reliable performance measurement. Diverse types of organizations can serve as an ACO, as long as they can meet the required criteria of accountability for health, quality, and costs of care over the full continuum of patient care.

The ACO model builds upon earlier models, especially those of the patient-centered medical home and bundled payment for a discrete episode of care. The ACO model goes further than the previous models by aligning payments, benefits, and other healthcare policies with measurable, meaningful progress in improving care while controlling cost increases.

As highlighted by the work of the Accountable Care Organization Learning Network (www.acolearningnetwork.org), the foundation of an ACO is clear, patient-focused aims of better overall health through higher quality and lower costs for patients; provider accountability through performance measures that are transparent; and payment reform that uses the measures to align and provide organizations that are focused on these aims directly and meaningfully. As health information technology, performance measurement, and effective medical practices continue to advance, the ability of organizations to meet the aims of ACOs is improved.

A basic feature of the ACO model is the establishment of a spending benchmark that is based on expected expenditures on the defined population. The benchmark established takes into consideration the health status and characteristics of the defined population. If the ACO can achieve the quality targets while slowing the growth in healthcare costs, then the ACO receives a portion (a share) of the savings from the payer. Medicare initially set the organization's share of the savings at 80%; that percentage now varies by payer. If preventive care, coordinated services, patient-centered care, and other quality-improvement strategies achieve better outcomes and lower resource use, then providers will receive bonuses to replace some of the upfront losses they may experience when restructuring to conform to the ACO model. Such payment reform should increase the sustainability of such services, as the financial incentives are aligned with the desired aims of the system. Another feature of the ACO model is that it reduces or eliminates incentives to expand service capacity that will be underutilized by its members.

ACOs have a number of key design features, regardless of their organizational structure. These features are (1) local accountability, (2) a legal structure with a governing board, (3) a focus on primary care, (4) adequate patient population size, (5) appropriate investments in improvements in the delivery system, (6) realistic and achievable opportunities for providers to realize shared savings, and (7) transparent and accessible performance measurements. These features are key to the success of the ACO model and will grow and become more sophisticated as experience and technical progress occur.

A major difference in the ACO model and previous efforts is that it combines care delivery and payment reform. However, change and results cannot be expected to occur overnight. It will take time and experimentation to identify and develop best practices, to redesign workflows in practice settings in order to assemble high-functioning teams, to improve performance measures, and to establish appropriate spending benchmarks. The initial expectations and values established should not be viewed as absolutes or permanent but as temporary benchmarks as the system evolves and more and better information becomes available.

Another key feature of the ACO model is the recognition of the need for local accountability in the system. Instead of establishing a national standard, it recognizes differences in populations in various locations and the diversity of practice types and organizational settings in the healthcare system. To be successful, the model must allow for variation in strategies undertaken to improve care and control costs, but it must establish boundaries to avoid claims of "uniqueness," which are designed to allow providers to continue to function and perform under current conditions. The focus must be on promoting value, not just on volume and intensity of services. The care must be coordinated across providers and settings to minimize duplication and excessive use. Many of these features are being incorporated into the changes occurring in the advanced ACO models and payment systems.

Currently, ACOs are providing care for over one-third of Medicare fee-for-service beneficiaries. A study by McWilliams, Hatfield, Landon, Hamed, and Chernew (2018) found that the first program year was associated with a mean reduction of $302 (3.1%) in total Medicare spending per beneficiary. The amount varied by type of ACO, with physician group ACOs achieving an average of $474 per beneficiary compared to $169 for hospital-integrated ACOs. Inclusive of bonus payments made for savings, the net saving to Medicare was $256.4 million

As the ACO model has evolved, Medicare has implemented the Pathways to Success program that requires ACOs to assume additional risk after 2 years of program participation. Presently, most ACOs participate in savings achieved but are not responsible for the risk for losses that occur. The new program will require ACOs to also accept the risk for losses that occur if the ACO does not meet the established target. As the ACO models and other financial payment systems and care delivery systems change and evolve, providers will continue to be asked to demonstrate the value of the services they perform.

The healthcare system is continuing to evolve, and the value-based payment models will continue to be a focus of that evolution. Bundled payments (or episode-based payments) will continue to expand as focus continues on the integration and coordination of healthcare services. For bundled payments to be successful, it is critical that clinically defined episodes of care can be defined and measured, since providers are paid on the basis of the expected costs of these episodes. Under a bundled payment system, a provider is paid the same for each episode of care in that category that is performed. If the costs are above that amount for an episode the provider suffers a loss. This use of an average payment for an episode recognizes that some episodes will be more expensive than others, but over time the differences should even out.

The amount of the bundled payment is established on what is expected to be required to provide all the care needed for that episode. Under this system, a provider will be underpaid if the patient is more severe than is considered in the pricing of the episode, and will be overpaid if the patient is less severe than is considered in the pricing of the episode. And so, in establishing the episode of care, it is important to incorporate various levels of severity in the pricing rate. Using appropriately established episode of care in the price structure should promote efficient care as revenue of the provider increases with the reduction in costs. To be effective however, the services included in the bundle of care needs to be clearly and appropriately defined, which is not an easy task in today's complex healthcare delivery system (Axene, 2019).

The current payment system is very complicated for the provider. For example, a single provider may have patients that are paid under a fee-for-service system, other patients that are paid under capitation, other patients paid under a bundled payment system, and yet other patients that are paid under a shared savings plan. These various payment methods increase the complexity and complications associated with management of the practice.

As payment methods continue to evolve, more focus is being placed on two-sided financial models in which providers not only share in the savings achieved but are also placed at risk for costs that exceed the expected amounts. These payment mechanisms focus on getting providers to make more efficient choices in the services they provide to their patients and to keep them healthy. They also put pressure on providers to educate their patients on ways to take care of themselves and not rely on the healthcare system for everything.

Finally, the healthcare system must include greater transparency for consumers. For consumers to make truly informed choices in their demand for healthcare services, they must have clear, reliable, valid, and understandable information on the overall quality, cost, and other performance aspects of providers within the system, and the system in general. Consumers need to have confidence in their providers and in the system that the most appropriate care is being provided and that they have the ability to determine the value of care available (Manahan, 2011).

Exercises

1. Explain the relationship between information asymmetry and health insurance market failure.
2. Explain why individual or small-group insurance tends to be more expensive than large-group insurance.
3. Explain the relationship between community rating and economic efficiency.
4. Contrast the incentives for resource use faced by a physician under a salary, under fee-for-service compensation, and under capitation.
5. Explain the problem presented by selection bias for research on the effects of managed care.
6. Describe the types of effects that the entry of managed care organizations into a market can have on other types of insurance providers.
7. Describe the potential effects that may be achieved by Accountable Care Organizations (ACOs) and Patient-Centered Medical Homes (PCMHs).
8. Explain how bundled (episode-based) payments impact the incentives to providers.

Bibliography

Accountable Care Organization Learning Network. (2011). *ACO toolkit*. Washington, DC: Engelberg Center for Health Care Reform, The Dartmouth Institute.

Amadeo, K. (2019a, April 16). 10 Obamacare pros and cons. *The Balance*. Retrieved from www.thebalance.com/10-obamacare-pros-and-cons/3306059

Amadeo, K. (2019b, May 30). Benefits of Obamacare. *The Balance*. Retrieved from www.thebalance.com/advantages-of-the-affordable-care-act/3306066

Amadeo, K. (2019c, June 25). What is wrong with Obamacare. *The Balance*. Retrieved from www.thebalance.com/what-is-wrong-with-obamacare/3306076

Axene, J. (2019, July 1). Paying healthcare providers: The impact of provider reimbursement on overall cost of care and treatment decisions. *Inspire*. Axene Health Partners. Retrieved from https://axenehp.com/paying-healthcare-providers-impact-provider-reimbursement-overall-cost-care-treatment-decisions/

Berchtold, P., Kunzi, B., & Busato, A. (2011). Differences of the quality of care experience: The perception of patients with either network or conventional health plans. *Family Practice*, 28(4), 406–413.

Berkowitz, S. A., & Miller, E. D. (2011). The individual mandate and patient-centered care. *JAMA, 306*(6), 648–649.

Bertakis, K. D., & Azari, R. (2011). Determinants and outcomes of patient-centered care. *Patient Education & Counseling, 85*, 46–52.

Butcher, L. (2011). Medical homes prepare the way for accountable care organizations. *Managed Care, 20*(10), 67–69.

Carecloud. (2019). Top 20 healthcare technology advances in 2018. *Continuum*. Retrieved from www.carecloud.com/continuum/top-20-healthcare-technology-advances/

Cogan, J. A., Jr. (2011). The Affordable Care Act's preventive services mandate: Breaking down the barriers to nationwide access to preventive services. *Journal of Law, Medicine & Ethics, 39*, 355–365.

Deom, M., Agoritsas, T., Bovier, P. A., & Perneger, T. V. (2010). What doctors think about the impact of managed care tools on quality of care, costs, autonomy, and relations with patients. *BMC Health Services Research, 10*, 331.

Dranove, D., Simon, C. J., & White, W. D. (1998). Determinants of managed care penetration. *Journal of Health Economics, 17*, 729–745.

Flieger, S. P. (2017). Implementing the patient-centered medical home in complex adaptive systems: Becoming a relationship-centered patient-centered medical home. *Health Care Management Review, 42*(2), 112–121.

Frank, R. G., & Welch, W. P. (1985). The competitive effects of HMOs: A review of the evidence. *Inquiry, 22*, 148–161.

Giacomini, M., Luft, H. S., & Robinson, J. C. (1995). Risk adjusting community rated health plan premiums. *Annual Review of Public Health, 16*, 401–430.

Hall, M. A. (1994). *Reforming private health insurance.* Washington, DC: American Enterprise Institute.

Hardcastle, L. E., Record, K. L., Jacobson, P. D., & Gostin, L. O. (2011). Improving the population's health: The Affordable Care Act and the importance of integration. *Journal of Law, Medicine & Ethics, 39,* 317–327.

Hill, S. C., & Wolfe, B. L. (1997). Testing the HMO competitive strategy: An analysis of its impact on medical care resources. *Journal of Health Economics, 16,* 261–286.

Jones, M. (2018, December 26). Healthcare: How technology impacts the healthcare industry. *Healthcare in America.* Retrieved from https://healthcareinamerica.us/healthcare-how-technology-impacts-the-healthcare-industry-b2ba6271c4b4

Kaiser Family Foundation. (2007, March). How changes in medical technology affect health care costs. *Snapshots: Health Care Costs.* Retrieved from http://www.kff.org/insurance/snapshot/chcm030807oth.cfm#back1

Kaiser Family Foundation. (2018). *Medicare delivery system reform: The evidence link.* San Francisco CA: Author.

Kolbasovsky, A. (2011). Strategies for measuring outcomes and ROI for managed care programs. Determining return on investment and improvement of outcomes is essential when new programs are being tried, but the research method must be chosen carefully. *Managed Care, 20*(11), 54–57.

Light, D. W. (1992). The practice and ethics of risk-rated health insurance. *JAMA, 267,* 2503–2508.

Manahan, B. (2011). The whole systems medicine of tomorrow: A half-century perspective. *Explore: The Journal of Science & Healing, 7*(4), 212–214.

McLaughlin, C. G. (1988). Market responses to HMOs: Price competition or rivalry? *Inquiry, 25,* 207–218.

McWilliams, J. M., Hatfield, L. A., Landon, B. E., Hamed, P., & Chernew, M. E. (2018). Re: Medicare spending after 3 years of the Medicare shared savings program. *JAMA, 320,* 1114–1130.

Peikes, D., Taylor, E., Dale, S., & Brown, R. (2018). *Evaluation of the comprehensive primary care initiative, 4th Annual Report.* Princeton, NJ: Mathematical Policy Research.

Reinhardt, U. E. (1993). An "all-American" health reform proposal. *Journal of American Health Policy, 3*(3), 11–17.

Stange, K. C., Nutting, P. A., Miller, W. L., Jaen, C. R., Crabtree, B.F., Flocke, S. A., & Gill, J. M. (2010). Defining and measuring the patient-centered medical home. *Journal of General Internal Medicine, 25*(6), 601–612.

Thorpe, K. E., Hendricks, A., Garnick, D., Donelan, K., & Newhouse, J. P. (1992). Reducing the number of uninsured by subsidizing employment-based health insurance. *JAMA, 267,* 945–948.

Vranceanu, A. M., & Ring, D. (2011). Factors associated with patient satisfaction. *Journal of Hand Surgery—American Volume, 36*(9), 1504–1508.

Answers to Odd-Numbered Exercises

Chapter 1: Introduction

1. Economics is the discipline that deals with the consequences of resource scarcity, and about making choices.

3. The three major tasks of economics are description, explanation, and evaluation. Description involves the identification, definition, and measurement of phenomena. Explanation involves conducting a cause-and-effect analysis. Evaluation involves judging or ranking alternative phenomena according to some standard or relative position of alternatives.

5. The slope of a geometric relation shows how much a change in one variable is associated with a given change in a related variable.

Chapter 2: Output of the Healthcare Sector

1. Medical care is a process during which certain inputs, or factors of production (e.g., healthcare provider services, medical instruments and equipment services, physical location and structure, and pharmaceuticals), are combined in varying quantities, often under a physician's supervision, to yield an output. Much of the difficulty in measuring the medical care process stems from the issue of defining the output of the healthcare system. If physician care is measured by the number of patient visits to a physician's office, then two cursory examinations count as two visits. But, one cursory examination followed by a more thorough examination involving a battery of tests also counts as two visits, even though more resources were used and a greater quantity of medical care was provided in the second case.

3. The World Health Organization defines health as "a complete state of physical, mental, and social well-being, and not merely the absence of illness or disease or infirmary." This is a very broad definition, and the characteristics of health suggested by it are not easy to pinpoint and measure. The definition stresses that there are three components of health, and even if a person is physically healthy, he or she can still be lacking in the other categories.

5. Unadjusted mortality rate does not consider such things as the age and sex of the population. If a population in one community is much younger than the population in another community, then comparing mortality (death) rates between the two communities would bias the results.

7. Health status has been shown to be positively influenced by medical care; however, as more medical care is provided to a given population, eventually additional units of medical care will improve their health at an increasingly lower rate. The "flat of the curve" describes the situation where the additional provision of medical care does not have a positive impact on health status.

Chapter 3: Economic Dimensions of the Healthcare System

1. An insured individual may still be responsible for deductibles, copayments, coinsurance, and costs that exceed the limits established by the insurance policy, and for healthcare services not covered by the insurance policy.

3. Medicare covers individuals 65 and older who have contributed to the Medicare program while working, and individuals with disabilities, end-stage renal disease, and Lou Gehrig disease.

5. Medicaid covers low-income populations who meet at least one categorical characteristic, including the aged (for services not covered by Medicare). There are no deductibles, but occasionally there are small copayments. There are no

premiums because low-income individuals could not afford them. Medicaid (in states not participating in the Medicaid expansion program) typically does not cover single individuals.

7. An individual does not enroll in an accountable care organization (the providers do) and there are no restrictions on individual's choice of providers. In a health maintenance organization, an individual must enroll in the HMO and in doing so accepts restrictions on his/her choice of providers in order to have the costs of services covered.

9. A cost-of-illness study measures the direct and indirect costs of illness for a population. Cost-of-illness studies can provide valuable information that can be used in budgeting decisions and in cost-effectiveness studies. Cost-of-illness studies focus on the economic component of trends in disease and consequently are useful for policymakers.

Chapter 4: Demand for Health and Medical Care

1. Demand is the relationship between price and quantity demanded. Quantity demanded is the amount consumers are willing and able to purchase at a certain price.

3. (A) The quantity demanded decreases with the increase in price; there is a movement along the original demand curve and not a shift in the demand curve with this change in the endogenous variable price. (B) The demand increases and there is an outward and to the right shift in the demand curve reflecting the increased number of consumers in the market. (C) The quantity demanded increases with the decrease in price; there is a movement along the original demand curve and not a shift in the demand curve with this change in the endogenous variable price. (D) The demand increases and there is an outward and to the right shift in the demand curve reflecting the increased number of health problems of consumers in the market. (E) The demand increases and the demand curve shifts outward and to the right as the substitute product (back surgery) becomes relatively more expensive than chiropractic services. (F) The demand increases as the price of the complement (radiographs) decreases, increasing the ability of the consumers to pay for more services. (G) The demand increases as the expected value of the services increases for the consumers now aware of the service; a change in tastes and preferences.

5. (A) There would be no impact on the demand for home care since the effective price to the consumer for nursing home care has remained unchanged with the government subsidy. (B) The quantity of home care demanded decreases with the increase in price from $12 to $15; there is a movement along the original demand curve and not a shift in the demand curve with this change in the endogenous variable price. (C) The demand increases and there is an outward and to the right shift in the demand curve reflecting the increased number of consumers in the market due to the increased number of people being discharged early from hospitals. (D) There is a movement along the original demand curve and not a shift in the demand curve with this increased productivity, which enables home care to be provided at a lower cost. (E) An increase in the percentage of low-income individuals in a given population reflects a lower income and so there is an inward and to the left shift in the demand curve reflecting the lower number of consumers in the market.

7. The three attributes of the quality of medical services are: (1) the structure of the resources provided, (2) the process of medical care, and (3) the outcomes or level of medical excellence of the services. Increased quality of medical care would lead to an increase in demand for medical services, cetera paribus, causing the demand curve to shift outward and to the right.

9. Information asymmetry occurs when the agent has better information than the principal. The principal cannot then effectively monitor the agent.

Chapter 5: Healthcare Production and Costs

1. Below are the values for total product (TP) and marginal product (MP) for Sweetgrass Radiology Labs.

Radiograph Technicians per Hour	Total Product (TP)	Marginal Product (MP)	Productivity
1	10	10	Increasing MP
2	26	16	Increasing MP
3	50	24	Increasing MP
4	74	24	Constant MP
5	94	20	Decreasing MP
6	100	6	Decreasing MP

3. The fixed costs total $8400 (office = $4000; phones = $400; secretary = $4000). The variable costs are as follows:

Variable Costs at 2700 Visits
Nurses 30 × $8000 = $240,000
Supplies $40 × 800 = $32,000
Total variable costs = $240,000 + $32,000 = $272,000
Total costs = $272,000 + $8400 = $280,400
Variable Costs at 3150 Visits

Currently, each nurse sees 30 patients a month or 900 visits per month (900 patients divided by 30 nurses = 30 patients per nurse). To increase the number of visits to 3150 (or to 1050 patients), CHC would need to hire 5 additional nurses (450 additional visits divided by 90 visits per nurse).

Nurses 35 × $8000 = $280,000
Supplies $40 × 1050 = $42,000
Total variable costs = $280,000 + $42,000 = $322,000
Total fixed costs = $8400 (the same as under original conditions)
Total costs = $322,000 + $8400 = $330,400

5. Fixed costs = $6000 a month for rent and utilities. Variable costs are:

Physician = $150/hour × 200 hours = $30,000
Nurse = $45/hour × 200 hours = $9000
Secretary = $30/hour × 200 hours = $6000
Supplies = $30/patient × 3000 patients = $90,000
Total variable costs = $30,000 + $9000 + $6000 + $90,000 = $135,000
Total costs = $6000 + $135,000 = $141,000

Chapter 6: Behavior of Supply

1. Dr. Kailikorn has indicated that he would be willing and able to provide twice as many procedures as the 1000 booked so his supply would be 2000 operations.

3. a) The marginal cost for each level of output is provided in the following table

Quantity	Total Cost (TC)	Marginal Cost (MC)
0	20	–
1	30	$10
2	60	$30
3	90	$30
4	150	$60
5	230	$80
6	330	$100

b) The maximum profit position will be at 3 units of output with a profit of $60 at this point when price per visit is $50, as illustrated in the following table.

Quantity	Total Costs (TC)	Total Revenue (TR)	Profit
0	$20	$0	–$20
1	$30	$50	$20
2	$50	$100	$50
3	$90	$150	$60
4	$150	$200	$50
5	$230	$250	$20
6	$330	$300	–$30

c) The maximum profit position will be at 5 units of output with a profit of $220 at this point when price per visit is $90, as illustrated in the following table.

Quantity	Total Costs (TC)	Total Revenue (TR)	Profit
0	$20	$0	–$20
1	$30	$90	$60
2	$50	$180	$130
3	$90	$270	$180
4	$150	$360	$210
5	$230	$450	$220
6	$330	$540	$210

5. Given the following cost schedule

Days of Care Supplied	Total Cost
0	$200
1	400
2	800
3	1400

Days of Care Supplied	Total Cost
4	2200
5	3200
6	4400

a) If the price per day is $440, then the quantity supplied would be 2 days of care with a profit of $80, as illustrated in the following table.

Quantity	Total Costs (TC)	Total Revenue (TR)	Profit
0	$200	$0	-$200
1	$400	$440	$40
2	$800	$880	$80
3	$1400	$1320	-$80
4	$2200	$1760	-$440
5	$3200	$2200	-$1000
6	$4400	$2640	-$1760

b) If the price per day is $640, then the quantity supplied would be 3 days of care with a profit of $520, as illustrated in the following table.

Quantity	Total Costs (TC)	Total Revenue (TR)	Profit
0	$200	$0	-$200
1	$400	$640	$240
2	$800	$1280	$480
3	$1400	$1920	$520
4	$2200	$2560	$360
5	$3200	$3200	$0
6	$4400	$3840	-$560

c) If the price per day is $900, then the quantity supplied would be 4 days of care with a profit of $1400, as illustrated in the following table.

Quantity	Total Costs (TC)	Total Revenue (TR)	Profit
0	$200	$0	-$200
1	$400	$900	$500

2	$800	$1800	$1000
3	$1400	$2700	$1300
4	$2200	$3600	$1400
5	$3200	$4500	$1300
6	$4400	$5400	$1000

7. Given the supply curve for radiographs by a radiology practice, the curve will shift as follows:

a) An increase in the wages of radiological technicians will cause supply to decrease, causing a movement in the supply curve upward and to the left.

b) A reduction in productivity will cause supply to decrease, causing a movement in the supply curve upward and to the left.

c) A decrease in the wages of technicians will cause supply to increase, causing a movement in the supply curve downward and to the right.

d) An increase in the price of radiographs will cause supply to increase, causing a movement in the supply curve downward and to the right.

e) An increase in the quality of services at a higher cost will cause supply to decrease, causing a movement in the supply curve upward and to the left.

f) An increase in the price of film will cause supply to decrease, causing a movement in the supply curve upward and to the left.

g) An increase in the number of patients with multiple and rare problems will cause supply to increase, causing a movement in the supply curve downward and to the right.

Chapter 7: Provider Payment

1. Four types of physician reimbursement are (1) fee for services, (2) per case, (3) per capita, and (4) salary. Fee-for-service payment encourages an increase in services, visits, and patients. Per case payment encourages a reduction in services per visit and an increase in visits and patients. Per capita payment encourages a reduction in services and visits and an increase

in patients. With a salary, the physician does not have a direct financial incentive to change treatment patterns because he/she does not face a financial risk, other than possible future salary increases. Under a salaried system, however, the physician does not have an incentive to increase the number of patients seen during office hours..

3. Resource-based relative value scale (RBRVS) is a fee-for-service system based on a detailed analysis of time costs, operating costs (overhead), and professional liability insurance costs. Implementation of the system led to a reduction in surgical fees relative to fees for nonsurgical services, which then led to a reduction in surgical services and an increase in nonsurgical services.

5. In prospective reimbursement, payment is based on predetermined rates. Payment can be made on the basis of services, days, and cases.

7. The likely effect of each of the hospital payment systems is illustrated in the following table:

Hospital Payment System	Effect on Relative Risk of Insurers	Effect on Relative Risk of Hospitals
Retrospective cost payment	High degree of risk	No risk
Prospective fee for service	Moderate degree of risk	Low degree of risk
Per diem fees	High degree of risk	Low degree of risk
Per case	Low to moderate degree of risk	Moderate to high degree of risk
Per case + outlier adjustment	Moderate degree of risk	Moderate degree of risk

9. Nursing homes can be funded on a per diem basis, either using a flat rate or a resource utilization adjusted rate taking into consideration the characteristics of the residents.

Chapter 8: Competitive Markets

1. Predicted effects
   a) Price and quantity increase (demand curve shifts upward and to the right).
   b) Price falls and quantity increases (demand curve shifts upward and to the right).
   c) Price increases and quantity increases (demand curve shifts upward and to the right).
   d) Price and quantity increase (demand curve shifts downward and to the left).
   e) Price and quantity decrease (demand curve shifts downward and to the left).

3. The FPL made $2.8 million in profits with an $8 million investment. Its return on capital (35%) is greater than in other industries. This higher rate of return means that capital will be attracted to this industry. As a result, supply will increase and price and profits will fall over time.

5. Given the information provided in the graph, 300 days of hospital care are demanded at all rates since the price is zero to consumers. At a rate of $450 per day, 200 days are supplied by the hospitals. At a rate of $600 per day, 300 days of care are supplied. At a rate of $450 per day, funding is $90,000 and 200 days are utilized. At a rate of $600 per day, funding is $180,000, and total utilization is 300 days.

Chapter 9: Market Power in Health Care

1. The answers are contained in the following table:

Price in Dollars	Quantity of Visits Demanded	Total Revenue	Marginal Revenue
$200	0	–	–
180	1	$180	$180
160	2	320	140
140	3	420	100
120	4	480	60
100	5	500	20
80	6	480	–20

At a marginal cost of $70 per visit, the monopolist will supply up to the point where marginal cost (MC) is above or equal to marginal revenue (MR). This is at a volume of three and a price of $140. To supply the fourth visit would generate a marginal revenue of only $60, while the marginal cost is above that at $70.

3. The information is provided in the following table:

Demand Schedule A (Medicaid)				Demand Schedule B (Private Insurance)			
Price	Number of Visits	Total Revenue	Marginal Revenue	Price	Number of Visits	Total Revenue	Marginal Revenue
$200	1	$200	$200	$200	6	$1200	$1200
180	2	360	160	180	7	1260	60
160	3	480	120	160	8	1280	20
140	4	560	80	140	9	1260	20
120	5	600	40	120	10	1200	–60

The marginal cost for both providers is $75 per visit.

The price in each market should be set where MR is closest to being equal to MC. This is $140 and four visits for Group A where the marginal revenue is $80 and the marginal cost is $75; the marginal revenue is only $40 for the fifth visit, which is below the marginal cost of $75. This is $200 and one visits for Group B where the marginal revenue is $1200 and the marginal cost is $75; the marginal revenue is only $60 for the second visit and the marginal cost is $75.

5. The information is provided in the following table:

Supply Price	Product Supplied	Total Cost	Marginal Cost	Demand Price	Nurses Demanded
$20	1	$20	$20	$200	1
40	2	80	60	180	2
60	3	180	100	160	3
80	4	320	140	140	4
100	5	500	180	120	5
120	6	720	220	100	6
				80	7
				60	8

The monopsonist will hire up to four nurses, at which point the marginal value of a nurse ($140) reflected in the demand price of $140 equals the marginal cost ($140) of hiring the additional nurse. If the monopsonist hired the fifth nurse, the marginal cost would be $180, but the demand price would be below it at only $120.

7. The consumers in the market may be influenced by the physicians to purchase more health care than they would without the influence of the physician. In other words, the physicians could increase the elasticity of the demand curve through supplier-induced demand.

Chapter 10: Health Insurance

1. The answers to each subquestion are as follows:
   a) With no insurance, the expected utility = (0.2 × 84.4) + (0.8 × 100) = 96.88. With insurance, the expected utility is 98.8 since insurance is $300, which would bring her wealth to $9700. The individual should purchase insurance.
   b) At a price of $600, expected utility is 95.8, which is the utility of $9400, or $10,000 − 600. This is less than a utility of 96.88, which is the expected utility if no insurance were bought. She would not buy insurance.

c) If she got sick, and had no insurance, her wealth level would be $8000 and utility would be 57.0 units. The expected utility without insurance would be 91.4 ($-0.2 \times 57 + 0.8 \times 100$). This is less than the utility of 95.8 which is the utility if she buys insurance. She would therefore buy insurance.

d) Mrs. Smith is risk averse.

3. The insurance benefit the employer purchases for the individual can be considered part of the individual's compensation package, which also includes the individual's salary. Since the insurance benefit is not taxed, at a tax rate of 30%, the price to the individual is $3500, or $5000 × $(1 - 0.3)$. The other $1500 would go to pay taxes if the individual took the $5000 in cash.

5. The answers to each subquestion are as follows:
   a) For healthy individuals, the expected utility with no insurance is 0.2 (89.0) + 0.8 (100) = 97.8 since the cost of healthcare services is $1000 if the healthy individual becomes ill. The cost of insurance under a community rating would be $300, so the expected utility for healthy individuals with insurance is based on the utility of wealth of $9700 or expected utility of 98.8, which is greater than the utility of 97.8 without insurance. A healthy person should, therefore, buy insurance. For unhealthy persons, the cost of healthcare services is $2000 if the unhealthy individual becomes ill, so the expected utility with no insurance for the unhealthy individual is 0.2 (57.0) + 0.8 (100) = 91.4. The cost of insurance under a community rating would also be $300 for the unhealthy individual, so the expected utility for unhealthy individuals with insurance is based on the utility of wealth of $9700 or expected utility of 98.8, which is greater than the utility of 91.4 without insurance. An unhealthy person should buy insurance.
   b) For healthy persons, the utility with no insurance = 0.2 (89.0) + 0.8 (100) = 97.8.

The expected utility with the cost of insurance of $200 and no expected additional out-of-pocket cost for healthy individuals with insurance is based on the utility of wealth of $9800 or expected utility of 99.4, which is greater than the utility of 97.8 without insurance. A healthy person should buy insurance. The total expenditure for each healthy individual in the low-cost plan is $200 or a total of $100,000 for the group of 500 healthy individuals. For unhealthy persons, the utility with no insurance = 0.2 (57.0) + 0.8 (100) = 91.4. The utility with insurance under the low-cost plan for unhealthy individuals is 0.2 (84.4) + 0.8 (100) = 96.88. An unhealthy person should buy insurance. The total expenditure for each unhealthy individual in the low-cost plan is $200 premium plus an additional $1000 out of pocket for medical expenses not covered by insurance for a total of $1200 per individual or $600,000 for the 500 unhealthy individuals.

7. Under a utilization management program, administrative costs would increase since the insurance company now has to monitor the providers to ensure that they are adhering to the utilization requirements. Since the utilization management program results in less utilization of services by consumers, the claims payout falls. However, despite the improvement in utilization management in terms of reducing utilization, the added administrative costs could be enough to push the total costs higher than they were before the implementation of the program. The final results depend on whether the reduction in utilization saves more costs than are incurred in managing the system.

Chapter 11: The Labor Market

1. The relevant data for this exercise are contained in the following table:

Number of Nurses	Number of Clinic Visits	Total Revenue	Value of the Marginal Product (Marginal Revenue)	Total Costs	(Wage per Nurse) Marginal Costs
1	12	$300	$300	$200	$200
2	22	$550	$250	$400	$200
3	30	$750	$200	$600	$200
4	36	$900	$150	$800	$200
5	40	$1000	$100	$1000	$200

Midwest will hire additional nurses up to the point where the wage (Marginal Cost) equals the value of the marginal product (Marginal Revenue). In the original case the quantity hired will be three. If Midwest adds $15 to the compensation of nurses, then the marginal cost becomes $215 instead of the $200 in the table above and Midwest will only hire two nurses since the value of the marginal product is $250 at two nurses and only $200 at three nurses.

3. The following answers are for the demand curve for labor in a clinic corresponding to the indicated event:

   a) There is no effect on the market demand curve when the wage falls, but there is a movement down the curve.

   b) The demand curve shifts outward and to the right with the increase in productivity.

   c) The demand curve shifts outward and to the right with the increase in the price of clinic visits since that increases revenue.

   d) There is no effect on the curve when the clinic hires more workers, there is a movement on the demand curve.

   e) The demand curve shifts outward and to the right with the increase in productivity per worker.

   f) The demand curve shifts inward and to the left since output of the nurse in terms of number of patients decreases with the production of higher quality care.

5. The introduction of health insurance as a benefit will cause the supply curve (relating wage rates and labor supplied) to shift downward and to the right, if insurance is valued equally with wages. The curve will shift parallel to the original curve by the amount of the premium paid by the employer.

7. The impact of poor health will be to lower the wages of these employees since they are less productive in the market because of absenteeism and presenteeism.

9. Organizations have a number of reasons for budgeting. These include such things as controlling activities, coordinating activities, communicating important objectives to everyone in the organization, motivating personnel's performance, and providing a measurement of results. Budgets can be used to either instill fear in managers or help the organization become efficient and effective.

Chapter 12: Economic Evaluation of Health Services

1. The evaluation concept to be used in this case is cost-effectiveness analysis (CEA). CEA is used when it is anticipated that the outcomes of the interventions may vary (in this case both severity and survival rate are anticipated to vary), but that the outcomes of the diabetes therapy alternatives can be expressed in common units. The differences in cost and outcomes are compared using a ratio of costs to benefits.

3. The additional costs involved with the new intervention were $1600 hospital costs, $600 for the drug, $40 nursing time, $20 in supplies for a total of $2260. The mortality rate was 20 deaths per 100 (rate of 0.2) with the drug and 24 per 100 (rate of 0.24) without the drug. The cost-effectiveness ratio is calculated using the following formula:

$$CE = (C2 - C1) / (Q2 - Q1)$$
$$= (\$2,260 - 0) / (0.24 - 0.20)$$
$$= \$56,500 \text{ per life saved.}$$

5. The outcome measure is considered to be a holistic one and is defined as the number of lives saved. The effectiveness measure of the drug, calculated as the difference in deaths per 1000 people, is equal to 10 fewer deaths per 1000 people with the use of the new drug.

Chapter 13: Value Judgments and Economic Evaluation

1. In a world of completely selfish individuals, the conditions that must be met in order for the healthcare market to be at an optimal level of output is for the marginal social values of medical care, which coincide with marginal private valuations in a world of completely selfish individuals, to equal the marginal social cost.

3. In a society with two persons, if one is altruistic and values the other's use of medical care, the socially optimal quantity of medical care that is produced will occur where the marginal social value for all individuals equals marginal cost. This optimal quantity incorporates each individual's

private valuations as well as his or her external valuations for the quantity consumed by the second person who may be poor, needy, sick, etc.

5. No, a freely competitive market without philanthropy will not yield a socially optimal output when there are consumption externalities because the private market only ensures that each person obtains health care in relation to his or her own valuations and associated costs. If there are consumption externalities, there may be room for increases in social valuations through the philanthropic transfer of funds.

7. Some of the goals of health policy include the following: (1) to achieve quality of care, (2) to achieve technical efficiency through low production costs and high quality of output, (3) to achieve levels of population health status, (4) to ensure an adequate supply of resources to provide care at an efficient level, and (5) to achieve economic efficiency.

Chapter 14: Financing Health Care

1. Out-of-pocket expenditures account for 10.47%, government for 55.63%, and private insurance for 33.90% of total healthcare expenses.

3. The government tax subsidy on insurance will increase the demand for insurance; consumers will purchase more since the price to them has been decreased.

5. A payroll tax is a tax on employment (wage) income. Payroll taxes lead to a reduction in employment and wages since the employer considers the tax to be part of the compensation paid to employees. A tax increases the cost of production to the employer.

7. The following discussion outlines the impact of each method of financing on individuals according to their income cohort (group):
   a) An income tax is a direct tax levied against the income (wages) of the individual. Since a percentage is applied to total taxable income, the income tax paid rises as income rises. The income tax is the most progressive (least regressive) way of financing insurance.
   b) A sales tax is an indirect tax and is levied against the price of goods and services purchased. Typically, lower income cohorts are unable to save some of their income and so

the tax is applied to their entire income. As income increases, individuals are typically able to save a greater percentage of their income and so the tax is applied to a smaller percentage of their income that is spent on goods and services.
   c) A payroll tax is a tax on employment income (wages). Most payroll taxes set an upper limit on the amount of income to which the tax will apply. The payroll tax will have the same impact on each income cohort until it reaches the income limit cohort. Once the limit is reached, the impact will begin to decline.
   d) Insurance premiums typically use the community rating when based in place of employment. The community rating says that the same amount (not rate) is charged to each individual. This means that individuals in the lowest income cohort will pay the same price as individuals in the highest income cohort. The insurance premium does not reflect the risk of an individual becoming ill and so the low-risk individuals will subsidize the high-risk individuals, regardless of income, possibly transferring resources from low-income cohorts to high-income cohorts. Insurance premiums are the most regressive (least progressive) way of financing insurance.

9. Bundled payments is a payment method based on the costs expected to be incurred in the provision of a clinically defined episode of care, adjusted for severity and complexity of a patient's condition. Bundled payments are viewed as a blend of fee-for-service and capitation payments, discouraging the provision of unnecessary care and encouraging the coordination of care across providers, but not penalizing providers who care for sicker patients in their practice. The goal of bundled payment is to reduce fragmentation of care, thereby improving quality and reducing costs. The use of bundled payments should encourage providers within the system to reorganize how care is delivered so that it is coordinated and responsive to the needs of patients. Under a bundled payment system, the services that are required by patients during a single illness or a course of treatment for a chronic disease are defined across providers and settings—the services are bundled into a single package of services. Once the required services are defined, a target price is established for the bundle. This target price reflects the total amount

that will be paid for the episode of care, and all providers involved in the provision of services are covered under that price. This comprehensive price provides an incentive for the coordination of care in order to keep the costs of producing the services below the price established. Within the provider network, decisions have to be made on how to allocate the global revenue among the participating providers rendering services to the patient.

Chapter 15: Public Health Insurance

1. Medicare is a national health insurance program for a subset of the U.S. population. It covers older persons (age 65 and older) who have contributed to Social Security for at least 40 quarters, Railroad Retirement, or federal retirement programs. It also covers certain disabled individuals, persons with end-stage renal disease, and persons with amyotrophic lateral sclerosis (Lou Gehrig disease).

    Medicare consists of four parts: Part A, Hospital Insurance; Part B, Supplemental Medical Insurance; Part C, Medicare Advantage; and Part D, Prescription Drugs. Part A, Hospital Insurance, covers inpatient hospital services, limited skilled-nursing facility services for rehabilitation, home health care, and hospice services.

    Part B, Supplemental Medical Insurance, covers medical necessary physician services, outpatient services, home health services, preventive services, ambulance services, clinical laboratory services, durable medical equipment (DME), kidney supply and services, outpatient, inpatient, and partial hospitalization for mental health services, and diagnostic tests. In addition, it covers an annual comprehensive wellness visit and personalized prevention plan.

    Part C, Medicare Advantage, must cover all of the medically necessary services that Original Medicare covers, although Original Medicare still covers the cost of hospice care, some new Medicare benefits, and some costs of clinical research studies. In addition, most Medicare Advantage plans offer coverage for items not covered under Original Medicare, such as vision, hearing, dental, and some wellness programs like gym memberships. Many of the plans cover other health-related services that promote health and wellness. Most

include Medicare prescription drug (Part D) coverage.

Part D, Prescription Drugs—each Part D drug plan under Medicare is required to provide at least a standard level of coverage set by Medicare. Plans are permitted to vary the list of prescription drugs they cover (their formulary) and how they place drugs in two different "tiers" on their formulary. These formularies cover both generic and brand-name prescription drugs. The formularies are required to include at least two drugs in the most commonly prescribed categories and classes, but can select which specific drugs are covered. Beginning in 2019, drug plans that meet certain requirements can immediately remove brand-name drugs from the formularies and replace them with new generic drugs or change the cost of coverage rules for brand names when adding new generic drugs.

3. Medicaid is a joint federal-state partnership health insurance program that covers both working and jobless families and children, pregnant women, individuals with a variety of physical and mental conditions, and elderly individuals. The federal government defines minimum requirements that states must meet, but the states have broad authority to establish eligibility criteria, benefits covered, provider payments, delivery systems, and a number of other conditions for their program. As a result, the percentage of the population covered across states varies widely.

    Medicaid covers a broad array of services, both mandatory and optional. The federal government mandates each state offer a specific set of services in order to participate in the program. The federal government also allows states to cover additional optional services under the Medicaid allowable services. These optional services qualify for the same federal match as the mandated services. The specific optional services covered vary across states.

5. Medigap is private insurance that can be purchased by Medicare beneficiaries to cover gaps in coverage due to Medicare premiums, deductibles, and copayments.

7. The following are potential policies Medicare could pursue:
    a) Medicare can increase the scope of the program by eliminating the "doughnut hole" in Part D. This would have an effect on the affordability goal and the adequacy goal.

b) Medicare can increase premiums, which would affect the equity goal.

c) Medicare can drastically reduce provider payments, which would decrease participation by providers in the program; not feasible.

d) Medicare can increase copayments, which would affect the equity goal.

e) Medicare can introduce managed care for everyone, which might not be acceptable to the population.

Chapter 16: Regulation and Antitrust Policy in Health Care

1. The physician is sometimes described as a "double agent" because the physician acts as an agent for two principals: the patient and the insurer.

3. Patent rights allow pharmaceutical companies a substantial amount of time to recover the investment made in the development of drugs (the development of a single drug can take many years and millions of dollars in investment).

5. Two largest hospitals are proposing a merger.
   a) HHI = $\Sigma(MS)2$, where MS is each firm's market share.

   Pre-merger = $(40^2 + 40^2 + 20^2) = (1600 + 1600 + 400) = 3600$

   Post-merger is based on two hospitals, one with 80%, one with 20% of market

   Post-merger = $(80^2 + 20^2) = (6400 + 400) = 6800$

   The change between pre-merger and post-merger is 3200 (6800 – 3600)
   b) The high post-merger HHI of 6800 is well above the 2500 that the agency regards as being highly concentrated. The merger would also produce an increase in the HHI above 100, which potentially raises significant competitive concerns.

7. A public good or service is one that has the characteristics of being nonrivalous and nonexcludable. The nonrivalous characteristic means that the consumption of the good or service by an individual does not reduce the amount available for consumption by another individual. The nonexcludable characteristic means that an individual cannot be excluded from using the good or service.

A problem encountered in the provision of a public good in the free market arises from the free rider phenomenon. A free rider is an individual who receives the benefits of the good or service without paying for it. As a result, the good or service may be underproduced. For goods that the consumption by one individual does not prevent simultaneous consumption by another and when it is very difficult if not impossible to prevent individuals who have not paid for the good or service from having access to it, then the free market lacks adequate features to ensure inefficiencies do not occur in its production and consumption.

Chapter 17: Reform of the Healthcare Market

1. Information asymmetry is when different parties of a transaction have unequal amounts of information. If insurers lack sufficient information to determine consumer risk, then they will set prices at the group average. Low-risk persons may drop out of the market, leaving higher risk persons in the market. Rates (or premiums) will spiral upward and the market may disappear, even though some persons would be willing to buy insurance and there are potential suppliers who would provide it at rates acceptable to the consumers (if the risks could be adequately determined).

3. Community rating hinders economic efficiency in two ways. One, it discourages individuals from engaging in health promotion activities when the social costs would warrant them to do so. As a result, individuals who do engage in the activities do not experience cost savings. One innovation in response to this is a mandate requiring that all individuals purchase insurance. Two, community rating hinders economic efficiency by encouraging insurers to seek out lower risk individuals, causing individuals who normally buy insurance not to purchase it and eventually leading to a disappearance of the market. A response to this is the use of risk rating so that individuals are assigned to groups and charged a premium based on risks.

5. Comparisons between members of managed care and of traditional insurance groups have been researched. It was found that managed care members seemed to use fewer resources than the comparison group of individuals. This could be due to selection bias, however, if people joining managed

care differ from and are healthier than the population of people with traditional insurance. If this the case, then it wouldn't be possible to conclude that the observed difference in resource utilization represented greater efficiency.

7. The foundation of an ACO is clear, patient-focused aims of better overall health through higher quality and lower costs for patients; provider accountability through performance measures that are transparent; and payment reform that uses the measures to align and provide organizations that are focused on these aims directly and meaningfully. Presently, most ACOs participate in savings achieved but are not responsible for the risk for losses that occur. The new program will require ACOs to also accept the risk for losses that occur if the ACO does not meet the established target.

The patient-centered medical home (PCMH) program is a model of primary care that is patient-centered, comprehensive, team-based, integrated and coordinated, accessible, and focused on quality and safety. The patient-centered medical home model is based on the fundamental tenets of primary care. It has been shown that systems with a focus on primary care have better quality, lower cost, less inequality in health care and health, and better population health when compared with systems based on other approaches to health care.

Glossary of Health Economics Terms

absolute advantage The ability of a given amount of resources to produce more of some goods or services in one industry or organization than in another one.

abuse (health care) Excessive, unnecessary, or improper treatment, including failure to provide medically necessary care.

access Potential and actual entry of a population into the healthcare delivery system (U.S. Congress, 1988).

accountability Duty to provide evidence necessary to establish confidence that the activity for which one is responsible is performed and described transparently the way the activity has been performed to all concerned.

Accountable Care Organization (ACO) A group of doctors, hospitals, and other healthcare providers who come together voluntarily to give coordinated high-quality care to their Medicare patients (https://www.cms.gov /Medicare/Medicare-Fee-for-Service-Payment/ACO/index .html?redirect=/ACO/).

accountable care plan Form of health plan proposed in the 1990s as part of the managed competition approach to health care, accountable for meeting federal requirements for providing a defined set of standardized services.

accreditation Process performed by a nongovernmental agency to evaluate an institution or education program to determine if a set of standards has been met.

activities of daily living (ADL) Activities that are typically done for oneself, such as eating, dressing, brushing teeth, etc.; the ADL scale assigns numerical scores according to the degree of physical functioning an individual can attain in each of six categories: bathing, dressing, toileting, feeding, transferring between locations, and continence (Katz, Ford, Moskowitz, Jackson, & Jaffe, 1963).

acuity Level or severity of an illness.

acute care Inpatient diagnostic and short-term treatment of patients.

adjusted community rate Term used in Medicare risk contracts to indicate the premium to be charged for providing exactly the same Medicare-covered benefits to a community-rated group, adjusted to allow for greater intensity and frequency of utilization by Medicare recipients.

administered price Price set by the seller or payer instead of by impersonal market forces.

admission Formal acceptance of a patient by a hospital or other healthcare institution in order to provide care to that patient.

adverse drug event Harm (illness or injury) resulting from the use or administration of a drug or medication.

adverse selection Based on the ability of consumers to gauge their risk of needing healthcare services more accurately than the insurance company, and to act on the information asymmetry they possess; the systematic selection by high-risk consumers of insurance plans with greater degrees of coverage so that the insurers who offer these plans end up with insureds who incur greater than normal costs.

advocacy Attempt to persuade regarding the rightness of a cause or point of view regarding an issue.

affiliation Number of arrangements among providers outlining relationships and individual responsibilities.

agency (agent) A group or individual who has been delegated authority to make decisions and perform activities on behalf of those doing the delegating; physicians are often said to act as agents for their patients, indicating that the physicians make decisions about treatments based on their knowledge.

aggregate demand Total desired purchases by all buyers of goods or services produced.

aggregate supply Total desired sales by all producers of goods or services.

algorithm Set of rules for carrying out a process or the calculation of a statistic.

allocative efficiency No reorganization of production or consumption could make one person better off without making someone else worse off.

all-payer system A system of reimbursing providers in which all separate insurers coordinate to set uniform payment policies. Individual providers will then receive the same reimbursement from different insurers for cases with similar characteristics.

alternate level of care (ALC) A level of care other than the appropriate one, such as that given to a non-acute-treatment patient occupying an acute-care bed.

ambulatory care Care rendered to individuals under their own cognizance any time when they are not resident in an institution.

ambulatory care groups (ACGs) A case-mix classification system incorporating related ambulatory care visits, based on ICD-9-CM diagnostic codes and patient age and gender (Starfield, Weiner, Mumford, & Steinwachs, 1991).

ambulatory visit groups (AVGs) A classification system by which ambulatory care visits with associated procedures are classified into similar resource-using groups based on diagnosis, procedure, age, and gender.

ancillary services Hospital services other than room and board (nursing services are included as part of room and board).

antikickback statute Federal legislation making it a felony for an individual to receive or offer a bribe, or kickback, in exchange for a referral from another person in any federally financed healthcare program.

antitrust Laws seeking to prevent monopolies or unfair competition in a market, or other activities that unreasonably restrain trade.

any willing provider State laws requiring a managed care organization to grant participation to any provider who is legally qualified as a practitioner and who is willing to become a member of the organization.

APACHE III System designed to predict risk of dying in a hospital, generally used to measure the severity of illness of intensive care unit (ICU) patients.

appropriateness of care Degree to which tests, medications, procedures, education, and other healthcare services are clearly indicated, adequate, not excessive, and provided in the setting most appropriate to meet the needs of the patient.

arc elasticity Measured by using the average of the original price and the new price and the average of the original and new quantities.

area wage adjustment Part of the prospective payment formula allowing for differences in wage scales in different parts of the country.

assignment of benefits Voluntary action by an insured beneficiary to have insurance benefits paid directly to the provider of services.

asymmetric information An imbalance of information between buyers and sellers of a service, by which one group is better informed than the other.

atypical patients Patients who exhibit patterns of care different from typical cases, either because they do not complete a full and successful course of treatment in a single institution or because their length of stay exceeds the statistical trim point.

autonomy Right of an individual to make decisions for his or her health or life.

availability The supply of services, generally in relation to the demand for the services.

average adjusted per capita cost (AAPCC) An estimate of the average cost incurred by Medicare per beneficiary in the fee-for-service system, adjusted by county for geographic cost differences related to age, gender, disability status, Medicaid eligibility, and institutional status.

average cost (AC) The unit cost for a selected volume of output; total cost divided by total quantity of output. The average cost is equal to the average variable cost plus the average fixed cost.

average fixed cost (AFC) The unit fixed cost for a specific volume of output. The average fixed cost is equal to the total fixed cost divided by the volume of output.

average length of stay See **length of stay**.

average product (AP) Total product divided by number of units used in its production.

average revenue (AR) Total revenue divided by number of units (quantity) sold.

average variable cost (AVC) The unit variable cost for a specific volume of output; total variable cost divided by quantity of output.

baby boomers Individuals born in the United States from 1946 to 1964.

balance billing Practice of physicians to charge patients the difference between their charges and the amount paid by the insurance company for the service.

Balanced Budget Act of 1997 (BBA) Federal law enacting many changes in health care, including the creation of the State Children's Health Insurance Program (S-CHIP), as well as changed design to extend the Medicare Trust Fund's financial life and created the Medicare + Choice program, now called the Medicare Advantage program.

basis of payment The unit of output in terms for which the provider is paid; this can be on any of a per day of care, per service provided, per case, or per person (capitation).

bed capacity The number of patients a hospital can house.

bed days The number of days in a period that beds are available; in a year, bed days are the number of regularly maintained available beds multiplied by 365.

behavioral health Umbrella term including mental health and substance abuse; used to distinguish services provided for physical health.

benchmark Reference point for each element being monitored; used to compare performance or outcomes of an institution or a provider against the defined measure or best practice.

benefit (1) Money, care, or other services that an individual is entitled to receive because of insurance coverage; (2) the compensation of labor that is additional to wages (e.g., health insurance, life insurance, pension rights, etc.).

benefit cost The relationship between the dollar impact of an intervention and its opportunity cost. It can be expressed as a ratio (benefits divided by costs) or as a net value (benefits minus costs).

benefit-cost ratio approach Compares projects on the basis of the average benefit per unit cost; in this approach, the project with the greatest ratio of benefits to costs is selected.

biased selection The deliberate choice, by a provider or insurer, of a group of patients (insureds) with preselected characteristics associated with low utilization of health care.

brand-name drug A drug or pharmaceutical product sold by a pharmaceutical company under a specific name or trademark and that is protected by a patent.

break-even point Volume of activity where revenues and expenses are equal.

budget Simply a financial plan for a given period of time; a method of answering the question: "What do I think it will cost me to do what I want to do?"

budget neutrality Requirement that payment under a new system cannot be larger or smaller than under the previous system.

bundled payment Also known as episode-based payment, case rate, package pricing, or global payment; it is simply a single payment made for all healthcare services that a patient requires related to a specific course of treatment or condition over a period of time from all providers involved; the providers involved in the treatment are not paid for each discrete service, interaction, or procedure.

bundling Grouping goods and services together into a package for delivery or payment.

burden With reference to a tax, the reduction in real income resulting from the tax (Due, 1957, p. 6).

cafeteria plan Allows employees to choose from a menu of different healthcare coverage and provider options.

capacity A measure of the output that can be reached when existing resources are fully and efficiently used; output corresponds to the firm's minimum short-run average total cost.

capital Human, physical, and financial means of production, usually long-term assets that are primarily fixed and not bought and sold in the course of operations; capital resources are not totally consumed in the current production cycle.

capitalist economy When capital is predominately owned privately rather than by the state or government.

capitation A payment system in which the entity financially responsible for the patients' healthcare services receives a fixed periodic sum for each patient (per capita) that covers the costs of utilization by the patient; the sum can be adjusted for specific patient characteristics, such as age and gender.

cartel Organization of producers who agree to act as a single seller in order to maximize joint profits.

case management A collection of organized activities to identify high-cost patients as early as possible, locate and assess alternative treatment methods, and manage healthcare benefits for these patients in a cost-effective manner (Scheffler, Sullivan, & Ko, 1991); sometimes used interchangeably with care management and disease management.

case mix Grouping of patients according to characteristics (age, gender, diagnoses, treatments, severity of illness, etc.) and then determining the proportion of the total patients falling into each group.

case-mix groups (CMGs) A Canadian system for classifying hospital inpatients into groups using similar quantities of resources according to selected patient characteristics such as diagnosis, procedure, age, and comorbidity; CMGs are maintained by the Canadian Institute for Health Information.

case-mix index An index or measure of the average level of resource requirements for a group of cases sorted and weighted according to type of case; the weights represent the estimated resource use for each type of case.

causal factors of demand Income, tastes and preferences, prices of other goods and services, expectations, and health status.

causal factors of supply Technology, input prices, governmental policies, substitutes and complements, and goals and expectations.

causal relation The value of one economic variable changes and results in the value of a second economic variable changing.

certificate-of-need regulation The basic assumption underlying CON regulation is that excess capacity stemming from overbuilding of healthcare facilities results in healthcare price inflation; price inflation can occur when a facility cannot fill its beds and fixed costs must be met through higher charges for the beds that are used.

ceteris paribus Other things being equal.

change agent Individual whose efforts facilitate change in an organization.

change in demand Increase or decrease in the quantity demanded at each possible price of the good or service represented by a shift in the entire demand curve.

change in quantity demanded Increase or decrease in the specific quantity bought at a specified price, represented by a movement along a given demand curve.

change in quantity supplied Increase or decrease in the specific quantity sold at a specified price, represented by a movement along a given supply curve.

change in supply Increase or decrease in the quantity supplied at each possible price of the goods or services, represented by a shift in the entire supply curve.

charges A price set for a product by the supplier; charges may not equal cash received, because some payers may receive a discount or fail to pay.

charity care Healthcare services provided free of charge to those who do not have the ability to pay for care.

chart of accounts A listing that accumulates the revenues and expenses according to the unit that has the responsibility for producing the revenue and incurring the expenses.

cherry picking (also called cream skimming) Practice by insurers of selling policies only to low-risk individuals.

Children's Health Insurance Program (CHIP) To assist states in providing insurance coverage to low-income children who were not eligible for Medicaid but couldn't afford private insurance.

chronic Illness that lasts a long time and usually without prospect of immediate change for either improvement or deterioration.

churning Practice of discharging a patient from the hospital and readmitting the patient for what is really a single episode of care in order to increase payment.

cognitive services Activities of a health professional other than the performance of a procedure.

coinsurance A system of provider payment in which the patient is responsible for a portion/percentage of the payment, and the insurer or third party is responsible for the rest.

collusion Overt or covert, explicit or tacit, agreement among suppliers to act jointly in their common interests.

community care Care provided in a noninstitutional setting, including in the home or in the patient's "neighborhood."

community rating A method of setting insurance premiums for healthcare coverage. In this method, all insurers in the group pay the same premium, regardless of their risk-related characteristics, such as age or health problems.

comorbidity A disease or condition that is present at the same time as the principal disease or condition of the patient.

comparative advantage Ability of one supplier to produce goods or services at a lower cost than other suppliers.

competition A state of competition exists in a market if no single firm or consumer is large enough to influence the market price; this state usually occurs if there are many buyers and sellers in the market.

competitive price The price at which demand and supply are in equilibrium in a competitive market.

complements Two goods or services that are consumed together, such as surgeons' services and operating room services; the economic relevance of complementarity is that a change in the direct price of a complement will cause a shift in the demand curve of the other service.

complex adaptive system Collection of individual components possessing the freedom to act in ways that are not always predictable and whose actions are interconnected.

complications Adverse patient conditions that arise during the process of medical care.

concentration (market) The extent to which market activity is confined to a limited number of firms.

concierge physician practice (also called boutique medicine) Arrangement between healthcare provider and a patient in which the patient pays a retainer fee to the provider and, in return, is provided a special class of care and services.

concurrent review A process of ongoing review while the patient is undergoing treatment in the hospital and of certifying the length of stay that is appropriate for the approved admission (Scheffler et al., 1991).

conspiracy of silence Alleged tacit agreement among health professionals not to testify against one another in malpractice lawsuits.

consumer-driven health plan Option designed to influence consumer behavior, typically offering a cost-sharing health plan in conjunction with discretionary healthcare dollars (high-deductible health plan combined with a health savings account).

consumerism A view that health care should be directly driven by the interests of consumers.

consumer's surplus The difference between what an individual is willing to pay for a given quantity of goods or services and what is actually paid. This is equal to the area under the demand curve between no consumption and that specified quantity minus the amount paid for all the units (price times quantity).

consumption The use of goods or services to satisfy current wants.

contingent valuation The valuation that a person would place on a service if he/she had the option of having it available.

continuum of care The entire spectrum of specialized health, rehabilitative, and residential services available to the frail and chronically ill. The services focus on the social, residential, rehabilitative, and supportive needs of individuals, as well as needs that are essentially medical in nature (Department of Health and Human Services, 1994).

contract costs The costs of reaching an agreement with the provider or buyer as to what services are to be provided.

conversion factor Dollar amount for one base unit in the relative value scale or the diagnosis-related group.

copayments Out-of-pocket payments for health services made by users at the time a service is rendered.

core services In Canada, health services that must be available to every resident of a province (Saskatchewan Health, 1993) (see also **insured services**); also, the set of services that must be provided by U.S. hospitals if they are to be eligible for registration with the American Hospital Association.

cost The expense incurred (resources used) in producing goods and services. See **opportunity cost** and **money cost**.

cost–benefit evaluation (also called benefit–cost evaluation) Used to place a monetary value on the benefits of the outcomes; in the analysis, both the resources used and the benefits gained are usually expressed in monetary terms, since monetary values are common measure across multiple types of projects.

cost-consequence evaluation Compares the costs of the program or intervention with its consequences; unlike the other four types of economic evaluation, cost-consequence analysis does not summarize outcomes into a single result or financial determination.

cost curve The relationship between cost and volume of output. It can be specified in terms of total costs, average or unit costs, and marginal costs. See **long-run cost curve** and **short-run cost curve**.

cost effectiveness The relationship between the additional cost and the additional health outcome (expressed in physical terms) of one intervention compared with another.

cost-effectiveness evaluation Used when it is anticipated that the outcomes of the interventions may vary, but that the outcomes of the alternatives can be expressed in some common unit.

cost function A behavioral relationship between cost (viewed from either a marginal, average, or total perspective) and the variables that influence cost, including volume of output, quality of output, input prices, and variables affecting organizational efficiency. See **cost curve**, **long-run cost curve**, and **short-run cost curve**.

cost-minimization evaluation Used when the alternative interventions have equal effects; used to determine the least costly alternative when it has been determined that the results (or outcomes) of either of the alternatives will be the same.

cost sharing The joint payment or sharing of a price by the consumer and the payer (insurer).

cost shifting The charging of different prices for differentially insured patients, usually including the subsidization of care for another group of patients for which the costs are not covered and for nonpaying patients.

cost-to-charge ratio The total amount of money required to operate a hospital, divided by the sum of the revenues received from patient care and all other operating revenues.

cost utility The relationship between the additional cost and the additional health outcome (expressed in terms of a utility index) of one intervention compared with another.

cost-utility evaluation A specific type of cost-effectiveness analysis, which refers to the subjective level of well-being expressed by individuals in different states of health; measures the costs of various interventions in terms of the achievement of the desired outcomes.

Critical Access Hospital (CAH) Program Medicare's Rural Hospital Flexibility Program, designed to assist rural communities preserve access to primary care and emergency services by paying rural hospitals on a cost-plus basis and having different operating requirements for these hospitals, providing the hospitals meet certain conditions.

critical care See **intensive care**.

cross-sectional comparison Measures the output of the good or service among different groups at the same time.

Current Procedural Terminology (CPT) A classification of procedures and services, primarily for physicians, widely used for coding in billing and payment for physician services.

customary fee Refers to fees charged by all physicians in the community.

customary, prevailing, reasonable charge (CPR) The charge that is the lowest of the following: actual charge made for the service, the provider's customary (usual) charge for the service, or the fee prevailing in the community for the service; also called usual, customary, and reasonable charge (UCR).

day procedure groups (DPGs) A classification system for ambulatory patients in which patients are assigned to classes according to principal procedures that use similar resources; the DPG system was developed from New York's PAS system and is used by the Canadian Institute for Health Information.

deadweight loss The loss of economic efficiency in terms of utility for consumers or producers such that the optimal or allocative efficiency is not achieved in the market exchange.

deductible A fixed amount that a consumer must spend out of pocket before insurance coverage begins; for example, if the deductible is $200, the individual must pay for the first $200 of medical expenditures out of pocket before the insurance company begins to pay its share of the remaining costs.

defensive medicine Provision of services, mainly diagnostic services, in anticipation of defending against a possible lawsuit alleging malpractice.

defined benefit Type of health insurance in which specific benefits are promised to the purchaser (employee).

defined contribution Type of health insurance in which the purchaser (employee) of the insurance is provided a specific amount for the insurance premium.

delagatory or top-down method A value system imposed on the members of society by a higher entity.

demand Consumer willingness and ability to purchase alternative quantities of services at various specified prices, represented by the position of the demand curve; the quantity demanded at any specific price, all other causal factors held constant.

demand curve (schedule) A graph or schedule indicating the quantities of a service that an individual or group is willing to purchase at different prices of that service, all other factors (income, tastes and preferences, other prices, expectations) held constant.

derived demand A good or service that is desired or wanted, not for its own sake, but for its contribution to another good or service; for example, the demand for a physician visit is derived from our demand for better health, not for the direct utility of a physician visit.

descriptive economics Involves the identification, definition, and measurement of phenomena.

diagnosis A determination of the specific physical or mental ailment of an individual.

diagnosis-related groups (DRGs) A system of classifying hospital inpatients into groups using similar quantities of resources according to selected characteristics, such as diagnoses, procedure, age, and any complications or comorbidities; DRGs were used for hospital reimbursement in the U.S. Medicare system (Fetter, 1992) (see MS-DRGs for current classification system).

diminishing marginal rate of substitution The marginal rate of substitution changes systematically as the amounts of two goods or services being consumed vary.

direct cost (1) In social cost accounting, the cost of all resources incurred by providers of health care; usually refers to paid resources; (2) in hospital cost accounting, the cost of resources (doctors, nurses, lab techs) that are directly involved in the provision of care, but overhead costs are excluded.

direct price See **out-of-pocket price.**

direct regulation Refers to intervention in markets by regulatory agencies to control price, quantity, or quality by direct action, such as instituting price controls, establishing professional licensure requirements, or assessing and regulating the quality of services.

direct teaching costs In hospital care, the costs in a teaching hospital that can be directly traced to educational rather than patient care functions; these include resident and intern salaries.

discharge The formal release of a patient from a hospital or physician's care.

discharge planning The process of assessing needs and making sure arrangements are made outside the hospital to receive the patient upon discharge and ensuring appropriate continuity of care is provided.

discount (time discount) A constant applied to future costs and benefits in order to value them as equivalent to costs and benefits occurring in the present period.

disease prevention See **prevention**

disequilibrium A state in which a market is not in equilibrium (demand and supply are not equal). As a result of a shift in demand or supply, a market will be in *dynamic* disequilibrium until the price and quantity adjust to the new equilibrium levels. A state of *static* disequilibrium can be permanent if there is some barrier (e.g., government price

control, monopoly power) that permanently maintains the price at a level above or below that of equilibrium.

disruptive innovation New technology or processes that upset current conditions, but in such a way that progress, in terms of better results or lower costs, is the final result.

distributive justice Principles of ethics used to allocate resources that are limited in supply; many different approaches are available, such as egalitarianism, desert-based principle, libertarianism, difference principle, resource-based principle, welfare-based principle.

doctor–patient relationship Legal term for relationship between a patient and a healthcare provider that gives rise to legal obligations.

doughnut hole Gap in Medicare Part D prescription drug coverage.

DRG See **diagnosis-related groups**.

DRG cost weight Weight assigned to each DRG to reflect the DRG's use of resources relative to the cost of the average Medicare patient; the average Medicare patient's cost, when multiplied by the DRG cost weight, gives the price for the DRG.

DRG creep Change in the distribution of patients among DRGs without a real change in the distribution of patients treated in the hospital.

dual eligible Individual qualified for both Medicare and Medicaid coverage.

economic behavior Involves attaining or attempting to attain goods and services.

economic cost See **opportunity cost**.

economic efficiency Least costly method of producing an output.

economic evaluation The practice of assessing changes in outcomes due to an intervention and the resources used to achieve the results.

economic flow A flow will summarize a transaction in which a service or good is exchanged for money.

economic rent Surplus of total earnings over amount required to prevent a factor from transferring to another use.

economic system Way in which goods and services are produced, distributed, and consumed.

economic variable An economically relevant phenomenon whose value or magnitude may vary.

economics The discipline that deals with the consequences of resource scarcity, and about making choices.

economies of scale Reductions in operating costs associated with larger-scale operations.

economies of scope Reductions in the operating costs of two or more related services (e.g., home care and hospital care) associated with joint production (e.g., production of both services by the same organization).

effectiveness The relationship between an intervention and its health outcome, usually measured in physical units (e.g., life years saved); some definitions specify that effectiveness is a measure of the ability of an intervention to bring about an outcome under actual practice conditions.

efficacy The relationship between an intervention and its health outcome under ideal (usually experimental) clinical conditions.

efficiency Relationship between amount of output and the amount of effort: (1) technical efficiency is a measure of how close a given combination of resources is to producing a maximum amount of output; (2) allocative or economic efficiency is a measure of how close a given combination of resources is to yielding maximum consumer satisfaction.

elasticity of demand The quantity of a service demanded in response to the out-of-pocket price of a service or product; elasticity is calculated by dividing the percentage change in the product demanded by the percentage change in the direct price (see point and arc elasticities for specific methods).

elasticity of supply Measure of the responsiveness of quantity of goods or services supplied to a change in the market price, and calculated by dividing percentage change in quantity supplied by the percentage change in market price (see point and arc elasticities for specific methods).

electronic health record (or electronic medical record) A digital version of the paper chart of a patient's medical and treatment history, making information available instantly and securely.

emergency care Involves immediate decision making and action to prevent death or any further disability for patients in a health crisis.

encounter A single visit to a provider (sometimes used as an output measure).

endogenous variable Variable that is explained within a theory (e.g., price is the endogenous variable in the theory of demand and theory of supply).

enforcement costs The costs of ensuring that the provider meets the agreed criteria.

enrollee Person covered (receives benefits) under a contract for care.

entry barrier Natural or created impediment to entry into an industry.

episode of care A series of temporarily contiguous healthcare services related to treatment of a given spell of illness, or provided in response to a specific request by the patient or other relevant entity (Hornbrook, Hurtado, & Johnson, 1985, p. 171).

episode of illness A single unbroken interval of time during which the patient suffers from a continuous spell of signs and/or symptoms that are perceived as sickness or ill-health (Hornbrook et al., 1985, p. 170).

equilibrium A situation in which all forces are in balance so there is no tendency to change: (1) *consumer equilibrium* occurs where the individual consuming the unit has acquired a composition of goods that gives the unit its maximum attainable satisfaction (utility) given the constraints (prices, incomes) it faces; (2) *producer or provider equilibrium* occurs when the firm is producing the level of output that achieves its objectives (e.g., maximum profits, maximum output); (3) *market or competitive equilibrium* occurs when all buyers and sellers simultaneously achieve their maximized positions; demand and supply are therefore in balance at these determined levels of price and quantity.

equity Fairness (e.g., in the provision of health care). See **horizontal equity** and **vertical equity**.

evaluative economics Involves judging or ranking alternative phenomena according to some standard or relative position of alternatives.

evidence-based medicine Using current best information in making decisions regarding care of individual patients.

excess profits Earnings in excess of normal returns; defined as profits greater than the amount required to cover the opportunity costs of the resources invested in the firm.

exogenous variable Variable that influences endogenous variables in a theory but is itself determined by factors outside the theory.

experience rating A method of setting health premiums for healthcare coverage. In this method, each insured in the group pays a premium that is based on his or her risk-related characteristics.

explanatory economics Involves explaining and predicting certain phenomena.

explicit Specifically stated conditions.

extra billing Billing for an insured health service rendered to an insured person by a medical practitioner in an amount in addition to any amount paid for that service by the provincial or territorial health insurance plan (Canada Health Act, 1984).

extra-welfarism Tries to maximize health, which is done by choosing all medical procedures that are more cost-effective than a certain threshold.

externalities Effects, good or bad, that occur to parties not directly involved in the production or consumption of goods or services.

False Claims Act Covers individuals and groups that defraud government programs.

factors of production See **resources**.

fee Charge for a service provided.

fee-for-service payment Payment for each item or service provided.

fee schedule List of prices for specific procedures and services; the schedule may be negotiated between provider and payer or set externally.

final goods Goods that are not used as inputs by other firms.

firm A self-contained organization that engages in the production or provision of a service or product; the production can occur in more than one facility. See **plant**.

fixed costs Costs that remain the same despite changes in the volume of output.

fixed inputs Inputs that, within a selected range, do not vary with output. Examples include office space and major equipment.

flat-of-the-curve medicine Medical care that has no impact on health status. The reference is to the curve relating medical care inputs to health status output; eventually, if medical care is provided in large enough quantities, its additional effectiveness is hypothesized to be zero (i.e., the output will be constant and the curve will be flat).

flexible spending account (FSA) Account managed by employer allowing employees to set aside pretax funds for medical, dental, legal, and daycare services.

Food and Drug Administration (FDA) Responsible for protecting the public's health by assuring the safety, efficacy, and security of human and veterinary drugs, biological products, food supply, cosmetics, and products that emit radiation; the FDA also provides science-based information to the public.

formulary List of pharmaceutical products covered by a health plan.

fraud Obtaining goods or services or payment by intentional false statements.

free rider An individual who receives the benefits of a good or service without paying for it.

freedom of choice Policy permitting individuals to select their own physician or hospital.

full cost The cost that a provider incurs in producing services. The total cost covers *all* inputs, direct and indirect, used in the production of the services.

funding A payment made to a provider to cover expenses for services rendered. The funding is not necessarily related to the costs incurred for specific patients or services.

gag rule Practice employed by health plans to forbid physicians to tell patients about alternative, more expensive forms of treatment that are not covered or authorized by the plan.

gaming Manipulating the system in an illegal or unethical way.

gaps Services not covered by insurance.

gatekeeper Person responsible for determining services to be provided to a person and coordinating the provision of appropriate care.

generic drugs Medication that has exactly the same active ingredient as the brand-name drug and yields the same therapeutic effect; it is the same in dosing, safety, strength, quality, the way it works, the way it is taken, and the way it should be used; however, generic drugs do not need to contain the same inactive ingredients as the brand-name product.

global budget A fixed annual operating grant paid to a provider that is to cover all services (regardless of location) provided to all patients who are treated; it encompasses all sources of payment.

global fee Single fee charged for certain medical services, such as pregnancy and delivery, instead of a fee charged for each service or procedure.

graphic analysis The purpose is to illustrate visually relations between economic variables.

gross domestic product (GDP) The money amount of all final goods and services (consumer, investment, and government) produced within defined geographical boundaries during a defined period of time. A standard measure of relative health expenditures for a given state, province, or country is total health spending divided by GDP.

gross national product (GNP) The money amount of all final goods and services produced by residents of a country during a defined period of time, regardless of where the actual production took place.

group model HMO A health maintenance organization in which the HMO contracts with an independent group practice to provide care for its members; the contractual arrangements are usually on a per capita basis.

group practice A medical practice in which several practitioners share some inputs, such as office staff and space.

health (1) A complete state of physical, mental, and social well-being, and not merely the absence of disease or illness (World Health Organization, 1948); (2) a state characterized by anatomic integrity; ability to perform personally valued family, work, and community roles; ability to deal with physical, biologic, and social stress; a feeling of well-being; and freedom from the risk of untimely disease (Stokes et al, 1982).

health care A range of services and products whose end purpose is the preservation or enhancement of health.

health economics Branch of economics dealing with the provision, delivery, and use of healthcare goods and services.

health insurance The payment for the expected costs of a group resulting from medical utilization based on the expected expenses incurred by the group. The payment can be based on community or experience rating; health insurance is designed to reduce the risk of financial loss from the occurrence of an illness or accident event.

health insurance exchanges Also known as a **health insurance marketplace;** it is a key provision of the

Affordable Care Act, established to provide a selection of competing private health insurance providers, each offering different qualified plans.

Health Insurance Portability and Accountability Act of 1996 (HIPAA) Federal legislation whose primary function is to provide continuity of healthcare coverage; it also imposed protection of patient privacy.

health insurance purchasing cooperative (HIPC) An insurance organization that acts as a broker between payers of health insurance (households, businesses, governments) and healthcare providers; the HIPC sets standards for healthcare services and seeks competitive bids for these services, and consumers can then select from among the competing providers.

health maintenance organization (HMO) An organization in which a provider or management group takes on the responsibility for providing health services to a specific group of enrollees in exchange for a set annual fee for each enrollee; the HMO can be the provider or it can contract for services with outside providers.

health plan An organization that acts as an insurer for an enrolled group of members (Prospective Payment Assessment Commission, 1993).

health promotion Education and/or other supportive services that will assist individuals or groups to adopt healthy behaviors and/or reduce health risks, increase self-care skills, improve management of common minor ailments, use healthcare services effectively, and/or improve understanding of medical procedures and therapeutic regimens (American Hospital Association, 1991).

health-related quality of life (HRQOL) A measure of health status that can incorporate physical, emotional, social, and role functioning; pain; and many other factors; it is usually based on the responses of patients to questions in professionally devised instruments.

health savings account (HSA) Replaced the medical savings account and is available to anyone who has a qualified high-deductible health plan and is not covered by other health insurance; contributions up to a defined amount are tax deductible, and cash in the account is available to pay for qualified health expenditures.

health status State of health of an individual or population.

health technology All procedures, devices, equipment, and drugs used in the maintenance, restoration, and promotion of health.

health technology assessment A comprehensive form of policy research that looks at the technical, clinical, economic, and social consequences of the introduction and use of health technology.

Herfindahl Index (also called Herfindahl-Hirschman Index, or HHI) A measure of market concentration, computed as the sum of the square of firms' market shares, where market share (MS) is an individual firm's output divided by the total output in the market ($HHI = \Sigma(MS_i)^2$).

high-deductible health plan Health insurance with a very high deductible for which the insured individual is responsible.

home care Care provided in the home for a wide variety of purposes, including health maintenance, preventive care, and substitution for acute care (Hollander & Pallan, 1995). See also **home support**.

home support Home- and community-based long-term care services provided by persons other than professionals, such as nurses or rehabilitation therapists (Hollander & Pallan, 1995).

horizontal equity Fairness in the treatment of individuals who are at the same level with regard to some scale (e.g., people who are equally wealthy or have the same degree of health).

horizontal integration The combining under one management or ownership of two or more previously independent producers of the same type of service.

hospice A combination of services for terminally ill patients and their caregivers that is based on a humanistic philosophy of care.

hospital-acquired condition reduction program Under the Medicare program, hospitals will incur a 1% payment reduction if they rank in the worst performing quartile (25%) of all applicable hospitals, relative to the national average, of conditions acquired during the applicable period and on all the hospital's discharges for the specified fiscal year.

hospital census Number of patients in a hospital at a given point in time.

human capital Capitalized value of productive investments in individuals.

human capital approach A method of valuing outcomes that is based on lost productivity.

implicit A part of, but not specifically stated.

inappropriate care See **appropriateness of care**.

incentive Reward for desired behavior.

incidence Number of new events occurring in a defined period of time.

income effect Effect of a change in real income on quantity demanded.

income elasticity of demand Measure of the responsiveness (sensitivity) of quantity demanded to a change in income, calculated by percentage change in quantity demanded divided by percentage change in income.

income tax Levied on all sources of income.

increasing returns When output increases more in proportion to input as the scale of a firm's production increases.

incremental cost The additional cost resulting from a change in output by one or more than one unit.

incremental cost-effectiveness ratio (ICER) Assesses the difference between cost and effectiveness of two different events or interventions for the same condition; ICER is typically used to compare a new approach to an old approach of treating a disease or problem.

indemnity A type of insurance contract in which the insurer pays for care received up to a fixed amount per episode of illness.

independent practice association (IPA) A type of HMO that contracts with independent physician practices to provide health care for the enrollees; payment to providers is usually on a fee-for-service basis.

indifference curve Curve showing all combinations of two goods or services that provide an equal amount of satisfaction and between which the consumer is indifferent.

indigent An individual who cannot pay for his or her own care.

indirect cost (1) In social cost accounting, the cost of time lost due to illness (i.e., resources that are not directly paid for). (2) In hospital cost accounting, the cost of resources not directly related to patient care.

indirect regulation Refers to regulatory activities that affect price, quantity, or quality by enforcing the competitive behavior of firms in the market or by changing the structure of the market.

indirect teaching costs The additional costs that a teaching hospital incurs in the process of training interns and residents; these costs cannot be measured directly because they are inseparably joined with treatment costs.

inelastic demand For a given percentage change in price, there is a smaller percentage change in quantity demanded.

inferior good Goods or services for which income elasticity is negative; as income increases, quantity demanded of the goods or services decreases.

informed consent Legal permission to provide a treatment or to release information.

inpatient care Care provided to individuals lodged within a healthcare facility.

inputs See **resources**.

insurance Method of paying for specific types of losses that may occur; a contract between one party, the insurer, and another party, the insured; an economic device transferring the financial consequences of risk from an individual to a company and reducing the uncertainty of risk through pooling of the risk across many individuals (National Association of Insurance Commissioners, August 26, 2019).

intensity of care The amount of resources and services embodied in a unit of care (e.g., a day of hospitalization, a hospital stay, or a physician visit).

intensive care Care provided to patients with life-threatening conditions who require intensive treatment and continuous monitoring.

intermediate care facility (ICF) A facility providing a lower level of nursing care than a skilled nursing facility; Medicare no longer pays for ICF-level care.

intermediate product Outputs that are used as inputs by other producers in another stage of production.

International Classification of Diseases, Injuries, and Causes of Death, Tenth Revision (ICD-10) A comprehensive disease coding system developed by the World Health Organization.

International Classification of Diseases, Injuries, and Causes of Death, Tenth Revision, Clinical Modification (ICD-10-CM) A two-part medical information coding system used in abstracting systems and for classifying patients for DRGs. The first part consists of a comprehensive list of diseases with corresponding codes compatible with the World Health Organization list of disease codes. The second part contains procedure codes that are independent of the disease codes. ICD-10-CM was developed in the United States based on the World Health Organization system, and is the U.S. coding standard. Some Canadian provinces also use ICD-10-CM diagnosis and procedure codes.

intervention A task or set of tasks performed by a health professional with the object of influencing health status by interrupting or changing the course of events in progress.

inventory Stock of raw materials, goods in process, and finished goods held by firms to mitigate effects of short-term fluctuations in production or sales.

investment The employment of physical or human capital to create the conditions for further production.

investor-owned Formerly known as for-profit; these organizations attempt to maximize profits and produce at the minimum point on their long-run average cost curve.

joint venture Business arrangement to share profits, losses, and control in health care, often between a hospital and physicians.

labor market The institution by which workers and employers come together to engage in the production of output.

law of diminishing returns If increasing quantities of a variable factor are applied to a given quantity of fixed factors, the marginal product and average product of the variable factor will eventually decrease.

leading health indicators Set of 10 key determinants that influence health and are used to measure the health of the nation (US Department of Health and Human Services, 2000).

length of stay Number of days an individual remains in an institution.

life expectancy Estimate of how much longer an individual with a given characteristic may be expected to live.

loading charge The portion of an insurance premium that is over and above the amount expected to cover payment for insured services.

long run A period over which all inputs can be increased, including capital stock and specialized labor.

long-run cost curve The relation between the cost of production and volume of output or scale of plant for a period during which all inputs, including capital equipment, have sufficient time to vary.

long-term care Services that address the health, social, and personal care needs of individuals who, for one reason or another, have never developed or have lost the capacity for self-care; these services may be continuous or intermittent, but it is generally presumed that they will be delivered indefinitely.

malpractice Loss or injury to a patient resulting from failure of care or skill by a professional, leading to legal liability.

managed care Any system of health service payment or delivery arrangements in which the health plan attempts to control or coordinate the use of health services by its enrolled members in order to contain health expenditures, improve quality, or both; arrangements often involve a defined delivery system of providers who have some form of contractual arrangements with the plan (Physician Payment Review Commission, 1994).

managed care plan Organization providing managed care.

managed competition A manner of funneling payments for health services from a collective insurance fund to competing providers (Enthoven, 1993; Reinhardt, 1993).

mandate A legal requirement that certain actions be carried out; for example, the requirement that businesses provide health insurance coverage to their employees.

mandatory assignment Requirement for physicians to accept Medicare payment as payment in full for their services.

marginal cost (MC) The change in cost resulting from a change in output by one unit; because fixed costs do not change with output, marginal cost is related only to variable cost.

marginal productivity The additional output due to the application of one or more units of an input or resource, holding all other inputs constant; marginal productivity can be increasing, constant, or diminishing.

marginal rate of substitution In consumption, how much more of one product or service must be provided to compensate for giving up one unit of another product or service, if the level of satisfaction is to remain constant; in production, how much more of one factor of production must be used to compensate for the use of one less unit of another factor of production, if production is to remain constant.

marginal revenue (MR) The additional revenue that a firm obtains from selling one more unit of a service.

marginal value product The money value of additional output that is produced by one extra unit of an input (e.g., labor).

market A network of buyers and sellers whose interaction determines the price and quantity traded of goods and services; a set of arrangements that brings buyers (demanders) and sellers (suppliers) together, although especially in today's environment, a market should not be thought of as a physical location.

market clearing price Price at which quantity demanded equals quantity supplied: the equilibrium price.

market equilibrium The quantity demanded by buyers is just equal to the quantity supplied by the sellers; buyers are satisfied with the quantities they purchase at the established price and sellers are satisfied with the quantities they sell at the established price and are making the maximum profit.

market failure The incentives/disincentives present in the market do not lead to rational, market clearing outcomes for the market.

market power Refers to the ability of one participant in a market to influence the terms and conditions by which exchanges occur in the market.

market structure Those organizational characteristics of a market that determine the relationship of sellers to sellers, buyers to buyers, and sellers to buyers.

Medicaid A federally aided, state-administered program that provides medical assistance to certain low-income people.

Medicaid expansion Under the health reform law, the categorical exclusion of adults under 65 without dependent children would end, expanding Medicaid eligibility to reach adults under 65 with federal subsidy of most of the costs to states; participation in Medicaid expansion was voluntary.

medical care A component of health care; a process or activity, guided by medical practitioners, in which certain inputs or factors of production (e.g., physician services, medical instruments, and pharmaceuticals) are combined in varying quantities to yield an output (medical care services) or outcome (health status); it is the totality of diagnostic efforts and treatment involved in the care of patients.

medical devices Apparatus, instrument, or machine used for diagnosis, treatment, or prevention that does not depend upon chemical action on or within the body (distinguished from a drug).

medical harm Physical injury resulting from, or contributed to by, medical care (or the absence of medical care) and requiring additional monitoring, treatment, hospitalization, or results in death (Conway, Federico, Stewart, & Campbell, 2011).

medical loss ratio (MLR) Percentage of insurance premium that must be paid out to care for patients.

medically necessary A medical service that a health professional has determined to be medically required, or indicated, for the diagnosis or treatment of a patient in a particular instance, and not mainly for the convenience of patient or provider.

Medicare (1) In the United States, a nationwide, federally administered program that covers hospital, physician care, some related services, and prescription drugs for eligible persons age 65 and older, persons receiving Social Security disability insurance payments, and persons with end-stage renal disease or Lou Gehrig disease; (2) in Canada, the health insurance system that is jointly financed by the federal and provincial governments and administered by the provincial governments.

Medicare Advantage (formerly Medicare + choice) A program of benefits for Medicare beneficiaries that provides choice among different types of health plans, including capitation coverage.

Medicare Severity Diagnosis-Related Group (MS-DRG) The main patient characteristics now incorporated in the determination of the classification of the patient are the principal diagnosis, up to 25 additional diagnoses, and up to 25 procedures performed during the stay and in a small number of cases, classification is also based on the age, sex, and discharge status of the patient; there are now three levels of severity: MCC—Major Complication/Comorbidity, which reflect the highest level of severity; CC—Complication/Comorbidity, which is the next level of severity; and Non-CC—Non-Complication/Comorbidity, which do not significantly affect severity of illness and resource use.

medication error A failure in the process of drug administration that violates one of the following: right medication, right dosage, right patient, right time, or right route of administration.

medigap A class of insurance policies designed to cover gaps in coverage left by Medicare, such as deductibles, coinsurance, copayments, and gaps in coverage.

merit good or service One that is judged to have value that an individual or society should have based on some concept of need rather than on the willingness and ability of individuals to pay for the good or service in the market.

model Allows drawing inferences about the relations that might be expected to occur when specific underlying conditions are present.

money cost Expenditures incurred (paid out) for a given volume of output.

monitoring costs The costs of identifying the desired outcomes, collecting data on these outcomes, and determining whether the outcomes have been achieved.

monopolistic competition A state of monopolistic competition exists in a market if there are many sellers, but each is able to achieve a certain degree of customer loyalty and thus, has some influence over price.

monopoly A state of monopoly exists in a market if there is a single supplier; the supplier will then have control over prices in the market.

monopoly demand curve The monopoly demand curve is downward (negative) sloping, since the monopolist, unlike in a competitive market, faces trade-off between price and quantity.

monopsony A single buyer in a market; the monopsonist generally uses market power to achieve a satisfactory price

moral hazard The risk to an insurer that its insureds will increase their consumption of insured services because of the reduction in the out-of-pocket price resulting from the insurance coverage; moral hazard occurs when health insurance coverage causes individuals to take greater risk with their health or to consume more health care than they would if they did not have health insurance.

morbidity Illness, injury, or other than normal health; the morbidity rate is the rate of illness or injury in a population.

mortality Death; the mortality rate is the number of individuals who died divided by those at risk.

most responsible diagnosis The ICD-10 code identifying the disease or condition considered by the physician to be most responsible for the patient's stay in the institution; in a case in which multiple diseases or conditions may be classified as most responsible, it is the one responsible for the greatest length of stay (Juurlink et al., 2006). (This is the Canadian coding convention; for the U.S. convention, see **principal diagnosis**.)

multiproduct firm A firm that produces a variety of products with different specifications (e.g., types of medical services).

natural monopoly Industry characterized by sufficiently large economies of scale to supply the entire market demand.

need A quantity of services that an expert (doctor, planner, etc.) judges that a patient or group of patients ought to have in order to achieve a desired level of health status (Boulding, 1966).

net-benefit approach Compares projects on the basis of the excess of benefits to costs; net benefits of each intervention are calculated by subtracting its total costs from its total benefits and the net benefits are then compared to determine the greatest value of net benefit.

network An entity providing comprehensive, integrated health services to a defined population of individuals; historically, a network was associated with a health maintenance organization composed of several different medical groups under contract to provide care to enrollees; currently, it refers to a broader set of arrangements than just HMOs.

noncausal relation While the value of two variables has changed, the change in one value did not cause the change in the second variable.

noncompliance Failure or refusal of a patient to take medications as instructed or follow through on recommended or prescribed therapy.

nonexcludable characteristic An individual cannot be excluded from using the good or service available.

nonpatient revenue Unearned revenue, such as a grant or subsidy, sale from a gift shop, etc., that is unrelated to the amount of patient care produced.

nonrivalous characteristic The consumption of the good or service by an individual does not reduce the amount available for consumption by another individual.

normal demand curve A demand curve for a normal good or service slopes downward and to the right.

normal good There is a direct relationship between price and quantity; a good for which income elasticity is positive; the higher the income, the greater the quantity of the goods or services demanded.

normal profits Opportunity cost of capital and risk-taking needed to keep the investors and owners in the industry.

normative economics Expresses value or normative judgments about economic fairness or what the outcome of the economy or goals of public policy should be.

not for profit A not-for-profit organization has as its prime purpose the provision of services to a specified population rather than the earning of profits for shareholders; the term "not-for-profit" organization is being replaced with "tax-exempt organization" to decrease confusion regarding the role of normal profits in the organization and its mislabeling as nonprofit. Every organization must make some profit if it is to survive and grow in the long run.

nursing home An institution providing supervised, personal care for people who are not ill enough to require hospitalization in an acute care or auxiliary hospital, but who require assistance with the activities of daily living.

oligopoly Industry that contains only a few firms, at least one of which produces a significant portion of the industry's total output and new entrants have difficulty establishing a place in the market.

open access plan The beneficiary or member of a health plan can go directly to a healthcare specialist without going through a gatekeeper.

open enrollment period A limited time period during which individuals are given the opportunity to enroll in a health insurance plan without medical screening and without regard to health status.

opportunity cost The value of the alternative use of resources that was highest valued but not selected. With some exceptions (e.g., when resources are overpaid), this equals the market value of all resources used to produce a given volume of output.

outlier A patient who has a long length of stay (or a long length of treatment) or generates unusually high costs, compared with other patients with the same diagnosis.

out of area Beyond the geographical service area of a managed care plan, and those providers that are not participating in the plan; services of these providers are usually covered only for emergency or urgent care.

out of plan Either providers or services that are not part of the enrollee's health plan.

out-of-pocket price The price that is directly paid for healthcare services by the consumer and is not subsequently recovered from an insurer or government; the out-of-pocket price is the burden that falls directly on the consumer as a result of his or her use of medical care.

outpatient care Hospital-provided care that does not involve an overnight stay.

output The goods and services that result from the process of production; an activity or process during which a patient is treated or "cared for" by healthcare resources with the object of improving the patient's health.

overhead costs Costs that are involved in the administration of the organization, such as utilities, rent, management, etc.

Pareto-optimality Situation in which it is not possible to reallocate production or consumption activities to make someone better off without simultaneously making someone else worse off.

participatory or bottom-up decision making The views of the members of the community or society play a role in the decision-making process.

patent Government authority or license conferring a right or title for a set period, especially the sole right to exclude others from making, using, or selling an invention.

pathway-to-success program Overhauled the original shared-savings program and sped up the process of requiring Accountable Care Organizations (ACOs) to take on real risk, but also offered ACOs the flexibility needed to coordinate care and innovate.

patient Person who is receiving services from a healthcare provider.

patient care Totality of diagnostic, treatment, and preventive services provided to an individual to meet their physical, mental, social, and spiritual needs.

patient-centered care Care that takes into consideration the patient's preferences, values, lifestyle, family, and friends; care approached from the patient's point of view.

patient-centered medical home A team-based model of care led by a personal physician who provides continuous and coordinated care throughout a patient's lifetime to maximize health outcomes.

patient days The number of days that patients are under inpatient hospital or nursing-home care during a year.

patient-driven payment method (PDPM) Medicare system that incorporates a case mix classification almost exclusively based on verifiable nursing home resident characteristics, not volumes of services provided; this system adjusts five different case mix components reflecting the varied needs and characteristics of a nursing home resident's care, which is then combined with the non-case mix components resulting in the full SNF PPS per diem rate for the resident.

patient empowerment Enabling individuals to control their own health and healthcare decisions.

Patient Protection and Affordable Care Act On March 23, 2010, President Obama signed the Patient Protection and Affordable Care Act; the law put in place comprehensive health insurance reforms that rolled out over 4 years and beyond, with most changes taking place by 2014. Challenges have been lodged against the bill, including the elimination of mandated health insurance.

patient safety Protection of patients from injury and illness during the provision of healthcare services.

pay for performance (P4P) Model of payment for healthcare services designed to provide incentives to providers to improve quality and reduce costs, either through payment of bonuses for meeting a target or through withholding payments for failure to meet a target.

payroll tax Levied on income from salary and wages.

peer review Review of performance by individuals from the same discipline and with essentially equal qualifications (peers).

per capita payment A fixed annual payment per person made to a provider or health maintenance organization; the totality of payments is intended to cover the cost of care for all enrollees during the year.

per-case payment The provider is paid a fixed amount for each type of case treated.

per diem payment A flat-rate payment to a hospital or other institution for each day the patient is an inpatient in the institution.

perfect competition Market structure in which all firms are price takers and in which there is freedom of entry into and exit from the industry.

perspective The viewpoint (of the person or group) with respect to which economic assessment is taken.

plant A single facility engaged in production. See **firm**.

point elasticity Measure of the responsiveness of quantity to price at a particular point on the demand curve; it is calculated by measuring the change in the original price and quantity compared to the change in the new price and quantity.

point of diminishing average productivity Level of output at which average product reaches a maximum.

point of diminishing marginal productivity Level of output at which marginal product reaches maximum.

point-of-service plan (POS) A health maintenance organization plan that allows members to use providers not on the organization's panel at the time (and each time) service is needed; to gain access to such providers, the members must pay an added premium or additional out-of-pocket payment.

population Group of individuals occupying a specified area at the same time.

portability Ability of a beneficiary to move from one employer to another without loss of benefits or having to go through a waiting period for coverage.

positive economics Concerned with the development and testing of factual statements about the world which are verifiable and objective.

potential years of life lost (PYLL) Sum of years that a group of individuals would have lived had they not died prematurely.

preadmission certification The prospective review and evaluation of proposed elective hospital admissions using acceptable medical criteria as the standard for determining the appropriateness of the site or level of care and certifying the length of stay required (Scheffler et al., 1991).

predatory pricing Practice by insurers of giving low premiums to a low-risk small group or individual and then raising premiums when the insured file claims; also called churning the books.

preexisting condition Physical or mental condition discovered before an individual applies for health insurance, often leading to insurance company denying coverage for the individual or condition, or requiring a waiting period before the condition is covered.

preferred provider organization (PPO) An arrangement in which a group of health providers agrees to provide services to a defined group of patients at an agreed-upon rate for each service (Ermann et al., 1986).

premature mortality The difference between expected age of death and the actual age of death as a measure of life-years lost prematurely.

premium The payment made to an insurance company in return for insurance coverage.

prepaid group practice (PGP) A group practice that charges patients on an annual per capita basis and bears the risk for providing the insured services.

present on admission (POA) A diagnosis, condition, disease, or cause of injury that an individual had at time of admission to the hospital.

prevalence Number of events or cases present in a given population at a given time.

prevention Any intervention that reduces the likelihood that a disease or disorder will affect an individual or that interrupts or slows the progress of the disorder (Spitzer, 1990).

preventive medicine That aspect of the physician's practice in which he applies, to individual patients, the knowledge and techniques from medical, social, and behavioral science to promote and maintain health and well-being and prevent disease or its progression (Hilleboe, 1971; Last, 1988).

price An amount of money paid or received per unit of a service or good.

price ceiling A government-imposed maximum permitted price at which a good or service may be sold.

price discrimination The charging of different prices for the same product to different customers, made possible by the inability of consumers to resell the product to each other; the charging of different prices is usually due to the existence of different demand conditions for different groups of customers; different elasticities of demand must exist.

price fixing Two or more competitors agree on prices.

price floor A government-imposed minimum permitted price at which goods or services may be sold.

price taker A supplier that has no influence over the price of the goods or services it sells; the supplier can alter its rate of production and sales without significantly impacting the market price of its product.

primary care A type of medical care that emphasizes first-contact care and assumes ongoing responsibility for the patient in health maintenance and therapy for illness; primary care is comprehensive in scope and includes overall coordination of treatment of the patient's health problems.

primary prevention Reduces the likelihood that a particular disease or disorder will develop in a person.

principal The person in whose interests an agent is contracted to act.

principal–agent relationship The relationship or arrangement exists when one entity or individual (called the agent) acts on behalf of another individual or entity (called the principal).

principal diagnosis The U.S. coding convention in which the diagnosis that, after investigation, is found to have been responsible for the patient's admission to the hospital; for example, if a patient is admitted to the hospital for a minor TURP (transuretheral resection of the prostate) procedure, and it is discovered he has carcinoma of the lung, the prostate diagnosis would be the one coded under this convention. (For the Canadian convention, see **most responsible diagnosis**.)

principle of substitution Method of production will change if the relative prices of inputs change, with relatively more of the less expensive input and relatively less of the more expensive input being used.

procedure An operative or nonoperative intervention.

producer surplus The difference between the total amount that producers receive for all units sold and the total variable cost of producing the goods or services.

product differentiation Existence of similar, but not identical, products sold by a single industry.

production The act of combining resources to yield output; production involves the creation or addition of utility, which is the want-satisfying capacity of a good or service.

production function A quantitative relationship expressing how outputs vary when the quantity of inputs changes; also called **production relation**.

production possibility boundary Curve that shows alternative combinations of goods and services that can be attained if all available resources are used; the boundary between attainable and unattainable output combinations.

productivity The ratio of physical inputs to physical outputs. The inputs can be one single input (e.g., labor), with others held constant, or all inputs combined.

productivity efficiency Production of any output at the lowest attainable cost for that level of output.

products of ambulatory care (PACs) An ambulatory care classification system developed in New York State primarily for the funding of nonsurgical, nonemergency ambulatory care visits, based on body parts and purpose of visit (Tenan, 1988).

products of ambulatory surgery (PASs) An ambulatory surgery classification system developed in New York State for funding ambulatory surgery procedures, based on similar resource-using procedures (Kelley et al., 1990).

profit Total revenue minus total cost; accounting profit is defined as total revenue for a period's sales minus costs matched to those sales and economic profit is defined as total revenue minus economic or opportunity costs.

progressive tax Tax that takes a higher percentage of income the higher the level of income.

prospective payment Payment to providers based on predetermined rates unrelated to current or past costs of the individual provider.

provider A supplier of healthcare services.

public good or service One that has the characteristics of nonrivalous and nonexcludable.

public health The combination of science, practical skills, and beliefs that is directed to the maintenance and improvement of the health of all the population; it is one of the efforts organized by society to protect, promote, and restore the people's health through collective or social actions (Last, 1988).

quality-adjusted life year (QALY) A numerical assessment of the proportion of an individual's state of full health experienced over a year; QALY values generally range from 0 (assigned to death) to 1 (full health), although certain states of health can be valued at less than 0 and QALY values can be directly derived from individuals' utility measurements or can be based on existing values of health states.

quality of care The degree to which the process of medical care increases the probability of outcomes desired by patients and reduces the probability of undesired outcomes, given the state of medical knowledge (U.S. Congress, 1988).

quality of life (QOL) The degree to which an individual enjoys everything; it has been defined, by a philosopher, as the possession and enjoyment of all the real goods in the right order and proportion and for nonphilosophers, see **health-related quality of life (HRQOL)** or **health status** for terms only slightly less stratospheric.

quality of life-years lived The average number of healthy years a person can expect to live.

quantity demanded The quantity of goods or services that an individual or group is willing to buy at one specific rate during a specified time; a change in quantity demanded refers to a movement along a given demand curve in response to a change in price.

quantity exchanged The identical amount of goods or services that individuals actually purchase and producers actually sell in some time period.

quantity supplied The amount of goods or services a supplier or market is willing to supply at any one price during a specified time; a change in quantity supplied refers to a movement along a given supply curve in response to a change in price.

rate The price per unit charged by an institution for its services.

rate of return The ratio of net profits earned by a firm to total invested capital.

rate review Review by a regulatory agency of a budget and financial picture in order to determine the reasonableness of the proposed rate change.

rate setting The setting of institutional prices by a paying or regulatory agency.

rationing Process of making choices regarding who will receive scarce resources.

real income Income expressed in terms of the purchasing power of money income; the quantity of goods and services that can be purchased with money income.

reasonable fee Refers to allowances for particular extenuating circumstances when the fee charged deviates from the usual or customary fee charged.

referral Sending of a patient by one physician (the referring physician) to another physician (or some other service), either for consultation or for care.

refined diagnosis-related groups (RDRGs) Also called **refined group numbers (RGNs)** A classification system in which resource-use patterns and secondary diagnoses are used to refine the assignment of patients to severity classes (RDRGs).

regression analysis Quantitative measure of the systematic relationship among two or more variables.

regressive tax Tax that takes a lower percentage of income the higher the level of income.

regulation (1) A law or rule imposing government or government-mandated standards and significant economic responsibilities on individuals or organizations outside the government establishment; (2) the process carried out by government or mandated agencies through such means as setting or approving prices, rates, fares, profits, interest rates, and wages; awarding licenses, certificates, and permits; devising safety rules; setting quality levels; enacting public disclosure of financial information regulations; and enacting prohibitions against price, racial, religious, or sexual discrimination (Khemani & Shapiro, 1993).

reimbursement The payment made by an insurer to a provider for specific services provided to an insured patient; reimbursement is usually associated with payments based on a service-by-service, or patient-by-patient basis.

relative price Ratio of the money price of one product or service to the money price of another product or service; a ratio of two absolute prices.

relative value A value placed on a specific unit of service (e.g., a follow-up office visit, a blood test, or an inpatient cholecystectomy) expressed in relation to some standard (e.g., a minute of lab test time or physician care).

resource allocation Distribution of an economy's (or firm's, industry's) scarce resources of land, labor, and capital among alternative uses.

resource-based relative value scale (RBRVS) A resource-weighted service-classification system that aims at setting resource weights according to the total relative cost of each service, including "psychological" costs of the provider, time costs, and training costs.

resource-intensive weights (RIW) Canadian relative weightings for inpatient groups. RIWs combine Canadian length-of-stay and U.S. cost-per-day data to form hybrid cost-per-case weights; separate weights are calculated for "typical" and "atypical" cases.

resources The means used in producing services, which can include physical capital (beds and equipment) and the mental and physical aspects of human capital (physicians, nurses, etc.); also called *inputs* and *factors of production*.

resource utilization groups (RUGs) The classification is based on a set of hierarchical groups related to levels and types of services (rehabilitation, extensive services, special care, clinically complex cases, impaired cognition, behavioral problems, and reduced physical functioning) and, within these hierarchical groups, scores on the activities of daily living (ADL) scale are incorporated.

retrospective payment Payment to a provider for services provided based on actual costs incurred by the provider. Since the payment is based on costs incurred, the amount to be paid must be determined after the service has been provided (i.e., retrospectively).

retrospective review A review of claims after the episode of care is concluded and the claim is submitted to the insurer (Scheffler et al., 1991).

returns to scale The relationship between total output and scale of operations, which are measured as proportional increases in all resources; because all resources are allowed to increase in proportion, this is a long-run relationship.

revenue Income earned from the provision of services; gross revenues equal income earned overall, while net revenues equal income earned minus costs or expenses.

risk Uncertainty as to loss; in the case of health care, the loss can be due to the cost of medical treatment or other losses arising from illness; risk can be objective (relative variations between the difference between actual and probable losses) and subjective (psychological uncertainty relating to the occurrence of an event) (Howarth, 1988); see also **risk averse**, **risk neutral**, and **risk taker**.

risk averse A person is said to be risk averse if losses of a given amount create more disutility than the utility that comes from gains of the same amount (and so losses will tend to be avoided).

risk factor Behavior or condition that, based on evidence or theory, is thought to directly influence the level of a specific health problem.

risk neutral A person is said to be risk neutral if he or she values losses and gains of the same amount equally.

risk pooling The sharing of the costs incurred by members of a population; the payment method can vary but will not be based on the risk of individuals.

risk taker A person is said to be a risk taker if, for that person, the utility of gains is greater than the disutility of losses of equal value; a risk taker is therefore predisposed to gamble.

safe harbor Assurance that a certain specified behavior or action will not result in civil or criminal penalties when done in a specified way.

safe harbor regulation Describes certain acts or behaviors that will not be illegal under a specific law, even though they might otherwise be illegal.

safety net provider Provider obligated to provide health care to patients whether or not they are able to pay for the services.

sales tax Levied on a good or service sold in the market.

scarce good Good or service for which the quantity demanded is greater than the quantity supplied.

scarcity A deficiency in the quantity and/or quality of available goods and services compared with the amounts that people desire.

search cost The costs of determining specifications of the services needed and the prices of these services.

second surgical opinion Patients are sometimes required to get a second or even a third consulting opinion for specified nonemergency surgical procedures (Scheffler et al., 1991).

secondary care Specialist-referred care for conditions of a relatively low level of complication and risk; secondary care can be provided in an office or hospital and can be diagnostic or therapeutic.

secondary prevention Interrupts or minimizes the progress of a disease or irreversible damage from a disease by early detection and treatment;

selective contracting A procedure whereby an insurer can legally exclude providers from its list of participating providers (Melnick & Zwanzinger, 1988, p. 2669).

self-insurance Assumption of risk by an individual or entity by setting aside own resources instead of purchasing an insurance policy.

sensitivity analysis Determining the extent to which the conclusions or results of a model depend on the model's assumptions.

severity of illness Gravity of a patient's illness.

severity score Mathematical score that expresses the severity of illness of a patient according to a predefined method.

shared-savings program A Medicare program that establishes financial incentives for Accountable Care Organizations (ACOs) to provide coordinated, well-integrated care across all types of providers; emphasis in this program is placed on moving away from the fee-for-service chassis that rewarded volume and, instead, rewards value and outcome by placing the provider at financial risk for the care required by a specific patient population.

shortage An excess of demand over supply at a given price.

short run A period in which all of the inputs cannot be adjusted (increased or reduced) and those inputs that cannot be adjusted are called "fixed" and include capital stock; *short run* also refers to lengths of time insufficient for new firms to enter a market or industry.

short-run cost curve The relation between cost and volume of production of a plant during a short adjustment period in which only some inputs are variable (and the rest are fixed); short-run cost curves reflect the law of diminishing returns.

side effect Effect of a drug or treatment that is other than the intended, desired effect.

sign-out case A patient who leaves the hospital against medical advice.

single-payer system A reimbursement system in which there is a single payer or one dominant payer.

sin tax Tax on goods, services, or activities that are allegedly harmful, such as a tax on tobacco products.

single-product firm A production unit that produces a single, homogeneous product.

skilled nursing facility (SNF) A facility that provides skilled nursing care to residents who do not need acute hospital care but who do need inpatient professional nursing care and other social and health needs.

sliding fee scale High-income patients pay higher prices than low-income patients for the same service; or patients with insurance pay a different price than patients with another insurance or no insurance.

slope The slope of a geometric relation shows how much of a change in one variable is associated with a given change in a related variable; it can be expressed as the magnitude or sensitivity of response.

social benefit Contribution that an activity makes to society's welfare.

social cost The cost to all members of society of any activity or service; it can be the sum of private and external costs or of direct and indirect costs and is also viewed as the value of the best alternative use of the resources available to society as valued by society.

social welfare The well-being of the entire society; not the same as standard of living but is more concerned with the quality of life that includes such factors as the quality of the environment (air, soil, water), level of crime, extent of drug abuse, availability of essential social services, as well as religious and spiritual aspects of life.

social welfare loss The lost welfare to society as a result of too much or too little production and consumption of a good or resource.

solo practice A single physician medical practice.

sound organizational structure The authority and lines of responsibility in the organization are clearly defined.

specialization of labor Organization of production in which individual workers specialize in the production of particular goods or services (and satisfy their wants and needs by trading) rather than producing everything they consume.

staff model HMO A health maintenance organization whose practitioner staff are employees of the health plan; usually the practitioners are paid on a salary rather than fee-for-service basis.

standardized mortality rate (SMR) A single mortality rate for a large group of individuals who are in different age and gender categories; the total rate for the entire group is made up of the rates in different age and gender subgroups, which are weighted or averaged according to a given structure of a standard population (e.g., the population of an entire country or the population in a base year).

stop-loss insurance Insurance purchased to pay a health plan or a group of providers for costs of care for individual patients or a panel of patients over a ceiling amount; designed to protect against catastrophic claims; sets an upper limit on the amount that will have to be paid.

substitutes Goods or services that compete with each other, such as aspirin and Tylenol; the direct price of one of the substitutes will cause a shift in the demand curve for the other.

substitution effect The shift from one product to another as a result of a price change, after compensating for any increase or reduction in real income that accrues from the price change.

supplier-induced demand The amount of shift in the demand for services resulting from the suppliers' influence on consumers' tastes (intensity of desire for the services).

supply A supply curve; the quantity supplied at each price.

supply curve (1) For a single firm, the quantity the firm is willing to supply of a service at alternative prices of the commodity; (2) for the market, the relationship between the quantity that all firms are willing to supply and alternative prices of the service.

supply function (1) For a single provider, a quantitative relationship between the quantity the supplier is willing to supply and a series of variables that influence the supplier's behavior, such as price, technology, case mix, quality, and input prices; (2) for a market, the quantitative relationship between the quantity that all suppliers in the market are willing to supply and a series of variables that influence all of the suppliers' behaviors, including price, technology, case mix, quality, input prices, and the number of suppliers in the market.

surplus (1) For a tax-exempt firm, total revenue minus total expense (the counterpart of profit for a investor-owned firm); (2) for a market, the excess of quantity supplied over quantity demanded at a given price.

tastes Consumer preferences for goods and services expressed in terms of an index of satisfaction or utility; taste is a catchall concept for everything other than prices and incomes that affect demand, including health status, age, gender, level of education, and so on.

tax-exempt organization Tax-exempt designation indicates that these organizations do not pay taxes on the profits generated through the provision of goods and services or on the properties they own; formerly known as not-for-profit.

technology See **health technology**.

technology assessment See **health technology assessment**.

tertiary care Highly specialized care administered to patients who have complicated conditions or require high-risk pharmaceutical treatments or surgery; tertiary care is provided in a setting that houses high-technology services, specialists and subspecialists, and intensive care and other highly specialized services.

tertiary prevention Slows the progress of the disease and reduces the resultant disability through treatment of established diseases

third-party payment Payment by a private insurer or government to a medical provider for care given to a patient.

time cost The value of time required to conduct an activity; this variable has two components: value per unit of time and time actually spent in the activity, where value per unit of time is taken as equivalent to lost earnings or the value placed on forgone leisure activities.

time series comparison Measures the output of the same good or service at different times.

total costs (TC) The sum of fixed and variable costs; all of the costs required to produce a specified level of output.

total fixed costs (TFC) All of the fixed costs required to produce a specified level of output.

total product The total amount of output produced.

total variable costs (TVC) All of the variable costs required to produce a specified level of output.

transaction costs The costs of reaching an agreement and coordinating activity among participants in a market; these include the costs of *searching* for potential buyers or sellers and for product quality and cost, *negotiating* an agreement, *monitoring* that the agreement conditions are met, and *enforcing* the terms of the agreement.

transfer case A hospital inpatient who is admitted from or discharged to another institution.

transfer payment A payment made to an individual or institution that does not arise out of current productive activity.

trim point A point, calculated using a statistical formula, applied to all lengths of stays (or cost per case) within a single DRG (or CMG) in order to separate outlier cases from the rest.

typical patient A patient who receives a full, successful course of treatment in a single institution and is discharged when he or she no longer requires acute-care services.

unit costs Costs per unit of output, equal to total costs divided by total output.

usual fee Refers to the usual or typical fee charged by the billing physician.

utility Represents the amount of satisfaction that an individual receives from possessing or consuming a good or service, and can be measured as (1) an index comparing various levels of an individual's satisfaction with alternative quantities of specified goods, services, or situations under certainty and the index that allows the quantification of differences between the levels is called *cardinal utility* (Pigou, 1932); (2) a ranking of alternative bundles of goods and services under certainty, on the basis of better, equal, or worse, with no indication as to *degrees* of satisfaction (ordinal utility); or (3) a ranking of alternative risky situations on the basis of an individual's own preferences regarding probabilities (von Neumann-Morgenstern utility) (Torrance et al., 1996).

utility possibility frontier Represents all allocations that are efficient and shows the level of satisfaction that each person achieves when he/she has traded to an efficient outcome, on the contract curve; shows the maximum amount of one person's utility given each level of utility attained by all others in society.

utilization The actual use of services by consumers (the services must be demanded and supplied).

utilization management A set of techniques used by or on behalf of purchasers of healthcare benefits to manage healthcare costs by influencing patient care decision making through case-by-case assessments of the appropriateness of care prior to provision (Institute of Medicine, 1991).

utilization review (UR) Examination and evaluation of the efficiency and appropriateness of any healthcare service that has already been provided.

value-added Reflects the position that an activity performed on a given product or service has increased its value.

value-added tax (VAT) Tax imposed on goods and services at each stage of production.

value-based purchasing Obtaining the highest quality health care at the most reasonable price; links payment for care to the quality of care and rewards cost-effective practices.

value-driven health care Healthcare system in which price and quality are made visible (transparent) so purchasers of care can make choices based on value.

value judgment A pronouncement that states or implies that something is desirable (or undesirable) and is not derived from any technical or objective data but instead from considerations of ultimate value, that is, ethical considerations (Nath, 1969).

variable costs Costs that change in response to changes in output; variable costs can be expressed as total, average, or marginal.

variable inputs Inputs that can vary in quantity during a specified time period.

vertical equity Fairness in the treatment of individuals who are at different levels with regard to some scale (e.g., people who fall into different income classes).

vertical integration The combining under one management of activities at different stages of the production process.

virtual merger Loosely defined concept in which healthcare organizations agree to cooperate in some areas in which they had previously competed.

volume The number of cases (or other service units) provided.

wants Consumer tastes or desires; desires that can be satisfied by the consumption of a good, service, or leisure activity.

wealth Sum of all the valuable assets owned minus liabilities.

willingness-to-pay approach A method of valuing an outcome that is based on the consumer's own preferences.

windfall profits Change in profits that arises out of an unanticipated change in market conditions.

work–leisure tradeoff The tradeoff between working more hours and earning a wage for an extra hour versus the extra benefit received for consuming an extra hour of leisure; the work–leisure theory illustrates the possible trade-off between potential uses of an individual's time, in which each combination results in the same level of utility (satisfaction) to the individual.

x-inefficiency Use of resources at a lower level of productivity than is possible, even if they are allocated efficiently, so that the economy is at a point inside its production possibility curve.

Bibliography

Accountable Care Organizations (ACO). Retrieved from https://www.cms.gov/Medicare/Medicare-Fee-for-Service-Payment/ACO/index.html?redirect=/ACO/

American Hospital Association. (1991). *AHA Guide.* Chicago, IL: Author.

Boulding, K. E. (1966). The concept of need for health services. *Milbank Memorial Fund Quarterly, 44*(4), 202–223.

Canada Health Act, R.S.C. 1984, C-6 (1984). Published by the Minister of Justice.

Conway, J., Federico, F., Stewart, K., & Campbell, M. (2011). *Respectful management of serious clinical adverse events* (2nd ed.). *IHI Innovation Series white paper.* Cambridge, MA: Institute for Healthcare Improvement.

Due, J. F. (1957). *Government finance: Economics of the public sector.* Homewood, IL: Richard D. Irwin, Inc.

Enthoven, A. C. (1993a). Achieving effective cost control in comprehensive health care reform. The Jackson Hole "managed care managed competition" approach. *Health Pac Bulletin, 23*(1), 13–15.

Enthoven, A. C. (1993b). The history and principles of managed competition. *Health Affairs, 12 Suppl,* 24–28.

Ermann, D., deLissovoy, G., Gabel, J., & Rice, T. (1986). Preferred provider organizations: issues for employers. *Health Care Management Review, 11*(4), 26–36.

Fetter, R. B. (1992). Hospital payment based on diagnosis-related groups. *Journal of the Society for Health Systems, 3*(4), 4–15.

Fries, B. E., Schneider, D. P., Foley, W. J., Gavazzi, M., Burke, R., & Cornelius, E. (1994). Refining a case-mix measure for nursing homes: Resource utilization groups (RUG-III). *Medical Care, 32*(7), 668–685.

Hilleboe, H. E. (1971). Modern concepts of prevention in community health. *American Journal of Public Health, 61*(5), 1000–1006.

Hollander, M. J., & Pallan, P. (1995). The British Columbia Continuing Care system: Service delivery and resource planning. *Aging-Clinical & Experimental Research, 7*(2), 94–109.

Hornbrook, M. C., Hurtado, A. V., & Johnson, R. E. (1985). Health care episodes: Definition, measurement and use. *Medical Care Review, 42*(2), 163–218.

Howarth, C. I. (1988). The relationship between objective risk, subjective risk and behaviour. *Ergonomics, 31*(4), 527–535.

Juurlink, D., Preyra, C., Croxford, R., Chong, A., Austin, P., Tu, J., & Laupacis, A. (2006). *A Canadian Institute for health information discharge abstract database: A validation study.* Toronto, ON: Institute for Clinical Evaluative Sciences.

Katz, S., Ford, A. B., Moskowitz, R. W., Jackson, B. A., & Jaffe, M. W. (1963). Studies of illness in the aged. *JAMA, 185,* 914–919.

Kelley, S. W., Donnelly, J. H., & Skinner, S. J. (1990). Consumer participation in service production and delivery. *Journal of Retailing, 66*(3), 315–336.

Khemani, R. S., & Shapiro, D. M. (1993). *Glossary of industrial organisation economics and competition law.* Geneva: Directorate for Financial, Fiscal and Enterprise Affairs, OECD.

Last, J. M. (1988). The future of health in Canada. *Canadian Journal of Public Health. Revue Canadienne de Sante Publique, 79*(3), 147–149.

Melnick, G. A., & Zwanziger, J. (1988). Hospital behaviour under competition and cost-containment policies. The California experience, 1980 to 1985. *JAMA, 260*(18), 2669–2675.

Nath, S. K. (1969). *A reappraisal of welfare economics.* London, England: Routledge and Kegan Paul.

National Association of Insurance Commissioners. (2019, August 08). *Glossary of insurance terms.* Retrieved from https://www.naic.org/consumer_glossary.htm#1

Pigou, A. C. (1932). *The economics of welfare.* London, England: Macmillan & Co.

Preamble to the Constitution of the World Health Organization as adopted by the International Health Conference, New York, 19–22 June, 1946; signed on 22 July 1946 by the representatives of 61 States (Official Records of the World Health Organization, no. 2, p. 100) and entered into force on 7 April 1948.

Prospective Payment Assessment Commission. (1993). *Report and recommendations to the congress.* Washington, DC: Author.

Reinhardt, U. E. (1993). Comment on the Jackson Hole initiatives for a twenty-first century American health care system. *Health Economics, 2*(1), 7–14.

Saskatchewan Statutes (1993). The Occupational Health and Safety Act, 1993. Chapter 0-1.1 of the Statutes of Saskatchewan, Canada.

Scheffler, R. M., Sullivan, S. D., & Ko, T. H. (1991). The impact of Blue Cross and Blue Shield Plan utilization management programs, 1980–1988. *Inquiry, 28*(3), 263–275.

Spitzer, P. G. (1990). Building a model for the development of better healthcare systems. *Health Informatics, 7*(12), 42, 44.

Starfield, B., Weiner, J., Mumford, L., & Steinwachs, D. (1991). Ambulatory care groups: A categorization of diagnoses for research and management. *Health Services Research, 26*(1), 53–74.

Stokes, J. III, Noren, J., & Shindell, S. (1982). Definition of terms and concepts applicable to clinical preventive medicine. *Journal of Community Health, 8*(1), 33–41.

Torrance, G. W., Feeny, D. H., Furlong, W. J., Barr, R. D., Zhang, Y., & Wang, Q. (1996). Multiattribute utility function for a comprehensive health status classification system: Health utilities index mark 2. *Medical Care, 34*(7), 702–722.

US Congress, Office of Technology Assessment. (1988). *The quality of medical care: Information for consumers,* OTA-I-I-386. Washington, DC: US Government Printing Office.

US Department of Health and Human Services. (1994). *Public financing of long-term care: Federal and state roles.* Washington, DC: Office of the Assistant Secretary for Planning and Evaluation.

US Department of Health and Human Services. (2000). *Healthy people 2010: Understanding and improving health.* 2nd ed. Washington, DC: US Government Printing Office.

Index

NOTE: Page references in italics refer to figures, graphs, tables, etc.